Instructor's Resource Manual
for
MEDICAL-SURGICAL NURSING

Critical Thinking in Client Care

LeMone—Burke

Instructor's Resource Manual for

MEDICAL-SURGICAL NURSING

Critical Thinking in Client Care

FOURTH EDITION

NANCY H. WRIGHT, RN, BS, CNOR
PROFESSOR OF NURSING
VIRGINIA COLLEGE
BIRMINGHAM, ALABAMA

PAMELA FOWLER, MSN, BSN
ASSISTANT PROFESSOR OF NURSING
ROGERS STATE UNIVERSITY
CLAREMORE, OKLAHOMA

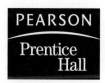

PEARSON

Prentice Hall

Upper Saddle River, New Jersey 07458

Pearson Education Ltd.
Pearson Education Singapore, Pte. Ltd.
Pearson Education Canada, Ltd.
Pearson Education—Japan
Pearson Education Australia PTY, Limited

Pearson Education North Asia Ltd.
Pearson Educación de Mexico, S.A. de C.V.
Pearson Education Malaysia, Pte. Ltd.
Pearson Education, Inc., Upper Saddle River, New Jersey

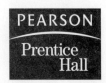

10 9 8 7 6 5 4 3 2 1
ISBN-10: 0-13-198572-8
ISBN-13: 978-0-13-198572-8

CONTENTS

PREFACE

Medical-Surgical Nursing, 4th edition was written to provide the knowledge and skills needed to care for adult clients, promote health, facilitate recovery from illness and injury, and provide support when coping with disability or loss. This accompanying **Instructor's Resource Manual** is designed to support your teaching in today's challenging environment, and to reduce your preparation time for class. It will help you to provide an optimal learning experience for your students and their many learning needs.

Each chapter in the Instructor's Resource Manual (IRM) is thoroughly integrated with the corresponding chapter in the textbook *Medical-Surgical Nursing, 4th edition* by LeMone and Burke. Chapters are organized by learning outcomes, and the teaching unit flows from these outcomes. You will find the following features to support the objectives:

- The Concepts for Lecture in this manual may be used in their entirety for class presentation or they may be merged with the classroom activities for a mixture of teaching styles that will meet the needs of students with various learning styles.

- The Lecture Outlines can be found on your Instructor's Resource DVD-ROM in PowerPoint.

- Suggestions for Classroom and Clinical Experiences attempt to go beyond the traditional activities that have been the mainstay of nursing education for many years.

- The Resource Library identifies for you—the instructor—all the specific media resources and activities available for that chapter on the Prentice Hall Nursing MediaLink DVD-ROM, Companion Website, and Instructor's Resource DVD-ROM. Chapter by chapter, the Resource Library helps you decide what resources from these media sources to use to enhance your course and your students' ability to apply concepts from the book into practice.

This IRM also contains a brand new "Strategies for Success" module written by Sandra DeYoung. Included in this module are Learning Theories, Planning for Instruction, How to Use Effective Pedagogies, Assessing Learning, and more! There is also a guide on "Teaching Medical-Surgical Nursing to Students who Speak English as a Nonnative Language." This tool is intended to guide you in reaching across cultural barriers to train nurses.

Finally, the following additional resources are also available to accompany this textbook. For more information or sample copies, please contact your Prentice Hall Sales Representative.

- **Study Guide (ISBN: 0-13-198570-1)**—This study guide incorporates strategies for students to focus their study and increase comprehension of nursing care concepts. It contains a variety of activities such as multiple choice, fill-in-the-blank, case studies, and more.

- **Prentice Hall Nursing MediaLink DVD-ROM**—This DVD-ROM is packaged with the textbook. It provides an interactive study program that allows students to practice answering NCLEX®-style questions with rationales for right and wrong answers. It also contains an audio glossary, animations and video tutorials, and a link to the Companion Website (an Internet connection is required). Note: A Prentice Hall Nursing MediaLink CD-ROM version is available for purchase on *www.MyPearsonStore.com*.

- **Companion Website** *www.prenhall.com/lemone*—This on-line Study Guide is designed to help students apply the concepts presented in the book. Each chapter-specific module features Learning Outcomes, NCLEX® Review Questions with rationales, Chapter Outlines for lecture notes, Case Studies, Critical Thinking WebLinks, Audio Glossary, and more.

- **Instructor's Resource DVD-ROM (ISBN: 0-13-198569-8)**—This cross-platform DVD-ROM provides text slides and illustrations in PowerPoint for use in classroom lectures. It also contains an electronic test bank, and animations and video clips from the student DVD-ROM. This supplement is available to faculty upon adoption of the textbook. Note: An Instructor's Resource CD-ROM is also available upon request.

It is our hope that the information provided in this manual will decrease your class preparation time and optimize the learning experience for your students.

Teaching Medical-Surgical Nursing to Students who Speak English as a Nonnative Language

We are fortunate to have so many multinational and multilingual nursing students in the United States in the 21st century. As our classrooms become more diverse, there are additional challenges to communication, but we in the nursing education community are ready. Our goal is to educate competent and caring nurses to serve the health needs of our diverse communities.

We know that ENNL students experience higher attrition rates than their native English-speaking counterparts. This is a complex problem. However, there are teaching strategies that have helped many students be successful.

The first step toward developing success strategies is understanding language proficiency. Language proficiency has four interdependent components. Each component is pertinent to nursing education.

Reading is the first aspect of language. Any nursing student will tell you that there are volumes to read in nursing education. Even native English speakers find the reading load heavy. People tend to read more slowly in their nonnative language. They also tend to recall less. Nonnative speakers often spend inordinate amounts of time on reading assignments. These students also tend to take longer to process exam questions.

Listening is the second component of language. Learning from lectures can be challenging. Some students are more proficient at reading English than listening to it. It is not uncommon for ENNL students to understand medical terminology, but to become confused by social references, slang, or idiomatic expressions used in class. The spoken language of the teacher may be different in accent or even vocabulary from that experienced by immigrant students in their language education. ENNL students may not even hear certain sounds that are not present in their native languages. The generic drug names amoxicillin and ampicillin may sound the same. Asian languages do not have gender-specific personal pronouns (he, she, him, her, etc.). Asian students may become confused when the teacher is describing a case study that involves people of different genders.

Speaking is the third component of language proficiency. People who speak with an accent are often self-conscious about it. They may hesitate to voice their questions or to engage in discussion. Vicious cycles of self-defeating behavior can occur in which a student hesitates to speak; this results in decreased speaking skills, which results in more hesitation to speak. Students may develop sufficient anxiety about speaking that their academic outcomes are affected. Students tend to form study groups with others who have common first languages. Opportunities to practice English are therefore reduced, and communication errors are perpetuated. When the teacher divides students into small groups for projects, ENNL students often do not participate as much as others. If these students are anxious about speaking, they may withdraw from classroom participation. ENNL students may feel rejected by other students in a small group situation when their input is not sought or understood.

The fourth aspect of language is *writing*. Spelling and syntax errors are common when writing a nonnative language. Teachers often respond to student writing assignments with feedback that is too vague to provide a basis for correction or improvement by ENNL students. When it comes to writing lecture notes, these students are at risk of missing important details because they may not pick up the teacher's cues about what is important. They might miss information when they spend extra time translating a word or concept to understand it, or they might just take more time to write what is being said.

Another major issue faced by ENNL nursing students is the culture of the learning environment. International students were often educated in settings where students took a passive role in the classroom. They may have learned that faculty should be respected, not questioned. Memorizing facts may have been emphasized. It may be a shock to them to discover that the nursing faculty expect assertive students who ask questions and think critically. These expectations cannot be achieved unless students understand them.

Finally, the European-American culture, which forms the context for nursing practice, creates challenges. Because they are immersed in Euro-American culture and the culture of nursing, faculty may not see the potential sources of misunderstanding. For example, if a teacher writes a test question about what foods are allowed on a soft diet, a student who understands therapeutic diets may miss the question if s/he does not recognize the names of the food choices. Nursing issues with an especially high culture connection are: food, behavior, law, ethics, parenting, games, or choosing the right thing to say. These topics are well-represented in psychiatric nursing, which makes it a difficult subject for ENNL students.

MINIMIZING CULTURE BIAS ON NURSING EXAMS

Our goal is not really to eliminate culture from nursing or from nursing education. Nursing exists in a culture-dependent context. Our goal is to practice transcultural nursing and to teach nursing without undue culture bias.

Sometimes our nursing exam questions will relate to culture-based expectations for nursing action. The way to make these questions fair is to teach transcultural nursing and to clarify the cultural expectations of a nursing student in the Euro-American-dominated healthcare system.

Students must learn the cultural aspects of the profession before they can practice appropriately within it. Like other cultures, the professional culture of nursing has its own language (medical terminology and nursing diagnosis, of course). We have our own accepted way of dress, our own implements, skills, taboos, celebrations, and behavior. The values accepted by our culture are delineated in the ANA Code of Ethics, and are passed down to our students during nursing education.

It is usually clear to nursing educators that students are not initially aware of all the aspects of the professional culture, and that these must be taught. The social context of nursing seems more obvious to educators, and is often overlooked in nursing education. Some aspects of the social context of nursing were mentioned above (food, games, social activities, relationships, behavior, what to say in certain situations). Students must also learn these social behaviors and attitudes if they are to function fully in nursing. If they do not already know about American hospital foods, what to say when someone dies, how to communicate with an authority figure, or what game to play with a 5-year-old child, they must learn these things in nursing school.

Try for yourself the following test. It was written without teaching you the cultural expectations first.

CULTURE BIASED TEST

1. Following radiation therapy, an African-American client has been told to avoid using her usual hair care product due to its petroleum content. Which product should the nurse recommend that she use instead?
   A. Royal Crown hair treatment
   B. Dax Wave and Curl
   C. Long Aid Curl Activator Gel
   D. Wave Pomade

2. A Jewish client is hospitalized for pregnancy-induced hypertension during Yom Kippur. How should the nurse help this client meet her religious needs based on the tradition of this holy day?
   A. Order meals without meat-milk combinations.
   B. Ask a family member to bring a serving of *Marror* for the client.
   C. Encourage her to fast from sunrise to sunset.
   D. Remind her that she is exempt from fasting.

3. Based on the Puerto Rican concept of *compadrazco*, who is considered part of the immediate family and responsible for care of children?
   A. Parents, grandparents, aunts, uncles, cousins, and godparents
   B. Mother and father, older siblings
   C. Mother, father, any blood relative
   D. Parents and chosen friends (*compadres*) who are given the honor of child care responsibility

4. A 60-year-old Vietnamese immigrant client on a general diet is awake at 11:00 p.m. on a summer night. What is the best choice of food for the nurse to offer to this client?
   A. Warm milk
   B. Hot tea
   C. Ice cream
   D. Iced tea

5. Which of the following positions is contraindicated for a client recovering from a total hip replacement?
   A. Side-lying using an abductor pillow
   B. Standing
   C. Walking to the restroom using a walker
   D. Sitting in a low recliner

When you took this test, did it seem unfair? It was intended to test nursing behaviors that were based on culture-specific situations. Your immigrant and ENNL students are likely to face questions like these on every exam.

Item #1 is about hair care products for black hair. Option C is the only one that does not contain petroleum products. Students could know this, if they were given the information before the exam. Otherwise, the item is culture-biased.

Item #2 is about the Jewish holiday Yom Kippur. To celebrate this holiday, it is customary to fast from sunrise to sunset, but people who are sick, such as the client in the question, are exempted from fasting. This is only unfair if students did not have access to the information.

Item #3 expects you to know about *compadrazco*, in which parents, grandparents, aunts, uncles, cousins, and godparents are all considered immediate family. This can be an important point if you are responsible for visiting policies in a pediatrics unit.

Item #4 tests knowledge about the preferred drink for an immigrant Vietnamese client. Many people in Asia feel comforted by hot drinks and find cold drinks to be unsettling.

Item #5 does not seem as biased as the others. If you understand total hip precautions, it is a fairly simple question, unless you have never heard of a "low recliner." An ENNL student who missed this question said, "I saw the chairs in clinical called 'geri chairs' and I know that the client cannot bend more than 90 degrees, but 'low recliner' was confusing to me. I imagined someone lying down (reclining) and I think this would not dislocate the prosthesis."

The best way to avoid culture bias on exams is to know what you are testing. It is acceptable to test about hip precautions, but not really fair to test about the names of furniture. The same is true of foods. Test about therapeutic diets, but not about the recipes (an African immigrant student advised us to say "egg-based food" instead of "custard").

Behavior in social and professional situations is especially culture-bound. Behavior-based questions are common on nursing exams. Make behavior expectations explicit. Especially when a student is expected to act in a way that would be inappropriate in his or her social culture, these are very difficult questions. For example, we expect nurses to act assertively with physicians and clients. It is inappropriate for many Asian students to question their elders. When a client is their elder, these students will choose the option that preserves respect for the client over one that provides teaching. We must make our expectations very clear.

Finally, talk with your ENNL and immigrant students after your exams. They can provide a wealth of information about what confused them or what was ambiguous. Discuss your findings with your colleagues and improve your exams. Ultimately your exams will be more clear and more valid.

SUCCESS STRATEGIES

The following strategies were developed originally to help ENNL students. An interesting revelation is that they also help native English speakers who have learning styles that are not conducive to learning by lecture, who read slowly, or have learning disabilities or other academic challenges.

STRATEGIES FOR PROMOTING ENNL STUDENT SUCCESS

1. You cannot decrease the reading assignment because some students read slowly, but you can help students prioritize the most important areas.
2. Allow adequate time for testing. The NCLEX® is not a 1-minute-per-question test anymore. Usually 1.5 hours is adequate for a 50-item multiple-choice exam.
3. Allow students to tape lectures if they want to. You might have lectures audiotaped and put in the library for student access.
4. Speak clearly. Mumbling and rapid, anxious speech are difficult to understand. If you have a problem with clarity, provide handouts that contain the critical points. Provide the handouts anyway. You want to teach and test nursing knowledge, not note-taking skills.
5. Avoid slang and idiomatic expressions. This is hard to do, but you can do it with practice. When you do use slang, explain it. This is especially important on exams. When in doubt about whether a word is confusing, think about what the dictionary definition would be, and if there are two meanings, use another word.
6. Allow the use of translation dictionaries on exams. You can say that students must tell you what they are looking up, so they cannot find medical terminology that is part of the test.
7. Be aware of cultural issues when you are writing exams. Of course you will test on culture-specific issues, but be sure you are testing what you want to test (the student's knowledge of diets, not of recipes).
8. Feel free to use medical terminology; after all, this is nursing school. However, when you use an important new term, write it on the board so students can spell it correctly in their notes.
9. In clinical, make the implied explicit. It seems obvious that safety is the priority, but if a student thinks the priority is respecting her elders, when an elderly client with a new hip replacement demands to get out of bed, there could be a disaster.
10. Hire a student who takes clear and accurate lecture notes to post his/her notes for use by ENNL and other students. The students will still attend class and take their own notes, but will have this resource to fill in the details that they miss.
11. Spell out abbreviations (SOA).
12. Many international students learned to speak English in the British style. If something would be confusing to a British person, they will find it confusing.
13. Provide opportunities for students to discuss what they are learning with other students and faculty. A faculty member might hold a weekly discussion group in which students bring questions. It can be interesting to find a student who has no trouble tracing the path of a red cell from the heart to the portal vein, but has difficulty understanding what Cream of Wheat is (for example, the student may say, "I thought it was a stalk of grain in a bowl with cream poured on it").
14. Make it clear that questions are encouraged. When a student is not asking, and you think they may not understand, ask the student after class if s/he has questions. Make it easier for students to approach you by being approachable. Learn their names, and learn to pronounce them correctly. Hearing you try to pronounce their name might be humorous for them, and it will validate how difficult it is to speak other languages.
15. Take another look at basing grades on class participation. You may be putting inordinate demands on the ENNL students. Of course nurses must learn to work with others, but the nurse who talks most is not necessarily the best.
16. Be a role model for communication skills. You might even say in class when you talk about communication that if you respect a person who is trying to communicate with you, you will persist until you understand the message. Say, "Please repeat that," or "I think you said to put a chicken on my head, is that correct?" or "You want me to do what with the textbook?" It may be considered socially rude to ask people to repeat themselves. Make it clear that this is not a social situation. In the professional role, we are responsible for effective communication. We cannot get away with smiling and nodding our heads.
17. In clinical, if a student has an accent that is difficult for the staff to understand, discuss clarification techniques (see #16) to the student and staff member. Make it explicit that it is acceptable for the student to ask questions and for the staff to ask for clarification.
18. If your college has a writing center where students can receive feedback on grammar and style before submitting papers, have students use it. If you are not so fortunate, view papers as a rough draft instead of a final product. Give specific feedback about what to correct and allow students to resubmit.
19. Make any services that are available to ENNL students available to all students (such as group discussions and notes). These services may meet the learning needs of many students while preventing the attitude that "they are different and they get something I don't."
20. Faculty attitudes are the most important determinant of a successful program to promote the success of ENNL nursing students. Talk with other faculty about the controversial issues. Create an organized program with a consistent approach among the faculty. The rewards will be worth the work.

Strategies for Success

Sandra DeYoung, EdD, RN
William Paterson University
Wayne, New Jersey

Improving Our Teaching

Every faculty member wants to be a good teacher, and every teacher wants the students to learn. In particular, we want to achieve the student learning outcomes that our educational institutions say we must achieve. How can we best meet both goals? We cannot just teach as we were taught. We have to learn a variety of teaching methods and investigate best practices in pedagogy. We also have to learn how to measure student learning outcomes in practical and efficient ways. The next few pages will introduce you to principles of good teaching and ways to evaluate learning. Keep in mind that this is only an introduction. For a more extensive study of these principles and pedagogies, you might consult the resources listed at the end of this introduction.

Learning Theory

In order to improve our teaching, we must have some familiarity with learning theory. Nurses who come into educational roles without psychology of learning courses in their background should read at least an introductory-level book on learning theories. You should, for example, know something about stages and types of learning, how information is stored in memory and how it is retrieved, and how knowledge is transferred from one situation to another.

Behaviorist Theories

Behaviorist theories are not in as much favor today as they were 25 years ago, but they still help to explain simple learning. Conditioning and reinforcement are concepts with which most educators are familiar. Conditioning explains how we learn some simple movements and behaviors that result in desired outcomes, such as a nurse responding when an alarm sounds on a ventilator. Reinforcement refers to the fact that behavior which is rewarded or reinforced tends to reoccur. Therefore, reinforcement is a powerful tool in the hands of an educator.

Cognitive Learning Theories

Cognitive learning theories are much more sophisticated. They deal with how we process information by perceiving, remembering, and storing information. All of these processes are a part of learning. One of the most useful concepts in cognitive theory is that of mental schemata.

Schemata (plural) are units of knowledge that are stored in memory. For example, nurses must develop a schema related to aseptic technique. Once a schema is stored in memory, related information can be built on it.

For instance, changing a dressing is easier to learn if the learner already has a schema for asepsis.

Metacognition is another concept identified in cognitive theories. This concept refers to thinking about one's thinking. To help learners who are having difficulty mastering certain material, you might ask them to think about how they learn best and help them evaluate whether they really understand the material.

Transfer of learning occurs when a learner takes information from the situation in which it is learned and applies it to a new situation. Transfer is most likely to occur if the information was learned well in the first place, if it can be retrieved from memory, and if the new situation is similar to the original learning situation. Educators can teach for transfer by pointing out to students how a concept is applied in several situations so that learners know the concept is not an isolated one, and the students begin to look for similar patterns in new situations.

Adult Learning Theories

Adult learning theories help to explain how learning takes place differently for adults than for children. Adults usually need to know the practical applications for the information they are given. They also want to see how it fits with their life experiences. When teaching adults, nurse educators need to keep in mind adult motivation for learning.

Learning Style Theories

Learning style theories abound. Research has shown that some learners are visually oriented, some are more auditory or tactile learners, some are individualistic and learn best alone, others learn best by collaboration, some deal well with abstract concepts, and others learn better with concrete information. Measurement instruments that can determine preferred learning styles are readily available. Although not many educators actually measure their students' learning styles, they should keep learning styles in mind when they plan their instruction.

Planning for Instruction

With some background knowledge of how students learn, the nurse educator can begin to plan the learning experiences. Planning includes developing objectives, selecting content, choosing pedagogies, selecting assignments, and planning for assessment of learning. All nurse educators come to the teaching process already knowing how to write objectives. Objectives can be written in the cognitive, psychomotor, and affective domains of learning. In the cognitive domain, they can be written at the knowledge, comprehension, application, analysis, and synthesis levels of complexity. The critical aspect of objectives is to keep referring to them as you plan your lesson or course. They will help you focus on the "need to know" versus the "nice to know" material. They will help you decide which assignments will be most suitable, and they will guide your development of evaluation tools.

SELECTING ASSIGNMENTS

Selecting and developing out-of-class assignments calls for creativity. You may use instructor's manuals such as this for ideas for assignments or you may also develop your own. To encourage learning through writing, you can assign short analysis papers, position papers, or clinical journals, all of which promote critical thinking. Nursing care plans of various lengths and complexity may be assigned. You may create reading guides with questions to help students read their textbooks analytically. You might also ask students to interview or observe people to achieve various objectives.

USING EFFECTIVE PEDAGOGIES

Selecting teaching methods or pedagogies takes considerable time. You must consider what you are trying to achieve. To teach facts, you may choose to lecture or assign a computer tutorial. To change attitudes or motivate learners, you may use discussion, role-playing, or gaming. Developing critical thinking may be done effectively using critical-thinking exercises, concept maps, group projects, or problem-based learning. There are traditional pedagogies, activity-based pedagogies, and technology-based pedagogies.

TRADITIONAL PEDAGOGIES

Traditional pedagogies include lecture, discussion, and questioning. Lecturing is an efficient way to convey a great deal of information to large groups of people. However, the lecture creates passive learning. Learners just sit and listen (or not) and do not interact with the information or the lecturer. Research has shown that students learn more from active learning techniques (i.e., from being able to talk about, manipulate, deduce, or synthesize information). If you are going to lecture, it would be wise to intersperse lecture with discussion and questioning.

Discussion gives students an opportunity to analyze and think critically about information that they have read or were given in a lecture. By discussing key concepts and issues, they can learn the applicability of the concepts and see how they can transfer to varied situations. Discussions can be formal or informal, but they generally work best if they are planned. For a formal discussion, students must be held accountable for preparing for it. The teacher becomes a facilitator by giving an opening statement or question, guiding the discussion to keep it focused, giving everyone a chance to participate, and summarizing at the end.

Questioning is a skill that develops over time. The first principle to learn is that you have to give students time to answer. Most teachers wait only 1 second before either repeating the question or answering it themselves. You should wait at least 3 to 5 seconds before doing anything, to allow students time to think and prepare a thoughtful answer. Research has revealed that most instructor-posed questions are at a very low level (lower-order), eliciting recall of facts. But questioning can be used to develop critical thinking if it is planned. Higher-order questions are those that require students to interpret information, to apply it to different situations, to think about relationships between concepts, or to assess a situation. If you ask higher-order questions during your classes or clinical experiences, students will rise to the occasion and will be challenged to provide thoughtful answers.

ACTIVITY-BASED PEDAGOGIES

Activity-based teaching strategies include cooperative learning, simulations, games, problem-based learning, and self-learning modules, among others. Cooperative learning is an old pedagogy that has received more research support than any other method. This approach involves learners working together and being responsible for the learning of group members as well as their own learning. Cooperative learning groups can be informal, such as out-of-class study groups, or they can be formally structured in-class groups. The groups may serve to solve problems, develop projects, or discuss previously taught content.

Simulations are exercises that can help students to learn in an environment that is low risk or risk-free. Students can learn decision making, for example, in a setting where no one is hurt if the decision is the wrong one. Simulations in skill laboratories are frequently used to teach psychomotor skills. Simulations can be written (case studies), acted out (role-playing), computer-based (clinical decision-making scenarios), or complex technology-based (active simulation manikins).

Games can help motivate people to learn. Factual content that requires memorization (such as medical terminology) can be turned into word games such as crossword puzzles or word searches. More complex games can teach problem solving or can apply previously learned information. Board games or simulation games can be used for these purposes.

Problem-based learning (PBL) provides students with real-life problems that they must research and analyze and then develop possible solutions. PBL is a group activity. The instructor presents the students with a brief problem statement. The student group makes lists of what they know and don't know about the problem. They decide what information they must collect in order to further understand the problem. As they collect the information and analyze it, they further refine the problem and begin to investigate possible solutions. The educator serves as a facilitator and resource during the learning process and helps keep the group focused.

Self-learning modules are a means of self-paced learning. They can be used to teach segments of a course or an entire course or curriculum. Modules should be built around a single concept. For example, you might design a module for a skill lab based on aseptic technique, or you could develop a module for a classroom course around the concept of airway impairment. Each module contains components such as an introduction, instructions on how to use the module, objectives, a pretest, learning activities, and a posttest. Learning activities within a module should address various learning styles. For example, you should try to include activities that appeal to visual learners and tactile learners, conceptual learners and abstract learners, and individual learners and collaborative learners. Those activities could be readings, audiovisuals, computer programs, group discussion, or skills practice. The educator develops and tests the module and then acts as facilitator and evaluator as learners work through the module.

TECHNOLOGY-BASED PEDAGOGIES

Technology-based pedagogies include computer simulations and tutorials, internet use, and distance learning applications. Computer simulations include decision-making software in which a clinical situation is enacted and students are asked to work through the nursing process to solve problems and achieve positive outcomes. They also include simulation games such as SimCity, which can be a useful tool in teaching community health principles. Computer tutorials are useful for individual remedial work such as medication calculations or practice in answering multiple-choice test questions.

The internet is a rich resource for classroom use and for out-of-class assignments. There are hundreds of websites that can be accessed for health-related information. Students need to be taught how to evaluate the worth of these websites. The criteria they should apply to this evaluation include identifying the intended audience, the currency of the information, the author's credentials or the affiliated organization, and content accuracy. Students may not know how to identify online journal sources compared to other websites. It is worth spending time, therefore, teaching students how to use the internet before giving them such assignments. If your classroom is internet access enabled, you can visually demonstrate how to identify and use appropriate websites. For example, if you want students to find relevant information for diabetic teaching, you can show them the differing value of information from official diabetes associations versus pharmaceutical sites versus chat rooms or public forums.

You may be using this instructor's manual in a distance learning course. Distance learning takes the forms of interactive television classes, webcasting, or online courses. In any form of distance learning, students are learning via the technology, but they are also learning about technology and becoming familiar with several computer applications. Those applications may include synchronous and asynchronous applications, streaming video, and multimedia functions.

ASSESSING LEARNING

You can assess or evaluate learning in a number of ways. Your first decision is whether you are just trying to get informal, ungraded feedback on how well students are learning in your class, or whether you are evaluating the students for the purpose of assigning a grade. Following are a number of techniques that can be used for one or both purposes.

CLASSROOM ASSESSMENT TECHNIQUES

Classroom assessment techniques (CATs) are short, quick, ungraded, in-class assessments used to gauge students' learning during or at the end of class. Getting frequent feedback on students' understanding helps educators to know if they are on the right track and if students are benefiting from the planned instruction. If you wait until you give a formal quiz or examination, you may have waited too long to help some students who are struggling with the material. The most popular CAT is probably the *minute paper*. This technique involves asking students to write down, in 1 or 2 minutes, usually at the end of class, what was the most important thing they learned that day or what points remain unclear. A related technique is the *muddiest point*, in which you ask the class to write down what the "muddiest" part of the class was for them. In nursing, *application cards* can be especially useful. After teaching about a particular concept or body of knowledge, and before you talk about the applications of the information, ask the students to fill out an index card with one possible clinical application of the information. This technique fosters application and critical thinking. Always leave class time during the following session to give feedback on the CAT results.

Another means of doing a quick assessment of learning in the classroom is the use of a *classroom (or student) response system*, sometimes called *clicker* technology. By the use of radio frequency technology, a laptop computer, a projector, and student remote controls (the clickers), an instructor can pose a written question on the screen and ask students to use their clickers to select the correct answer. The answers are then tallied and can be projected as a graph of results on the screen. This technology permits quick assessment of student understanding of critical information and keeps students active during a lecture. Classroom response systems are often made available by publishers in conjunction with their textbooks.

TESTS AND EXAMINATIONS

Tests and examinations are also used to assess or evaluate learning. Tests should be planned carefully to measure whether learning objectives have been met. You should form a test plan in which you decide the number of test items to include for each objective as well as the complexity of the items. Just as objectives can be written at the knowledge through synthesis levels of knowing, test items can be written at each level, too. Some types of items lend themselves to the lower levels of knowing, such as true-false and matching items, while multiple-choice and essay questions can be used to test higher levels.

TRUE-FALSE QUESTIONS

True-false questions are used simply to determine if the student can identify the correctness of a fact or principle. This type of question should be used sparingly, because the student has a 50% chance of guessing the correct answer. Well-written true-false questions are clear and unambiguous.

The entire statement should be totally true or totally false. An example of a question that is ambiguous is:

(T F) A routine urinalysis specimen must be collected with clean technique and contain at least 100 mL.

The answer to this question is false because the specimen does not require 100 mL of volume. However, the clean technique part of the question is true. Because part of the statement is true and part is false, the question is misleading. A better question is:

(T F) A routine urinalysis specimen must be collected with clean technique.

True-false questions can be made more difficult by requiring the student to explain why the statement is true or false.

MATCHING QUESTIONS

Matching questions also test a low level of learning—that of knowledge. They are most useful for determining if students have learned definitions or equivalents of some type. They should be formatted in two columns, with the premise words or statements on the left and the definitions or responses on the right. You should have more responses than premises so that matching cannot be done simply by process of elimination. Instructions should be given that indicate if responses can be used more than once or even not used at all. An example of a matching question is:

Match the definition on the right with the suffix on the left. Definitions can be used only once or not at all.

_____ 1. –itis	a.	presence of
_____ 2. –stalsis	b.	abnormal flow
_____ 3. –rrhage	c.	inflammation
_____ 4. –iasis	d.	discharge or flow
_____ 5. –ectomy	e.	contraction
	f.	surgical removal of

MULTIPLE-CHOICE QUESTIONS

Multiple-choice questions can be written at the higher levels of knowing, from application through evaluation. At these higher levels they can test critical thinking. A multiple-choice question has two parts. The first part, the question, is also called the *stem*. The possible answers are called *options*. Among the options, the correct one is called the *answer*, while the incorrect options are termed *distractors*. You can word stems as questions or as incomplete statements that are completed by the options. For example, an item written as a question is:

WHAT IS A QUICK WAY TO ASSESS THE APPROXIMATE LITERACY LEVEL OF A PATIENT?

a. Pay attention to her vocabulary as she speaks.

b. Give her an instruction sheet to read.

c. Administer a literacy test.

d. Ask her whether she graduated from high school.

The same knowledge can be tested by a stem written as an incomplete statement:

A QUICK WAY TO ASSESS THE APPROXIMATE LITERACY LEVEL OF A PATIENT IS TO

a. pay attention to her vocabulary as she speaks.

b. give her an instruction sheet to read.

c. administer a literacy test.

d. ask her whether she graduated from high school.

Notice the differing formats of each item. When the stem is a question it is also a complete sentence, so each option should be capitalized because each is also a complete sentence and each ends with a period. When the stem is an incomplete statement, it does not end with a period, so the options that complete the statement do not begin with a capital letter but do end with a period. Stems should be kept as brief as possible to minimize reading time. Avoid negatively stated stems. For example, a poor stem would be:

WHICH OF THE FOLLOWING IS NOT A GOOD WAY TO ASSESS A PATIENT'S LITERACY LEVEL?

It is too easy for readers to miss the word *not* and therefore answer incorrectly. If you feel compelled to write negative stems occasionally, be sure to capitalize or underline the word *not*, or use the word *except* as in the following example:

ALL OF THE FOLLOWING ARE GOOD WAYS TO ASSESS A PATIENT'S LITERACY LEVEL EXCEPT

In this case, the reader is less likely to miss the negative word because of the sentence structure and also because the word *except* is capitalized.

Options usually vary from three to five in number. The more options you have, the more difficult the item. However, it is often difficult to write good distractors. Be sure that your options are grammatically consistent with the stem. Next is a test item in which all of the options do not fit grammatically with the stem:

THE LECTURE METHOD OF TEACHING IS BEST SUITED TO

a. when the audience already knows a lot about the topic.

b. large audiences.

c. times when you are in a hurry to cover your material and don't want to be interrupted.

d. young children.

Not only are the options grammatically inconsistent, they are also of varied lengths. Attempt to keep the options about the same length. The following restatement of the item corrects the problems with grammar and with length:

THE LECTURE METHOD OF TEACHING IS BEST SUITED TO

a. an audience that already knows the topic.

b. an audience that is very large.

c. times when you must cover your material quickly.

d. an audience of young children.

Distractors that make no sense should never be used. Instead, try to develop distractors that reflect incorrect ideas that some students might hold about a topic.

ESSAY QUESTIONS

Essay-type questions include short answer (restricted-response questions) and full essays (extended-response questions). These types of items can be used to test higher-order thinking. Extended-response essays are especially suited to testing analysis, synthesis, and evaluation levels of thinking. An example of an essay that might test these higher-order levels of thinking is:

Explain how exogenous cortisone products mimic a person's normal cortisol functions and why long-term cortisone administration leads to complications. Also explain how nursing assessment and intervention can help to reduce those complications.

The educator must plan how the essay is going to be graded before the test is given. An outline of required facts and concepts can be developed and points given to each. Then a decision must be made as to whether it is appropriate to give points for writing style, grammar, spelling, and so on.

TEST ITEM ANALYSIS

After a test is given, an analysis of objective items can be conducted. Two common analyses are *item difficulty* and *item discrimination.* Most instructors want to develop questions that are of moderate difficulty, with around half of the students selecting the correct answer. A mixture of fairly easy, moderate, and difficult questions can be used. The difficulty index can be calculated by dividing the number of students who answered the question correctly by the total number of students answering the question. The resulting fraction, converted to a percentage, gives an estimate of the difficulty, with lower percentages reflecting more difficult questions.

Item discrimination is an estimate of how well a particular item differentiates between students who generally know the material and those that don't. In other words, a discriminating item is one that most of the students who got high scores on the rest of the examination got right and most of the students who got low scores got wrong. The discrimination index can be calculated by computer software or by hand using a formula that can be found in tests and measurement textbooks.

HELPFUL RESOURCES

These few pages are but an introduction to teaching techniques. To be fully prepared for the educator role, you will need to enroll in formal courses on curriculum and teaching or do more self-learning on educational topics. For more information, you might consult the following print and web-based resources:

DeYoung, S. (2003). *Teaching Strategies for Nurse Educators.* Upper Saddle River, NJ: Prentice Hall.

Websites:

www.crlt.umich.edu/tstrategies/teachings.html

www.gmu.edu/facstaff/part-time/strategy.html

www.ic.arizona.edu/ic/edtech/strategy.html

CHAPTER 1
MEDICAL-SURGICAL NURSING

RESOURCE LIBRARY

 PRENTICE HALL NURSING MEDIALINK DVD-ROM

Audio Glossary
NCLEX-RN® Review

 COMPANION WEBSITE

Audio Glossary
NCLEX-RN® Review
Care Plan Activity: Nursing Process
Case Studies
  Advance Directive
  Critical Thinking in the Nursing Process
MediaLink Applications
  *Medication and Healthcare Needs Assist
   Programs*
  Nursing Code of Ethics
Links to Resources

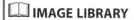 **IMAGE LIBRARY**

Figure 1.1 Steps of the nursing process.
Figure 1.2 The healthcare team discusses the individualized plan of care and outcomes.

Figure 1.3 The nurse's role as educator is an essential component of care.

LEARNING OUTCOME 1

Describe the core competencies for healthcare professionals: client-centered care, interdisciplinary teams, evidence-based practice, quality improvement, and informatics.

CONCEPTS FOR LECTURE

1. The core competencies are based on using communication, knowledge, technical skills, critical thinking, and values in clinical practice.
2. The nursing process allows for the inclusion of specific, individualized, and holistic activities in planning client-centered care for the client.
3. Interdisciplinary teams should communicate, collaborate, and cooperate to provide continuous care.
4. Evidence-based practice integrates the best research findings with clinical expertise and client values to provide optimum care.
5. Errors are identified and safety principles are implemented through the application of quality improvement measures.
6. Informatics is used to communicate, manage knowledge, decrease errors, and support critical thinking.

POWERPOINT LECTURE SLIDES

Core Competencies for Healthcare Professionals
- Provide client-centered care
- Work in interdisciplinary teams
- Use evidence-based practice
- Apply quality improvement
- Use informatics

SUGGESTIONS FOR CLASSROOM ACTIVITIES

- Discuss the core competencies and the relationship to excellent client care. Give examples of evidence-based practice.
- Show the video about the changing roles of nurses.

LEARNING OUTCOME 2

Apply the attitudes, mental habits, and skills necessary for critical thinking when using the nursing process in client care.

CONCEPTS FOR LECTURE

1. Thinking critically requires focused attention on attitudes and how they affect nursing actions.
2. The major critical thinking skills are divergent thinking, reasoning, clarifying, and reflection.

POWERPOINT LECTURE SLIDES

Attitudes, Mental Habits, and Skills for Critical Thinking
- Attitudes, mental habits, and skills
  - Think independently
  - Be willing to listen
  - Have empathy
  - Be fair-minded
  - Be disciplined
  - Be creative
- Types of critical thinking
  - Divergent thinking: weigh the importance of information
  - Reasoning: ability to discriminate between fact and guesses
  - Clarifying: noting similarities and differences to sift out unnecessary information
  - Reflection: comparing different situations with similar solutions

SUGGESTIONS FOR CLASSROOM ACTIVITIES

- Discuss the legal and ethical implications of nursing.

LEARNING OUTCOME 3

Explain the importance of nursing codes and standards as guidelines for clinical nursing practice.

CONCEPTS FOR LECTURE

1. Nurses encounter legal and ethical problems almost daily.
2. Nursing practice is structured by codes and standards that guide nursing practice and protect the public. Nurses are held to these standards in a court of law.
3. Codes of ethics provide a frame of reference for nursing behaviors.
4. The International Council of Nurses (ICN) code helps guide nurses in setting priorities, making judgments, and taking action when they face ethical dilemmas in clinical practice.
5. The ANA code defines nursing for the general public, guides behavior of nurses, and states principles of ethical concern.
6. Standards of Nursing Practice are criteria that can be used by a professional nurse and by the general public to measure quality of practice.

POWERPOINT LECTURE SLIDES

Nursing Codes and Standards
- Importance of nursing codes and standards
  - Guide nursing practice
  - Protect the public
- Code of ethics
  - Provides a frame of reference for nursing behaviors
- ICN code
  - Helps guide nurses
  - Setting priorities
  - Making judgments
  - Taking action when faced with ethical dilemmas
- ANA code
  - Defines nursing for general public
  - Guides behavior of nurses
  - States principles of ethical concern
- Standards of nursing practice
  - Provides criteria that can be used to measure quality of practice

LEARNING OUTCOME 4

Explain the activities and characteristics of the nurse as caregiver, educator, advocate, leader and manager, and researcher.

CONCEPTS FOR LECTURE

1. Medical-surgical nurses are not only caregivers but also educators, advocates, leaders and managers, and researchers.
2. Nurses are leaders and managers of client care within a variety of models of care delivery.
3. Critical pathways are used in conjunction with case management models and/or quality improvement efforts.
4. The nurse assumes these various roles to provide the best care and to promote client health.

POWERPOINT LECTURE SLIDES

Nursing Roles
- Caregiver
  - Acts both independently and collaboratively
  - Practices nursing as an art and a science
  - Provides comprehensive, individualized care
- Educator
  - Assesses client learning needs
  - Plans and implements teaching to meet needs
- Advocate
  - Speaks for the client
  - Protects the client's rights
- Leader/Manager
  - Manages time, people, client care
  - Delegates, evaluates
- Researcher
  - Identifies problems in client care
  - Develops interventions to meet client needs

CHAPTER 2
HEALTH AND ILLNESS IN THE ADULT CLIENT

RESOURCE LIBRARY

 PRENTICE HALL NURSING MEDIALINK DVD-ROM

Audio Glossary
NCLEX-RN® Review

 COMPANION WEBSITE

Audio Glossary
NCLEX-RN® Review
Care Plan Activity: Family-Centered Care in Chronic
  Illness
Case Studies
  Care Across the Lifespan
  Developing Teaching Programs
MediaLink Applications
Links to Resources

📖 IMAGE LIBRARY

Figure 2.2 The revised Food Guide Pyramid is designed to be used as a method of helping Americans make healthy food choices and be active every day.

Figure 2.3 The older adult population is increasing more rapidly than any other age group, making gerontologic nursing an integral component of medical-surgical nursing practice.

LEARNING OUTCOME 1

Define health, incorporating the health–illness continuum and concept of high-level wellness.

CONCEPTS FOR LECTURE

1. Health is defined as a state of complete physical, mental, and social well-being, not merely the absence of disease or infirmity.
2. The health–illness continuum is a dynamic process with high-level wellness at one extreme end of the continuum, and death at the opposite extreme.

POWERPOINT LECTURE SLIDES

Defining Health
- Health
  - Defined as a state of complete physical, mental, and social well-being, not merely the absence of disease or infirmity
- Health–illness continuum
  - Dynamic process
  - High-level wellness at one extreme
  - Death at opposite extreme

SUGGESTIONS FOR CLASSROOM ACTIVITIES

- Discuss wellness opportunities for yourself and family. What facilities are available?

SUGGESTIONS FOR CLINICAL ACTIVITIES

- Visit a wellness center.
- Ask a personal fitness trainer to speak to the class concerning wellness for all member of the family.

LEARNING OUTCOME 2

Explain factors affecting functional health status.

CONCEPTS FOR LECTURE

1. Different factors affect a person's health or wellness. These factors may promote health and wellness or become a risk factor.
2. Wellness is an integrated method of functioning.
3. A variety of factors can affect health, including: genetic makeup, cognitive abilities and educational level, self-concept, cultural background, age, gender, developmental level, lifestyle and environment, socioeconomic background, and geographic area.

POWERPOINT LECTURE SLIDES

Factors Affecting Health
- Genetic makeup
- Cognitive abilities and educational level
- Race, ethnicity, and cultural background
- Age, gender, and developmental level
- Lifestyle and environment
- Socioeconomic background
- Geographic area

SUGGESTIONS FOR CLASSROOM ACTIVITIES

- Discuss the effect that socioeconomic factors have on overall wellness.

SUGGESTIONS FOR CLINICAL ACTIVITIES

- If your hospital affiliate has a wellness center, visit the center and have students apply nursing implications to what they saw or learned.

LEARNING OUTCOME 3

Discuss the nurse's role in health promotion.

CONCEPTS FOR LECTURE

1. The nurse promotes health and wellness by teaching activities that maintain wellness.
2. The nurse also promotes health by following healthy practices and serving as a role model.

POWERPOINT LECTURE SLIDES

Nurse's Role in Health Promotion
- Teach clients activities that maintain wellness
- Follow health practices
- Serve as a role model

SUGGESTIONS FOR CLASSROOM ACTIVITIES

- Develop an educational poster or brochure that promotes wellness for children.

SUGGESTIONS FOR CLINICAL ACTIVITIES

- Visit a daycare center or preschool and teach a component of wellness to the students.

LEARNING OUTCOME 4

Describe characteristics of health, disease, and illness.

CONCEPTS FOR LECTURE

1. Health is defined as "a state of complete physical, mental, and social well-being, not merely the absence of disease or infirmity."
2. The characteristics of health needs to take into account the various levels of health a person may experience, or that a person may be clinically described as ill yet still defined oneself as well.
3. Disease is a medical term that describes alterations in structure or functions in the body.
4. Illness is a person's response to a disease.

POWERPOINT LECTURE SLIDES

Characteristics of Health, Disease, and Illness
- Health
  - State of complete physical, mental, and social well-being
  - Not merely the absence of disease or infirmity
- Disease
  - Medical term describing alterations in structure and/or functions in the body
- Illness
  - Response to disease

- Discuss why health is not just the absence of disease.

LEARNING OUTCOME 5

Describe illness behaviors and needs of the client with acute illness and chronic illness.

CONCEPTS FOR LECTURE

1. Illness behaviors are the way people cope with the alterations in health and function caused by a disease.
2. Illness behaviors are highly individualized and are based on gender, age, family values, economic status, culture, educational level, and mental status.
3. Clients with acute illness usually have a full recovery and return to normal pre-illness functioning.
4. Clients with a chronic illness may have many different lifelong pathologic and psychologic alterations in health.

POWERPOINT LECTURE SLIDES

Acute and Chronic Illness Behaviors and Needs
- Acute illness behaviors
  - Experience symptoms
  - Assume the sick role
  - Seek medical care
  - Assume a dependent role
  - Achieve recovery and rehabilitation
- Chronic illness needs
  - Try to live as normal a life as possible
  - Learn to adapt daily activities
  - Comply with medical treatment plan
  - Maintain a positive self-concept and a sense of hope
  - Maintain a feeling of being in control
  - Confront the inevitability of death

SUGGESTIONS FOR CLASSROOM ACTIVITIES

- Discuss the reactions of clients to disease. How does the client's culture and socioeconomic status affect this reaction?

SUGGESTIONS FOR CLINICAL ACTIVITIES

- Visit a long-term care facility. Assign students to care for long-term care clients.
- Discuss the differences in caring for acute clients versus long-term care clients.

LEARNING OUTCOME 6

Describe the primary, secondary, and tertiary levels of illness prevention.

CONCEPTS FOR LECTURE

1. The primary level of prevention includes generalized health promotion activities.
2. Specific actions that prevent or delay the occurrence of a disease are also part of the primary level of prevention.
3. Activities that emphasize early diagnosis and treatment of illness comprise the secondary level.
4. The tertiary level focuses on stopping the disease process and returning the client to a useful place in society.
5. The activities in the tertiary level of prevention revolve around rehabilitation.

POWERPOINT LECTURE SLIDES

Levels of Illness Prevention
- Primary level
  - Protect oneself against environmental risks
  - Eat nutritious foods
  - Avoid industrial hazards
  - Obey seatbelt and helmet laws
  - Obtain immunizations
- Secondary level
  - Health screenings
  - Self-exams for breast or testicular cancer
  - TB skin tests
  - Obtain specific treatment for illnesses
- Tertiary level
  - Obtain medical or surgical treatment for illness
  - Rehabilitation
  - Join work training program following illness or injury

SUGGESTIONS FOR CLASSROOM ACTIVITIES	SUGGESTIONS FOR CLINICAL ACTIVITIES
• Ask students to select a disease or condition and follow the disease through all three levels of wellness.	• Visit an occupational health clinic. Observe how clients prepare to return to work.

LEARNING OUTCOME 7

Compare and contrast the physical status, risks for alterations in health, assessment guidelines, and healthy behaviors of the young adult, middle adult, and older adult.

CONCEPTS FOR LECTURE

1. The young adult (ages 18–40) is at the peak of physical development between ages 18 to 25. The risk for alterations in health is from accidents, sexually transmitted disease, substance abuse, and physical or psychosocial stressors.

2. Assessment of the young adult should include assessing the achievement of significant developmental tasks.

3. Physical assessment should include the usual height, weight, and vital signs. During the health history the nurse should ask questions about substance abuse, sexual history, coping mechanisms, familial chronic illnesses, and family changes.

4. The young adult should have regular physical examinations, avoid risky behaviors, eat a well-balanced diet, and exercise regularly.

5. The middle adult (ages 40–65) has physical status and function similar to the young adult; however, many changes take place between these ages. Risks for alterations in health are obesity, cardiovascular disease, cancer, substance abuse, and physical and psychosocial stressors.

6. Assessment guidelines include assessing the achievement of significant developmental tasks in the middle adult.

7. Physical assessment should include all body systems, vital signs, and monitoring for risks and onset of cancer symptoms.

8. The middle adult behaviors should include self-examination for cancer, eating a healthy diet, and exercise.

9. The older adult period begins at age 65, but can be divided into further groups: the young-old (65–74), the middle-old (75–84), and the old-old (85 and over).

10. Risks for alterations in health are a sedentary lifestyle, cardiovascular disease, obesity, and injuries.

11. Assessment of the older adult should include assessing the achievement of significant developmental tasks.

12. The older adult behaviors should include protecting themselves from injury along with regular health assessments.

POWERPOINT LECTURE SLIDES

Meeting Health Needs of Adults
- Young adult
  - Risks for alterations in health
  - Injuries
  - Substance abuse
  - Sexually transmitted disease
  - Physical and psychosocial stressors
- Middle adult
  - Obesity
  - Cardiovascular disease
  - Cancer
  - Substance abuse
  - Physical and psychosocial stressors
- Older adult
  - Injuries
  - Pharmacologic effects
  - Physical and psychosocial stressors

SUGGESTIONS FOR CLASSROOM ACTIVITIES

- Identify some stressors that affect the 18–25 year old age group. How do these stress factors relate to the client's health status?
- Discuss the achievement goals for each age group discussed.
- Why and how would achievement or lack of achievement of these goals affect the client?

SUGGESTIONS FOR CLINICAL ACTIVITIES

- Assign students to work in a physician's office that specializes in family practice. These practices usually have a good cross-section of age groups.

LEARNING OUTCOME 8

Explain the definitions, functions, and developmental stages and tasks of the family.

CONCEPTS FOR LECTURE

1. Traditionally, the family is defined as a unit of people that are related by marriage, birth, or adoption.
2. The "family" to the client may not always be traditional. It can include persons who are friends, or even pets. The family is an integral part of the client's care.
3. The family has developmental stages and tasks. Each stage brings change that requires adaptation.

POWERPOINT LECTURE SLIDES

Family Functions and Developmental Stages
- Family functions
  - Interdependence
  - Maintaining boundaries
  - Adapting to change
  - Performing family tasks
- Developmental stages
  - Couple
  - Family with infants and preschoolers
  - Family with school-age children
  - Family with adolescents and young adults
  - Family with middle adults
  - Family with older adults
  - Family of a client with a chronic illness

SUGGESTIONS FOR CLASSROOM ACTIVITIES

- Discuss a "nontraditional" family. What are the different compositions?
- Form the students into small groups and have each group take a "family" group that is discussed in the text, and discuss the developmental tasks for each group.

CHAPTER 3
COMMUNITY-BASED AND HOME CARE OF THE ADULT CLIENT

RESOURCE LIBRARY

 PRENTICE HALL NURSING MEDIALINK DVD-ROM

Audio Glossary
NCLEX-RN® Review

 COMPANION WEBSITE

Audio Glossary
NCLEX-RN® Review
Care Plan Activity: Home Health Assessment
Case Study: Safety in the Home
MediaLink Application: Home Nursing Care Strategies
Links to Resources

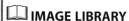 **IMAGE LIBRARY**

Figure 3.1 The home health nurse provides client and caregiver education.

Figure 3.2 Home visits offer opportunities to work on health promotion.

LEARNING OUTCOME 1
Differentiate community-based care from community health care.

CONCEPTS FOR LECTURE

1. Health care has become a managed care, community-based system. Hospitals are primarily acute care providers.
2. Communities are formed by the characteristics of the people who make up the community and the culture therein.
3. Nurses who provide community-based care must know the composition and characteristics of the clients with whom they will work.
4. Community-based health care is dependent upon many factors that comprise the community that it serves.

POWERPOINT LECTURE SLIDES

Community-Based Care and Healthcare Services
- Factors affecting community-based healthcare
  - Social support system
  - Community healthcare structure
  - Environmental factors
  - Economic resources
- Community-based healthcare services
  - Community centers and clinics
  - Day care programs
  - Parish nursing
  - Meals-on-Wheels

SUGGESTIONS FOR CLASSROOM ACTIVITIES

- Have students research community programs for inner-city and for rural health care.

SUGGESTIONS FOR CLINICAL ACTIVITIES

- Assign students to visit a home healthcare agency and accompany the registered nurse on a home visit.
- Create a nursing care plan for the client in a community-based setting.

LEARNING OUTCOME 2
Discuss selected factors affecting health in the community.

CONCEPTS FOR LECTURE

1. Many factors can affect the health of individuals in a community. These factors include social support systems, the community healthcare structure, environmental factors, and economic resources.

POWERPOINT LECTURE

Factors Affecting Health in the Community
- Social support systems
- Community healthcare structure
- Environmental factors
- Economic resources

2. Social support systems: A person's social support system consists of the people who lend assistance to meet financial, personal, physical, or emotional needs. In order to understand the community social structure, the nurse needs to know what support is available for health care for the client and family, including neighbors, friends, their church, organizations, self-help groups, and professional providers. The nurse also must know and respect the cultural and ethnic background of the community.

3. Community healthcare structure: The healthcare structure of a community has a direct effect on the health of the people who live and work within it. The size of the community often determines the type of services provided as well as the access to the services. Nurses who provide community-based care must know about public health services, the number and type of health screenings offered, the location and specialty of healthcare professionals within the community, and the availability and accessibility of services and supplies. Other factors to consider include facilities (e.g., day care and long-term care), housing, and the number and type of support agencies that provide assistance (e.g., housing, shelter, and food).

4. Environmental factors: The environment within which a person lives and works may have both helpful and harmful effects on health. Air and water quality differs across communities. Within the home, pollution may occur from such sources as molds, pesticides, and fumes from new carpet. The water source also varies, with water supplies coming from rivers, lakes, reservoirs, or wells. No matter the source, chemical runoff or bacteria may contaminate water. Household and community safety and health resource accessibility are also important. Nurses must consider lighting, street and sidewalk or road upkeep and conditions, effects of ice and snow, condition of stairs and floors, and usefulness and availability of bathroom facilities. Physical barriers to accessing community resources include lack of transportation, distance to services, and location of services.

5. Economic resources: Economic resources encompass the financial and insurance coverage that provide the means for health care within the community. As private medical insurance becomes more and more expensive, fewer citizens have it; and many U. S. citizens have no insurance at all.

SUGGESTIONS FOR CLASSROOM ACTIVITIES

- Explore the community facilities and services available in your area.

SUGGESTIONS FOR CLINICAL ACTIVITIES

- Visit community facilities and services in your area that provide healthcare assistance.

LEARNING OUTCOME 3

Describe services and settings for healthcare consumers receiving community-based and home care.

CONCEPTS FOR LECTURE

1. Many services are available to the healthcare consumer in the community-based setting. Selected examples include community centers and clinics, daycare programs, parish nursing, and Meals-on-Wheels.
2. Home care encompasses both health and social services provided to the chronically ill, disabled, or recovering person in his or her own home. Home care is usually provided when a person needs help that cannot be provided by a family member or friend. The services provided in the home may include professional nursing care, care provided by home care aides, physical therapy, speech therapy, occupational therapy, medical social worker services, and nutritional services. Clients who receive home care services are usually under the care of a physician, and the focus of care is treatment or rehabilitation. Registered nurses or licensed practical nurses provide nursing care based on physician orders.
3. An interdisciplinary team may need to be involved to assist the community care nurse in directing clients to the services available.

POWERPOINT LECTURE SLIDES

Community-Based and Home Care Settings and Services
- Community-based care
  - Settings
    - Satellite hospital-based clinic
    - Community-based clinic
    - Senior centers
    - Daycare programs
  - Services
    - Social support system: family, friend, neighbors
    - Economic resources such as private insurance, Medicare, Medicaid
    - Meals-on-Wheels
- Home care
  - Health and social services provided to chronically ill, disabled, or recovering person
  - Services may include professional nursing care, physical therapy, speech therapy, occupation therapy, and nutritional services

SUGGESTIONS FOR CLASSROOM ACTIVITIES

- Ask the class to find out the criteria for clients who need community assistance for healthcare assistance organizations.

SUGGESTIONS FOR CLINICAL ACTIVITIES

- Visit a senior center or senior daycare center.
- Ask a home health nurse to speak to the class about special needs in various communities.

LEARNING OUTCOME 4

Describe components for the home healthcare system, including agencies, clients, referrals, physicians, reimbursement, legal considerations, and nursing care.

CONCEPTS FOR LECTURE

1. Home health care is defined as services for recovering, disabled, or chronically ill people who are in need of treatment or support to function effectively in the home environment.
2. The home healthcare system encompasses both health and social services that are provided to a client in their own home.
3. Home health agencies may be either public or private, but all must meet uniform standards for licensing.
4. Clients in the home healthcare setting include both the person receiving care and the person's family.
5. Nursing care is provided to the home health client by a registered nurse or a licensed practical nurse.
6. Referrals for home care may come from anyone connected with the client.
7. Reimbursement sources pay for home health care. This can come from private insurance, Medicare, Medicaid, and private funding and other private sources.

POWERPOINT LECTURE SLIDES

Components for Home Healthcare Systems
- Clients
  - Clients who benefit from home health care may:
    - Be unable to live independently due to age or disability
    - Have chronic or debilitating disease
    - Be terminally ill and want to die with comfort and dignity at home
    - Not need acute care, but require additional assistance
    - Need short-term help for postoperative care
  - Family members also considered clients
- Types of home health agencies
  - Official or public agencies (tax funded)
  - Voluntary or private not-for-profit agencies
  - Private, proprietary agencies (for profit organizations, usually private pay)
  - Institution-based agencies (usually operate under a parent organization such as a hospital)

CONCEPTS FOR LECTURE *continued*

8. A physician must order home health care and must provide an approved treatment plan for the client.
9. The legal considerations in home care center around issues of privacy, confidentiality, and other legal issues.

POWERPOINT LECTURE SLIDES *continued*

- Referral sources
  - Nurse
  - Physician
  - Family members
  - Social worker
  - Discharge planner
  - Other
- Legal considerations
  - Privacy and confidentiality
  - Client's access to health information
  - Client's freedom from unreasonable restraint
  - Witnessing of documents
  - Informed consent and matters of negligence and/or malpractice

SUGGESTIONS FOR CLASSROOM ACTIVITIES

- Explore the legal and ethical responsibilities of home health nursing with regard to client privacy and family intervention.

SUGGESTIONS FOR CLINICAL ACTIVITIES

- Assign students to a home health agency and accompany a registered nurse on rounds to client's homes.

LEARNING OUTCOME 5

Compare and contrast the roles of the nurse providing home care with the roles of the nurse in medical-surgical nursing discussed in Chapter 1.

CONCEPTS FOR LECTURE

1. The nursing process in home care is no different from nursing care practiced in any other setting, with the exception of the implementation step.
2. The difference between nursing care in the home and in other settings is assessing how the home's unique environment affects the need or problem of the client.
3. Since few home health clients are referred with copies of their medical history, the home health nurse must try to obtain as complete a clinical picture as possible.
4. In the home, there are no colleagues present to consult, to assist, or to rely on for support. The nurse must learn to trust his or her theoretical and intuitive knowledge.
5. The role of the home care nurse is multifaceted.

POWERPOINT LECTURE SLIDES

Home Care Nursing Roles and Considerations
- Roles of the home care nurse
  - Advocate
  - Provider of direct care, not personal care
  - Educator
  - Coordinator of services
- Special considerations in home care nursing
  - Set boundaries
  - Establish rapport
  - Proceed slowly
  - Assess the home environment
  - Set priorities
  - Promote learning
  - Limit distractions
  - Remember: safety first
  - Be resourceful
  - Teach infection control
- The home care nurse
  - Main contact with the client's physician and all other providers involved in the treatment plan
  - Report client changes
  - Discuss responses
  - Develop and secure treatment plan revisions on an ongoing basis

SUGGESTIONS FOR CLASSROOM ACTIVITIES

- Have the students discuss safety issues in home care nursing.
- Discuss personal safety and safety for the client.

SUGGESTIONS FOR CLINICAL ACTIVITIES

- Discuss emergency procedures for a client in a home care setting.
- Create a nursing intervention plan for an emergency in the home.

LEARNING OUTCOME 6

Explain the purpose of rehabilitation in health care.

CONCEPTS FOR LECTURE

1. Rehabilitation nursing is based on a philosophy that each person has a unique set of strengths and abilities that can enable that person to live with dignity, self-worth, and independence.
2. Rehabilitation nursing care focuses on clients with chronic illnesses or impairments.
3. Rehabilitation promotes reintegration into the client's family and community through a team approach.
4. Assessment of the client and family is multifaceted.
5. Interventions to facilitate rehabilitation are revised to meet client and family needs as the client progresses toward reintegration.

POWERPOINT LECTURE SLIDES

Rehabilitation in Health Care
- Terminology
  - Impairment: disturbance in structure of function resulting from physiologic or psychological abnormalities
  - Disability: degree of observable and measurable impairment
  - Handicap: the total adjustment to disability that limits functioning at normal level
- Plan of care should include
  - Physical function
  - Mental health
  - Interpersonal relationships
  - Social interactions
  - Family support
  - Vocational status

SUGGESTIONS FOR CLASSROOM ACTIVITIES

- Discuss the differences between impairment, disability, and handicap.
- Create a plan of care for a young adult with a severe disability due to a closed head trauma.

SUGGESTIONS FOR CLINICAL ACTIVITIES

- Visit a home healthcare agency that specializes in rehabilitation clients.

CHAPTER 4
NURSING CARE OF CLIENTS HAVING SURGERY

RESOURCE LIBRARY

 PRENTICE HALL NURSING MEDIALINK DVD-ROM

Audio Glossary
NCLEX-RN® Review
Animation/Video
  Epidural Placement

 COMPANION WEBSITE

Audio Glossary
NCLEX-RN® Review
Care Plan Activity: Providing Postoperative Care
Case Study: The Circulating Nurse
MediaLink Applications
  Anesthesia and Outpatient Surgery
  Consent Forms
  Joint Replacement Patient Education Program
Links to Resources

IMAGE LIBRARY

Figure 4.1 Informed consent form.
Figure 4.2 A scrub nurse in the operating room.
Figure 4.3 Surgical attire.
Figure 4.4 Areas to be shaved.

Figure 4.5 Wound healing by primary, secondary, and tertiary intention.
Figure 4.6 Wound complications.

LEARNING OUTCOME 1

Discuss the differences and similarities between outpatient and inpatient surgery.

CONCEPTS FOR LECTURE

1. The complexity of the surgery and recovery and the expected disposition of the client following surgery will dictate whether the client will be an inpatient or outpatient.
2. Inpatient and outpatient surgeries are performed in the same operating room in many hospitals.
3. Freestanding facilities are not physically connected to a hospital.
4. Many surgeries are performed in the surgeon's office.
5. Increasingly complex surgeries on clients with complicated medical problems are now commonly performed on an outpatient basis.
6. Outpatient surgery potentially offers many advantages but also presents some disadvantages.

POWERPOINT LECTURE SLIDES

Outpatient and Inpatient Surgery
- Many surgeries are done on an outpatient basis
  - Cataract removal with or without lens implant
  - Hernia repairs
  - Biopsies
  - D&C
- Increasingly complex surgeries are being done on an outpatient basis
  - Endoscopic procedures
  - Arthroscopic procedures
- Outpatient surgery potentially has many advantages
  - Decreased cost
  - Reduced risk of hospital acquired infections
  - Less physiologic stress to the client and family
- Disadvantages to outpatient surgery
  - Less time for the nurses to assess, evaluate, and teach the client and family
  - Lack of opportunity for the nurse to assess for the risk of postoperative complications
  - Less time for adequate pain control prior to discharge

LEARNING OUTCOME 2

Describe the various classifications of surgical procedures.

CONCEPTS FOR LECTURE

1. The classification of surgical procedures includes diagnostic, ablative, constructive, reconstructive, palliative, and transplant.
2. Diagnostic surgery determines or confirms a diagnosis. An example would be a breast biopsy or a bronchoscopy.
3. Ablative surgery removes diseased tissue, an organ, or an extremity, such as an appendectomy or an amputation.
4. Constructive and reconstructive surgery builds tissues and organs that are absent due to a congenital anomaly. Palliative surgery rebuilds organs and tissues that have been damaged due to disease, as in some types of cancer.
5. Transplant surgery replaces organs or tissues to restore function or alleviate symptoms of a disease. An example of transplant surgery would be heart, lung, or liver transplants.

POWERPOINT LECTURE SLIDES

Classifications of Surgical Procedures
- Diagnostic
  - Determine or confirm a diagnosis
  - Examples:
    - Breast biopsy
    - Bronchoscopy
- Ablative
  - Remove diseased tissue, organ, or extremity
  - Examples:
    - Appendectomy
    - Amputation
- Constructive/Reconstructive
  - Build or rebuild tissue and organs that are damaged or absent
  - Examples:
    - Repair a cleft palate
    - Skin graft after a burn
    - Total joint replacement
- Palliative
  - Alleviate symptoms of a disease (not curative)
  - Example:
    - Bowel resection in client with terminal cancer
- Transplant
  - Replace organs/tissue to restore function
  - Examples:
    - Heart, lung, liver, kidney transplant

LEARNING OUTCOME 3

Identify diagnostic tests used in the perioperative period.

CONCEPTS FOR LECTURE

1. Diagnostic tests performed prior to surgery provide baseline data or detect problems that may place the client at additional risk during and after surgery.
2. Complete blood counts, coagulation studies and electrolyte counts, and urinalysis are the most commonly performed preoperative laboratory tests.
3. The history and physical may dictate other diagnostic tests that may be indicated.
4. In addition to laboratory tests, clients may require a chest x-ray or other radiologic procedures.
5. An electrocardiogram (EKG) may be required for clients over the age of 40, or who may have cardiovascular disease.
6. Pulmonary function tests may be required for clients who have chronic obstructive pulmonary disease.

POWERPOINT LECTURE SLIDES

Diagnostic Tests Used in the Perioperative Period
- Laboratory test to be performed prior to surgery
  - Complete blood count (CBC)
  - Electrolyte studies
  - Prothrombin time (PT)
  - Partial thromboplastin time (PTT)
  - Urinalysis
- Radiologic procedures
  - Chest x-ray
- Cardiac studies
  - Electrocardiogram (EKG)
  - Pulmonary function tests

SUGGESTIONS FOR CLASSROOM ACTIVITIES

- Review the normal laboratory values for common preoperative tests. Ask students what abnormal values would indicate and their impact on the nursing process.
- Bring a normal and abnormal chest x-ray to the classroom. Explain the differences between the two films.
- Discuss pulmonary function tests and their impact on anesthesia.

SUGGESTIONS FOR CLINICAL ACTIVITIES

- Have students observe a pulmonary function test. Ask a pulmonologist to discuss the findings.

LEARNING OUTCOME 4

Describe nursing implications for medications prescribed for the surgical client.

CONCEPTS FOR LECTURE

1. The client with nothing-by-mouth (NPO) orders requires careful analysis.
2. Potential drug interactions exist between anesthesia and certain medications.
3. Special consideration must be used when caring for the client with diabetes preoperatively.
4. It is vital to assess medications the client uses preoperatively, including over-the-counter medications, herbals, and illegal drugs.

POWERPOINT LECTURE

Nursing Implications for Medication Prescribed for the Surgical Client
- Nursing implications for the diabetic client
  - Insulin withheld
  - NPO status
  - Signs of hypoglycemia
- Assessment of all medications the client uses
  - Over the counter
  - Vitamins/herbal medications
  - Illegal drugs
  - Aspirin or other blood thinning medication

SUGGESTIONS FOR CLASSROOM ACTIVITIES

- Discuss the common over-the-counter medications and the nursing implications of a client who takes these drugs prior to surgery.
- What are the nursing implications of a client who takes illegal drugs prior to surgery?
- Discuss the nursing implications for a client who is an insulin-dependent, noncompliant diabetic prior to emergency surgery.
- Ask an anesthesiologist or nurse anesthetist to speak to the class about preoperative medications.

LEARNING OUTCOME 5

Provide appropriate nursing care for the client in the preoperative, intraoperative, and postoperative phases of surgery.

CONCEPTS FOR LECTURE

1. A thorough nursing assessment is needed to determine the most appropriate care for each client undergoing surgery.
2. In caring for the preoperative client, a nursing assessment should be made based on the information from the nursing history and physical assessment data.
3. The type of surgical procedure directs the assessment and intervention planned by the nurse.
4. The client and family will be anxious. Therapeutic communication can help the client and family identify fears and concerns.
5. Client teaching is essential in the preoperative period.
6. Preoperative client preparation includes completing the surgical checklist.
7. Intraoperative care begins when the client enters the operating room.
8. Circulating nurses and scrub nurses provide care for the client during this phase.
9. The postoperative phase begins when the client is transferred to the postanesthesia care unit (PACU).

POWERPOINT LECTURE SLIDES

Preoperative, Intraoperative, and Postoperative Nursing Care
- Preoperative nursing care
  - Nursing assessment
  - Client/family teaching
  - Preoperative surgical check list
- Intraoperative nursing care
  - Care is provided by a perioperative registered nurse
  - Main focus of intraoperative care is client safety
- Postoperative care
  - Begins in the PACU
  - Vital signs are monitored
  - Level of consciousness
  - Emotional support
  - Assessing and evaluating hydration status
  - Assess client pain level
- Care when the client is stable
  - PACU nurse communicates client status to floor nurse
  - Immediate assessment by the floor nurse upon client arrival to floor
  - Assess level of consciousness, vital signs, pain level
  - Assess IV fluids and any drainage tubes, including urinary catheter
  - Reassess according to hospital policy or more often if client condition dictates
  - Be constantly aware of any status changes in the immediate postoperative client to include vital sign changes, difficulty breathing, and excessive blood loss
  - Assess the postoperative client for deep vein thrombosis, pulmonary edema, and other complications that could occur after the immediate postoperative phase

SUGGESTIONS FOR CLASSROOM ACTIVITIES

- Role-play preoperative teaching for a preoperative client.
- Discuss postoperative complications in the newly postoperative client.
- Discuss the nursing implications for pulmonary embolism, shock, and deep vein thrombosis.

SUGGESTIONS FOR CLINICAL ACTIVITIES

- Observe in the operating room. Note the different roles that registered nurses play in the perioperative areas.

LEARNING OUTCOME 6

Identify variations in perioperative care for the older adult.

CONCEPTS FOR LECTURE

1. The older adult is at increased risk for postoperative complications due to physiological, cognitive, and psychosocial changes.
2. Nurses must be aware of the normal changes in the older client and modify nursing care accordingly.
3. Nursing interventions must include assessment of the integumentary system, sensory and perceptual issues, respiratory and cardiovascular systems, and gastrointestinal and genitourinary systems.
4. Frequent orientation may be needed.

POWERPOINT LECTURE SLIDES

Perioperative Care for the Older Adult
- Areas nurses should consider
  - Postoperative risks due to psychological, cognitive, and psychosocial changes
  - Integument—diminished skin integrity due to loss of subcutaneous fat, decreased oil production and hydration
  - Respiratory—decreased efficiency of cough reflex and aeration of lung fields
  - Sensory-perceptual—decline in vision and hearing
  - Cardiovascular—less efficient, decreased adaptation to stress
  - Gastrointestinal—decrease in motility
  - Genitourinary—decreased in efficiency for kidney; loss of bladder control
  - Cognitive-psychosocial—decreased reaction time, prone to delirium, and altered mental status

SUGGESTIONS FOR CLASSROOM ACTIVITIES

- Encourage discussion of how to care for older adult clients and the modifications that would need to be made for their care.

LEARNING OUTCOME 7

Describe principles of pain management specific to acute postoperative pain control.

CONCEPTS FOR LECTURE

1. Postoperative pain is to be expected.
2. It is neither realistic nor practical to eliminate postoperative pain completely.
3. Providing the client with postoperative pain relief facilitates coughing, turning, deep breathing, and earlier ambulation, which decrease postoperative complications.
4. Managing acute postoperative pain is an important nursing role. It involves cooperative efforts of the client, physician, and nurse.
5. Preoperatively, the client should learn how much pain to anticipate and what methods are available to control pain.
6. Various nonpharmacologic approaches to pain management are used alone or in combination to control acute postoperative pain.
7. Assess pain at various intervals using the 0–10 pain scale (0 equals no pain, 10 is unbearable pain) to assess pain relief.

POWERPOINT LECTURE SLIDES

Acute Postoperative Pain Management
- Guidelines for perioperative pain management (American Society of Anesthesiologists)
  - Education and training for healthcare providers
  - Monitoring of client outcomes
  - 24-hour availability of anesthesiologists providing perioperative pain management
  - Use of a dedicated pain management service
- Assess pain at various intervals using the 0–10 pain scale
  - 0 indicates no pain or discomfort, 10 indicates unbearable pain
  - Assess effectiveness of medication given for pain
  - Observe for drug reactions and side effects
  - Assess the need for changes in the dosage and/or frequency of medication administration

LEARNING OUTCOME 8

Use the nursing process as a framework for providing individualized care for the client undergoing surgery.

LECTURE CONCEPTS

1. Every pre- and postoperative client has unique problems that will affect the overall care.
2. When assessing the client, take into consideration age, predisposing conditions, health history, and psychosocial factors. Use this information to establish baseline data, identify physical needs, determine teaching needs and psychologic support for the client and family, and prioritize nursing care.
3. Assessing mental status and level of consciousness is another ongoing nursing responsibility, and the client may require repeated orientation to time, place, and person.
4. Be sure to assess information about use of over-the-counter medications including herbal supplements.
5. Immediate and continuing assessment is essential to detect and/or prevent complications.
6. The nurse must build the nursing process based on these individualized assessments.

POWERPOINT LECTURE SLIDES

Considerations When Providing Individualized Care
- Physical factors
  - Obesity
  - Age
  - Nutritional status
- Psychosocial factors
  - Family support
  - Coping mechanisms
  - Thought processes
- Health history
  - Cardiovascular status
  - Respiratory status
  - Metabolic status
  - Alcohol/tobacco usage

CHAPTER 5
NURSING CARE OF CLIENTS EXPERIENCING LOSS, GRIEF, AND DEATH

RESOURCE LIBRARY

 PRENTICE HALL NURSING MEDIALINK DVD-ROM

Audio Glossary
NCLEX-RN® Review

 COMPANION WEBSITE

Audio Glossary
NCLEX-RN® Review
Care Plan Activity: Anticipatory Grieving
Case Study: Do-Not-Resuscitate
MediaLink Applications
   DNR Regulations
   Explore Your Feelings about Death
   Grieving Process
   Hospice: Purpose and Benefits
Links to Resources

IMAGE LIBRARY

Figure 5.1 The nurse helps the client visualize the hospital room as a safe, comfortable place to die by surrounding the client with familiar pictures and objects.

Figure 5.2 Nurses who work with dying clients need support from their colleagues to work through their often overwhelming feelings of grief.

LEARNING OUTCOME 1

Differentiate loss, grief, and mourning.

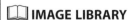

CONCEPTS FOR LECTURE

1. Loss may be defined as an actual or potential situation in which a valued object, person, body part, or emotion that was formerly present is lost or changed and can no longer be seen, felt, heard, known, or experienced.
2. Grief is the emotional response to loss and its accompanying changes.
3. Grieving may be thought of as the internal process the person uses to work through the response to loss.
4. Mourning describes the actions or expressions of the bereaved, including the symbols, clothing, and ceremonies that make up the outward manifestations of grief.

POWERPOINT LECTURE SLIDES

Loss
- An actual or potential situation in which a valued object, person, body part, or emotion that was formerly present is lost or changed and can no longer be seen, felt, heard, known, or experienced
- It may be temporary or permanent, complete or partial, objectively verifiable or perceived, physical or symbolic
- Only the person who experiences the loss can determine the meaning of the loss
- Loss always results in change
- The stress associated with the loss may be the precipitating factor leading to physiologic or psychologic change in the person or family
- The effective or ineffective resolution of feelings surrounding the loss determines the person's ability to deal with the resulting changes

Grief
- Grief is the emotional response to loss and its accompanying changes
- Grief as a response to loss is an inevitable dimension of the human experience

- The loss of a job, a role (e.g., the loss of the role of spouse, as occurs in divorce), a goal, body integrity, a loved one, or the impending loss of one's own life may trigger grief

Grieving
- May be thought of as the internal process the person uses to work through the response to loss

Mourning
- Describes the actions or expressions of the bereaved, including the symbols, clothing, and ceremonies that make up the outward manifestations of grief
- Both grieving and mourning are healthy responses to loss because they ultimately lead the person to invest energy in new relationships and to develop positive self-regard

---

SUGGESTIONS FOR CLASSROOM ACTIVITIES

- Ask the students to write an example of loss, grief, and mourning.

LEARNING OUTCOME 2

Compare and contrast theories of loss and grief.

CONCEPTS FOR LECTURE

1. The client's reaction to grief and loss is highly individualized.
2. Freud described the process of mourning as a gradual withdrawal from the lost object or person.
3. Bowlby believed the grieving process is initiated by a loss or separation. He divided the process into three phases which are protest, despair, and detachment.
4. Engel related the grief process with other methods of coping with stress. He describes three stages of the process. These stages include acute grief, restitution, and long-term grief.
5. The acute stage is initiated by shock and disbelief and is manifested by denial, which may help the person to cope with the overwhelming pain.
6. The acute stage is followed by a stage of restitution, in which the mourning is institutionalized.
7. Friends and family gather to support the grieving person through rituals dictated by the culture.
8. The mourner continues to feel a painful void and is preoccupied with thoughts of the loss. This stage lasts about 1 year, after which the mourner begins to come to terms with the loss and interest in people and activities are renewed.
9. Lindemann's research describes normal grief, anticipatory grieving, and morbid grief.
10. Caplan expanded the grief process to include surgery or childbirth.

POWERPOINT LECTURE SLIDES

Theories of Loss and Grief
- Freud: Psychoanalytic theory
  - Normal grieving is a withdrawal of attachment followed by readiness to make new attachments
  - Grief is a "nonpathologic condition" that reaches a state of completion after a period of inner labor
- Bowlby: Protest, despair, and detachment
  - Protest: lack of acceptance, crying, angry behavior
  - Despair: crying, sadness, disorganized behavior and thoughts as reality of the loss is recognized
  - Detachment: realization of loss, gradually relinquishes attachment, positive and negative aspects of the relationship are remembered, expressions of hopefulness and readiness to move forward
- Engel: Acute grief, restitution, and long-term grief
  - Acute grief: mourner experiences shock and disbelief
    - Denial
    - Pain, anger, guilt, and blame
    - Weeping openly or remaining stoic (cultural patterned behaviors)
  - Restitution: mourning is institutionalized
    - Family and friends gather to support the grieving person

11. Kübler-Ross identified distinct stages of grief and loss in death and dying. These stages are denial, anger, bargaining, depression, and acceptance.

  – Preoccupied with thoughts of loss
  – Stage lasts 1 year
  ○ Long-term grief: mourner comes to terms with loss and interests in people and activities are renewed
- Lindemann: Normal, anticipatory, and morbid grief
  ○ Normal grief
    – Somatic distress
    – Preoccupation with image of the diseased
    – Feelings of guilt
    – Hostile reactions
    – Loss of patterns of conduct
  ○ Anticipatory grieving
    – Predictable responses to an anticipated loss
  ○ Morbid grief
    – Delayed and dysfunctional reaction to loss
- Caplan: Stress and loss
  ○ Three factors influence ability to cope with loss
    – Psychic pain of the broken bond and the agony of coming to terms with the loss
    – Living without the assets and guidance of the lost person or resource
    – Reduced cognitive and problem-solving effectiveness
  ○ Process of building new attachments may occur if two elements present
    – Feelings of hope
    – Assumption of regular activities (ordinary living)
- Kübler-Ross: Stages of coping with loss
  ○ Anger: resists the loss; anger may be directed toward healthcare providers and family
  ○ Bargaining: attempts to postpone the loss
  ○ Depression: enters stage of depression as the full impact of the loss is realized
  ○ Acceptance: begins to come to terms with the loss and feels an air of hopefulness for the future

---

SUGGESTIONS FOR CLASSROOM ACTIVITIES

- Ask students to compare the similarities in the different studies that have been done on grief. Are the stages similar? How are the stages different?

LECTURE OUTCOME 3

Explain factors affecting responses to loss.

CONCEPTS FOR LECTURE

1. A variety of factors affect a person's responses to loss. These include age, social support, families, cultural and spiritual practices, and rituals of mourning.
2. The nurse must not place a value on the extent of the loss when assessing the need for support.

POWERPOINT LECTURE SLIDES

Factors Affecting Responses to Loss
- Age
- Social support
- Family
- Culture and spiritual practices

3. The reaction to loss is influenced by the age of the person who is experiencing the loss.
4. A social support system is important due to its potentially positive influence on the successful resolution of grief. Grieving can be painful and lonely.
5. The functional family usually rallies after the initial shock and disbelief. The family usually shifts roles, levels of responsibility, and ways of communicating.
6. The differences in cultural and spiritual beliefs are important considerations for the nurse when providing nursing care.
7. Spirituality is the core of human existence. When spiritual distress is relieved, the client can die more peacefully. The nurse may assess the client's needs by asking questions based on faith, influence, community, and address (FICA).
   - Faith: "What is your faith or belief?"
   - Influence: "How does your faith or spirituality influence your thoughts?"
   - Community: "Are you a part of a spiritual or religious community?"
   - Address: "Do you have any special needs or concerns? Is there someone you would like to speak to?"
8. Through rituals of mourning and ceremony, people symbolically express triumph over death and deny the fear of death.
9. The nurse needs to take time to analyze their own feelings related to loss and grief.
10. Factors that can interfere with successful grieving-include:
    - Perceived inability to share loss.
    - Lack of social recognition of the loss.
    - Ambivalent relationships prior to the loss.
    - Traumatic circumstances of the loss.

- Spiritual beliefs
  - Faith: What is your faith or belief?
  - Influence: How does your faith or spirituality influence your thoughts?
  - Community: Are you a part of a spiritual or religious community?
  - Address: Do you have any special needs or concerns? Is there someone you would like to speak to?
- Rituals of mourning
- Factors that can interfere with successful grieving
  - Perceived inability to share loss
  - Lack of social recognition of the loss
  - Ambivalent relationships prior to the loss
    – Traumatic circumstances of the loss

LEARNING OUTCOME 4

Discuss legal and ethical issues in end-of-life care.

CONCEPTS FOR LECTURE

1. Nursing care must ensure a peaceful death and incorporate high-quality end-of-life care as defined by the AACN competencies.
2. The Dying Person's Bill of Rights states that each person has the right to be cared for by caring, sensitive, and knowledgeable people.
3. Nurses must be aware of any advance directives, living wills, and other specific care requests.
4. A do-not-resuscitate order is written by the physician for the client who is near-death or has a terminal illness.
5. The term *euthanasia* comes from the Greek word for painless, easy death. Euthanasia is very controversial, and many times leaves the healthcare worker in a dilemma.

POWERPOINT LECTURE SLIDES

Legal and Ethical Issues in End-of-Life Care
- Examples of advanced directives
  - Living will: written directions concerning life-prolonging procedures
  - Healthcare surrogate: individual selected to make medical decisions
- Durable power of attorney: document delegating authority to make health, financial, and or legal decisions
- DNR order
  - Usually based on the wishes of the client and family
  - No cardiopulmonary resuscitation is to be performed
- Comfort measures only with goal of a comfortable death

LEARNING OUTCOME 5

Describe the philosophy and activities of hospice.

CONCEPTS FOR LECTURE

1. Hospice is a philosophy of care rather than a program of care.
2. Hospice is a comprehensive and coordinated care for clients with a limited life expectancy.
3. Hospice reaffirms that every client has the right to fully participate in the final stages of life. It is based on a philosophy of death with comfort and dignity, and encompasses biomedical, psychosocial, and spiritual aspects of the dying experience.

POWERPOINT LECTURE SLIDES

Hospice
- Philosophy rather than program
- Comprehensive and coordinated care for clients with limited life expectancy
- Supports a dignified and peaceful death
- Care focused on the physical, mental, and spiritual distress

CHAPTER 6
NURSING CARE OF CLIENTS WITH PROBLEMS OF SUBSTANCE ABUSE

RESOURCE LIBRARY

 PRENTICE HALL NURSING MEDIALINK DVD-ROM

Audio Glossary
NCLEX-RN® Review
Animation
  Cocaine

 COMPANION WEBSITE

Audio Glossary
NCLEX-RN® Review
Care Plan Activities
  Alcohol Withdrawal
  Tobacco Cessation
Case Study: Alcohol Withdrawal
MediaLink Applications
Links to Resources

IMAGE LIBRARY

Figure 6.1 Action of abusive substances at brain receptor sites.
Figure 6.2 Methamphetamine use by race/ethnicity: 2002, 2003, and 2004.
Figure 6.3 Methamphetamine use by gender and age: 2002, 2003, and 2004.

Figure 6.4 Methamphetamine use by state: 2002, 2003, and 2004.
Figure 6.5 Annual numbers of new nonmedical users of OxyContin, 1995–2003.
Figure 6.7 Assessment tool for alcohol withdrawal.

LEARNING OUTCOME 1

Explain risk factors associated with substance abuse.

CONCEPTS FOR LECTURE

1. Various risk factors help explain why one person becomes addicted while another does not.
2. Genetic factors include an apparent hereditary factor, especially in alcohol use and dependence.
3. Biological factors, such as low levels of dopamine and serotonin, are implicated in the development of alcohol dependency.
4. Psychological factors include attempts to explain substance abuse through a combination of psychoanalytic, behavioral, and family system theories.
5. Sociocultural factors include ethnic differences and religious background.
6. Many factors place a person at risk for substance abuse. No single cause can explain why one person develops a pattern of abuse and another does not.

POWERPOINT LECTURE SLIDES

Risk Factors for Substance Abuse
- Genetic factors
- Biological factors
- Psychologic factors
- Sociocultural factors
- No single cause is identified for substance abuse

SUGGESTIONS FOR CLASSROOM ACTIVITIES

- Research the internet for research and theories about substance abuse.

SUGGESTIONS FOR CLINICAL ACTIVITIES

- Ask a substance abuse counselor to speak to the class about substance abuse.

LEARNING OUTCOME 2

Recognize the signs and symptoms of potential substance abuse in coworkers.

CONCEPTS FOR LECTURE

1. The impaired nurse in the workplace displays warning signs of substance abuse.
2. The following are at-risk situations for the impaired nurse: easy access to prescription drugs, role strain, depression, and signs of alcohol or drug abuse.
3. The nurse has easy access to prescription drugs. Signs that indicate potential substance abuse include: inaccurate narcotic counts or frequent missing drugs; client complaints of ineffective pain control or denial of receiving pain medications; excessive "wasting" of drugs; volunteering to give medications to clients; or frequent trips to the bathroom.
4. The nurse can experience role strain. Signs that indicate potential substance abuse include: frequent tardiness or absenteeism, shoddy charting, client care judgment errors, erratic behavior, or an unkempt appearance.
5. The nurse can experience depression. Signs that indicate potential substance abuse include: irritability; inability to focus or concentrate; abrupt mood swings; taking long breaks; isolation; lethargy; apathy; or unexplained absences from assigned unit.
6. Signs of alcohol or drug use include: the smell of alcohol on breath; excessive use of perfumes, mouthwash or mints; slurred speech; reddened eyes; unsteady gait; flushed face; or wearing long sleeves in summer to cover up arms.
7. Signs of substance withdrawal include tremors, restlessness, sweating, watery eyes, runny nose, or stomach aches.

POWERPOINT LECTURE SLIDES

Signs of Potential Substance Abuse in Coworkers
- Easy access to prescription drugs
  - Inaccurate narcotic counts or frequent missing drugs
  - Client complaints of ineffective pain control or deny receiving pain meds
  - Excessive "wasting" of drugs
  - Volunteering to give medications to clients
  - Frequent trips to the bathroom
- Role strain
  - Frequent tardiness or absenteeism
  - Shoddy charting
  - Client care judgment errors erratic behavior, unkempt appearance
- Depression
  - Irritability, unable to focus or concentrate
  - Abrupt mood swings
  - Taking long breaks, isolation, lethargic, apathetic
  - Unexplained absences from assigned unit
- Signs of alcohol or drug use
  - Smell of alcohol on breath
  - Excessive use of perfumes, mouthwash, or mints
  - Slurred speech, reddened eyes, unsteady gait, flushed face
  - Wearing long sleeves in summer to cover up arms
- Signs of withdrawal
  - Tremors, restlessness, sweating
  - Watery eyes, runny nose, stomach aches

SUGGESTIONS FOR CLASSROOM ACTIVITIES

- Research the internet for new data and theories about factors that contribute to substance abuse.

SUGGESTIONS FOR CLINICAL ACTIVITIES

- Ask students to research the provisions and guidelines written by your state board of nursing for impaired nurses.

LEARNING OUTCOME 3

Describe common characteristics of substance abusers.

CONCEPTS FOR LECTURE

1. Many abusers have several characteristics in common; however, no addictive personality trait exists.
2. Drug abusers have a tendency toward more risky behaviors.
3. There is a tendency toward anxiety, anger, and low self-esteem in substance abusers.
4. Other abusers may suffer from social anxiety and use drugs or alcohol to "fit in."

POWERPOINT LECTURE SLIDES

Characteristics of Substance Abusers
- Compulsive preoccupation with obtaining the substance
- Loss of control over consumption
- Development of tolerance, dependence
- Impaired social /occupational functioning

SUGGESTIONS FOR CLASSROOM ACTIVITIES	SUGGESTIONS FOR CLINICAL ACTIVITIES
• Have the students identify addictive behaviors and risky behaviors.	• Assign students to an acute rehabilitation unit for chemical dependency.

LEARNING OUTCOME 4

Classify major addictive substances.

CONCEPTS FOR LECTURE

1. The following substances are listed as addictive: caffeine, nicotine, cannabis, central nervous system (CNS) depressants, alcohol, psychostimulants, opiates, and hallucinogens.
2. Caffeine is a stimulant that increases heart rate and is a diuretic. It is found in chocolate, coffee, tea, and many soft drinks. Consumption of 300 mg/day is considered safe, but over 600 mg/day is considered excessive.
3. Nicotine (a CNS stimulant) increases heart rate, gastric secretions, and causes vasoconstriction.
4. Cannabis' (marijuana) psychoactive component is THC.
5. Alcohol (a CNS depressant) is the most commonly used and abused substance in the United States.
6. People who abuse CNS depressants can develop a cross-tolerance with CNS stimulants.
7. Psychostimulants include cocaine and amphetamines.
8. Opiates include oxycodone HCL (oxycontin), hydrocodone bitartrate and acetaminophen (Vicodin), oxycodone and acetaminophen (Percocet), morphine (MS-Contin), meperidine (Demerol).
9. Hallucinogens are called psychedelics, e.g., PCP, LSD, or Ecstasy.

POWERPOINT LECTURE SLIDES

Major Addictive Substances
- Caffeine—stimulant
- Nicotine—CNS stimulant
- Cannabis—marijuana
- Alcohol—CNS depressant
- CNS depressants
- Psychostimulants—cocaine, amphetamines
- Opiates—OxyContin, Vicodin, Percocet, morphine, meperidine
- Hallucinogens—called psychedelics-PCP-LSD-ecstasy

SUGGESTIONS FOR CLASSROOM ACTIVITIES

- Ask students to investigate the newest, most popular street drugs in your area.
- Discuss what the usual age is for clients who use these drugs, and why they use the drugs.

LEARNING OUTCOME 5

Explain the effects of addictive substances on physiologic, cognitive, psychologic, and social well-being.

CONCEPTS FOR LECTURE

1. Anxiety and depressive disorders frequently occur with substance abuse. More than 90% of suicides have a depressive or substance abuse disorder.
2. Continued use of a substance usually persists despite adverse effects on the person's physical condition, psychologic health, and interpersonal relationships.
3. The human tendency to seek pleasure and avoid stress and pain is partially responsible for substance abuse.
4. The physiologic, cognitive, psychologic, and social well-being will vary depending on the addictive substance being used.

POWERPOINT LECTURE SLIDES

(The physiologic, cognitive, psychologic, and social well-being will vary depending on the addictive substance being used.)

Caffeine (consumed in large quantities) Causes
- Higher total cholesterol levels insomnia

Nicotine (initially)
- Increases respiration
- Mental alertness
- Cognitive ability

5. Caffeine, if consumed in large quantities, can also cause higher total cholesterol levels and insomnia.
6. Initially, nicotine increases respiration, mental alertness, and cognitive ability, but eventually it depresses these responses.
7. Physiologic effects of cannabis are dose related and can cause an increase in heart rate and bronchodilation in short-term use.
8. When used in moderation, certain types of alcohol can have positive physiologic effects by decreasing coronary artery disease and protecting against stroke. However, when consumed in excess, alcohol can severely diminish one's ability to function and will ultimately lead to life-threatening conditions.
9. Chronic users of barbiturates require progressively higher doses to achieve subjective effects as tolerance develops, but they develop little tolerance to respiratory depression.
10. Methamphetamine users in treatment have reported physical symptoms associated with the use of methamphetamine including weight loss, tachycardia, tachypnea, hyperthermia, insomnia, and muscular tremors.
11. Physical dependence occurs with long-term use of opiates. Initial withdrawal symptoms such as drug craving, lacrimation, rhinorrhea, yawning, and diaphoresis usually take 10 days to run their course, with the second phase of opiate withdrawal lasting for months with insomnia, irritability, fatigue, and potential GI hyperactivity and premature ejaculation as problems.
12. PCP is known for inducing violent behavior and for inducing negative physical reactions such as seizures, coma, and death.
13. The effects from inhaling organic solvents are similar to those of alcohol, with prolonged use leading to multiple toxicities and an increased risk for abusing other substances.

Nicotine Eventually Depresses These Responses

Cannabis
- Increase in heart rate
- Bronchodilation

Alcohol
- Can have positive physiologic effects by decreasing coronary artery disease and protecting against stroke
- When consumed in excess, alcohol can severely diminish one's ability to function and will ultimately lead to life-threatening conditions

Chronic Users of Barbiturates Require
- Progressively higher doses to achieve subjective effects as tolerance develops
- Develop little tolerance to respiratory depression

Methamphetamine
- Physical symptoms include weight loss, tachycardia, tachypnea, hyperthermia, insomnia, and muscular tremors

Opiates
- Initial withdrawal symptoms such as drug craving, lacrimation, rhinorrhea, yawning, and diaphoresis
- Second phase of opiate withdrawal lasting for months with insomnia, irritability, fatigue, and potential GI hyperactivity and premature ejaculation as problems

PCP
- Induces violent behavior
- Physical reactions such as seizures, coma, and death

Suggestions for Classroom Activities

- Lead a discussion about the effects of substance abuse on the family and community.

Suggestions for Clinical Activities

- Assign students to the chemical dependency unit to care for clients with addictive problems.

Learning Outcome 6

Support interdisciplinary care for the client with substance abuse problems, including diagnostic tests, emergency care for overdose, and treatment of withdrawal.

Concepts for Lecture

1. The effective treatment of substance abuse and dependence results from the efforts of an interdisciplinary team.

PowerPoint Lecture Slides

Emergency Care for Overdose
- Support airway
- Keep awake
- Induce vomiting treat for shock and cardiac arrest

2. Clients may be treated in an outpatient or inpatient facility.
3. Diagnostic testing is used to treat the substance abuse client. This includes both blood and urine tests that may be repeated frequently in the initial treatment stages.
4. Emergency care for the overdose client is a serious medical emergency. The client must be observed for signs of respiratory depression, because mechanical ventilation may be necessary.
5. Treatment is based on the severity of the symptoms and the drug that is being abused. Treatment includes: titrated detoxification with a similar drug, methadone for opiate abuse, and support for relief of symptoms.

- Administer narcotic antagonist if overdose is caused by an opiate

Withdrawal Signs
- Nausea, vomiting
- Seizures
- Anxiety
- Insomnia
- Lethargy
- Irritability
- Muscle cramps
- Diarrhea
- Chills/fever

Treatment Includes
- Titrated detoxification with like drug
- Methadone for opiate abuse
- Support for relief of symptoms

SUGGESTIONS FOR CLASSROOM ACTIVITIES

- Create a case study about a young adult who is admitted to the emergency department for an accidental drug overdose. Ask the class to describe and discuss the role and function of each interdisciplinary team member.

SUGGESTIONS FOR CLINICAL ACTIVITIES

- Visit an outpatient treatment facility.
- Develop a nursing care plan for a client with a chemical dependency.

LEARNING OUTCOME 7

Develop a framework for providing individualized nursing care for clients experiencing problems with substance abuse using the nursing process.

CONCEPTS FOR LECTURE

1. The nurse caring for a client with a substance abuse problem requires a nonjudgmental atmosphere that promotes trust and respect.
2. Nurses should provide health education material to the client about the psychologic and physiologic effects of substance abuse.
3. The nurse should encourage and support the client during periods of abstinence.
4. Assessment must include a history of the client's past substance abuse, medical and psychiatric history, and presence of psychosocial concerns.

POWERPOINT LECTURE SLIDES

Framework of Care for Client with Abuse Problems
- Requires nonjudgmental atmosphere
- Provide health education material
- Support clients during period of abstinence
- Assessment

SUGGESTIONS FOR CLASSROOM ACTIVITIES

- Ask students to develop an educational trifold pamphlet about the psychologic and physiologic effects of substance abuse.

SUGGESTIONS FOR CLINICAL ACTIVITIES

- Assign students to visit a group meeting of recovering clients.

CHAPTER 7
NURSING CARE OF CLIENTS EXPERIENCING DISASTERS

RESOURCE LIBRARY

 PRENTICE HALL NURSING MEDIALINK DVD-ROM

Audio Glossary
NCLEX-RN® Review

 COMPANION WEBSITE

Audio Glossary
NCLEX-RN® Review
Care Plan Activity: Clients Experiencing Disasters
Case Study: Disaster Scenario
MediaLink Applications
Links to Resources

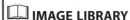 **IMAGE LIBRARY**

Figure 7.1 The stages of a disaster are cyclical.

Figure 7.2 The CDC's Mass Trauma Data Instrument.

LEARNING OUTCOME 1

Distinguish the difference between an emergency and a disaster.

CONCEPTS FOR LECTURE

1. An emergency encompasses an unforeseen combination of factors that need immediate action for victims who range in number from one to many.
2. Disasters may be natural or man-made. Disasters are defined as events that require extraordinary efforts beyond those needed to respond to everyday emergencies.

POWERPOINT LECTURE SLIDES

Disasters and Emergencies
- Types of disasters
  - Natural: caused by acts of nature or emerging diseases
  - Man-made: may be accidental or intentional
- Types of emergencies
  - Multiple casualty incidents-complex emergencies
  - Mass casualty: more than 100 casualties

SUGGESTIONS FOR CLASSROOM ACTIVITIES

- Research on the internet the effects on health care for the clients who live on the Gulf Coast after Hurricane Katrina.

LEARNING OUTCOME 2

Describe the types of injuries or symptoms that are associated with biologic, chemical, or radiologic terrorism.

CONCEPTS FOR LECTURE

1. Detonation of a "dirty" bomb would disperse radioactive waste into the atmosphere and cause radiation sickness and DNA mutation.
2. Thermal burns are the most common mechanism that result in injury and death associated with nuclear detonation.
3. Flu-like symptoms may appear in the presence of biological exposure.
4. Chemical exposure injuries may range from minor to life-threatening, depending on exposure and type of chemical.

POWERPOINT LECTURE SLIDES

Types of Injuries or Symptoms Associated with Terrorism
- Dirty bomb blast: radiation sickness, DNA mutation
- Nuclear detonation: thermal burns/eye burn injuries
- Chemical: minor to life-threatening injuries
- Biological: flu-like symptoms

LEARNING OUTCOME 3

Evaluate nursing interventions for the treatment of injuries related to biologic, chemical, and radiologic terrorism.

CONCEPTS FOR LECTURE

1. Healthcare providers must be alert to the recognition, reporting, and treatment of high-priority biologic agents.
2. A disaster preparedness plan should be established in every healthcare facility that outlines the protocol and procedures to be taken with a suspected bioterrorism attack.
3. Hospital staff will alert the infection control nurse when subtle changes or trends in symptoms among clients are seen.
4. The public health department is also given these data.
5. When an unusual disease pattern presents itself, laboratories perform tests on cultures that would normally be discarded as contaminants.
6. The Centers for Disease Control and Prevention (CDC) have created detailed "Fact Sheets" about bioterrorism agents and diseases for healthcare providers.
7. During a disaster, nurses may be expected to perform triage.
8. A very basic triage system is to categorize or label victims needing the most support and emergency care as "red." Those less critical but still in need of transport to emergency centers for care are classified as "yellow." Victims who have minor injuries and do not warrant transport to an emergency center are categorized as "green." Victims who are least likely to survive or are already deceased are color coded as "black."
9. When there is a mass casualty event with greater than 100 victims, reverse triage may be instituted.
10. Reverse triage works on the principle of the greatest good for the greatest number.
11. Persons who are the most ambulatory and least injured would be transported or instructed to move quickly to the warm zone, away from the immediate accident site to get processed first.
12. The most victims with the greatest chance of survival could be saved most efficiently with limited resources.
13. Many emergency personnel will share the difficulty of making these decisions at disaster sites when the first inclination might be to rescue the most severely injured.
14. Triage is a continuous process in which priorities are reassigned as needed treatments, time, and the condition of the victims change. This process must balance human lives with the realities of the situation, such as supplies and personnel.

POWERPOINT LECTURE SLIDES

Nursing Interventions for Treatment of Injuries Related to Biologic, Chemical, and Radiologic Terrorism

• Healthcare providers must be alert to the recognition, reporting, and treatment of high-priority biologic agents
• A disaster preparedness plan should be established in every healthcare facility
• During a disaster, nurses may be expected to perform triage
• A very basic triage system is to categorize or label victims
  ○ Red = victims needing the most support and emergency care
  ○ Yellow = victims less critical but still in need of transport to emergency centers for care
  ○ Green = victims who have minor injuries and do not warrant transport to an emergency center
  ○ Black = victims who are least likely to survive or are already deceased
• When there is a mass casualty event with greater than 100 victims, reverse triage may be instituted
• Reverse triage works on the principle of the greatest good for the greatest number
• Persons who are the most ambulatory and least injured would be transported or instructed to move quickly to the warm zone, away from the immediate accident site to get processed first
• Triage is a continuous process in which priorities are reassigned as needed treatments, time, and the condition of the victims change. This process must balance human lives with the realities of the situation, such as supplies and personnel
• The triage role requires a person who is able to rapidly assess clients' conditions under stressful, often adverse conditions and assign a category
• It is imperative that nurses first know how to take care of themselves in order to assist others
• By educating oneself and being proactive in regular drills and practice of skills, nurses take an active role in helping others to save lives and fulfill an important obligation to society
• Applying basic first aid skills can be very helpful in immediate disaster relief efforts until emergency help can be obtained

15. The triage role requires a person who is able to rapidly assess clients' conditions under stressful, often adverse conditions and assign a category.
16. People react to disasters in a variety of ways, both physically and behaviorally.
17. The closer the person is to the area of impact and the longer the exposure, the greater the likelihood of a more severe reaction to the event.
18. It is imperative that nurses first know how to take care of themselves in order to assist others.
19. By educating oneself and being proactive in regular drills and practice of skills, nurses take an active role in helping others to save lives and fulfill an important obligation to society.
20. Applying basic first aid skills can be very helpful in immediate disaster relief efforts until emergency help can be obtained.
21. Roles of nurses in disasters include:
    a. Prepare selves, families, friends, and communities for disasters in conjunction with the local disaster preparedness plan.
    b. Continue educating self on various types of disasters and appropriate response.
    c. Provide emergency services with consideration of victims' abilities, deficits, culture, language, or special needs.
    d. Assist in the mobilization of healthcare personnel, food, water, shelter, medication, clothing, and other assistive devices.
    e. Collaborate with agencies in authority including local, state, and federal representatives to deploy resources based on the greatest good for the greatest number.
    f. Consider needs of victims including shelter both temporary and permanent, as well as psychologic, economic, legal, and spiritual factors.
    g. Become involved with local, state, and national disaster planning agencies to schedule regular meetings to continually review and modify disaster plans.

- Roles of nurses in disasters include:
  ○ Prepare selves, families, friends, and communities for disasters in conjunction with the local disaster preparedness plan
  ○ Continue educating self on various types of disasters and appropriate response
  ○ Provide emergency services with consideration of victims' abilities, deficits, culture, language, or special needs
  ○ Assist in the mobilization of healthcare personnel, food, water, shelter, medication, clothing, and other assistive devices
  ○ Collaborate with agencies in authority including local, state, and federal representatives to deploy resources based on the greatest good for the greatest number
  ○ Consider needs of victims including shelter both temporary and permanent, as well as psychologic, economic, legal, and spiritual factors
  ○ Become involved with local, state, and national disaster planning agencies to schedule regular meetings to continually review and modify disaster plans

---

SUGGESTIONS FOR CLASSROOM ACTIVITIES

- Have each student write a short summary of why it is important to have and practice a disaster policy.

SUGGESTIONS FOR CLINICAL ACTIVITIES

- Have each student review and practice the hospital's disaster policy.

LEARNING OUTCOME 4

Explain the rationale for reverse triage in disasters versus conventional triage in emergencies.

CONCEPTS FOR LECTURE

1. Conventional triage is done every day in every emergency department. The most seriously injured are treated first, and the minor injuries are treated last.

POWERPOINT LECTURE SLIDES

Reverse versus Conventional Triage
- Triage means sorting
- Conventional triage system categories
  ○ Red: those needing the most support and care

CONCEPTS FOR LECTURE *continued*

2. Reverse triage works on the principle of the greatest good for the greatest number of people. The victims who have the greatest chance of survival will be treated first, and the most seriously injured will be treated last.
3. Triage is a continuous process in which priorities change as the victim's condition changes.
4. Those assigned to triage are expected to function independently, but as part of a coordinated team effort.

POWERPOINT LECTURE SLIDES *continued*

- ○ Yellow: those less critical
- ○ Green: minor injuries
- ○ Black: dead and least likely to survive
- Reverse triage
  - ○ Used for mass casualties
  - ○ Least injured would be transported away from a scene first
  - ○ Minor injuries would be treated next
  - ○ Critical injuries treated after the minor injuries
  - ○ Most critical and severely injured would be treated last

SUGGESTIONS FOR CLASSROOM ACTIVITIES

- Ask students to discuss the aspects of reverse triage, and explore their feelings about treating the most severely injured last.

SUGGESTIONS FOR CLINICAL ACTIVITIES

- Have students participate in a mass casualty activity in your area or hospital. If none are available, do a "paper" disaster drill. What are the roles for each healthcare participant?

LEARNING OUTCOME 5

Discuss situations requiring the need for client isolation or client decontamination.

CONCEPTS FOR LECTURE

1. Situations that require the need for client isolation or decontamination include: persons suspected of having smallpox or other contagious diseases; and persons who were exposed to radioactivity.
2. Persons exposed to a chemical agent must be decontaminated so as not to spread the chemical contamination further and to decrease the impact of the substance on the client.

POWERPOINT LECTURE SLIDES

Situations Requiring Client Isolation or Decontamination

- Biological agents exposure: containment is essential; accomplished by isolation of the victim
- Radioactive exposure: will spread to other persons if the client is not isolated
- Chemical exposure: person must be decontaminated according to protocol prior to treatment

SUGGESTIONS FOR CLASSROOM ACTIVITIES

- Ask the class to identify different biologic agents and how the different agents affect the client.
- A client has been exposed to a dangerous chemical and has been transported to the emergency department by private car. How should the team care for this client and protect themselves?

LEARNING OUTCOME 6

Discuss the role of the nurse in disaster planning, response, and mitigation.

CONCEPTS FOR LECTURE

1. The general public looks to the nurse for information and trusts that a nurse's advice is true and accurate.
2. Nurses have a responsibility to be educated and to assimilate new skills and demands necessary to assist clients, families, and communities in preparing for and responding to disaster situations.
3. Nurses must know how to take care of themselves in order to take care of others.

POWERPOINT LECTURE SLIDES

Role of the Nurse in Disaster Planning, Response, and Mitigation

- Nurses must receive in-service education on biological, chemical, and radiological threats
- Nurses serve on disaster response and preparedness planning committees
- In a disaster, nurses may have to assume an expanded role due the shortage of physicians

LEARNING OUTCOME 7

Identify ways that nurses are able to provide care to clients with special considerations.

CONCEPTS FOR LECTURE

1. Many groups of clients will require special nursing intervention due to several factors including age, literacy, disease process, sensory deficit, and mobility.
2. The nurse must assess each individual's ability to cope with and recover from unexpected events.
3. Older adults need to determine the appropriateness of "sheltering in place" should there be an environmental event outside of their homes, or of being evacuated if they are unable to care for themselves for extended periods of time.
4. A current list of medications, doses, and times of administration should be kept in an easily accessible,-secure place.
5. The names and phone numbers of significant persons, relatives, those with power of attorney, healthcare providers, or any others to be notified in case of emergency should also be kept in an easily accessible place.
6. Discuss materials that should be considered essential in keeping with the person should evacuation to a shelter be necessary.
7. The immunocompromised population would be at greater risk for complications and death than the general population should a bioterrorist attack occur.
8. Bottled water should be ready so the client can avoid drinking water of questionable purity.
9. Persons who have sensory deficits, speech or language impairments, or who are illiterate must be assessed for the most effective means of communicating steps to be taken in the case of a disaster.
10. One cannot generalize that all people with hearing impairments or speech impairments will choose a particular means of communication. This may be an individual preference.
11. A multitude of communication means are available through technological support systems as well as written and visual cue boards.
12. The U.S. Department of Health and Human Services has estimated that 13% of the U.S. population experiences some form of activity limitation due to a chronic condition.
13. Many persons require the use of assistive technology devices (ATDs) to accommodate mobility and other impairments.

POWERPOINT LECTURE SLIDES

Special Considerations
- Older adults
  - Do not generalize their needs
  - Need to determine the "appropriateness" of staying in their own home during a disaster
  - List of medications, names of family members, attorney, and who to notify in case of emergency
  - Need list of allergies, special dietary information, name of healthcare provider, and any special equipment needed for ADL
- Immunocompromised
  - Assess client's knowledge level concerning drinking and dietary restrictions
- Sensory deficit, speech, or language impaired
  - Assess the most effective means of communication
- Mobility deficit
  - Assess the support services needed
- Non-English speaking
  - Assess the literacy of the client in their own language through the use of an interpreter or use visual aids
- Spiritual considerations
  - Religion is a source of comfort
  - Be sensitive to religious beliefs when concerning the human body and tissues

14. Careful planning must be in place in order to provide necessary support during and after a disaster. Arrangements must be made in advance to provide adequate numbers of volunteers or staff to assist when this group must be relocated or regrouped in a safe room or shelter.

15. The literacy of non-English-speaking clients should be assessed in both their own language and in English.

16. One cannot assume that individuals are literate in their own language.

17. The communication aids or disaster preparedness and response procedures should be practiced on a regular basis prior to an emergency.

18. The use of visual aids is very helpful.

19. Religion tends to be a source of comfort for those who are experiencing the threat of loss of life, property, or way of living.

20. Churches, synagogues, and clergy become active in supporting their congregations in times of disaster.

21. Religious leaders should be actively involved in community planning for disaster preparedness especially if certain religious considerations should be strictly followed.

22. Rescue personnel would need to be informed of specific religious obligations or rights to be able to be sensitive to the individual's religious beliefs and practices.

SUGGESTIONS FOR CLASSROOM ACTIVITIES

- Role-play with students to assess a client who does not speak English.
- Explore different religious cultures and the significance of the care of the remains.

CHAPTER 8
GENETIC IMPLICATIONS OF ADULT HEALTH NURSING

RESOURCE LIBRARY

 PRENTICE HALL NURSING MEDIALINK DVD-ROM

Audio Glossary
NCLEX-RN® Review
Animation
   Human Genome Project

 COMPANION WEBSITE

Audio Glossary
NCLEX-RN® Review
Care Plan Activity: Genetic Implications of Adult
   Health Nursing Care
Case Study: Genetic Implications
MediaLink Application: Create and Analyze a Family
   Pedigree
Links to Resources

IMAGE LIBRARY

Figure 8.1 Each cell nucleus throughout the body contains the genes, DNA, and chromosomes that make up the majority of an individual's genome.

Figure 8.2 A karyotype is a picture of an individual's chromosomes.

Figure 8.3 This Punnett square shows potential gene combinations (genotypes) and resulting phenotypes of children from parent genotypes with an autosomal dominant altered gene.

Figure 8.4 This Punnett square shows potential gene combinations (genotypes) and resulting phenotypes

of children from parent genotypes with an autosomal recessive altered gene.

Figure 8.5 These Punnett squares show potential gene combinations (genotypes) and resulting phenotypes of children from different parent genotypes with an X-linked recessive altered gene.

Figure 8.6 Selected standardized symbols for use in drawing a pedigree.

Figure 8.7 Sample three-generation pedigree.

LEARNING OUTCOME 1

Discuss the role of genetic concepts in health promotion and health maintenance.

CONCEPTS FOR LECTURE

1. Good health is associated with genes that function properly; when genes function improperly, disease or an increased risk for disease can result. The knowledge gained from the human genome research has, and will continue to have, a profound impact on the prevention, diagnosis, and treatment of genetic disorders and complex diseases.

2. A national interdisciplinary group known as the National Coalition for Health Professional Education in Genetics (NCHPEG) developed competencies to encourage healthcare providers to integrate genetic knowledge, skills, and attitudes while delivering care to clients.

POWERPOINT LECTURE SLIDES

Role of Genetic Concepts in Health Promotion and Maintenance
- The client will
  - Make informed decisions concerning genetic health issues
  - Accurately identify basic genetic concepts
  - Understand the influence of genetic factors in health promotion and maintenance
  - Understand the differences in medical and genetic tests
  - Understand social, legal, and ethical issues related to genetic testing

LEARNING OUTCOME 2

Apply knowledge of the principles of genetic transmission and risk factors for genetic disorders.

CONCEPTS FOR LECTURE

1. Nurses must have basic genetic knowledge to care for the needs of clients and their families with known or suspected genetic disease.
2. Through the application of fundamental genetic concepts, nurses can significantly improve the nursing care provided to clients.
3. The nurse must have knowledge of genes; how gene alterations are inherited is also important for nursing intervention and teaching the client who is at risk for, or who has, a known gene (DNA-based) condition.
4. Knowledge of the function and inheritance of genes are implicit in health promotion as well as health maintenance of the client and his or her family.

POWERPOINT LECTURE SLIDES

Applying Knowledge of Genetic Transmission
- Identify simple risk factors by obtaining a genetic family history and three-generation pedigree
- Incorporate genetic focus into physical assessment
- Assist the client and family to make informed decisions and lifestyle choices
- Be the client's advocate
- Educate the public, support legislative action that protects genetic information
- Evaluate the delivery of care
- Apply knowledge of the ethical, legal, and social implications of genetic information

LEARNING OUTCOME 3

Describe the significance of delivering genetic education and counseling follow-up in a professional manner.

CONCEPTS FOR LECTURE

1. Knowledge of genetic inheritance allows the nurse to not only offer and reinforce genetic information to clients and their families, but also to assist them in managing their care and making reproductive decisions.
2. The nurse must also convey to the client and family that a negative test result does not guarantee that the disease or condition may not develop in the future because environmental influences cannot be controlled.
3. The nurse must understand that genetic conditions may have life-altering implications for the client's children, grandchildren, and other siblings.
4. The nurse must understand that there are two classifications of genetic testing: screening and diagnostic. Screening predicts the probability of disease, and diagnostic confirms the presence of disease.

POWERPOINT LECTURE SLIDES

Basic Underlying Principles of Inheritance
- All genes are paired
- Only one gene of each pair is transmitted to an offspring
- One copy of each gene in the offspring comes from the mother and one from the father
- Categories of genetic testing
  - Screening: a positive screening notifies client of increased risk or probability of disease
  - Diagnostic: confirms the disease

LEARNING OUTCOME 4

Identify the implications of genetic advances on the role of nurses with particular attention to spiritual, cultural, ethical, legal, and social issues.

CONCEPTS FOR LECTURE

1. With the increasing availability of genetic testing, nurses have expressed concern that quality, accuracy, and reliability of genetic test results are not measured against any common standard.
2. Clients often have many unreliable sources of information about genetic testing. The nurse can assist clients to make informed decisions that are based on factual information.
3. The nurse is also responsible for alerting the client of their right for making an informed decision prior to any genetic testing with consideration of the special circumstances that arise from the family, culture, and community life.
4. Nurses have a responsibility to fully educate clients about the multiple issues related to genetic testing, so the client will have full knowledge, confidentiality, and act autonomously.
5. Confidentiality and privacy is an integral part of care delivery for all nurses. The issue of genetic testing is very far-reaching. The results can have impact on insurance coverage, employment, and family and cultural values.
6. Cultural and religious beliefs and values must be assessed by the nurse prior to educating the client about genetic testing.

POWERPOINT LECTURE SLIDES

Implications of Genetic Advances on the Nurse's Role
- Provide the client with reliable information
- Assist the client in making an informed decision by educating the client concerning the outcomes of the testing
- Assure the client concerning confidentiality and the rights and responsibilities of those who have access to the information
- Assess the client's coping mechanisms

LEARNING OUTCOME 5

Identify the significance of recent advances in human genetics and the impact on healthcare delivery.

CONCEPTS FOR LECTURE

1. Nurses have always taken the role of educator for the client and family. The nurse is still an essential part of this component.
2. As more information about the genetic revolution becomes available to consumers—in areas such as pharmacogenomics, gene transfer, ethics, genetic engineering, and stem cell research—the role of nurses remains not only vital, but is growing enormously.

POWERPOINT LECTURE SLIDES

Impact of Genetic Advances on Healthcare Delivery
- Nurse's role as educator for client, family, community
- Role of the nurse grows enormously as more information about genetics becomes available
- Nurses must remain educated, informed, knowledgeable, and read to discuss trends and changes in genetic research

3. Nurses must remain educated, informed, knowledgeable, and ready to discuss trends and changes in genetic research with their clients.

SUGGESTIONS FOR CLASSROOM ACTIVITIES

• Research the role of a genetic nurse. Where are these special nurses employed? Is there a professional organization for registered nurses who are genetic specialists?

CHAPTER 9
NURSING CARE OF CLIENTS EXPERIENCING PAIN

RESOURCE LIBRARY

💿 PRENTICE HALL NURSING MEDIALINK DVD-ROM

Audio Glossary
NCLEX-RN® Review
Animation/Video
  Epidural Placement
  Morphine
  Naproxen
  Reflex Arc

📖 IMAGE LIBRARY

Figure 9.1 *A*, Cutaneous nociceptors generate pain impulses that travel via A-delta and C fibers to the spinal cord's dorsal horn. *B*, Secondary neurons in dorsal horn pass impulses across spinal cord to anterior spinothalamic tract. *C*, Slow pain impulses ascend to the thalamus, while fast pain impulses ascend to the cerebral cortex.

Figure 9.2 *A*, Pain impulse causes presynaptic neuron to release burst of neurotransmitters across synapse. *B*, Inhibitory neuron releases endorphins, which bind to presynaptic opiate receptors.

Figure 9.3 The spinal cord component of the gate-control theory.

🌐 COMPANION WEBSITE

Audio Glossary
NCLEX-RN® Review
Care Plan Activity: The Client in Pain
Case Study: Assessing the Client in Pain
MediaLink Applications
Links to Resources

Figure 9.4 Referred pain is the result of the convergence of sensory nerves from certain areas of the body before they enter the brain for interpretation.

Figure 9.6 The transdermal patch administers medication in predictable doses.

Figure 9.8 Surgical procedures are used to treat severe pain that does not respond to other types of management.

Figure 9.11 Examples of commonly used pain scales.

LEARNING OUTCOME 1

Describe the neurophysiology of pain.

CONCEPTS FOR LECTURE

1. The peripheral nervous system is composed of two types of neurons: sensory and motor. Pain is perceived through the sensory neurons and motor neurons respond to the pain.
2. Nociceptors are nerve receptors for pain. They are located throughout the body except in the brain.
3. The pain pathway is a complex mechanism that transmits pain impulses throughout the body in a highly sophisticated manner.
4. Cutaneous pain is transmitted through small afferent A-delta and even smaller C nerve fibers to the spinal cord.
5. A-delta fibers are myelinated and transmit impulses rapidly. They produce sharp, well-defined pain sensations,

POWERPOINT LECTURE SLIDES

Pain Pathway
- A-delta fibers: transmit pain quickly, associated with acute pain
- C fibers: transmit pain more slowly, diffuse burning pain and chronic pain
- Inhibitory mechanisms: the analgesia system stimulates a pain inhibitory center in the dorsal horns of the spinal cord (the exact mechanism is unknown)
- Endorphins: naturally occurring opioid peptides present in the neurons in the brain

    such as those that result from cuts, electric shocks, or the impact of a blow.

6. A-delta fibers are associated with acute pain.

7. C fibers are not myelinated and thus transmit pain impulses more slowly.

8. The pain from deep body structures (such as muscles and viscera) is primarily transmitted by C fibers, producing diffuse burning or aching sensations.

9. C fibers are associated with chronic pain.

10. Both A-delta and C fibers are involved in most injuries.

11. Secondary neurons transmit the impulses from the afferent neurons through the dorsal horn of the spinal cord, where they synapse in the substantia gelatinosa. The impulses then cross over to the anterior and lateral spinothalamic tracts.

12. The impulses ascend the anterior and lateral spinothalamic tracts and pass through the medulla and midbrain to the thalamus.

13. In the thalamus and cerebral cortex, the pain impulses are perceived, described, localized, and interpreted, and a response is formulated. A noxious impulse becomes pain when the sensation reaches conscious levels and is perceived and evaluated by the person experiencing the sensation.

14. Some pain impulses ascend along the paleospinothalamic tract in the medial section of the spinal cord. These impulses enter the reticular formation and the limbic systems, which integrate emotional and cognitive responses to pain.

15. Interconnections in the autonomic nervous system may also cause an autonomic response to the pain.

16. Deep nociceptors often converge on the same spinal neuron, resulting in pain that is experienced in a part of the body other than its origin.

SUGGESTIONS FOR CLASSROOM ACTIVITIES

• Review the anatomy and physiology of pain receptors.

LEARNING OUTCOME 2

Compare and contrast definitions and characteristics of acute, chronic, breakthrough, central, phantom, and psychogenic pain.

CONCEPTS FOR LECTURE

1. Acute pain has a sudden onset, and usually results from tissue injury from trauma, surgery, or inflammation.

2. The three major types of acute pain are as follows: somatic pain, visceral pain, and referred pain.

3. Somatic pain arises from nerve receptors originating in the skin or close to the surface of the body. It may be sharp and well localized, or dull and diffuse. It is often accompanied by nausea and vomiting.

4. Visceral pain arises from body organs. It is dull and poorly localized. It is also associated with nausea and vomiting, hypotension, and restlessness. It often radiates

POWERPOINT LECTURE SLIDES

Acute, Chronic, Central, Phantom, and Psychogenic Pain
- Acute pain
  - Somatic pain
    - May be sharp or diffused
    - May be accompanied by nausea and vomiting
  - Visceral pain
    - Arises from the body organs
    - Usually dull and poorly localized
    - May be referred or may radiate

or is referred. It may be described as cramping, intermittent pain, or colicky pain.

5. Referred pain is pain that is perceived in an area distant from the site of the stimuli.

6. Chronic pain is prolonged pain that usually lasts longer than six months and is not always associated with an identifiable cause. Chronic pain has a much more complex and poorly-understood cause.

7. Chronic pain can be subdivided into four categories: recurrent acute pain, ongoing time-limited pain, chronic nonmalignant pain, chronic intractable nonmalignant pain syndrome.

8. Recurrent acute pain is characterized by relatively well-defined episodes of pain interspersed with pain-free episodes.

9. Ongoing time-limited pain is identified by a defined time period.

10. Chronic nonmalignant pain is non–life-threatening pain that nevertheless persists beyond the expected time for healing.

11. Chronic intractable nonmalignant pain syndrome is similar to simple chronic nonmalignant pain but is characterized by the person's inability to cope well with the pain and sometimes by physical, social, and/or psychologic disability resulting from the pain.

12. There are also common chronic pain conditions which include: neuralgias, complex regional pain syndrome, hyperesthesias or hyperalgesias, and myofascial pain syndrome.

13. Central pain is related to a lesion in the brain that produces bursts of impulses that are perceived as pain.

14. Phantom pain is a syndrome that occurs after a limb has been amputated.

15. The client experiences pain in the missing body part even though he or she is completely mentally aware that it is gone. This pain may include itching, tingling, or pressure sensations, or it may be more severe, including burning or stabbing sensations.

16. Psychogenic pain is experienced in the absence of any diagnosed physiologic cause or event.

17. Psychogenic pain is real, and may in turn lead to physiologic changes, such as muscle tension, which may produce further pain.

- ○ Referred pain
  - – Perceived in an area distant from the site of the stimuli
- • Chronic pain
  - ○ Recurrent acute pain
    - – Well-defined episodes of pain
    - – Migraine headaches, sickle cell crisis
  - ○ Ongoing time-limited pain
    - – Persists for a definite time period
    - – Ends with control of the disease, rehabilitation, or death
  - ○ Chronic nonmalignant pain
    - – Not life-threatening but persists past expected time for healing
  - ○ Chronic intractable nonmalignant pain syndrome
    - – Client unable to cope well with the pain
    - – Pain may be mild to severe
    - – The pain itself becomes the pathologic process
- • Central pain
  - ○ May be caused by a vascular lesion, tumor, or inflammation
- • Phantom pain
  - ○ Thought to be due to stimulation of severed nerves at the amputation site
- • Psychogenic pain
  - ○ Involves a long history of severe pain
  - ○ Pain is real and can lead to physiologic changes

SUGGESTIONS FOR CLASSROOM ACTIVITIES

- Compare and contrast the differences between chronic, acute, and phantom pain.

SUGGESTIONS FOR CLINICAL ACTIVITIES

- Ask a pain management physician or nurse to speak to the class.

LEARNING OUTCOME 3

Discuss factors affecting individualized responses to pain.

CONCEPTS FOR LECTURE

1. The individualized response to pain is shaped by multiple and interacting factors:
   - Age: There are many misconceptions about pain in the older adult.
   - Sociocultural influences: Each person's response to pain is strongly influenced by the family, community, and culture.
   - Emotional status influences pain.
   - Past experiences with pain: If pain in childhood was handled by supportive adults, the client will usually have a healthy attitude toward pain. If the pain was handled with indifference or exaggerated emotions, the person's future pain can be exaggerated or denied.
   - The meaning associated with the pain influences the experience of pain; e.g., childbirth pain vs. organ removal for cancer.
   - Lack of knowledge can negatively impact the management of pain.
2. It is important to remember that pain behaviors are not an objective indicator of the amount of pain present for any client.

POWERPOINT LECTURE SLIDES

Factors Affecting Pain Response
- Age
- Sociocultural influences
- Emotional status
- Past experiences with pain
- Meaning associated with the pain
- Lack of knowledge

SUGGESTIONS FOR CLASSROOM ACTIVITIES

- Ask students how they perceive pain.

SUGGESTIONS FOR CLINICAL ACTIVITIES

- Develop a nursing care plan for clients in chronic pain.
- Assign students to care for clients with chronic pain.

LEARNING OUTCOME 4

Clarify myths and misconceptions about pain.

CONCEPTS FOR LECTURE

1. There are many misconceptions about pain and pain management that are common among both healthcare providers and clients.
   - Pain is a result, not a cause.
   - Chronic pain is really a masked form of depression.
   - Narcotic medication is too risky to be used for chronic pain.
   - It is best to wait until a client has pain before giving medication.
   - Many clients lie about the existence or severity of pain.
   - Pain relief interferes with diagnosis.
   - Postoperative pain is best treated with intramuscular injections.

POWERPOINT LECTURE SLIDES

Myths and Misconceptions Concerning Pain
- Pain is a result, not a cause
- Chronic pain is really a masked form of depression
- Narcotic medication is too risky to be used for chronic pain
- It is best to wait until a client has pain before giving medication
- Many client's lie about the existence or severity of pain
- Pain relief interferes with diagnosis

LEARNING OUTCOME 5

Discuss interdisciplinary care for the client in pain, including medications, surgery, transcutaneous electrical nerve stimulation, and complementary therapies.

CONCEPTS FOR LECTURE

1. Effective pain relief comes from collaboration among healthcare providers. Pain clinics use a multidisciplinary approach to managing chronic pain.
2. Medications may be used effectively in conjunction with other therapies. When medications are used as recommended, there is little or no risk of addiction.
3. Medication is the most common approach to pain management.
4. A variety of drugs with many kinds of delivery systems are available. These drugs include nonnarcotic analgesics, nonsteroidal anti-inflammatory drugs (NSAIDs), narcotics, synthetic narcotics, antidepressants, and local anesthetic agents.
5. In addition to administering the prescribed medications, the nurse may act independently in choosing the dosage and timing.
6. The nurse is also responsible for assessing the side effects of the medications, evaluating the medication's effectiveness, and providing client teaching.
7. The nurse's roles in pain relief are those of client advocate and direct caregiver.
8. The route of administration significantly affects how much of the medication is needed to relieve pain.
9. Surgery is performed usually after all other measures have failed.
10. Surgical procedures are used to treat severe pain that does not respond to other types of management. They include cordotomy, neurectomy, sympathectomy, and rhizotomy.
11. A transcutaneous electrical nerve stimulation (TENS) unit consists of a low-voltage transmitter connected by wires to electrodes placed by the client as directed by the physical therapist.
12. Complementary therapies are used with other treatments and usually are practiced only by care providers with special training.
13. Complementary therapies include: acupuncture, biofeedback, hypnotism, relaxation, distraction, and cutaneous stimulation.

POWERPOINT LECTURE SLIDES

Collaborative Care for Pain
- Medications
  - NSAIDs: analgesic, antipyretic, and anti-inflammatory action
  - Narcotics: opioids
  - Antidepressants: act on the retention of serotonin, thus inhibiting the pain sensation
  - Anticonvulsants: used for headache and neuropathic pain
  - Local anesthetics: blocks the transmission of nerve impulses, therefore blocking pain
- Surgery
  - Cordotomy: an incision into the anterolateral tracts of the spinal cord to interrupt the transmission of pain
  - Neurectomy: removal of part of the nerve
  - Sympathectomy: destruction of the ganglia by incision or injection
  - Rhizotomy: surgical severing of the dorsal spinal roots
  - Transcutaneous electrical nerve stimulation (TENS): electrodes stimulate the A-beta touch fibers to close the "pain" gate
- Complementary therapies
  - Acupuncture
  - Biofeedback
  - Hypnotism
  - Relaxation
  - Distraction
  - Cutaneous stimulation

LEARNING OUTCOME 6

Use the nursing process as a framework for providing individualized nursing care for clients experiencing pain.

CONCEPTS FOR LECTURE

1. Assess the client's pain level by asking to rate the pain on a scale of 1–10.
2. Establish a nursing diagnosis based on the nursing history and assessment.
3. Determine the level of sedation the client with tolerate.
4. Teach the client and family nonpharmacologic methods of pain management, such as relaxation, distraction, and cutaneous stimulation.
5. Provide comfort measures, such as changing positions, back massage, oral care, skin care, and changing bed linens.
6. Provide client and family teaching, and make referrals if necessary to assist with coping, financial resources, and home care.
7. Plan and implement a care plan based on all modalities of pain management. Educate the client about different types of methods of pain management.
8. Therapies may include traditional pharmacologic agents as well as herbs, vitamins, and other dietary supplements; nutritional counseling; psychotherapy; biofeedback; hypnosis; acupuncture; massage; and other treatments.
9. Evaluate the client's response to the care plan.
10. Predictable physiologic changes occur in the presence of acute pain. These may include muscle tension; tachycardia; rapid, shallow respirations; increased blood pressure; dilated pupils; sweating; and pallor. Over time, however, the body adapts to the pain stimulus, and these physiologic changes may be extinguished in clients with chronic pain.
11. Some behaviors are so typical of people in pain that the behaviors are referred to as *pain behaviors*. They include bracing or guarding the painful part, taking medication, crying, moaning, grimacing, withdrawing from activity and socialization, becoming immobile, talking about pain, holding the painful area, breathing with increased effort, exhibiting a sad facial expression, and being restless.
12. Behavioral responses to pain may or may not coincide with the client's report of pain and are not very reliable cues to the pain experience.
13. Clients may also use pain as a mechanism to gain attention from family and healthcare providers.

POWERPOINT LECTURE SLIDES

Nursing Process for Clients with Pain
- Assess the client's pain level
- Establish a nursing diagnosis
- Plan and implement a care plan
- Educate the client
- Evaluate the client's response to the care plan

SUGGESTIONS FOR CLASSROOM ACTIVITIES

- Develop a plan of care for a client with the nursing diagnosis of Risk of Constipation.

SUGGESTIONS FOR CLINICAL ACTIVITIES

- Assign students to work in the pain management clinic or visit a pain management center.

CHAPTER 10
NURSING OF CLIENTS WITH ALTERED FLUID, ELECTROLYTE, AND ACID-BASE BALANCE

RESOURCE LIBRARY

PRENTICE HALL NURSING MEDIALINK DVD-ROM

Audio Glossary
NCLEX-RN© Review
Animations
   Acid–Base Balance
   Fluid Balance
   Furosemide
   Membrane Transport

COMPANION WEBSITE

Audio Glossary
NCLEX-RN© Review
Care Plan Activities
   Fluid Volume Deficit
   Hypocalcemia
Case Studies
   Third Spacing
   Hypernatremia
MediaLink Applications
   Metabolic Acidosis and Type 1 Diabetes
   Alterations in Electrolytes, Medications, Fluid
    Volumes
Links to Resources

IMAGE LIBRARY

Figure 10.1 The major fluid compartments of the body.

Figure 10.3 Osmosis.

Figure 10.4 The effect of tonicity on red b lood cells.

Figure 10.5 Diffusion.

Figure 10.6 Fluid balance between the intravascular and interstitial spaces is maintained in the capillary beds by a balance of filtration at the arterial end and osmotic draw at the venous end.

Figure 10.7 The sodium-potassium pump.

Figure 10.8 Factors stimulating water intake through the thirst mechanism.

Figure 10.9 The renin–angiotensin–aldosterone system.

Figure 10.10 Antidiuretic hormone (ADH) release and effect.

Figure 10.11 The effects of changes in potassium levels on the electrocardiogram (ECG).

Figure 10.12 Low calcium levels (hypocalcemia) trigger the release of parathyroid hormone (PTH), increasing calcium ion levels through stimulation of bones, kidneys, and intestines.

Figure 10.13 *A*, Positive Chvostek's sign. *B*, Positive Trousseau's sign.

Figure 10.14 The normal ratio of bicarbonate to carbonic acid is 20:1.

Figure 10.15 Metabolic acid–base imbalances.

Figure 10.16 Respiratory acid–base imbalances.

LEARNING OUTCOME 1

Describe the functions and regulatory mechanisms that maintain water and electrolyte balance in the body.

CONCEPTS FOR LECTURE

1. Fluid and electrolyte balance in the body involves regulatory mechanisms that maintain homeostasis.
2. Water is the primary component of body fluids.
3. Total body water constitutes about 60% of the total body weight, but this amount varies with age, gender, and the amount of body fat.
4. The average fluid intake and output usually is about 2500 mL over a 24-hour period.

POWERPOINT LECTURE SLIDES

Maintaining Water and Electrolyte Balance in the Body

- **Osmosis:** water moves across a selectively permeable membrane from an area of lower concentration to an area of higher concentration
- **Diffusion:** molecules move from an area of high concentration to lower concentration

5. Urine production and excretion account for most water loss. The average daily urine output is 1500 mL in adults. At least 400 mL of highly concentrated urine per day is required to excrete metabolic wastes produced by the body.
6. The body also contains electrolytes that are charged particles called ions.
7. Body fluid is classified by its location inside or outside of cells. Intracellular fluid (ICF) is found within cells. It accounts for approximately 40% of total body weight.
8. Extracellular fluid (ECF) is located outside of cells. It accounts for approximately 20% of the total body weight.
9. Four chemical and physiologic processes control the movement of fluid, electrolytes, and other molecules across membranes between the intracellular and interstitial space and plasma. These processes are osmosis, diffusion, filtration, and active transport. Osmosis: water moves across a selectively permeable membrane from an area of lower concentration to an area of higher concentration. Diffusion: molecules move from an area of high concentration to lower concentration. Filtration: occurs across capillary membranes from an area of high hydrostatic pressure to lower hydrostatic pressure. Active Transport: molecules move across cell membranes against a concentration gradient (this movement requires energy).

- **Filtration:** occurs across capillary membranes from an area of high hydrostatic pressure to lower hydrostatic pressure
- **Active transport:** molecules move across cell membranes against a concentration gradient (this movement requires energy)

SUGGESTIONS FOR CLASSROOM ACTIVITIES

- View a DVD about fluid and electrolyte balance.

SUGGESTIONS FOR CLINICAL ACTIVITIES

- Assign students to care for clients with fluid deficits, including preoperative clients, postoperative clients, and clients with nausea and vomiting.

LEARNING OUTCOME 2

Compare and contrast the causes, effects, and care of the client with fluid volume or electrolyte imbalance.

CONCEPTS FOR LECTURE

1. The most common cause of fluid volume deficit is excessive loss of gastrointestinal fluids from vomiting, diarrhea, gastrointestinal suctioning, intestinal fistulas, and intestinal drainage.
2. Other causes of fluid losses include: excessive renal losses of water and sodium from diuretic therapy, renal disorders, or endocrine disorders, water and sodium losses during sweating from excessive exercise or increased environmental temperature, hemorrhage, chronic abuse of laxatives and/or enemas, inadequate fluid intake may result from lack of access to fluids, inability to request or to swallow fluids, oral trauma, or altered thirst mechanisms.
3. Fluid volume deficit can develop slowly or very rapidly.
4. The older adult client is more at risk for fluid deficit due to self limiting fluids (fear of incontinence), physical

POWERPOINT LECTURE SLIDES

Causes and Care of Client with Fluid Volume or Electrolyte Imbalance
- Causes of fluid loss
  ○ Vomiting, diarrhea
  ○ Gastrointestinal suctioning, intestinal fistulas, and intestinal drainage
  ○ Diuretic therapy, renal disorders, endocrine disorders
  ○ Sweating from excessive exercise, increased environmental temperature
  ○ Hemorrhage
  ○ Chronic abuse of laxatives
- Cause of fluid loss in the older adult
  ○ Self-limiting fluids (fear of incontinence)
  ○ Physical disabilities
  ○ Cognitive impairments
  ○ Older adults without air conditioning

disabilities, cognitive impairments, and lack of air conditioning.

5. Nurses are responsible for identifying clients at risk for fluid volume deficit, initiating and carrying out measures to prevent and treat fluid volume deficit, and monitoring the effects of therapy. Treatment for fluid volume deficit (FVD) includes oral, intravenous, or enteral routes and management of the effects and prevent further complications by monitoring intake, assessing lab values, and observing vital signs and skin integrity.

- Treatment for fluid volume deficit (FVD)
  - Oral, intravenous, or enteral routes
  - Manage the effects and prevent further complications by monitoring intake, assessing lab values, and observing vital signs and skin integrity

---

SUGGESTIONS FOR CLASSROOM ACTIVITIES

- Discuss methods to encourage a client with a fluid deficit to increase fluid intake.

SUGGESTIONS FOR CLINICAL ACTIVITIES

- Assign students to geriatric clients. These clients often have fluid deficits.
- Develop a care plan about increasing the fluid intake for this type of client.

LEARNING OUTCOME 3

Explain the pathophysiology and manifestations of imbalances of sodium, potassium, calcium, magnesium, and phosphorus.

CONCEPTS FOR LECTURE

1. Sodium imbalances affect the osmolality of extracellular fluid (ECF) and water distribution between fluid compartments. When sodium levels are low (as in hyponatremia) water is drawn into the cells, which causes them to swell; high levels of sodium (as in hypernatremia) draw water out of the cells. Early manifestations of hyponatremia include muscle cramps, weakness, and fatigue from its effects on muscle cells. Gastrointestinal function is affected, causing anorexia, nausea and vomiting, abdominal cramping, and diarrhea. Neurologic manifestations progress rapidly when the serum sodium level falls below 120 mEq/L and include headache, depression, dulled sensorium, personality changes, irritability, lethargy, hyperreflexia, muscle twitching, and tremors. If serum sodium falls to very low levels, convulsions and coma are likely to occur.

2. Most potassium is found within the cells or intracellular fluid (ICF). Low potassium levels (hypokalemia), or high potassium levels (hyperkalemia), can have adverse affects on cardiac and nervous tissue. Hypokalemia affects the transmission of nerve impulses, interfering with the contractility of smooth, skeletal, and cardiac muscle, as well as the regulation and transmission of cardiac impulses. Characteristic electrocardiogram (ECG) changes of hypokalemia include flattened or inverted T waves, the development of U waves, and a depressed ST segment. Hypokalemia affects both the resting membrane potential and intracellular enzymes in skeletal and smooth muscle cells. This causes skeletal muscle weakness and slowed peristalsis of the gastrointestinal tract.

POWERPOINT LECTURE SLIDES

Manifestations of Imbalances

- Hyponatremia
  - Muscle cramps, weakness, fatigue
  - Dulled sensorium, irritability, personality changes
- Hypernatremia
  - Most serious effects are seen in the brain
  - Lethargy, weakness, irritability can progress to seizures, coma, and death
- Hypokalemia
  - EKG changes (flattened or inverted T waves)
  - Skeletal muscle weakness
- Hyperkalemia
  - Cardiac arrest
  - Paresthesias
  - Abdominal cramping
- Hypocalcemia
  - Tetany, paresthesias, muscle spasms
  - Hypotension
  - Anxiety, confusion, psychosis
- Hypercalcemia
  - Muscle weakness, fatigue
  - Personality changes
  - Anorexia, nausea, vomiting
- Hypomagnesemia
  - Muscle weakness and tremors
  - Dysphasia
  - Tachycardia hypertension
  - Mood and personality changes
- Hypermagnesemia
  - Depressed deep tendon reflexes
  - Hypotension
  - Respiratory depression

3. Calcium levels are regulated by the interaction of three hormones: parathyroid hormone, calcitonin, and calcitriol. Manifestations of hypercalcemia can include muscle weakness and fatigue, as well as gastrointestinal manifestations such as anorexia, nausea, vomiting, and constipation. Central nervous system (CNS) effects may include confusion, lethargy, behavior or personality changes, and coma. Cardiovascular effects include dysrhythmias, ECG changes, and possible hypertension. Hypercalcemia causes polyuria and, as a result, increased thirst. Hypercalcemic crisis, an acute increase in the serum calcium level, can lead to cardiac arrest.

4. Magnesium deficiency usually occurs along with low serum potassium and calcium levels. The primary cause of hypomagnesemia is chronic alcoholism.

5. Neuromuscular manifestations of hypomagnesemia include tremors, hyperreactive reflexes, positive Chvostek's and Trousseau's signs, tetany, paresthesias, and seizures. CNS effects include confusion, mood changes (apathy, depression, agitation), hallucinations, and possible psychoses. An increased heart rate, ventricular dysrhythmias, cardiac arrest and sudden death may occur. Gastrointestinal manifestations include nausea, vomiting, anorexia, diarrhea, and abdominal distention.

6. Phosphate is the primary intracellular ion. Levels may vary with age, gender, and diet. Phosphate is essential to the production of ATP.

7. Severe hypophosphatemia affects virtually every major organ system some include: muscle pain and tenderness, muscle weakness and paresthesias, confusion, manifestations of hypophosphatemia, muscle spasms, tetany, and soft tissue calcifications.

- Hypophosphatemia
  - Muscle pain and tenderness
  - Muscle weakness and paresthesias
  - Confusion
  - Manifestations of hypophosphatemia
  - Muscle spasms, tetany
  - Soft tissue calcifications

SUGGESTIONS FOR CLASSROOM ACTIVITIES

- Discuss different laboratory values for electrolyte imbalances. What symptoms might the client display?

SUGGESTIONS FOR CLINICAL ACTIVITIES

- Assign student to clients with lab values consistent with hypokalemia, hyponatremia, and other imbalances.

LEARNING OUTCOME 4

Describe the causes and effects of acid–base imbalances.

CONCEPTS FOR LECTURE

1. Homeostasis and optimal cellular function require maintenance of the hydrogen ion concentration of body fluids within a narrow range. As the hydrogen ion concentration falls, the pH rises and the solution becomes more alkaline or basic.

2. Three systems work together in the body to maintain the pH despite continuous acid production: buffers, the respiratory system, and the renal system.

3. Buffers are substances that prevent major changes in pH by removing or releasing hydrogen ions.

POWERPOINT LECTURE SLIDES

Acid–Base Disorders
- **Acidosis:** hydrogen ion concentration above normal (pH below 7.35)
- **Alkalosis:** hydrogen ion concentration below normal (pH above 7.45)
- **Metabolic acidosis:** bicarbonate is decreased in relation to the amount of acid
- **Metabolic alkalosis:** excess of bicarbonate in relation to the amount of hydrogen ion

CONCEPTS FOR LECTURE *continued*

4. The respiratory system and the respiratory center of the brain regulate carbonic acid in the body by eliminating or retaining carbon dioxide.
5. The renal system is responsible for the long-term regulation of acid–base balance in the body.
6. Acid–base imbalances fall into two major categories: acidosis and alkalosis. Acidosis occurs when the hydrogen ion concentration increases above normal (pH below 7.35). Alkalosis occurs when the hydrogen ion concentration falls below normal (pH above 7.45). Acid–base imbalances are further classified as metabolic or respiratory disorders.
7. Acid–base disorders include: acidosis—hydrogen ion concentration above normal (pH below 7.35); alkalosis: hydrogen ion concentration below normal (pH above 7.45); metabolic acidosis—bicarbonate is decreased in relation to the amount of acid; metabolic alkalosis—excess of bicarbonate in relation to the amount of hydrogen ion; respiratory acidosis—CO_2 is retained, caused by sudden failure of ventilation due to chest trauma, aspiration of foreign body, acute pneumonia, and overdose of narcotics or sedatives; respiratory alkalosis—CO_2 is blown off, caused by mechanical ventilation and anxiety with hyperventilation.

POWERPOINT LECTURE SLIDES *continued*

- **Respiratory acidosis:** CO_2 is retained, caused by sudden failure of ventilation due to chest trauma, aspiration of foreign body, acute pneumonia, and overdose of narcotics or sedatives
- **Respiratory alkalosis:** CO_2 is blown off, caused by mechanical ventilation and anxiety with hyperventilation

SUGGESTIONS FOR CLASSROOM ACTIVITIES

- Explain a positive Chvostek's sign and Trousseau's sign.

SUGGESTIONS FOR CLINICAL ACTIVITIES

- Assign students to clients who are experiencing an acid–base disorder.

CHAPTER 11
NURSING CARE OF CLIENTS EXPERIENCING TRAUMA AND SHOCK

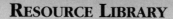

RESOURCE LIBRARY

 PRENTICE HALL NURSING MEDIALINK DVD-ROM

Audio Glossary
NCLEX-RN® Review
Animation/Video
  Administering Blood
  Hypovolemic Shock
  Trauma Injuries

 COMPANION WEBSITE

Audio Glossary
NCLEX-RN® Review
Care Plan Activity: Clients Experiencing Trauma and
  Shock
Case Studies
  A Client Experiencing Trauma
  Identifying Types of Shock
MediaLink Applications
  Injury Prevention
  Organ Donation
  Shock
Links to Resources

IMAGE LIBRARY

Figure 11.1 Placement of an oral endotracheal tube (ETT) for intubation.

Figure 11.2 A needle thoracostomy may be used in the emergency treatment of a tension pneumothorax.

Figure 11.3 The major pressure points used for the control of bleeding.

Figure 11.4 Traumatic injuries to the skin include *A*, contusion; *B*, abrasion; *C*, puncture wound; *D*, laceration.

Figure 11.5 Immobilization of the cervical spine at the scene of the accident is essential to prevent further injury to the spinal cord.

Figure 11.6 Flight nurses provide initial assessment, stabilization, and support for clients with trauma.

Figure 11.7 A kinetic continuous rotation bed provides a means of turning the client with multiple injuries to decrease the hazards of immobility.

Figure 11.8 The stages of hypovolemic shock.

Figure 11.9 The client in shock should be positioned with the lower extremities elevated approximately 20 degrees (knees straight), trunk horizontal, and the head elevated about 10 degrees.

LEARNING OUTCOME 1

Define the word *trauma*.

CONCEPTS FOR LECTURE

1. Trauma is defined as injury to human tissues and organs resulting from the transfer of energy from the environment.
2. In the past the term trauma has been associated with the word accident. Accident means that the injury occurred without intent, a result of random chance.
3. Intentional and nonintentional trauma encompass a variety of injuries resulting from motor vehicle crashes, pedestrian injuries, gunshot wounds, falls, violence toward others, or self-inflicted violence.
4. Trauma usually occurs suddenly, leaving the client and family with little time to prepare for its consequences.

POWERPOINT LECTURE SLIDES

Trauma
- Trauma: injury to human tissues and organs resulting from the abnormal transfer of energy from the environment
- Usually occurs suddenly
- Kills more people between the ages of 1 and 44 than any other disease or illness and 62% of all deaths from ages 15–24 are due to trauma
- May alter the client's previous way of life, potentially affecting independence, mobility, cognitive thinking, and appearance

5. Injuries, disabilities, and deaths that result from trauma constitute a major healthcare challenge.
6. Trauma kills more people between the ages of 1 and 44 than any other disease or illness and 62% of all deaths from ages 15–24 are due to trauma.
7. Trauma may alter the client's previous way of life, potentially affecting independence, mobility, cognitive thinking, and appearance.

SUGGESTIONS FOR CLASSROOM ACTIVITIES

• Using the internet, research the types of trauma that cause deaths in the different age groups.

SUGGESTIONS FOR CLINICAL ACTIVITIES

• Assign students to work in the emergency department.
• Assign students to care for a trauma client in the intensive care unit.

LEARNING OUTCOME 2

Describe the components and types of trauma.

CONCEPTS FOR LECTURE

1. Trauma results from an abnormal exchange of energy between a host (person or group) and a mechanism (energy source) in a predisposing environment.
2. Multiple factors influence the host's potential for injury: age, sex, race, economic status, preexisting illness, and the use of substances such as street drugs or alcohol.
3. The mechanism may be mechanical, gravitational, thermal, electrical, physical, or chemical.
4. Intention is also a component in trauma and shock. Gunshot and stab wounds are examples of intentional injuries.
5. The final component of trauma is environmental, such as weather or occupation.
6. There are several types of trauma: minor, multiple, blunt, penetrating, and inhalation:
   • Minor: injury to a single part or system of the body; may be treated in a physicians office
   • Multiple trauma: serious multisystem injuries; usually due to motor vehicle accident
   • Blunt trauma: causes multiple injuries through shearing, compression, and crushing
   • Penetrating trauma: foreign object enters the body through gunshot wounds, stab wounds, and impalement
   • Inhalation: gas, steam

POWERPOINT LECTURE SLIDES

Components and Types of Trauma
• Trauma results from abnormal exchange of energy between a host, a mechanism, and a predisposing environment
• Factors influencing the host
  ○ Age
  ○ Sex
  ○ Race
  ○ Economic status
  ○ Preexisting illness
  ○ Abuse
• Mechanisms
  ○ Mechanical
  ○ Gravitational
  ○ Thermal
  ○ Electrical
  ○ Physical
  ○ Chemical
  ○ Environmental
  ○ Weather-related
  ○ Occupational
• Types of trauma
  ○ Minor
  ○ Multiple trauma
  ○ Blunt trauma
  ○ Penetrating trauma
  ○ Inhalation

SUGGESTIONS FOR CLASSROOM ACTIVITIES

• Explore why factors such as age, race, and economic status affect clients experiencing trauma and shock.

SUGGESTIONS FOR CLINICAL ACTIVITIES

• Set up a scenario for caring for a client experiencing multiple trauma. Ask students to develop a nursing care plan for this client.

LEARNING OUTCOME 3

Describe the result of energy transfer to the human body.

CONCEPTS FOR LECTURE

1. Trauma is classified as blunt or penetrating. Results are different due to the type of trauma and the amount and type of energy transfer.
2. Blunt trauma has no communication between the damaged tissue and the outside environment. It is caused by various forces including deceleration (a decrease in the speed of a moving object), acceleration (an increase in the speed of a moving object), shearing (forces occurring across a plane, with structures slipping across each other), compression, and crushing.
3. Blunt forces often cause multiple injuries that can affect the head, spinal cord, bones, thorax, and abdomen.
4. Penetrating trauma includes gunshot, stab wounds, and impalement. Structures commonly affected include the brain, lungs, heart, liver, spleen, the intestines, and the vascular system. Examples of penetrating trauma are gunshot or stab wounds and impalement.

POWERPOINT LECTURE SLIDES

Result of Energy Transfer to the Body
- **Blunt trauma:** causes multiple injuries to the head, spine, thorax, and abdomen
- **Penetrating trauma:** affects the brain, lungs, liver, spleen, intestines, and vascular system

SUGGESTIONS FOR CLASSROOM ACTIVITIES

- List types of penetrating trauma and instruments that are used in penetrating trauma.
- List objects that are used in blunt trauma.
- Discuss rapid deceleration injuries.

SUGGESTIONS FOR CLINICAL ACTIVITIES

- Assign students to observe the triage nurse in the emergency department.

LEARNING OUTCOME 4

Discuss causes, effects, and initial management of trauma.

CONCEPTS FOR LECTURE

1. Because of the seriousness of trauma, it is important to assess and initiate care rapidly.
2. Assessment of the airway is the highest priority in the trauma client.
3. Airway management in the trauma client requires special considerations. It is important to identify any potential obstruction from the tongue, loose teeth, foreign bodies, bleeding, secretions, vomitus, or edema. It is also important to determine if there are any of the following: closed head injury, maxillofacial trauma, direct airway trauma, cervical spine injury, burns, and hemorrhage.
4. Clients with burns often have airway compromise and require aggressive management. Secure an airway soon due to upper airway edema.
5. Tension pneumothorax is life-threatening and requires immediate attention.
6. Hemorrhage may result from blunt or penetrating trauma.
7. Assess the integumentary system for trauma to underlying structures.

POWERPOINT LECTURE SLIDES

Management of Trauma
- Effects of traumatic injury
  - Airway obstruction
    - Closed head trauma
    - Maxillofacial trauma
    - Direct airway trauma
    - Cervical spine injury
    - Burns
  - Tension pneumothorax
    - Air enters the plural space collapsing the lung and displacing the mediastinal contents
    - May require a needle thoracostomy
  - Hemorrhage
    - Assess and control hemorrhage with direct pressure
    - Discover the cause and extent of the injury
  - Integumentary effects
    - Contusions
    - Abrasions
    - Puncture wounds
    - Lacerations
    - Avulsion

8. Direct trauma to the abdominal cavity can lacerate and compress the solid organs and cause burst injuries to the hollow organs.
9. Musculoskeletal injuries are usually not a high priority, except in life- or limb-threatening injuries.
10. Neurologic injuries are usually caused by blunt trauma. Falls, sports injuries, and assault are sources of neurologic injuries.
11. Multiple organ dysfunction syndrome (MODS) is a common complication of severe injury. This is the result of an uncontrolled inflammatory response to severe injury or illness.

○ Abdominal effects
  – Immediate threat is hemorrhage, later threat is peritonitis
○ Musculoskeletal effects
  – May provide clues to the presence of other serious injuries (a fractured clavicle may indicated a thoracic injury)
○ Neurologic effects
  – Blunt trauma to the head causes neurological injuries
○ Multiple organ dysfunction syndromes (MODS)
  – Progressive impairment of two or more organ systems
○ Effects on the family

SUGGESTIONS FOR CLASSROOM ACTIVITIES

- Demonstrate endotracheal intubation. Discuss airway management in trauma clients.

SUGGESTIONS FOR CLINICAL ACTIVITIES

- Assign students to clients with endotracheal tubes.
- Assign students to care for clients with chest tubes.

LEARNING OUTCOME 5

Discuss diagnostic tests used in assessing clients experiencing trauma and shock.

CONCEPTS FOR LECTURE

1. Diagnostic tests that are ordered depend on the type of injury the client has sustained.
2. Tests that may be ordered for victims of trauma include the following:
   - Blood type and cross match
   - Blood alcohol level
   - Urine drug screen
   - Pregnancy test for any woman of childbearing age
   - Focused assessment by sonography in trauma (FAST) exam
   - Diagnostic peritoneal lavage
   - Computerized tomography (CT) scans
   - Magnetic resonance imaging (MRI) scans.

POWERPOINT LECTURE SLIDES

Diagnostic Tests for Assessing Trauma and Shock
- Blood type and crossmatch
- CBC, ABG
- Blood alcohol level
- Urine drug screen
- Pregnancy test
- Focused assessment by sonography in trauma (FAST)
- Diagnostic peritoneal lavage
- CT scan
- MRI

SUGGESTIONS FOR CLASSROOM ACTIVITIES

- Discuss what lab tests would be on a "trauma panel" and why.

SUGGESTIONS FOR CLINICAL ACTIVITIES

- Assign students to the emergency department to observe the trauma team.
- Discuss the duties of each member of a trauma team.

LEARNING OUTCOME 6

Describe collaborative interventions for clients experiencing trauma and shock, including medications, blood transfusions, and intravenous fluids.

CONCEPTS FOR LECTURE

1. The administration of medications and other interventions such as intravenous fluids and blood products depends upon the extent and type of injury sustained.

POWERPOINT LECTURE SLIDES

Interventions for Clients Experiencing Trauma and Shock
- Medications
  ○ Inotropic: increases cardiac contractility

- Inotropic medications: increase cardiac contractility
- Vasopressors: used to treat neurogenic, septic, or anaphylactic shock
- Opioids: used to treat pain
- Immunizations: tetanus prophylaxis

2. Blood and blood components increase the intravascular volume and increase the amount of hemoglobin needed to carry oxygen to the cells.
   - Red blood cells (RBCs): replace oxygen-carrying capabilities
   - Platelets: administered for continued hemorrhage
   - Whole blood products: replace blood volume
   - Albumin: expands blood volume
3. Intravenous fluids are used to expand fluid volume and to maintain venous access.
   - Ringer's lactate solution: replaces electrolyte deficits and creates increased circulating volume
   - Normal saline is compatible with the administration of blood.

- ○ Vasopressors: used to treat neurogenic, septic, or anaphylactic shock
- ○ Opioids: used to treat pain
- ○ Immunizations: tetanus prophylaxis
- Blood transfusions and blood products
  - ○ RBCs: replacement of oxygen carrying capabilities
  - ○ Platelets: given for continued hemorrhage
  - ○ Whole blood: replaces blood volume
  - ○ Albumin: expands blood volume
- Intravenous fluids
  - ○ Ringer's lactate: replaces electrolyte deficits, increases circulating volume
  - ○ Normal saline compatible with administration of blood

SUGGESTIONS FOR CLASSROOM ACTIVITIES

- Discuss reactions to blood transfusions.
- Discuss steps that should be taken if a client who is receiving a blood transfusion begins to show signs of a possible reaction.
- What steps are taken in the blood bank to ensure that the donor blood matches the client's blood?

SUGGESTIONS FOR CLINICAL ACTIVITIES

- Visit the hospital blood bank or local blood collection agency.
- Ask a healthcare provider who is employed in the blood bank to speak to the class about cross matching procedures.

LEARNING OUTCOME 7

Discuss organ donation and forensic implications of traumatic injury or death.

CONCEPTS FOR LECTURE

1. The Uniform Anatomical Gift Act requires that people be informed of their options for organ donation.
2. Most people can be organ donors with a few exceptions.
3. Once brain death has been established, the family needs to be allowed time to process and make decisions about organ donation.
4. Some religious and cultural groups have constraints or issues that forbid organ donation.
5. Many injuries, especially penetrating injuries, are caused by circumstances that require legal investigation. The nurse must be aware of the need to identify, store, and properly transfer potential evidence for medical legal investigations.

POWERPOINT LECTURE STATUS

Organ Donation
- Uniform anatomical gift act
- Most people can be organ donors
- Organ donation can occur once brain death established
- Exceptions for organ donation
  - ○ Currently abuse intravenous drugs
  - ○ Preexisting untreated infections
  - ○ Any malignancy other than primary brain tumor
  - ○ Have active TB

SUGGESTIONS FOR CLASSROOM ACTIVITIES

- Ask a healthcare provider who works for a local or regional organ and tissue bank to speak to the class.
- Invite a pathologist or coroner to speak to the class about the care of forensic evidence.

LEARNING OUTCOME 8

Discuss cellular homeostasis and basic hemodynamics.

CONCEPTS FOR LECTURE

1. Homeostatic regulation is maintained primarily by the cardiovascular system and depends on four physiologic components:
   - Cardiac output sufficient to meet bodily needs
   - An uncompromised vascular system
   - Sufficient blood volume and blood pressure to maintain adequate blood flow
   - Tissues that are able to extract and use oxygen delivered through the capillaries
2. When tissue perfusion is inadequate, normal cellular metabolism cannot be maintained.
3. If inadequate tissue perfusion is severe enough or of long duration, hypoxia and cellular death occur.

POWERPOINT LECTURE SLIDES

Cellular Homoeostasis and Basic Hemodynamics
- Homeostatic regulation maintained primarily by cardiovascular system
- Four physiologic components
  - Sufficient cardiac output
  - Uncompromised vascular system
  - Sufficient blood volume and blood pressure
  - Tissues that are able to extract and use oxygen

SUGGESTIONS FOR CLINICAL ACTIVITIES

- Have each student figure their clients' cardiac output using this formula:
  $CO = SV \times HR$

SUGGESTIONS FOR CLASSROOM ACTIVITIES

- An understanding of basic hemodynamics is necessary to understand the pathophysiology of shock. Ask the students to write a short paragraph about basic hemodynamics.

LEARNING OUTCOME 9

Discuss the risk factors, etiologies, and pathophysiologies of hypovolemic shock, cardiogenic shock, obstructive shock, and distributive shock.

CONCEPTS FOR LECTURE

1. Shock is defined as a systemic imbalance between oxygen supply and demand.
2. Shock is identified according to its underlying cause.
3. Hypovolemic shock is caused by a decrease in intravascular volume of 15% or more. As a result, stroke volume, cardiac output, and blood pressure drop.
4. Cardiogenic shock occurs when the heart's pumping ability is compromised to the point that it cannot maintain cardiac output and adequate tissue perfusion. Myocardial infarction is the most common cause of cardiogenic shock.
5. Obstructive shock is caused by an obstruction in the heart or great vessels.
6. Distributive shock combines several types of shock that result from widespread vasodilation and decreased peripheral resistance.

POWERPOINT LECTURE SLIDES

Types of Shock
- Hypovolemic shock
  - Affects all body systems
  - Most common type of shock
- Cardiogenic shock
  - Loss of pumping action of the heart
- Obstructive shock
  - Impaired diastolic filling (pericardial tamponade, pneumothorax)
- Distributive shock
  - Also known as vasogenic shock
  - Blood volume does not change, hypovolemic results

SUGGESTIONS FOR CLASSROOM ACTIVITIES

- Have each student write a short synopsis of each type of shock.

SUGGESTIONS FOR CLINICAL ACTIVITIES

- Have the students develop a care plan for a client in shock.

LEARNING OUTCOME 10

Use the nursing process as a framework for providing individualized care to clients experiencing trauma and shock.

CONCEPTS FOR LECTURE

1. Accessing, establishing, and maintaining an airway is the most critical nursing intervention.
2. Establish a baseline assessment of the client in shock.
3. Prevent further progression of shock by assessment, monitoring, and intervention.
4. Assess and monitor overall tissue perfusion.
5. Assess and meet the psychosocial needs of the client.
6. Provide comfort measures and reduce stimuli that can cause increased anxiety in the client.

POWERPOINT LECTURE SLIDES

Nursing Process
- Access, establish, and maintain an airway
- Establish a baseline assessment
- Prevent further progression
- Assess and monitor overall tissue perfusion
- Assess and meet psychosocial needs
- Provide comfort measures and reduce stimuli

SUGGESTIONS FOR CLASSROOM ACTIVITIES

- Create a nursing care plan based on individual types of shock.

SUGGESTIONS FOR CLINICAL ACTIVITIES

- Amplify and amend the nursing care plan that was created in the classroom and apply to the client in the intensive care unit (ICU) who is assigned to the student.

CHAPTER 12
NURSING CARE OF CLIENTS WITH INFECTIONS

RESOURCE LIBRARY

 PRENTICE HALL NURSING MEDIALINK DVD-ROM

Audio Glossary
NCLEX-RN® Review
Animation/Videos
  Inflammatory Response
  Penicillin
  White Blood Cells

 COMPANION WEBSITE

Audio Glossary
NCLEX-RN® Review
Care Plan Activity: Postoperative Infection
Case Study: The Client with an Infection
MediaLink Applications
  Antibiotic-Resistant Organisms
  Hospital-Acquired Infections
Links to Resources

📖 IMAGE LIBRARY

Figure 12.1 The development and differentiation of leukocytes from hemocytoblasts.
Figure 12.2 The development and differentiation of lymphocytes from the lymphoid stem cell (lymphoblasts).
Figure 12.3 The lymphoid system: the central organs of the thymus and bone marrow, and the peripheral organs, including the spleen, tonsils, lymph nodes, and Peyer's patches.
Figure 12.4 The process of leukocyte emigration at the site of inflammation.
Figure 12.5 The process of phagocytosis.

Figure 12.6 Antibody-mediated (humoral) immunity.
Figure 12.7 An antibody molecule.
Figure 12.8 Antigen–antibody binding.
Figure 12.9 Antibody production in the primary and secondary responses of the antibody-mediated immune response.
Figure 12.10 Cellular immune response.
Figure 12.11 Lymph nodes that may be assessed by palpation.
Figure 12.12 The chain of infection.
Figure 12.13 Neutrophils by stage of maturity and normal distribution in the blood.

LEARNING OUTCOME 1

Discuss the components and functions of the immune system and the immune response.

CONCEPTS FOR LECTURE

1. The immune system is a complex and intricate network of specialized cells, tissues, and organs.
2. The immune system consists of molecules, cells, and organs that produce the immune response.
3. Cells and tissues of the immune system include; leukocytes, granulocytes, neutrophils, eosinophils, basophils, monocytes and macrophages, lymphocytes, T cells, B cells, NK (natural killer) cells, lymphoid tissues, primary or central lymphoid structures; bone marrow and thymus gland, secondary or peripheral lymphoid structures; lymph nodes, spleen, tonsils, intestinal lymphoid tissue, and lymphoid tissue in other organs.
4. The thymus and bone marrow, in which T cells and B cells mature, are considered central lymphoid organs. The spleen, lymph nodes, tonsils, and other peripheral lymphoid tissue are peripheral lymphoid organs.

POWERPOINT LECTURE SLIDES

Components of the Immune System and the Immune Response
- Cells of the immune system
  ○ Leukocytes
    – Granulocytes
      · Neutrophils
      · Eosinophils
      · Basophils
    – Monocytes and macrophages
    – Lymphocytes
      · T cells
      · B cells
      · NK (natural killer cells)
- Lymphoid tissue
  ○ Primary of central lymphoid structures
    – Bone marrow, thymus gland

5. The immune system is activated by injury or disease. When the inflammatory process is unable to destroy invading organisms or toxins, the immune response is activated.
6. When these first-line defenses are breached, resulting tissue damage or foreign material entering the body induces a nonspecific immune response known as inflammation. Inflammation is an adaptive response to injury that brings fluid, dissolved substances, and blood cells into the interstitial tissues where the invasion or damage has occurred.
7. The introduction of antigens into the body causes a more specific reaction than the nonspecific inflammatory response. On the first exposure to an antigen, a change occurs in the host, resulting in a specific and rapid response following subsequent exposures. This specific response is known as the immune response.

- ○ Secondary or peripheral lymphoid structures
  - – Lymph nodes, spleen, tonsils, intestinal lymphoid tissue, lymphoid tissue in other organs
- • Immune Response
  - ○ Activated by injury or disease
  - ○ Activated when the inflammatory process is unable to destroy invading organisms

SUGGESTIONS FOR CLASSROOM ACTIVITIES

- • Review the anatomy and physiology of the immune system.
- • View a video about the immune system.

LEARNING OUTCOME 2

Compare antibody-mediated and cell-mediated immune responses.

CONCEPTS FOR LECTURE

1. Antibody-mediated immune response is produced by B lymphocytes (B cells).
2. B cells are activated by contact with an antigen or antigens. The B cell then proliferates and differentiates into antibody-producing plasma cells and memory cells.
3. An antibody is an immunoglobulin molecule with the ability to bind to and inactivate a specific antigen. Immunoglobulins comprise the gamma globulin portion of the blood proteins.
4. Many antigens cannot stimulate the antibody-mediated response because they live inside the body's cells. Viruses and mycobacteria are examples of these antigens.
5. The immune response that provides protection against these antigens is the cell-mediated immune response called cellular immunity. T cells initiate this type of immune response. There are two major classes of T cells. These are effector cells (cytotoxic cells, or killer T cells) and regulator cells (helper T cells and suppressor T cells).

POWERPOINT LECTURE SLIDES

Antibody-mediated and cell-mediated immune responses
- • Antibody-mediated immune response
  - ○ B cells link with and inactivate antigens by one of the following processes
    - – Phagocytosis of the antigen by neutrophils
    - – Precipitation
    - – Neutralization
    - – Lysis
    - – Agglutination
    - – Opsonization
- • Cell-mediated immune response
  - ○ Two major classes of T cells
    - – Effector cells (cytotoxic cells, or killer T cells)
    - – Regulator cells (helper T cells and suppressor T cells)

SUGGESTIONS FOR CLASSROOM ACTIVITIES

- • Review and discuss the roles of killer T cells and suppressor T cells.

LEARNING OUTCOME 3

Describe the pathophysiology of wound healing, inflammation, and infection.

CONCEPTS FOR LECTURE

1. The tissue damage that evokes an inflammatory response may be caused by specific or nonspecific antigens.
2. The causes of inflammation include the following; mechanical injuries, physical damage, chemical injury, microorganisms, extreme heat or cold, hypersensitivity response, ischemic damage, or trauma.
3. Infection occurs when an organism is able to colonize and multiply within a host.
4. For a microorganism to cause infection, it must have disease causing potential (virulence), be transmitted from its reservoir, and gain entry into a susceptible host. This is known as the chain of infection. The chain of Infection includes an etiologic agent (microorganism), reservoir (source), portal of exit from reservoir, method of transmission, portal of entry to susceptible host, and susceptible host.
5. Inflammation and wound healing are highly metabolic processes that may be affected by a number of factors. These factors include: malnutrition, vitamin deficiency, tissue hypoxia, impaired blood supply, impaired immunity, and inflammation processes.

POWERPOINT LECTURE SLIDES

Inflammation, Infection, and Wound Healing
- Causes of inflammation
  - Mechanical injuries
  - Physical damage
  - Chemical injury
  - Microorganisms
  - Extreme heat or cold
  - Hypersensitivity response
  - Ischemic damage or trauma
- Chain of infection
  - Etiologic agent (microorganism)
  - Reservoir (source)
  - Portal of exit from reservoir
  - Method of transmission
  - Portal of entry to susceptible host
  - Susceptible host
- Factors affecting wound healing
  - Malnutrition
  - Vitamin deficiency
  - Tissue hypoxia
  - Impaired blood supply
  - Impaired immunity and inflammation processes

SUGGESTIONS FOR CLASSROOM ACTIVITIES

- Discuss the chain of infection and how the chain could be disrupted.
- Ask students to devise an educational poster for pre-school children that teaches methods of preventing the spread of pathogens.
- Discuss the factors of wound healing.

SUGGESTIONS FOR CLINICAL ACTIVITIES

- Visit a school to teach preventative measures to stop the spread of pathogens that cause colds and flu.
- Assign students to clients who have a wound that is not healing properly.

LEARNING OUTCOME 4

Identify factors responsible for nosocomial infections.

CONCEPTS FOR LECTURE

1. Nosocomial infections are acquired in a healthcare setting. Also known as healthcare associated infections (HAIs), nosocomial infections account for an estimated 2 million infections, 90,000 deaths, and $4.5 billion in excess healthcare costs annually.
2. Clients who enter the hospital are the least able to mount immune defenses to infection.
3. Effective hand washing is the single most important measure in infection control.

POWERPOINT LECTURE SLIDES

Factors Responsible for Nosocomial Infections
- Immune-impaired client
- Antibiotic therapy has altered natural defense mechanisms
- Chemotherapy, corticosteroids, radiation therapy
- Invasive procedures
- Pneumonia associated with ICU admission

SUGGESTIONS FOR CLASSROOM ACTIVITIES

- Research the internet for data about HAIs. What are the most commonly-occurring infections?
- Ask the infection control nurse to speak to the class about the role of the infection control nurse.

SUGGESTIONS FOR CLINICAL ACTIVITIES

- Make rounds with the infection control nurse. Observe how the data is collected.

LEARNING OUTCOME 5

Use the nursing process as a framework to provide individualized care to clients with inflammation and infection.

CONCEPTS FOR LECTURE

1. Assess the client's pain level and provide comfort measures.
2. Provide teaching for client and family to prevent further spread of disease.
3. Evaluate the client's health history for chronic disease.
4. Monitor the client's vital signs, including temperature, blood pressure and pulse, and respirations.
5. Assess the client's wound or inflammatory process.

POWERPOINT LECTURE SLIDES

Nursing Process
- Assess pain level
- Provide comfort measures
- Provide teaching for client and family
- Evaluate health history for chronic disease
- Monitor vital signs
- Assess wound or inflammatory process

SUGGESTIONS FOR CLASSROOM ACTIVITIES

- Develop a nursing care plan that includes education for the family of a diabetic client with a foot ulcer.

SUGGESTIONS FOR CLINICAL ACTIVITIES

- While caring for a client with a chronic wound, develop a teaching plan for the family.

CHAPTER 13
NURSING CARE OF CLIENTS WITH ALTERED IMMUNITY

RESOURCE LIBRARY

💿 PRENTICE HALL NURSING MEDIALINK DVD-ROM

Audio Glossary
NCLEX-RN® Review
Crossword Puzzle: The Immune System
Animation/Video
  Histamine
  Immune System
  Immune System in the Older Adult

📖 IMAGE LIBRARY

Figure 13.1 Type I IgE-mediated hypersensitivity response.
Figure 13.2 Type II cytotoxic hypersensitivity response.
Figure 13.3 Type III immune complex–mediated hypersensitivity response.
Figure 13.4 Type IV delayed hypersensitivity response.
Figure 13.6 Sites of action of immunosuppressive agents.

🌐 COMPANION WEBSITE

Audio Glossary
NCLEX-RN® Review
Care Plan Activity: A Client with AIDS
Case Study: HIV Prevention
MediaLink Application: At Risk for HIV/AIDS
Links to Resources

Figure 13.7 How HIV infects and destroys CD4 cells.
Figure 13.8 The progression of HIV infection.
Figure 13.10 Kaposi's sarcoma lesions.
Figure 13.11 This nurse is disposing of a needle and syringe in a special container, a necessary practice to avoid the transmission of HIV through needle sticks with contaminated needles.

LEARNING OUTCOME 1

Review normal anatomy and physiology of the immune system.

CONCEPTS FOR LECTURE

1. The immune system contains lymphocytes and lymphatic tissue.
2. The effectiveness of the immune system depends on the system's ability to differentiate between "self" and "non-self" properties.
3. When the immune system fails to recognize self, autoimmune disorders may ensue.
4. The antibody-mediated immune response is accomplished by activating the B cells and T cells.
5. Cell-mediated immunity acts at the cellular level by attaching the antigens directly.
6. The immune function declines with aging, although the many mechanisms that cause this are not known.

POWERPOINT LECTURE SLIDES

Anatomy and Physiology of the Immune System
- Contains lymphocytes and lymphatic tissue
- Effectiveness depends on systems ability to differentiate between "self" and "non-self" properties
- Autoimmune disorders occur when immune system fails to recognize itself
- Antibody-mediated immune response
- Cell-mediated immunity
- Declines with aging

SUGGESTIONS FOR CLASSROOM ACTIVITIES

- Research autoimmune diseases that are listed in the text, and create a nursing care plan for one of the diseases.

SUGGESTIONS FOR CLINICAL ACTIVITIES

- Assign students to clients with immunosuppression.

LEARNING OUTCOME 2

Describe the four types of hypersensitivity reactions.

CONCEPTS FOR LECTURE

1. Hypersensitivity is an altered immune response to an antigen that results in harm to the client.
2. Reactions are classified by the type of immune response that occurs on contact with the antigen.
3. Common hypersensitivity reactions, such as allergic asthma, allergic rhinitis (hay fever), allergic conjunctivitis, hives, and anaphylactic shock, are typical of type I or IgE-mediated hypersensitivity. This type of hypersensitivity response is triggered when an allergen interacts with IgE bound to mast cells and basophils. The antigen–antibody complex prompts release of histamine and other chemical mediators, complement, acetylcholine, kinins, and chemotactic factors.
4. A hemolytic transfusion reaction to blood of an incompatible type is characteristic of a type II or cytotoxic hypersensitivity reaction. IgG or IgM type antibodies are formed to a cell-bound antigen such as the ABO or Rh antigen. When these antibodies bind with the antigen, the complement cascade is activated, resulting in destruction of the target cell.
5. Type III hypersensitivity reactions result from the formation of IgG or IgM antibody–antigen immune complexes in the circulation. When these complexes are deposited in vessel walls and extravascular tissues, complement is activated and chemical mediators of inflammation such as histamine are released. Chemotactic factors attract neutrophils to the site of inflammation. When neutrophils attempt to phagocytize the immune complexes, lysosomal enzymes are released, increasing tissue damage.
6. Type IV reactions differ from other hypersensitivity responses in two ways. First, these reactions are cell-mediated rather than antibody-mediated, involving T cells of the immune system. Second, type IV reactions are delayed rather than immediate, developing 24 to 48 hours after exposure to the antigen. Contact dermatitis is a classic example of a type IV reaction.

POWERPOINT LECTURE SLIDES

Four Types of Hypersensitivity Reactions
- Type I: IgE-mediated hypersensitivity
  - Allergic asthma
  - Allergic rhinitis (hay fever)
  - Anaphylactic shock
- Type II: cytotoxic hypersensitivity
  - Blood transfusion reaction
- Type III: immune complex–mediated hypersensitivity
  - IgG or IgM antibody–antigen immune complexes
  - Histamine release
- Type IV: delayed hypersensitivity
  - Cell-mediated, not antibody-mediated
  - Reactions are delayed, developing 24–48 hours later

SUGGESTIONS FOR CLASSROOM ACTIVITIES

- Discuss the reaction chain due to a type II cytotoxic hypersensitivity.

SUGGESTIONS FOR CLINICAL ACTIVITIES

- Ask an allergy specialist or an allergy nurse to speak to the class.
- Assign students to visit a physician's office that specializes in allergies.

LEARNING OUTCOME 3

Discuss the pathophysiology of autoimmune disorders and tissue transplant rejection.

CONCEPTS FOR LECTURE

1. When self-recognition is impaired and immune defenses are directed against normal host tissue, the result is an autoimmune disorder. The mechanism that causes the immune system to not recognize host tissue as a foreign antigen is not clear.

2. Transplant success is closely related to obtaining an organ with tissue antigens as close to those of the recipient as possible. Matching the human leukocyte antigen (HLA) type of the donor and recipient as closely as possible decreases the potential for rejection of the transplanted organ or tissue.

3. Tissue typing is used to determine the histocompatibility and to decrease the possibility of transplant rejection.

4. Tissue rejection:
   - Hyperacute tissue rejection: occurs immediately to 2–3 days posttransplant or blood transfusion
   - Active tissue rejection: occurs within four days (three in most) posttransplant; this type of rejection is the most common and treatable
   - Chronic tissue rejection: occurs within four months to one year posttransplant; is usually the result of antimediated immune response
   - Graft-versus-host disease (GVHD): occurs when there is no close match between donor and host; is a potentially fatal condition

POWERPOINT LECTURE SLIDES

Autoimmune Disorders and Tissue Transplant Rejection
- Factors that may cause autoimmune disorders
  - Release of "hidden" antigens
  - Chemical, physical, or biologic changes in host tissue
  - An antigen whose properties closely resemble those of host tissue
  - Defect in normal cellular immune functions
  - Slow growing mycobacteria
- Tissue match terminology
  - Autograft: transplant of the client's own tissue
  - Isograft: tissue from identical twin
  - Allograft: graft between members of the same species
  - Xenograft: transplant from a different species
- Tissue rejection
  - Hyperacute tissue rejection
  - Active tissue rejection
  - Chronic tissue rejection
  - Graft-versus-host disease (GVHD)

SUGGESTIONS FOR CLASSROOM ACTIVITIES

- Discuss the history of transplants and how transplants have evolved to the current rates of successful transplantation.

SUGGESTIONS FOR CLINICAL ACTIVITIES

- Invite a speaker from the local tissue bank to speak to the class.

LEARNING OUTCOME 4

Discuss the characteristics of immunodeficiencies.

CONCEPTS FOR LECTURE

1. Disorders of impaired system responses may be congenital or acquired. The client demonstrates an unusual susceptibility to infection. When the antibody-mediated response is primarily affected, the client is at risk for severe and chronic bacterial infections.

2. Immunodeficiency is most severe when the antibody-mediated and cell-mediated responses are impaired.

3. Most immunodeficiency diseases are genetically determined and are rare. They affect children more than adults.

POWERPOINT LECTURE SLIDES

Characteristics of Immunodeficiencies
- May be congenital or acquired
- Unusual susceptibility to infection
- Most severe when the antibody-mediated and cell-mediated responses are impaired
- Genetically determined and rare
- Affecting children more than adults

LEARNING OUTCOME 5

Identify laboratory and diagnostic tests used to diagnose and monitor immune response.

CONCEPTS FOR LECTURE

1. To identify possible allergens or hypersensitivity reactions, laboratory tests may be ordered:
   - White blood cell (WBC) count with differential: detects high levels of circulating eosinophils.
   - Radioallergosorbent test (RAST): measures the amount of IgE that is directed toward specific allergens
   - Blood type and crossmatch: ordered prior to any transfusion
   - Indirect Coombs' test: detects the presence of circulating antibodies
   - Direct Combs' test: detects antibodies on the client's RBC that damage and destroy cells
   - Immune complex assays: detects the presence of circulating immune complexes
   - Complement assays: detects immune complex disorders
   - Prick (epicutaneous or puncture test): diluted allergic extract is placed on skin then the skin is pricked through it
   - Intradermal: an allergen is injected under skin to make a wheal
   - Patch: a one-inch patch is impregnated with allergen
   - Food allergy testing: client is asked to keep a food diary

POWERPOINT LECTURE SLIDES

Laboratory and Diagnostic Tests for Immune Response
- WBC count with differential
- Radioallergosorbent test (RAST)
- Blood type and crossmatch
- Indirect Coombs' test
- Direct Coombs' test
- Immune complex assays
- Complement assays
- Skin tests
  - Prick (epicutaneous or puncture test)
  - Intradermal
  - Patch
  - Food allergy

LEARNING OUTCOME 6

Describe pharmacologic and other collaborative therapies used in treating clients with altered immunity.

CONCEPTS FOR LECTURE

1. Various approaches are used in the treatment of the client with altered immunity when the activities of daily living are disrupted.
2. Nursing care is directed toward prevention and early intervention.
3. Immunotherapy, also called hyposensitization or desensitization, consists of injecting an extract of the allergen(s) in gradually increasing doses. Immunotherapy is used primarily for allergic rhinitis or asthma related to

POWERPOINT LECTURE SLIDES

Pharmacologic and Collaborative Therapies for Altered Immunity
- **Immunotherapy:** desensitization
- **Antihistamines:** used in type 1 responses
- **Epinephrine:** anaphylaxis
- **Corticosteroids:** used for anti-inflammatory effects
- **Plasmapheresis:** removes harmful components from the plasma

inhaled allergens. It has also been shown to be effective in preventing anaphylactic responses to insect venom. With weekly or biweekly subcutaneous injections of the allergen, the client develops IgG antibodies to the allergen that appear to block effectively the allergic IgE-mediated response. Once a therapy plateau is reached, injections are continued indefinitely either monthly or bimonthly.

4. Antihistamines are the major class of drugs used in treating the symptoms of hypersensitivity responses, type I in particular. They are also useful to some extent in relieving manifestations (such as urticaria) of some type II and type III reactions.

5. The immediate treatment for anaphylaxis is parenteral epinephrine, an adrenergic agonist (sympathomimetic) drug that has both vasoconstricting and bronchodilating effects. These qualities, combined with its rapid action, make epinephrine ideal for treating an anaphylactic reaction.

6. Glucocorticoids (corticosteroids) are used in both systemic and topical forms for many types of hypersensitivity responses. Their anti-inflammatory effects, rather than their immunosuppressive effects, are of most benefit. A short course of corticosteroid therapy is often used for severe asthma, allergic contact dermatitis, and some immune-complex disorders. Corticosteroids in topical forms or delivered by inhaler may be used for longer periods of time with few side effects; however, systemic absorption can occur.

7. Plasmapheresis, removal of harmful components in the plasma, may be used to treat immune complex responses such as glomerulonephritis and Goodpasture's syndrome. Plasma and the glomerular-damaging antibody–antigen complexes are removed by passing the client's blood through a blood cell separator. The RBCs are then returned to the client along with an equal amount of albumin or human plasma. This procedure is usually done in a series rather than as a one-time treatment. It is not without risk, and informed consent is required. Potential complications of plasmapheresis include those associated with intravenous catheters, shifts in fluid balance, and alteration of blood clotting.

SUGGESTIONS FOR CLASSROOM ACTIVITIES

- Develop a nursing care plan for a client who has altered immunity.

SUGGESTIONS FOR CLINICAL ACTIVITIES

- Demonstrate the technique for administering intradermal injections.

LEARNING OUTCOME 7

Correlate the pathophysiological alterations with the manifestations of HIV/AIDS infection.

CONCEPTS FOR LECTURE

1. The human immunodeficiency virus was isolated in 1984. It then became apparent that AIDS was the final, fatal stage of HIV infection.

2. HIV is a retrovirus, which means that it carries its genetic information in RNA. Upon entry into the body, the virus infects cells that have the CD4 antigen.

3. The clinical manifestations of HIV infection range from no symptoms to severe immunodeficiency with multiple opportunistic infections and cancers. Typical manifestations include fever, sore throat, arthralgias and myalgias, headache, rash, and lymphadenopathy. The client may also experience nausea, vomiting, and abdominal cramping. The client often attributes this initial manifestation of HIV infection to a common viral illness such as influenza, upper respiratory infection, or stomach virus.

4. Following this acute illness, clients enter a long-lasting asymptomatic period. Although the virus is present and can be transmitted to others, the infected host has few or no symptoms.

5. The move from asymptomatic disease or persistent lymphadenopathy to AIDS is often not clearly defined. The client may complain of general malaise, fever, fatigue, night sweats, and involuntary weight loss. Persistent skin dryness and rash may be a problem. Diarrhea is common, as are oral lesions such as hairy leukoplakia, candidiasis, and gingival inflammation and ulceration.

6. The development of advanced HIV infection typically occurs 10–11 years after initial infection. This varies according to viral load, rate of disease progress, and development of resistance to antiviral therapy.

POWERPOINT LECTURE SLIDES

Manifestations of HIV/AIDS
- Early clinical manifestations of HIV/AIDS
  - Flu and mononucleosis type symptoms
  - Persistent generalized lymphadenopathy
  - General malaise, fever, fatigue, night sweats, involuntary weight loss
- Later clinical manifestations of HIV/AIDS
  - Dementia and neurologic effects
  - Opportunistic infections
  - Pneumocystis carinii pneumonia
  - Tuberculosis
  - Candidiasis
  - Wasting syndrome
  - Kaposi's sarcoma
  - Lymphoma

SUGGESTIONS FOR CLASSROOM ACTIVITIES

- Develop a nursing care plan for teaching a client and his family about HIV.

SUGGESTIONS FOR CLINICAL ACTIVITIES

- Visit an immunosuppressed client care unit or community clinic.

LEARNING OUTCOME 8

Use the nursing process as a framework to provide individualized care to clients with altered immune responses.

CONCEPTS FOR LECTURE

1. The goal of care for the client with altered immune response is to prevent opportunistic infections and disease.

2. Coping mechanisms in the client with immune deficiency must be assessed.

3. Nutritional status must be monitored, especially in clients with HIV.

4. Assess family and community support for HIV clients.

POWERPOINT LECTURE SLIDES

Nursing Process for Care of Client with Altered Immune Responses
- Goal to prevent opportunistic infections
- Assess coping mechanisms
- Monitor nutritional status
- Assess family and community support

Suggestions for Classroom Activities

- Discuss preventative measures to protect those clients who are immunosuppressed to prevent opportunistic infections.
- Ask the hospital dietitian to speak to the class about the nutritional challenges that face a client who is immunosuppressed.

Suggestions for Clinical Activities

- Assign students to a client who is immunosuppressed. Discuss the measures that should be taken to prevent opportunistic infections.
- Visit the AIDS/HIV clinic.

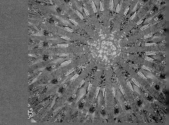

CHAPTER 14
NURSING CARE OF CLIENTS WITH CANCER

RESOURCE LIBRARY

 PRENTICE HALL NURSING MEDIALINK DVD-ROM

Audio Glossary
NCLEX-RN© Review
Animation/Video
  Cancer
  Cell Division
  Mini-infusion Pumps

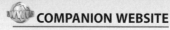 **COMPANION WEBSITE**

Audio Glossary
NCLEX-RN© Review
Care Plan Activity: Weight Loss and Chemotherapy
Case Studies
  Cancer Therapies
  Pain Management
MediaLink Applications
  Cancer Research
  Interpreting Lab Results
Links to Resources

IMAGE LIBRARY

Figure 14.1 Interaction of factors that promote cancer.
Figure 14.2 How cancer cells invade normal tissue.
Figure 14.3 Metastasis through the bloodstream.
Figure 14.4 Cachectic person.

Figure 14.5 Chemotherapeutic drugs useful in each phase of the cell cycle.
Figure 14.6 Vascular access devices.
Figure 14.7 The superior vena cava syndrome.

LEARNING OUTCOME 1

Define cancer and differentiate benign from malignant neoplasms.

CONCEPTS FOR LECTURE

1. Cancer is a group of complex diseases with various manifestations that depend on which body system is affected and the type of tumor cells. Cancer results when normal cells mutate into abnormal cells.
2. A neoplasm is a mass of new tissue (a collection of cells) that grows independently of its surrounding structures and has no physiologic purpose. The term neoplasm is often used interchangeably with tumor, from the Latin word meaning "swelling."
3. Neoplasms typically are classified as benign or malignant on the basis of their potential to damage the body and on their growth characteristics.
4. Benign neoplasms do not usually result in invasion and destruction of tissue.
5. Benign neoplasms are localized growths. They form a solid mass, have well-defined borders, and frequently are encapsulated.
6. Malignant neoplasms grow aggressively and do not respond to the body's homeostatic controls. Malignant neoplasms are not cohesive, and present with an irregular shape. Instead of slowly crowding other tissues aside, malignant neoplasms cut through surrounding tissues, causing bleeding, inflammation, and necrosis

POWERPOINT LECTURE SLIDES

Comparison of Benign and Malignant Neoplasms
- Benign
  - Local
  - Cohesive
  - Well-defined borders
  - Pushes other tissue out of the way
  - Slow growth
  - Encapsulated
  - Easily removed
  - Does not recur
- Malignant
  - Invasive
  - Noncohesive
  - Does not stop at tissue border
  - Invades and destroys surrounding tissues
  - Rapid growth
  - Metastasizes to distant sites
  - Not always easy to remove
  - Can recur

(tissue death) as they grow. Healthcare professionals are referring to a malignant neoplasm when they use the term cancer.

SUGGESTIONS FOR CLASSROOM ACTIVITIES	SUGGESTIONS FOR CLINICAL ACTIVITIES
• Discuss the role of the American Cancer Society and its role in public education, fund raising, and raising awareness.	• Ask students to participate in a local or national fund raiser for cancer research, such as the Susan G. Komen Foundation for breast cancer research.

LEARNING OUTCOME 2

Describe the theories of carcinogenesis.

CONCEPTS FOR LECTURE

1. The theory of cellular mutation suggests that carcinogens cause mutations in cellular DNA. It is believed that the carcinogenic process has three stages: initiation, promotion, and progression:
   • Initiation stage: involves permanent damage in the cellular DNA as a result of exposure to a carcinogen (e.g., radiation, chemicals) that was not repaired or had a defective repair
   • Promotion stage: may last for years and includes conditions, such as smoking or alcohol use, that act repeatedly on the already-affected cells
   • Progression stage: further inherited changes acquired during the cell replication develop into a cancer
2. Oncogenes are genes that promote cell proliferation and are capable of triggering cancerous characteristics. A decrease in the body's immune surveillance may allow the expression of oncogenes; this can occur during times of stress or in response to certain carcinogens.
3. Tumor suppressor genes normally suppress oncogenes. They can become inactive by deletion or mutation. Inherited cancers have been associated with tumor suppressor genes.
4. Central to these theories are two important concepts about the etiology of cancer. First, damaged DNA, whether inherited or from external sources, sets up the necessary initial step for cancer to occur. Second, impairment of the human immune system, from whatever cause, lessens its ability to destroy abnormal cells.

POWERPOINT LECTURE SLIDES

Theories of Carcinogenesis
• Cellular mutation
  ○ Suggests carcinogens cause mutations in cellular DNA
  ○ Three stages
    – Initiation stage
    – Promotion stage
    – Progression stage
• Oncogenes
  ○ Promote cell proliferation
  ○ Capable of triggering cancerous characteristics
• Tumor suppressor genes
  ○ Normally suppress oncogenes
  ○ Become inactive by deletion or mutation
  ○ Associated with inherited cancers

SUGGESTIONS FOR CLASSROOM ACTIVITIES

• Have each student write a short paper about the theories of carcinogenesis.

LEARNING OUTCOME 3

Explain and discuss known carcinogens and identify risk factors for cancer.

CONCEPTS FOR LECTURE

1. A number of agents are known to cause cancer or are strongly linked to certain kinds of cancers. These known carcinogens include viruses, drugs, hormones, and chemical and physical agents.
2. Carcinogens are grouped into two categories: genotoxic, which cause mutations and alter DNA; and promoter substances that cause biologic effects.
3. Although everyone comes into contact with a vast number of substances that are considered carcinogenic, not everyone develops cancer.
4. Other factors, such as genetic predisposition, impairment of the immune response, and repeated exposure to the carcinogen, are necessary for a cancer to develop.
5. Risk factors make an individual or a population vulnerable to a specific disease or other unhealthy outcome. Risk factors can be divided into those that are controllable and those that are not controllable. Knowledge and assessment of risk factors are especially important in counseling clients and families about measures to prevent cancer.
6. Risk factors include: heredity, age, gender, poverty, stress, diet, occupation, infection, tobacco use, alcohol use, recreational drug use, obesity, and sun exposure.

POWERPOINT LECTURE SLIDES

Known Carcinogens and Risk Factors for Cancer
- Known carcinogens
  - Viruses
  - Drugs and hormones
  - Chemical agents
  - Physical agents (solar radiation, radon gas, water polluted by nuclear waste)
- Risk factors
  - Heredity
  - Age
  - Gender
  - Poverty
  - Stress
  - Diet
  - Occupation
  - Infection
  - Tobacco use
  - Alcohol use
  - Recreational drug use
  - Obesity
  - Sun exposure

SUGGESTIONS FOR CLASSROOM ACTIVITIES

- Ask students to identify risk factors in their environment such as pollution and second-hand smoke.
- Discuss the risk factors in the students' life that can be changed. What risk factors cannot be changed?

SUGGESTIONS FOR CLINICAL ACTIVITIES

- Ask students to assess their own and their families' risk factors for cancer.

LEARNING OUTCOME 4

Compare the mechanisms and characteristics of normal cells with those of malignant cells.

CONCEPTS FOR LECTURE

1. A neoplasm is a mass of new tissue that grows independently of its surrounding structures and has no physiologic purpose.
2. Benign neoplasms are localized growths. They form a solid mass, have well-defined borders, and are frequently encapsulated.
3. Malignant neoplasms grow aggressively and do not respond to the body's homeostatic controls.
4. Malignant cells travel through the bloodstream and lymphatic system to invade other tissues.
5. If unchecked, malignant cells eventually destroy their host.

POWERPOINT LECTURE SLIDES

Characteristics of Malignant Cells
- Loss of regulation of the rate of mitosis
- Loss of specialization and differentiation
- Loss of contact inhibition
- Progressive acquisition of cancerous phenotype
- Irreversibility
- Altered cell structure
- Simplified metabolic activities
- Transplantability (metastasis)
- Ability to promote their own survival

LEARNING OUTCOME 5

Describe physical and psychological effects of cancer.

CONCEPTS FOR LECTURE

1. Nursing care of clients with cancer is related to the generalized effects of cancer on the body and the side effects of the treatments.
2. Physiological effects of the cancer may vary with the type and location of the cancer; however, certain effects are usually observed.
3. Disruption of function
   • Physiologic functioning can be upset by obstruction or pressure. Obstruction or pressure can cause anoxia and necrosis of surrounding tissues, which in turn cause a loss of function of the involved organ or tissue.
4. Hematologic alterations can impair the normal function of blood cells.
5. Infection
   • When a tumor grows near the surface of the body, it may erode through to the surface, thus breaking down the natural defenses of intact skin and mucous membranes and providing a site for the entry of microorganisms.
6. Hemorrhage
   • Tumor erosion through blood vessels can cause extensive bleeding, giving rise to severe anemia. Hemorrhage can be serious enough to cause life-threatening hypovolemic shock.
7. Anorexia (cachexia syndrome)
   • A characteristic feature of cancer is the wasted appearance of its victims, called cachexia. In many cases, unexplained rapid weight loss is the first symptom that brings the client to a healthcare provider. This can be due to a variety of problems associated with cancer, such as pain, infection, depression, or the side effects of chemotherapy and radiation. Usually, however, the emaciation, malnutrition, and loss of energy are attributed to the anorexia-cachexia syndrome.
8. Paraneoplastic syndromes are indirect effects of cancer. They may be early warning signs of cancer or indicate complications or return of a malignancy. The most frequently occurring paraneoplastic syndromes are endocrine, occurring when cancers set up ectopic sites of hormone production.

POWERPOINT LECTURE SLIDES

Physical and Psychological Effects of Cancer
  • Disruption of function
  • Hematologic alterations
  • Infection
  • Hemorrhage
  • Anorexia (cachexia syndrome)
  • Paraneoplastic syndromes
  • Acute and chronic pain
  • Physical stress
  • Psychological stress

9. Cancer pain can be divided into two main categories, acute and chronic, with subgroupings.
   - Acute pain has a well-defined pattern of onset, exhibits common signs and symptoms, and is often identified with hyperactivity of the autonomic system.
   - Chronic pain, which lasts more than 6 months, frequently lacks the objective manifestations of acute pain, primarily because the autonomic nervous system adapts to this chronic stress. Unfortunately, chronic pain often results in personality changes, alterations in functional abilities, and lifestyle disruptions that can seriously affect compliance with treatment and the quality of life.
10. Physical Stress
    - When the immune system discovers a neoplasm, it tries to destroy it using the resources of the body. The body mounts an all-out assault on the foreign invader, calling on many resources (i.e., hormones, enzymes, protein).
11. Psychological Stress
    - People confronted with the diagnosis of cancer exhibit a variety of psychologic and emotional responses.
    - These responses could include: guilt, fear, isolation, anger, powerlessness, hopelessness, body image concerns, sexual dysfunction, and grief.

SUGGESTIONS FOR CLASSROOM ACTIVITIES

- Assign different forms of cancer to each student. Ask the student to research the symptoms, pathology, and course of the disease.

SUGGESTIONS FOR CLINICAL ACTIVITIES

- Assign students to clients with a malignancy.

LEARNING OUTCOME 6

Describe and compare laboratory and diagnostic tests for cancer.

CONCEPTS FOR LECTURE

1. Several procedures and diagnostic tests are used to diagnose cancer.
   - X-ray imaging, computed tomography (CT), ultrasonography, and magnetic resonance imaging (MRI) can locate abnormal tissues or tumors
   - Only microscopic histologic examination of the tissue reveals the type of cell
   - Lab Tests (CBC, ALT, AST, CEA, PSA)
   - Tumor Marker
2. Tissue is recovered for examination by several means: biopsy, shedded cells, collections of secretions, and blood tests.
3. Some investigation shows a communication between chemical mediators and the emotional centers of the brain.

POWERPOINT LECTURE SLIDES

Laboratory and Diagnostic Tests for Cancer
- Grading and staging
- Cytologic examination
- Tumor marker
- Ongoing imaging (X-ray, CT scan, MRI, ultrasonography, nuclear imaging, PET scan)
- Direct visualization (endoscopy, sigmoidoscopy, bronchoscopy)
- Lab tests (CBC, ALT, AST, CEA, PSA)

LEARNING OUTCOME 7

Discuss the role of chemotherapy in cancer treatment and classify chemotherapeutic agents.

CONCEPTS FOR LECTURE

1. Chemotherapy involves the use of cytotoxic medications to cure some cancers, such as leukemias, lymphoma, and some solid tumors. Chemotherapy also may be used in conjunction with biotherapy.
2. Chemotherapy disrupts the cell cycle in various phases of metabolism.
3. Chemotherapeutic agents can be classified either by the effects of the agent on the cell or by the pharmacologic properties of the agent.
   - Alkylating agents: creates defects in the tumor DNA
   - Antimetabolites: phase-specific
   - Antitumor antibiotics: disrupt DNA replication and RNA transcription, create free radicals
   - Mitotic inhibitors: prevent cell division in the M phase
   - Hormones and hormone antagonists: hormones (corticosteroids) alter cellular function and growth

POWERPOINT LECTURE SLIDES

Chemotherapy Roles and Chemotherapeutic Agents
- Chemotherapy roles
  - Involves use of cytotoxic medications
  - May be used in conjunction with biotherapy
  - Disrupts the cell cycle
  - Classified by effect of agent or by pharmacologic properties
- Chemotherapeutic agents
  - *Alkylating agents:* Creates defects in the tumor DNA
  - *Antimetabolites:* Phase-specific
  - *Antitumor antibiotics:* Disrupt DNA replication and RNA transcription, create free radicals
  - *Mitotic inhibitors:* Prevent cell division in the M phase
  - *Hormones and hormone antagonists:* Hormones (corticosteroids) alter cellular function and growth

LEARNING OUTCOME 8

Discuss the role of surgery, radiation therapy, and biotherapy in the treatment of cancer.

CONCEPTS FOR LECTURE

1. Surgery was once considered the only treatment for cancer before the mechanisms of cancer were understood. Today, surgery remains an important approach in cancer care. Surgical resection is used for diagnosis and staging of more than 90% of all cancers and for primary treatment of more than 60% of cancers. The goals of surgery have also expanded to include prophylaxis, diagnosis, treatment, reconstruction, and palliation.
2. Radiation therapy is still the treatment of choice for some tumors or by some oncologists. Radiation may be used to kill the tumor, reduce its size, decrease pain, or relieve obstruction. Lymph nodes and adjacent tissues are irradiated when beginning metastasis is suspected.

POWERPOINT LECTURE SLIDES

Surgery, Radiation Therapy, and Biotherapy in Cancer Treatment
- Surgical interventions
  - *Prophylactic surgery:* Removes tissue for organs that are likely to develop cancer
  - *Diagnostic surgery:* Ensures histologic diagnosis
  - *Primary treatment:* Remove the entire tumor and involved tissue
- Radiation therapy
  - *Teletherapy:* External radiation
  - *Brachytherapy:* Radioactive material is placed directly into or adjacent to the tumor

CONCEPTS FOR LECTURE *continued*

Radiation therapy consists of delivering ionizing radiations of gamma and X-rays in one of two ways: teletherapy or brachytherapy.

3. Biotherapy modifies the biological processes that result in malignant cells primarily through enhancing the person's own immune response. Currently, biotherapy is used for both hematological malignancies, such as lymphoma and hairy cell leukemia, and solid tumors, such as renal cancer and melanoma.

POWERPOINT LECTURE SLIDES *continued*

- Biotherapy
  - Modifies the biologic processes that result in malignant cells

SUGGESTIONS FOR CLASSROOM ACTIVITIES

- Separate the students into groups. Assign the three methods of cancer treatment: surgery, radiation, and chemical therapy. Ask students to present their research to the class.

SUGGESTIONS FOR CLINICAL ACTIVITIES

- Assign students to the operating room, oncology radiation therapy, and chemotherapy centers.

LEARNING OUTCOME 9

Identify causes and discuss the nursing interventions for common oncologic emergencies.

CONCEPTS FOR LECTURE

1. When caring for a family member with cancer, the family is naturally anxious about emergency care. The family should be instructed about what to do in case of an emergency, and how to tell the difference between an emergency and a nonemergent condition.

2. Nurses may encounter a number of emergency situations in caring for a client with cancer. These emergencies require astute observation, accurate judgments, and rapid action once the problem is identified.
   - Malignant pericardial effusion is an accumulation of excess fluid in the pericardial sac that compresses the heart, restricts heart movement, and results in a cardiac tamponade.
   - The superior vena cava can be compressed by mediastinal tumors or adjacent thoracic tumors. The most common cause is small-cell or squamous-cell lung cancers. Occasionally the problem is caused by thrombus around a central venous catheter that then plugs up the vena cava, resulting in obstruction and backup of the blood flowing into the superior vena cava.
   - Clients with intra-abdominal, retroperitoneal, or pelvic malignancies, such as prostate, cervical, or bladder cancers, may experience obstruction of the bladder neck or the ureters.
   - Tumor necrosis, immune deficiency, antineoplastic therapy malnutrition, and comorbid conditions can lead to the development of sepsis.
   - Spinal cord compression is most commonly associated with pressure from expanding tumors of the breast, lung, or prostate; lymphoma; or metastatic disease.

POWERPOINT LECTURE SLIDES

Nursing Interventions for Common Oncologic Emergencies
- Nursing care
  - Assess frequently for signs and symptoms of organ obstruction
  - Provide guidelines to help clients and the family to recognize serious problems
  - Monitor lab values
  - Assess current eating patterns and evaluate degree of malnutrition
  - Assess and evaluate skin for loss of integrity
- Managing oncologic emergencies
  - Pericardial effusions and neoplastic cardiac tamponade
  - Hypotension
  - Tachycardia
  - Tachypnea
  - Cyanosis
  - Increased anxiety and restlessness

- Tumor lysis syndrome (TLS) is a life-threatening emergency for clients with cancer. TLS is characterized by a combination of two or more metabolic abnormalities, including hyperuricemia, hyperphosphatemia, hyperkalemia, and/or hypocalcemia.

SUGGESTIONS FOR CLASSROOM ACTIVITIES

- Discuss the differences between emergent and nonemergent situations that can happen to homecare clients. Develop an emergency plan for the family to follow.

LEARNING OUTCOME 10

Design an appropriate care plan for clients with cancer and their families regarding cancer diagnosis, treatment, and coping strategies.

CONCEPTS FOR LECTURE

1. Nursing care goals should focus on the whole client and everyone involved in the client's support system from initial diagnosis to the end result of the disease process.
2. When performing client or family teaching, involve the client while teaching the family and significant caregivers. Write the teaching plan down for the client and family for quick reference.
3. Many diagnoses are pertinent to clients with cancer; this section addresses only the most common diagnoses.

   Anxiety
   - Assess the client's level of anxiety (moderate, severe, or panic)
   - Establish a therapeutic relationship (warm, empathetic, nonjudgmental)
   - Encourage client to express feelings
   - Review and encourage appropriate coping strategies, discourage inappropriate coping strategies such as repressing anger or alcohol use
   - Identify community resources that can help client manage anxiety (hot lines, support groups)

   Disturbed body image
   - Observe and evaluate interaction with others
   - Encourage verbalization of feelings
   - Assist the client and others in coping with changes in appearance

   Anticipatory grieving
   - A response to a loss that has not occurred yet
   - Answer questions about loss honestly
   - Encourage client to make final arrangements
   - Encourage client to participate in activities he or she enjoys as long as possible

   Risk for infection
   - Encourage client to eat a high protein diet
   - Monitor vital signs
   - Protect skin and mucous membranes

POWERPOINT LECTURE SLIDES

Nursing Diagnosis and Interventions for Clients with Cancer
- Anxiety
  - Assess the client's level of anxiety (moderate, severe, or panic)
  - Establish a therapeutic relationship (warm, empathetic, nonjudgmental)
  - Encourage client to express feelings
  - Review and encourage appropriate coping strategies, discourage inappropriate coping strategies such as repressing anger or alcohol use
  - Identify community resources that can help client manage anxiety (hot lines, support groups)
- Disturbed body image
  - Observe and evaluate interaction with others
  - Encourage verbalization of feelings
  - Assist the client and others in coping with changes in appearance
- Anticipatory grieving
  - A response to a loss that has not occurred yet
  - Answer questions about loss honestly
  - Encourage client to make final arrangements
  - Encourage client to participate in activities he or she enjoys as long as possible
- Risk for infection
  - Encourage client to eat a high protein diet
  - Monitor vital signs
  - Protect skin and mucous membranes
- Risk for injury
  - Assess for signs and symptoms indicating problems with organ obstruction
  - Teach how to differentiate minor from serious problems
  - Monitor laboratory values

Risk for injury
- Assess for signs and symptoms indicating problems with organ obstruction
- Teach how to differentiate minor from serious problems
- Monitor laboratory values

Pain management
- Evaluate level of pain
- Establish a plan of combination of nonnarcotic drugs with other adjunct medications

- Pain management
  - Evaluate level of pain
  - Establish a plan of combination of nonnarcotic drugs with other adjunct medications

SUGGESTIONS FOR CLASSROOM ACTIVITIES

- Create a plan of care for a client who has been diagnosed with cancer and is in the early stages, then modify the plan for the end stage.

SUGGESTIONS FOR CLINICAL ACTIVITIES

- Ask a hospice nurse to speak to the class about care of the end-stage cancer client.

CHAPTER 15
ASSESSING CLIENTS WITH INTEGUMENTARY DISORDERS

RESOURCE LIBRARY

PRENTICE HALL NURSING MEDIALINK DVD-ROM

Audio Glossary
NCLEX-RN® Review

COMPANION WEBSITE

Audio Glossary
NCLEX-RN® Review
Care Plan Activity: Integumentary Disorders
Case Studies
   Assessing a Rash
   Skin Assessment for a Client with a Bacterial Infection
MediaLink Applications
   Moles
   Skin Cancer
Links to Resources

IMAGE LIBRARY

Figure 15.1 Anatomy of the skin.
Figure 15.2 Anatomy of a hair follicle.
Figure 15.3 Anatomy of a nail (frontal and side views).
Figure 15.4 Tenting in an older client.

Figure 15.5 *A*, Degrees of pitting in edema.
B, 4+ pitting.
Figure 15.6 *A*, Assessing clubbing of the nails.
B, Hand with nail clubbing.
Figure 15.7 Spoon-shaped nails.

LEARNING OUTCOME 1

Describe the anatomy, physiology, and functions of the skin, hair, and nails.

CONCEPTS FOR LECTURE

1. The skin is the largest organ in the body and consists of two regions: the epidermis and the dermis.
2. The epidermis is the outermost surface of the skin and consists of epithelial cells.
3. The dermis is the second or deepest layer of the skin.
4. The glands of the skin are sebaceous glands or oil glands, sudoriferous or sweat glands, and ceruminous glands.
   - Sebaceous glands are found all over the body except on the palms and soles. These glands secrete an oily substance called **sebum.** Sebum also protects the body from infection by killing bacteria.
   - Eccrine sweat glands are more numerous on the forehead, palms, and soles. The gland itself is located in the dermis. Sweat, the secretion of the eccrine glands, is composed mostly of water but also contains sodium, antibodies, small amounts of metabolic wastes, lactic acid, and vitamin C.
   - Most apocrine sweat glands are located in the axillary, anal, and genital areas. The secretions from apocrine glands are similar to those of sweat

POWERPOINT LECTURE SLIDES

The Skin
- Anatomy of the skin
  - Epidermis
    - 4–5 layers depending on location
    - Stratum basale (contains cells producing melanin and keratinocytes)
  - Dermis
    - Richly supplied with blood cells, nerve fibers, and lymphatic vessels
    - Most hair follicles, sebaceous glands, and sweat glands located here
- Glands of the skin
  - Sebaceous glands
    - Found all over the body except hands and soles of feet
    - Secrete oily substance called sebum (softens and lubricates skin and hair)
    - Protects the body from infections by killing bacteria

glands, but they also contain fatty acids and proteins. Apocrine glands are a remnant of sexual scent glands.

- Ceruminous glands are modified apocrine sweat glands. Located in the skin of the external ear canal, they secrete yellow-brown waxy cerumen. This substance provides a sticky trap for foreign materials.

5. Hair is distributed over most of the body and has protective functions.
6. Nails, like hair, consist mostly of dead cells and also serves as protection for the distal digits on the fingers and toes.

- ○ Sweat glands
  - – Eccrine: forehead, palms, soles (sweat composed mostly of water)
  - – Apocrine: axillary, anal, and genital areas (sweat composed mostly of water and fatty acids)

SUGGESTIONS FOR CLASSROOM ACTIVITIES

- Review anatomy and physiology of the integumentary system.

LEARNING OUTCOME 2

Discuss factors that influence skin color.

CONCEPTS FOR LECTURE

1. The color of skin is the result of levels of pigmentation. Melanin is darker and produced in greater amounts in persons with dark skin.
2. Carotene, although found in most parts of the body where the stratum corneum is thickest, is also most abundant in the skin of persons of Asian ancestry.
3. Caucasian skin has very little melanin and is almost transparent. The circulating hemoglobin gives the skin a pinkish color.

POWERPOINT LECTURE SLIDES

Factors that Influence Skin Color
- Color is the result of levels of pigmentation
- Melanin is darker and produced in greater amounts in persons of dark skin
- Carotene abundant in the skin of persons of Asian ancestry
- Caucasian skin has very little melanin and is almost transparent
- Circulating hemoglobin gives the skin a pinkish color

SUGGESTIONS FOR CLASSROOM ACTIVITIES

- Have each student bring in a variety of magazine clippings displaying a variety of skin colors. During class time compare the magazine clippings that were brought in.

SUGGESTIONS FOR CLINICAL ACTIVITIES

- Ask each student to share an occurrence when a client's skin color was influenced by emotions and/or illness.

LEARNING OUTCOME 3

Identify specific topics for a health history interview of the client with problems involving the skin, hair, and nails.

CONCEPTS FOR LECTURE

1. The assessment of the integumentary system begins with a health history interview to collect subjective data.
2. The interview should cover every facet of the client's activities of daily living: health perception, nutrition, elimination, activity and exercise, sleep and rest, cognition, self-perception, relationships, sexuality and reproduction, stress tolerance, and values and beliefs. See the Functional Health Pattern Interview in the student textbook.

POWERPOINT LECTURE SLIDES

Specific Topics for the Health History Interview
- Interview should cover
  - ○ Health perception
  - ○ Nutrition
  - ○ Elimination
  - ○ Activity and exercise
  - ○ Sleep and rest
  - ○ Cognition
  - ○ Self-perception

  ○ Relationships
  ○ Sexuality and reproduction
  ○ Stress tolerance
  ○ Values and beliefs

SUGGESTIONS FOR CLASSROOM ACTIVITIES

• Role-play taking a history from a client with a suspicious skin lesion.

LEARNING OUTCOME 4

Explain techniques for assessing the skin, hair, and nails.

CONCEPTS FOR LECTURE

1. Physical assessment of the skin, nails, and hair is conducted by inspection and palpation.
2. The examination should take place in a private area. The client should remove all clothes and put on a gown or use a drape.
3. Examine the hair by noting the color, quality, and any scalp lesions.
4. The nails should be assessed for color, splitting, shape, and contour.
5. Assess the skin for lesions, color, edema, and turgor.
6. Use standard precautions when examining a client's skin.
7. Use a ruler to measure any lesions.

POWERPOINT LECTURE SLIDES

Assessing the Skin, Nails, and Hair
  • Assessing skin problems
    ○ Onset, characteristics, and course
    ○ Severity
    ○ Precipitating and relieving factors
    ○ Timing and circumstances of associated symptoms
  • Assessing hair problems
    ○ Thinning or baldness
    ○ Excessive hair loss
    ○ Change in distribution of hair
    ○ Use of hair-care products
    ○ Diet and dieting
  • Assessing nails
    ○ Nail splitting or breakage
    ○ Discoloration
    ○ Infection
    ○ Diet
    ○ Exposure to chemicals

SUGGESTIONS FOR CLASSROOM ACTIVITIES

• Role-play examining the skin of a client with a rash. Ask questions based on the health history format.

SUGGESTIONS FOR CLINICAL ACTIVITIES

• Ask a dermatologist to speak to the class.

LEARNING OUTCOME 5

Compare and contrast normal and abnormal findings when conducting an assessment of the integumentary system.

CONCEPTS FOR LECTURE

1. The skin should be examined and assessed for both normal and abnormal findings.
2. Inspect skin color and note any odors coming from the skin. Skin should be even, and appropriate for age and race of the client, without foul odors. Inspect the skin for lesions and alterations, including calluses, scars, tattoos, and piercings. Include inspection of skin creases and folds.

POWERPOINT LECTURE SLIDES

Normal Finding for Integumentary System Assessment
  • Skin should be intact without abnormal lesions
  • Palpate skin temperature (skin should be warm)
  • Palpate skin texture (skin should be smooth)
  • Palpate skin moisture (skin should be dry)
  • Palpate skin turgor (skin fold should return rapidly to normal position)
  • Assess for edema (no edema should be present)

- Hair should be evenly distributed for client's gender, be of even texture, and the scalp should be free of lesions
- Nails should not be curved as in clubbing, the surface should be smooth, color even, and the nail should not be excessively thick

SUGGESTIONS FOR CLASSROOM ACTIVITIES

- Separate the class into two groups. Have one group discuss normal integumentary assessment findings and have the other group discuss abnormal integumentary assessment findings. Then have both groups share the information they discussed.

SUGGESTIONS FOR CLINICAL ACTIVITIES

- Have each student practice an integumentary assessment.

LEARNING OUTCOME 6

Describe normal variations in assessment findings for the older client.

CONCEPTS FOR LECTURE

1. Normal changes take place in the skin of older clients. The changes are usually benign.
2. Common Skin Lesions of Older Adults
   - **Skin tags:** Soft brown or flesh-colored benign papules
   - **Keratoses:** Horny growth of keratinocytes, may be seborrheic (benign) or actinic (premalignant)
   - **Lentigines ("liver spots"):** Brown or black benign macule with a defined border
   - **Angiomas (hemangioma):** Benign vascular tumors with dilated blood vessels, found in the middle to upper dermis
   - **Telangiectases:** Single dilated blood vessels, capillaries, or terminal arteries
   - **Venous lakes:** Small, dark blue, slightly raised benign papules
   - **Photoaging:** Wrinkling, mottling, pigmented areas, loss of elasticity, benign or malignant lesions

POWERPOINT LECTURE SLIDES

Common Skin Lesions of Older Adults
- Skin Tags
- Keratosis
- Lentigines (liver spots)
- Angiomas
- Telangiectases
- Venous lakes
- Photoaging

SUGGESTIONS FOR CLASSROOM ACTIVITIES

- Ask the students to do an evaluation of each other's skin. Be observant for moles, irregular shaped moles, and nail irregularities.

LEARNING OUTCOME 7

Identify abnormal findings that may indicate impairment of the integumentary system.

CONCEPTS FOR LECTURE

1. Abnormal findings of the integumentary system may be indicative of other disease processes in other organ systems.
2. Skin lesions are not normal. The following lesions indicate integumentary system impairment: pigmented,

POWERPOINT LECTURE SLIDES

Skin Lesions Indicative of Integumentary Impairment
- Pigmented (freckle, nevus, melanoma)
- Scaly (dermatitis, psoriasis)
- Pustular (acne vulgaris, folliculitis, candidiasis)

scaly, pustular, vesicular, nodular, weepy or crusted, figurate erythema, bullous, pruritic, or ulcerated.

- Vesicular (herpes simplex, herpes zoster, scabies)
- Nodular (warts, basal cell carcinoma, acne)
- Weepy, crusted (acute contact allergic dermatitis, impetigo)
- Figurate erythema (urticaria, cellulitis)
- Bullous (pemphigus, toxic epidermal necrolysis)
- Pruritic (xerosis, scabies, pediculosis)
- Ulcerated (pressure ulcer, skin cancer, herpes simplex)

SUGGESTIONS FOR CLASSROOM ACTIVITIES

- Discuss the treatment for the various integumentary conditions.

SUGGESTIONS FOR CLINICAL ACTIVITIES

- Visit a dermatologist's office and assist in caring for clients with integumentary disorders.

CHAPTER 16
NURSING CARE OF CLIENTS WITH INTEGUMENTARY DISORDERS

RESOURCE LIBRARY

 PRENTICE HALL NURSING MEDIALINK DVD-ROM

Audio Glossary
NCLEX Review
Animation/Video
  Pressure Ulcers

 COMPANION WEBSITE

Audio Glossary
NCLEX-RN® Review
Care Plan Activity: Pressure Ulcers
Case Study: Lesions and Pruritis
MediaLink Applications
Links to Resources

IMAGE LIBRARY

Figure 16.1 Keloids form as a result of deposits of excessive amounts of collagen during scar formation.

Figure 16.2 Nevi (moles) arise from melanocytes and are common in all adults.

Figure 16.3 The characteristic lesions of psoriasis are raised, red, round plaques covered with thick, silvery white scales.

Figure 16.4 The lesions of folliculitis are pustules surrounded by areas of erythema.

Figure 16.5 A furuncle (boil) is a deep, firm, red, painful nodule.

Figure 16.6 Cellulitis is a bacterial infection localized in the dermis and subcutaneous tissue.

Figure 16.7 Tinea pedis (athlete's foot) is a fungal infection that often occurs between the toes.

Figure 16.8 *Candida albicans*, a fungus, causes a skin infection characterized by erythema, pustules, and a typical white substance covering the area.

Figure 16.9 The common wart, caused by a virus, appears as a raised, dome-shaped lesion.

Figure 16.10 Herpes simplex is a viral infection of the skin and mucous membranes.

Figure 16.11 Herpes zoster is a viral infection of a dermatome section of the skin.

Figure 16.12 Dermatitis may be a response to allergens, infections, or chemicals.

Figure 16.13 Atopic dermatitis, or eczema, causes pruritus, resulting in lichenification, erythema, and scaling.

Figure 16.14 Acne vulgaris lesions include comedones, erythematous pustules, and cysts.

Figure 16.15 The effects of long-term sun exposure are illustrated in this epidermal skin lesion, called actinic keratosis.

Figure 16.16 A superficial basal cell cancer is characterized by erythema, ulcerations, and well-defined borders.

Figure 16.17 As a squamous cell cancer grows, it tends to invade surrounding tissue.

Figure 16.18 Malignant melanoma is a serious skin cancer that arises from melanocytes.

Figure 16.19 Clark's levels for staging measure the invasion of a melanoma from the epidermis to the subcutaneous tissue.

Figure 16.20 Skin depth of split-thickness and full-thickness grafts.

Figure 16.21 Alopecia (baldness) may be the result of scarring, disease, or genetic predisposition.

LEARNING OUTCOME 1

Describe the manifestations and nursing care of common skin problems and lesions.

CONCEPTS FOR LECTURE

1. Although considered minor in terms of healthcare, the integumentary system can be the source of a high level of discomfort for the client.
2. Common skin problems include: pruritis, dry skin, benign skin lesions and cysts, keloids, nevi, and angiomas. The client may also develop skin tags and psoriasis.

POWERPOINT LECTURE SLIDES

Common Skin Problems and Lesions
- Pruritis (Itching)
- Dry skin (Xerosis)
- Benign skin lesions and cysts
- Nevi (Moles)
- Angiomas
- Psoriasis (Chronic immune skin disorder)

SUGGESTIONS FOR CLASSROOM ACTIVITIES

- Discuss the cause and treatment of dry skin. What nursing interventions should be considered?
- Discuss the cardinal signs of a melanoma.

SUGGESTIONS FOR CLINICAL ACTIVITIES

- Observe in a dermatologist's office the treatment of skin disorders.

LEARNING OUTCOME 2

Compare and contrast the etiology, pathophysiology, interdisciplinary care, and nursing care of clients with infections and infestations, inflammatory disorders, and malignancies of the skin.

CONCEPTS FOR LECTURE

1. Although skin is usually resistant to infections and infestations, these disorders may result from a break in the skin surface, a virulent agent, or decreased resistance due to a compromised immune system.
2. The most common bacterial infections are caused by gram-positive *S. aureus* and beta hemolytic strep.
3. Bacterial infections of the skin may be primary or secondary. Diagnosis is made by identifying the causative organism.
4. Infestations are found in all socioeconomic classes and groups. The infestation is usually caused by lice or mites.
5. Inflammatory disorders of the skin are treated according to the disease and the causative factor.
6. The skin is a common site for malignant lesions. Causes may be from long-term sun exposure or environmental exposure.
7. Malignant melanomas arise from the melanocytes, and are increasing in incidence every year. This disease is ten times more common in fair-skinned people than in dark-skinned people. Diagnosis is made through biopsy.
8. The primary focus of nursing care is on preventing the spread of infection.
9. Instruct family and visitors to practice hand washing before and after client contact. Assess and teach the signs and symptoms of increasing infection.
10. Fungal infections are usually managed with nonprescription medications. The client should not share towels or wash cloths.
11. Pediculosis and scabies are treated according to the infestation. Nursing care focuses on teaching to prevent further infestation.
12. Nursing care for the client with a viral infection focuses on pain management, disturbed sleep patterns, and risk for infection.
13. Nursing care for nonmelanoma skin cancers involves teaching about prevention and cause of the lesions.
14. Nursing care for the client with malignant melanoma depends on whether the lesion is contained or is widespread with metastasis.

POWERPOINT LECTURE SLIDES

Disorders and Malignancies of the Skin
- Disorders of the skin
  - *Folliculitis:* Caused by *S. aureus*
  - *Furuncles (boils):* Spreads down the hair shaft
  - *Carbuncle:* Group of infected hair follicles
  - *Cellulitis:* Localized infection of the dermis and subcutaneous tissue
  - *Erysipelas:* Caused by group A strep
  - Fungal infections (candidiasis, tinea, ringworm)
  - *Pediculosis:* Caused by lice or mites
  - Viral infection (warts, herpes simplex, herpes zoster)
  - Dermatitis (contact and allergic)
  - Acne
- Malignant skin lesions
  - Premalignant lesions (actinic keratosis)
  - Nonmelanoma skin cancers (basal cell and squamous cell)
  - Malignant melanoma
- Nursing care
  - Prevent spread of infection
  - Family and visitor instruction
  - Teach the signs and symptoms of increasing infection

SUGGESTIONS FOR CLASSROOM ACTIVITIES

- Develop a teaching plan for clients to prevent the spread of infectious lesions.

LEARNING OUTCOME 3

Explain the risk factors for, the pathophysiology of, and nursing interventions to prevent and care for pressure ulcers.

CONCEPTS FOR LECTURE

1. Pressure ulcers are ischemic lesions of the skin caused by external pressure that impairs blood flow by shearing forces or from friction. When pressure is applied to skin over a bony prominence for more than two hours, ischemia and hypoxia can cause irreversible tissue damage.
2. Older adults, persons with limited mobility such as a para- or quadriplegic, are most susceptible to pressure ulcers.
3. For clients at risk for pressure ulcers, the goal is prevention.

POWERPOINT LECTURE SLIDES

Nursing Care for Pressure Ulcers
- Assess risk for impaired skin integrity
- Assess dietary intake
- Maintain client's current level of activity and mobility
- Maintain proper positioning

SUGGESTIONS FOR CLASSROOM ACTIVITIES

- Create a nursing care plan based on an 82-year-old homebound, wheelchair-bound stroke client.

SUGGESTIONS FOR CLINICAL ACTIVITIES

- Demonstrate proper skin care for the mobility-compromised client.

LEARNING OUTCOME 4

Discuss surgical options for excision of neoplasms, reconstruction of facial or body structures, and cosmetic procedures.

CONCEPTS FOR LECTURE

1. Scars, lesions, and wounds often cause embarrassment and alterations in body image. Removal of lesions may leave scars or areas of missing tissue.
2. The two divisions of plastic surgery are cosmetic and reconstructive surgeries. Cosmetic surgery enhances normal features, whereas reconstructive surgery improves the function or appearance of parts of the body damaged by trauma, disease, or birth defects.
3. Cosmetic surgery is also called aesthetic surgery. Some examples of cosmetic procedures are:
   - **Liposuction:** Aspirating fat from subcutaneous tissue
   - **Breast augmentation:** Increasing the size of the breast by implants
   - **Rhinoplasty:** Improve appearance of the nose
   - **Blepharoplasty:** Removes fat from upper and lower eyelid
   - **Rhytidectomy:** Face lift
4. Reconstructive procedures include:
   - **Skin grafts:** Detaching skin from a donor site and placing it on a recipient site
   - **Skin flap:** Tissue whose free end is moved from a donor site to a recipient site, for reconstruction or closure of large wounds

POWERPOINT LECTURE SLIDES

Cosmetic and Reconstructive Procedures
- Cosmetic procedures
  - *Liposuction:* Aspirating fat from subcutaneous tissue
  - *Breast augmentation:* Increasing the size of the breast by implants
  - *Rhinoplasty:* Improve appearance of the nose
  - *Blepharoplasty:* Removes fat from upper and lower eyelid
  - *Rhytidectomy:* Face lift
- Reconstructive procedures
  - *Skin grafts:* Detaching skin from a donor site and placing it on a recipient site
  - *Skin flap:* Tissue whose free end is moved from a donor site to a recipient site, for reconstruction or closure of large wounds

SUGGESTIONS FOR CLASSROOM ACTIVITIES	SUGGESTIONS FOR CLINICAL ACTIVITIES
• Discuss the differences between cosmetic and reconstructive procedures. • Create a care plan for a postoperative client who has had a flap reconstruction.	• Assign students to observe in surgery a reconstructive procedure. • Ask a plastic surgeon to speak to the class about reconstructive or cosmetic surgery.

LEARNING OUTCOME 5

Explain the pathophysiology of selected disorders of the hair and nails.

CONCEPTS FOR LECTURE

1. Disorders of the hair and nails are not serious threats to health, but they may cause embarrassment and a negative body image.
   • Hirsutism, also called hypertrichosis, is the appearance of excessive hair in normal and abnormal areas of the body in women. Hirsutism most often occurs in a male distribution (that is, on the upper lip, chin, abdomen, and chest) in women.
   • Alopecia is loss of hair, or baldness. Alopecia may result from scarring, various systemic diseases, or genetic predisposition.
   • Onycholysis is the separation of the distal nail plate from the nail bed. It occurs most often in the fingernails.
   • A paronychia is an infection of the cuticle of the fingernails or toenails. The disorder often follows a minor trauma and secondary infection with staphylococci, streptococci, or *Candida*.
   • Onychomycosis is a fungal or dermatophyte infection of the nail plate. The nail plate elevates and becomes yellow or white. Psoriasis infections of the nail plate cause the nails to pit.
   • Ingrown toenail (unguis incarnatus) results when the edge of the nail plate grows into the soft tissue of the toe. Pain and infection may occur.
2. Hair growth and patterns vary from person to person, and are determined largely by genetic inheritance.
3. Nail disorders may be due to systemic diseases, trauma, or allergies.

POWERPOINT LECTURE SLIDES

Disorders of the Hair and Nails
   • Hirsutism (hypertrichosis): appearance of excessive hair as a result of an increase in androgen level (testosterone)
   • Alopecia: loss of hair or baldness caused by medication, radiation, trauma
   • Onycholysis: separation of the nail bed caused by many factors
   • Paronychia: infection of the cuticle
   • Onychomycosis: fungal infection
   • Ingrown toenail

SUGGESTIONS FOR CLASSROOM ACTIVITIES

• Discuss the disease process that is common in clients who use nail salons. How can one prevent contracting an infection in a salon?

LEARNING OUTCOME 6

Discuss the effects and nursing implications of medications and treatments used to treat disorders of the integument.

CONCEPTS FOR LECTURE

1. The medication and interdisciplinary treatments for conditions of the integument are dependent upon the specialized disease process.
2. A variety of medications may be prescribed, many of which may be topical. The nursing care plan should involve teaching the proper application of topical medications.

POWERPOINT LECTURE SLIDES

Medications Used to Treat Skin Disorder
- Creams: moisturize the skin
- Ointments: lubricate the skin, retard water loss
- Lotions: moisturize and lubricate
- Anesthetics: relieve itching
- Antibiotics: treat infection
- Corticosteriods: suppress inflammation and relieve itching

SUGGESTIONS FOR CLASSROOM ACTIVITIES

- Discuss the proper method of application of topical medications.

CHAPTER 17
NURSING CARE OF CLIENTS WITH BURNS

RESOURCE LIBRARY

 PRENTICE HALL NURSING MEDIALINK DVD-ROM

Audio Glossary
NCLEX-RN© Review

 COMPANION WEBSITE

Audio Glossary
NCLEX-RN© Review
Care Plan Activities
  A Client Having a Skin Graft
  A Client with Burns
  Inhalation Injury
Case Studies
MediaLink Applications
Links to Resources

📖 IMAGE LIBRARY

Figure 17.1 Burn injury classification according to the depth of the burn.
Figure 17.2 Partial-thickness burn injury.
Figure 17.3 Burn contracture.
Figure 17.4 Full-thickness burn injury.
Figure 17.5 The "rule of nines" is one method for quickly estimating the percentage of TBSA affected by a burn injury.
Figure 17.6 The Lund and Browder burn assessment chart.
Figure 17.7 Effects of a severe burn on major body systems and metabolism.
Figure 17.8 The zones of injury.

Figure 17.9 The client's progression through the healthcare system during the emergent, acute, and rehabilitative stages of burn injury.
Figure 17.10 Escharotomy.
Figure 17.11 Skin grafting procedure.
Figure 17.12 Skin graft for burn injury (autograft).
Figure 17.13 Wound vacuum.
Figure 17.14 Closed method of dressing a burn.
Figure 17.15 The client may wear a custom-made elastic pressure garment for 6 months to a year postgraft.

LEARNING OUTCOME 1

Discuss the types and causative agents of burns.

CONCEPTS FOR LECTURE

1. A burn is an injury that results from exposure to heat, chemical, radiation, or electrical current. Although all four types can lead to generalized tissue damage and multisystem involvement, the causative agents and priority treatment measures are unique to each.
   - Thermal burns result from exposure to dry heat (flames) or moist heat (steam and hot liquids). They are the most common burn injuries and occur most often in children and older adults.
   - Chemical burns are caused by direct skin contact with acids, alkaline agents, or organic compounds. The severity of the chemical burn is related to the type of agent, the concentration of the agent, the mechanism of action, the duration of contact, and the amount of body surface area exposed.

POWERPOINT LECTURE SLIDES

Types and Causative Agents of Burns
- Thermal: open flame, steam, hot liquids
- Chemical: acids, strong alkalis, organic compounds
- Electrical: direct current, alternating current, lightening
- Radiation: solar, x-rays, radioactive agents

- The severity of electrical burns depends on the type and duration of current, and amount of voltage. Entry and exit wounds tend to be small, masking widespread tissue damage underneath the wound.
- Radiation burns are usually associated with sunburn or radiation treatment for cancer. These kinds of burns tend to be superficial, involving only the outermost layers of the epidermis.

2. Burns range in severity from a minor loss of small segments of the outermost layer of skin to a complex injury that involves all body systems.

SUGGESTIONS FOR CLASSROOM ACTIVITIES

- Review the layers of the skin.
- Discuss the types of thermal, chemical, electrical, and radiation burns.

LEARNING OUTCOME 2

Explain burn classification by depth and extent of injury.

CONCEPTS FOR LECTURE

1. Tissue damage from a burn is determined primarily by two factors: depth of burn and the extent of the burn (amount of body surface involved).

2. The depth of a burn injury is determined by the elements of the skin that have been damaged or destroyed. Burn depth results from a combination of the temperature of the burning agent and the length of contact.

3. Burns are classified as either superficial, partial thickness, or full thickness.
   - **Superficial burn** involves only the epidermal layer of the skin. Often results from damage from sunburn, ultraviolet light, minor flash injury (from a sudden ignition or explosion), or mild radiation burn associated with cancer treatment. The skin color ranges from pink to bright red, and there may be slight edema over the burned area.
   - **Partial-thickness burns** may be subdivided into superficial partial-thickness and deep partial-thickness burns. The classification depends on the depth of the burn.
     i. *Superficial partial-thickness burn* involves the entire dermis and the papillae of the dermis.
     ii. *Deep partial-thickness burn* also involves the entire dermis, but extends further into the dermis than a superficial partial-thickness burn.
   - **Full-thickness burn** involves all layers of the skin. It may extend into the subcutaneous fat, connective tissue, muscle, and bone. Full-thickness burns are caused by prolonged contact with flames, steam, chemicals, or high-voltage electric current.

POWERPOINT LECTURE SLIDES

Burn Injuries
- Characteristics of burns by depth
  - Superficial (epidermis): skin may be pink to red and dry
  - Partial thickness (epidermis and dermis): skin bright pink and blisters
  - Full thickness (epidermis, dermis, underlying tissues): skin appears waxy, dry, leathery, charred
- Classification of burn injuries
  - Minor burn injuries
    - Excludes electrical, inhalation, and complicated injuries such as trauma
    - Partial thickness burn of less than 15% of total body surface area
    - Full thickness burn of less than 2% of total body surface
  - Moderate burn injuries
    - Excludes electrical, inhalation, and complicated injuries such as trauma
    - Partial thickness burns of 15–25% of the total body surface
    - Full thickness burns of less than 10% of total body surface
  - Major burn injuries
    - Includes all burns of the hands, face, eyes, ears, feet, and perineum, all electrical injuries, multiple traumas, and all clients that are considered high risk
    - Partial thickness burns of greater than 25% of the total body surface
    - Full thickness burns of 10% or greater of the total body surface area

4. The "rule of nines" is used to estimate the extent of a burn by assigning percentages to different parts of the body.
5. A recognized system for describing a burn injury, developed by the American Burn Association, uses both the extent and depth of burn to classify burns as minor, moderate, or major.
   - Minor burn injuries
     - Excludes electrical, inhalation, and complicated injuries such as trauma
     - Partial thickness burn of less than 15% of total body surface area
     - Full thickness burn of less than 2% of total body surface
   - Moderate burn injuries
     - Excludes electrical, inhalation, and complicated injuries such as trauma
     - Partial thickness burns of 15–25% of the total body surface
     - Full thickness burns of less than 10% of total body surface
   - Major burn injuries
     - Includes all burns of the hands, face, eyes, ears, feet, and perineum, all electrical injuries, multiple traumas, and all clients that are considered high risk
     - Partial thickness burns of greater than 25% of the total body surface
     - Full thickness burns of 10% or greater of the total body surface area

SUGGESTIONS FOR CLASSROOM ACTIVITIES

- Discuss the "rule of nines."

LEARNING OUTCOME 3

Describe the pathophysiology, interdisciplinary care, and nursing care for the client with a minor burn.

CONCEPTS FOR LECTURE

1. Minor burn injuries consist of superficial burns that are not extensive, such as sunburns and scald burns.
   - Sunburns result from exposure to ultraviolet light. Such injuries, which tend to be superficial, are more commonly seen in clients with lighter skin. Because the skin remains intact, the manifestations in most cases are mild and are limited to pain, nausea, vomiting, skin redness, chills, and headache.
   - Minor scald burns result from exposure to moist heat and involve superficial and superficial partial-thickness burns of less than 15% of TBSA. The goals of therapy are to prevent wound contamination and to promote healing.
2. A minor burn injury is usually treated in an outpatient facility. The goal of therapy is to promote wound

POWERPOINT LECTURE SLIDES

Minor Burns
- Sunburn
  - Exposure to ultraviolet light
  - More commonly seen in light skinned clients
- Scald burn
  - Exposure to moist heat
  - Involves superficial and partial thickness
  - Superficial burns of less than 15% of TBSA

healing, eliminate discomfort, maintain mobility, and prevent infection.

Interdisciplinary and nursing care involves administering tetanus toxoid vaccine as necessary, eliminating discomfort, maintaining mobility, and preventing infection.

3. Proper use of sunscreen and limiting sun exposure to the less hazardous hours of the day (before 10 A.M. and after 3 P.M.) can prevent sunburn.

4. The nurse teaches the client with a scald burn to apply antibiotic solutions and light dressings and to maintain adequate nutritional intake. Mild analgesics may be ordered to help the client carry out activities of daily living. Tetanus toxoid is administered as appropriate.

SUGGESTIONS FOR CLASSROOM ACTIVITIES

- Discuss the scenario of an emergency department nurse working in a resort area and caring for clients with severe sunburns.
- Devise a pamphlet that educates the public about the danger of sunburns.

LEARNING OUTCOME 4

Discuss the systemic pathophysiologic effects of a major burn and the stages of burn wound healing.

CONCEPTS FOR LECTURE

1. The pathophysiologic changes that result from major burn injuries involve all body systems. Extensive loss of skin can result in massive infection, fluid and electrolyte imbalances, and hypothermia. Persons who inhale the products of combustion compromise respiratory function.

2. Cardiac dysrhythmias and circulatory failure are common manifestations of serious burn injuries.

3. A profound catabolic state dramatically increases caloric expenditure and nutritional deficiencies.

4. An alteration in gastrointestinal motility predisposes the client to developing paralytic ileus, and hyperacidity leads to gastric and duodenal ulcerations.

5. Dehydration slows glomerular filtration rates and renal clearance of toxic wastes and may lead to acute renal failure.

6. Overall body metabolism is profoundly altered.

7. The basal metabolic rate (BMR) significantly increases, reaching twice the normal rate. Body weight and heat drop dramatically. Total energy expenditure may exceed 100% of normal BMR. Hypermetabolism persists until after wound closure has been accomplished and may reappear if complications occur.

8. Burn wound healing is a slow process that involves the phases of wound healing: inflammation, proliferation, and remodeling. The following physiologic events occur:
   - Inflammation. Following the injury, platelets come in contact with the damaged tissue. Fibrin is deposited,

POWERPOINT LECTURE SLIDES

Pathophysiologic Effects of a Major Burn
- Can involve all body systems
- Extensive loss of skin can result in massive infection, fluid and electrolyte imbalances, and hypothermia
- Cardiac dysrhythmias and circulatory failure
- Profound catabolic state
- Alteration in gastrointestinal motility
- Dehydration
- Overall body metabolism is profoundly altered
- Burn wound healing
  - Inflammation
  - Proliferation
  - Remodeling

trapping further platelets, and a thrombus is formed. The thrombus, combined with local vasoconstriction, leads to hemostasis, which walls off the wound from the systemic circulation. Local vasodilation and an increase in capillary permeability follow hemostasis. Neutrophils infiltrate the wound and peak in about 24 hours, and then monocytes predominate. The monocytes are converted into macrophages, which consume pathogens and dead tissue, and also secrete various growth factors. These growth factors stimulate the proliferation of fibroblasts and a deposit of a provisional wound matrix.

- Proliferation. Within 2 to 3 days postburn, fibroblasts are the major cell within the wound. Their number peaks at about 14 days after the injury. Granulation tissue begins to form, with complete reepithelialization occurring during this stage. Epithelial cells cover the wound as each cell stretches across the wound surface to join with other epithelial cell sheets or the other side of the wound. The proliferation phase lasts until complete reepithelialization occurs, by epithelial cell migration, surgical intervention, or a combination of the two.
- Remodeling. This phase may last for years. Collagen fibers, laid down during the proliferative phase, are reorganized into more compact areas. Scars contract and fade in color. In normal healing following a minor burn injury, the newly formed skin closely resembles its neighboring tissue. However, when a burn injury extends into the dermal layer of skin, two types of excessive scar may develop. A hypertrophic scar is an overgrowth of dermal tissue that remains within the boundaries of the wound. A keloid is a scar that extends beyond the boundaries of the original wound. People with dark skin are at greater risk for hypertrophic scars and keloids.

SUGGESTIONS FOR CLASSROOM ACTIVITIES

- What are the emergent nursing interventions for a client with moderate burns? Severe burns?
- Prepare a nursing care plan for a client with a major burn over his legs and perineum.

SUGGESTIONS FOR CLINICAL ACTIVITIES

- If access to a burn unit or burn patients is available, assign students to provide care to clients.

LEARNING OUTCOME 5

Explain the interdisciplinary care and nursing implications necessary during the emergent/resuscitative stage, the acute stage, and the rehabilitative stage of a major burn.

CONCEPTS FOR LECTURE

1. The burn team consists of the nurse, physician, physical therapist, dietitian, and social worker. The team meets regularly to discuss progress and to determine the most effective regimen of care.

POWERPOINT LECTURE SLIDES

Burn Stages
- Emergent/Resuscitative stage
  - From onset of injury through successful fluid resuscitation

2. The clinical course of treatment for the burn client is divided into three stages: the emergent/resuscitative stage, the acute stage, and the rehabilitive stage.

    - The emergent/resuscitative stage lasts from the onset of injury through successful fluid resuscitation. Healthcare workers estimate the extent of burn injury, institute first-aid measures, and implement fluid resuscitation therapies. The client is assessed for shock and evidence of respiratory distress. If indicated, intravenous lines are inserted, and the client may be prophylactically intubated. Healthcare workers also determine whether the client is to be transported to a burn center for the complex intervention strategies of the professional, interdisciplinary burn team.

    - The acute stage begins with the start of diuresis and ends with closure of the burn wound (either by natural healing or by using skin grafts). During this stage, wound care management, nutritional therapies, and measures to control infectious processes are initiated. Hydrotherapy and excision and grafting of full-thickness wounds are performed as soon as possible after injury. Enteral and parenteral nutritional interventions are started early in the treatment plan to address caloric needs resulting from extensive energy expenditure. Measures to combat infection are implemented during this stage, including the administration of topical and systemic antimicrobial agents. Pain management constitutes a significant segment of the nursing care plan throughout the clinical course of the burn-injured client. The administration of narcotic pharmaceutical agents must precede all invasive procedures to maximize client comfort and to reduce the anxieties associated with wound debridement and intensive physical therapy.

    - The rehabilitative stage begins with wound closure and ends when the client returns to the highest level of health restoration, which may take years. During this stage, the primary focus is the biopsychosocial adjustment of the client, specifically the prevention of contractures and scars and the client's successful resumption of work, family, and social roles through physical, vocational, occupational, and psychosocial rehabilitation. The client is taught to perform range-of-motion exercises to enhance mobility and to support injured joints.

- ○ Healthcare workers estimate extent of burn injury
- ○ Institute first aid measures
- ○ Client may be intubated
- Acute stage
  - ○ Begins with start of diuresis and ends with closure of the wound, either by natural healing or by using skin grafts
- Rehabilitative stage
  - ○ Begins with wound closure and ends when client returns to highest level of health restoration, which may take years

---

SUGGESTIONS FOR CLASSROOM ACTIVITIES

- Create a nursing care plan for all three stages of recovery from a major burn.

SUGGESTIONS FOR CLINICAL ACTIVITIES

- Assign a student to care for a client with a major burn injury.

Chapter 18
Assessing Clients with Endocrine Disorders

Resource Library

PRENTICE HALL NURSING MEDIALINK DVD-ROM

Audio Glossary
NCLEX-RN® Review

COMPANION WEBSITE

Audio Glossary
NCLEX-RN® Review
Care Plan Activity: Type 2 Diabetes
Case Studies
   Assessing a Client for Hypocalcemia
   Endocrine Assessment
MediaLink Application: Endocrine Hormones
Links to Resources

IMAGE LIBRARY

Figure 18.1 Location of the major endocrine glands.
Figure 18.2 Location of the pituitary gland.
Figure 18.3 Actions of the major hormones of the anterior pituitary.
Figure 18.4 The thyroid gland.
Figure 18.5 Location of the adrenal glands.

Figure 18.6 Negative feedback.
Figure 18.7 Examples of three mechanisms of hormone release: *A*, hormonal; *B*, humoral; or *C*, neural.
Figure 18.8 Palpating the thyroid gland from behind the client.

Learning Outcome 1

Describe the anatomy and physiology of the endocrine glands.

Concepts for Lecture

1. The major endocrine organs are the pituitary gland, thyroid gland, parathyroid glands, pancreas, and gonads (reproductive glands).
2. The pituitary gland is located beneath the hypothalamus of the brain and has two parts. The pituitary is referred to as the master gland. The anterior pituitary secretes six hormones; the posterior pituitary secretes ADH and oxytocin.
3. The thyroid gland is anterior to the upper part of the trachea and interior to the larynx. The thyroid has two lobes and is connected by an isthmus. The thyroid secretes thyroid hormone (T4, T3) and calcitonin.
4. The parathyroid glands (4–6) are located in the thyroid gland.
5. Adrenal glands are located on top of the kidneys and are actually two glands, the adrenal medulla and adrenal cortex.
6. The pancreas is located behind the stomach between the spleen and duodenum and secretes thyroid hormone and calcitonin. It is both an endocrine gland and an exocrine gland.
7. The gonads are the testes in males and the ovaries in females. The hormones are important in regulating body growth and the onset of puberty.

PowerPoint Lecture Slides

Endocrine Glands
- Pituitary gland
- Thyroid gland
- Parathyroid glands
- Adrenal glands
- Pancreatic glands
- Reproductive glands

LEARNING OUTCOME 2

Explain the functions of the hormones secreted by the endocrine glands.

CONCEPTS FOR LECTURE

1. Hormones are chemical messengers secreted by the endocrine organs and transported throughout the body, where they exert their action on specific cells called target cells.
2. Hormones do not cause reactions directly but rather regulate tissue responses.
3. Hormones may produce either generalized effects or local effects.
4. Hormones are transported from endocrine gland cells to target cells in the body in one of four ways:
   • Endocrine glands release most hormones, including TH and insulin, into the bloodstream. Some hormones require a protein carrier.
   • Neurons release some hormones, such as epinephrine, into the bloodstream. This is called the neuroendocrine route.
   • The hypothalamus releases its hormones directly to target cells in the posterior pituitary by nerve cell extension.
   • With the paracrine method, released messengers diffuse through the interstitial fluid. This method of transport involves a number of hormonal peptides that are released throughout various organs and cells and act locally. An example is endorphins, which act to relieve pain.
5. Hormones that are released into the bloodstream circulate as either free, unbound molecules or as hormones attached to transport carriers.
6. Hormone receptors are complex molecular structures, located on or inside target cells. They act by binding to specific receptor sites located on the surfaces of the target cells.

POWERPOINT LECTURE SLIDES

Transportation of Hormones
  • Endocrine glands release most hormones into the bloodstream (some require a protein carrier)
  • Neurons release some hormones (epinephrine) into bloodstream (neuroendocrine route)
  • Hypothalamus releases hormones directly to target cells in posterior pituitary by nerve cell extension
  • Paracrine method: released messengers diffuse through interstitial fluid

LEARNING OUTCOME 3

Identify specific topics to consider during a health history interview of the client with health problems involving endocrine function.

CONCEPTS FOR LECTURE

1. The nurse must analyze the onset, characteristics and course, severity, precipitating and relieving factors, and any associated symptoms, and note the timing and circumstances.
2. The family may be able to provide information about changes in behavior and coping mechanisms.
3. Topics Covered in Health History Interview
   - Health perception and management: state of health, endocrine problems, use of drugs, alcohol, smoking, tested for high or low blood sugar
   - Nutritional: diet, fluid intake, weight changes, change in energy level, tolerance to heat and cold, difficulty swallowing, skin texture
   - Elimination: changes in bowel, bladder habits
   - Activity/exercise: describe physical activities, energy level
   - Sleep/rest: how many hours of sleep/night, problems sleeping, night sweats
   - Cognitive/perceptual: memory problems, restlessness, confusion, anxiety, vocal changes, visual changes, heart palpitations, abdominal pain, pain, stiffness in joints and/or muscles, headaches
   - Self-perception/self-concept: feelings about self, medications
   - Role/relationships: family history of endocrine disorders? Does this condition affect your relationship with others?
   - Sexuality/reproductive: affects on sexual activities and any changes that have occurred
   - Coping/stress tolerance: does stress make condition worse? Has condition made stress worse?
   - Value/belief: how do relationships or activities help you cope? How do cultural beliefs or practices affect how you care for yourself? Are there any specific treatments you would not use to treat this condition?

POWERPOINT LECTURE SLIDES

Topics Covered in Health History Interview
- Health perception and management: state of health, endocrine problems, use of drugs, alcohol, smoking
- Nutritional: diet, fluid intake, weight changes, change in energy level
- Elimination: changes in bowel, bladder habits
- Activity/exercise: describe physical activities, energy level
- Sleep/rest: how many hours of sleep/night, problems sleeping, night sweats
- Cognitive/perceptual: memory problems, restlessness, confusion, anxiety, vocal changes, visual changes, heart palpitations, abdominal pain, pain, stiffness in joints
- Self-perception/self-concept: feelings about self, medications
- Role/relationships: family history of endocrine disorders? Does this condition affect your relationship with others?
- Sexuality/reproductive: affects on sexual activities
- Coping/stress tolerance: does stress make condition worse? Has condition made stress worse?
- Value/belief: how do relationships or activities help you cope? How do cultural beliefs or practices affect how you care for yourself? Are there any specific treatments you would not use to treat this condition?

SUGGESTIONS FOR CLASSROOM ACTIVITIES

- Role-play using nursing diagnoses and interventions for selected endocrine disorders.

SUGGESTIONS FOR CLINICAL ACTIVITIES

- Assign students to care for clients with endocrine disorders.

LEARNING OUTCOME 4

Describe techniques for assessing the thyroid gland and the effects of altered endocrine function.

CONCEPTS FOR LECTURE

1. The thyroid gland is the only endocrine gland that can be palpated.
2. When examining the gland, stand behind the client, and palpate the thyroid gland. It should feel smooth and be uniform in size on both sides.

POWERPOINT LECTURE SLIDES

Disorders of the Thyroid Gland
- An enlarged thyroid may indicate Graves' disease or a goiter
- Exophthalmos (protruding eyes) seen in hyperthyroidism

3. A client with hypothyroidism may have the following assessment findings:
   - Rough, dry skin
   - Decreased reflexes
   - Dry, thick, brittle nails and hair
   - Peripheral neuropathy and paresthesias (altered sensations)
4. A client with hyperthyroidism may have the following assessment findings:
   - Smooth and flushed skin
   - Thin, brittle nails and thin, soft hair
   - Exophthalmos (protruding eyes)
   - Restlessness, anxious, disturbed sleep pattern
   - Increased reflexes
5. As a client ages, the parameters of normal lab values change.
   - Pituitary: decreased production of ACTH, TSH, FSH
   - Thyroid: decrease in gland activity
   - Adrenal medulla: increase secretion and level of norepinephrine
   - Pancreas: decreased absorption of fat soluble vitamins delayed and decreased insulin production

- Brittle nails, dry hair, hair loss indicative of hypothyroidism
- Restlessness, anxious, disturbed sleep pattern indicative of hyperthyroidism
- Age-related endocrine changes
  - Pituitary: decreased production of ACTH, TSH, FSH
  - Thyroid: decrease in gland activity
  - Adrenal medulla: increase secretion and level of norepinephrine
  - Pancreas: decreased absorption of fat soluble vitamins delayed and decreased insulin production

SUGGESTIONS FOR CLASSROOM ACTIVITIES

- Discuss clinical signs and symptoms of hypothyroidism and hyperthyroidism.

SUGGESTIONS FOR CLINICAL ACTIVITIES

- Assign students to care for preoperative or postoperative thyroidectomy clients.

LEARNING OUTCOME 5

Describe normal variations in assessment findings for the older adult.

CONCEPTS FOR LECTURE

1. Decreased ability to metabolize glucose with higher and more prolonged blood glucose levels may contribute to increased incidence of type 2 diabetes mellitus with aging (however, higher than normal blood glucose levels are not unusual in nondiabetic older adults).

POWERPOINT LECTURE SLIDES

Normal Variation
- Normal variation in assessment findings for the older adult
- Higher than normal blood glucose levels are not unusual in nondiabetic older adults

SUGGESTIONS FOR CLASSROOM ACTIVITIES

- Identify normal variations in assessment findings for the older adult.

LEARNING OUTCOME 6

Identify abnormal findings that may indicate malfunction of the glands of the endocrine system.

CONCEPTS FOR LECTURE

1. Diagnosis of endocrine disorders is based upon physical, laboratory, and radiologic findings.
2. The results of diagnostic tests of the endocrine system are used to support the diagnosis of a specific disease, to provide information to identify or modify the appropriate medication or therapy used to treat the

POWERPOINT LECTURE SLIDES

Diagnostic Tests to Assess the Structure and Function of the Glands of the Endocrine System
- Growth hormone—deficiency indicates dwarfism and excess indicates gigantism, acromegly
- MRI—identifies tumors of the pituitary and hypothalamus

disease, and to help nurses monitor the client's responses to treatment and nursing care interventions.

3. Diagnostic tests to assess the structure and function of the glands of the endocrine system are as follows:
   - Growth hormone—deficiency indicates dwarfism and excess indicates gigantism, acromegly
   - MRI—identifies tumors of the pituitary and hypothalamus
   - Thyroid stimulating hormone (TSH) differentiates between pituitary and thyroid causes of hypothyroidism
   - Thyronine-T4—aid in diagnosis of thyroid function
   - Triiodothyronine (T3)—compare T3 and T4 to diagnose thyroid disorder
   - T# RU—indirect measure of free thyroxin
   - Thyroid antibodies—identifies thyroid immune disease
   - Thyroid scan—evaluates nodules
   - Parathyroid hormone—identifies hypoparathyroidism or hyperparathyroidism
   - Fasting blood sugar—confirms diagnosis of diabetes mellitus
   - CT scan—identifies pancreatic tumors or cysts

- Thyroid Stimulating Hormone (TSH) differentiates between pituitary and thyroid causes of hypothyroidism
- Thyronine-T4—aid in diagnosis of thyroid function
- Triiodothyronine (T3)—compare T3 and T4 to diagnose thyroid disorder
- T# RU—indirect measure of free thyroxin
- Thyroid antibodies—identifies thyroid immune disease
- Thyroid scan—evaluates nodules
- Parathyroid hormone—identifies hypoparathyroidism or hyperparathyroidism
- Fasting blood sugar—confirms diagnosis of diabetes mellitus
- CT scan—identifies pancreatic tumors or cysts

SUGGESTIONS FOR CLASSROOM ACTIVITIES

- Identify nursing interventions for clients with abnormal laboratory findings.
- Discuss the possible interdisciplinary interventions for a client with thyroid nodules.

CHAPTER 19
NURSING CARE OF CLIENTS WITH ENDOCRINE DISORDERS

RESOURCE LIBRARY

 PRENTICE HALL NURSING MEDIALINK DVD-ROM

Audio Glossary
NCLEX-RN® Review

 COMPANION WEBSITE

Audio Glossary
NCLEX-RN® Review
Care Plan Activity: Cushing's Syndrome
Case Studies
  Compare and Contrast Endocrine Disorders
  Hyperthyroidism
MediaLink Application: Exophthalmos
Links to Resources

IMAGE LIBRARY

Figure 19.1 Exophthalmos in a client with Graves' disease.

Figure 19.2 Toxic multinodular goiter.

LEARNING OUTCOME 1

Apply knowledge of normal anatomy, physiology, and assessments of the thyroid, parathyroid, adrenal, and pituitary glands when providing nursing care for clients with endocrine disorders.

CONCEPTS FOR LECTURE

1. Clients with disorders of the endocrine system require nursing care for multiple problems. They often face exhausting diagnostic tests, changes in physical appearance and emotional responses, and permanent alterations in lifestyle.
2. Nursing care is directed toward meeting physiologic needs, providing education, and ensuring psychologic support for the client and family. A holistic approach to the complex needs of clients with these endocrine disorders is an essential component of nursing care.
3. In the adult, TH changes primarily affect metabolism, cardiovascular function, gastrointestinal function, and neuromuscular function. Thyroid disorders—both hyperthyroidism and hypothyroidism—are among the most common endocrine disorders.
4. Disorders of the parathyroid glands, hyperparathyroidism and hypoparathyroidism, are not as common as those of the thyroid gland.
5. Although disorders of the pituitary cause diverse and serious problems, they are not as common as disorders of other endocrine glands.

POWERPOINT LECTURE SLIDES

Nursing Care for Clients with Endocrine Disorders
- Directed toward
  - Meeting physiologic needs
  - Providing education
  - Ensuring psychologic support for client and family
- Holistic approach is essential

- Have each student research various holistic approaches for a client with an endocrine disorder.

- Have each student review a client's medical record for normal and abnormal assessment findings related to the endocrine system.

LEARNING OUTCOME 2

Compare and contrast the manifestations of disorders that result from hyperfunction and hypofunction of the thyroid, parathyroid, adrenal, and pituitary glands.

CONCEPTS FOR LECTURE

1. Hyperthyroidism (thyrotoxicosis) is the cause for increased metabolism and protein synthesis and affects all tissues in the body.

2. The client with hyperthyroidism may display increased weight loss, although they have an increased appetite, have hypermotile bowels and diarrhea. Other manifestations include heat intolerance, insomnia, palpitations, and increased sweating.

3. Hypothyroidism results when the gland produces insufficient amount of thyroid hormone (TH), which decreases the metabolic rate and also affects all body systems. Hypothyroidism may be primary, which is most common, or secondary. Hypothyroid clients may display decreased appetite, weight gain, dry skin, dyspnea, pallor, hoarseness, and muscle stiffness.

4. Hyperparathyroidism results from an increase in the secretion of parathyroid hormone, which regulates the normal serum level of calcium. The increase affects the kidneys and bones. Pathologic fractures and renal calculi are both symptoms of hyperparathyroidism.

5. Hypoparathyroidism results from abnormally low parathyroid hormone (PTH) levels. The most common cause is damage or removal during thyroid surgery. Reduced levels of PTH result in impaired renal tubular regulation of calcium and phosphate. Low calcium levels change neuromuscular activity, such as tetany, numbness, and tingling and neuromuscular irritability.

6. Disorders of the adrenal glands are the hyperfunction and hypofunction for the adrenal cortex and the hyperfunction of the adrenal medulla. Hypercortisolism (Cushing's syndrome) is a hyperfunction of the adrenal cortex that produces excessive amounts of circulating cortisol (ACTH). Manifestations of Cushing's syndrome are redistribution of body fat, fat pads under the clavicle, and a "buffalo hump." Easy bruising, poor wound healing, and frequent skin infections are also present. The client also has psychological manifestations that range from depression to psychosis.

7. Addison's disease is a disorder that results from destruction or dysfunction of the adrenal cortex. There is a chronic deficiency of cortisol, aldosterone, and adrenal androgens. Manifestations include postural hypotension, syncope, dizziness confusion, and neuromuscular irritability.

8. The client with pheochromocytoma (a tumor of the adrenal medulla) is at risk for paroxysmal hypertension

POWERPOINT LECTURE SLIDES

Hyperfunction and Hypofunction Disorders
- Hyperthyroidism: palpatations, increased sweating, increased appetite, weight loss
- Hypothyroidism: lethargy, weight gain, depression, dry skin
- Hyperparathyroidism: hypertension, psychosis, muscle weakness, renal calculi
- Hypoparathyroidism: tetany, muscle spasms; Arrhythmia: hyperactive reflexes
- Cushing's syndrome: weakness, easily bruised, poor wound healing, glycosuria

due to peripheral vascular constriction and increased cardiac output. Surgical intervention is the treatment of choice.

9. The most common cause of hyperpituitarism is a benign adenoma of the pituitary gland. Gigantism and acromegaly are both manifestations of hyperpituitarism. Conditions that cause hypopituitarism include tumors of the pituitary, surgical removal of the gland, radiation, infection, and trauma. Diabetes insipidus is often seen in clients with this condition.

SUGGESTIONS FOR CLASSROOM ACTIVITIES

- Discuss the symptoms of hyperthyroidism and hypothyroidism. Develop a nursing care plan for each of these clients.

SUGGESTIONS FOR CLINICAL ACTIVITIES

- Assign students to care for a client with parathyroid disease.

LEARNING OUTCOME 3

Explain the nursing implications for medications prescribed to treat disorders of the thyroid and adrenal glands.

CONCEPTS FOR LECTURE

1. Medications used to treat hyperthyroidism include iodine (SSKI, Lugol's solution, Thyro-Block, and Pima), which inhibits thyroid hormone (TH) synthesis and release. These medications are used only for short-term treatment.

2. The nurse should assess for hypersensitivity or allergy to iodine or shellfish prior to giving medication.

3. Antithyroid drugs include methimazole (Tapazole) and propylthiouracil (PTU, Propyl-thyracil), which inhibit TH production.

4. Nursing responsibilities for drugs that inhibit TH include monitoring for side effects such as pruritis rash, elevated temperature, anorexia, loss of taste, and menstrual changes. Also monitor for fatigue and weight gain.

5. Medications used in the treatment of hypothyroidism include Levothyroxine sodium (Synthroid), Liothyronine sodium (Cytomel), Levothyroxine sodium (Levothroid), and Liotrix (Euthroid).

6. Nursing responsibilities for medications that increase blood levels of TH include giving medication 1 hour prior to eating or at least 2 hours after eating. Thyroid medications potentiate the effect of anticoagulant drugs. Monitor client for minor bruising, bleeding gums, and blood in the urine. Also monitor the client for coronary insufficiency, chest pain, dyspnea, and tachycardia.

7. Long-term medication therapy for hyperparathyroidism involves medications such as alendronate (Fosamax) and zoledronate (Zometa) inhibit bone resorption. Nursing implications include educating the client to avoid over-the-counter (OTC) medications with calcium, drink fluids, and to remain active.

POWERPOINT LECTURE SLIDES

Nursing Implications for Selected Endocrine Medications
- Hyperthyroidism medications: assess for hypersensitivity to iodine or shellfish prior to giving medication
- Antithyroid drugs: monitor for side effects such as pruritis rash, elevated temperature, anorexia, loss of taste, menstrual changes, fatigue, and weight gain
- Hypothyroidism treatments
  - Administer 1 hour prior to eating or at least 2 hours after eating
  - Monitor for minor bruising, bleeding gums, and blood in the urine
  - Monitor for coronary insufficiency, chest pain, dyspnea, and tachycardia
- Hyperparathyroidism therapy: education to avoid OTC medications with calcium, drink fluids, and remain active

---

8. Medication therapy for hypoparathyroidism includes increased dietary calcium, supplemental calcium, and vitamin D therapy.
9. Drugs used for the treatment of Cushing's syndrome are mitotane (Lysodren), which suppresses activity of the adrenal cortex; aminogluthemide (Cytadren) and ketoconazole (Nizoral) which inhibit cortisol synthesis; and somatostatin, which suppresses ACTH.
10. The primary treatment for Addison's disease is cortisol replacement. Nursing implications are the same as those for clients who receive cortisol replacement therapy.

SUGGESTIONS FOR CLASSROOM ACTIVITIES

- Ask students to create drug cards for the most frequently prescribed endocrine medications.
- Develop nursing care plans for clients with selected endocrine disorders.

SUGGESTIONS FOR CLINICAL ACTIVITIES

- Have each student review a client's medical record and locate medications prescribed to treat disorders of the thyroid and adrenal glands.

LEARNING OUTCOME 4

Provide appropriate nursing care for the client before and after a subtotal thyroidectomy and an adrenalectomy.

CONCEPTS FOR LECTURE

1. Antithyroid medications must be administered prior to surgery to decrease the vascularity of the gland, thereby reducing the chance of hemorrhage.
2. Client teaching should include supporting the neck postoperatively to increase comfort and to decrease straining of the suture line.
3. Teach the client effective coughing and deep breathing exercises.
4. Reassure the client about the scar, and encourage client to verbalize any concerns or questions.
5. Postoperative care includes providing comfort measures, assessing pain, and placing the client in the semi-Fowler's position.
6. Assess the client for complications, such as hemorrhage, respiratory distress, laryngeal nerve damage, and tetany. The tracheotomy tray should be at the bedside in case an emergency tracheotomy must be performed.
7. Nursing care for the preoperative client who is having an adrenalectomy should include a dietary consultation because of the catabolism that is caused by glucocorticoid excess.
8. Use careful medical and surgical asepsis due to the increased risk of infection.
9. Teach the client to turn, cough, and deep-breathe.
10. Postoperative care includes taking and recording vital signs, and monitoring intake and output, especially during the first 48 hours. Addisonian crisis and hypovolemic shock may occur.

POWERPOINT LECTURE SLIDES

Nursing Care
- Client teaching to support the neck postoperatively, to increase comfort and to decrease straining of the suture line
- Teaching effective coughing and deep breathing exercises
- Reassurance concerning the scar
- Encourage verbalization of concerns
- Postoperative care
  - Comfort measures
  - Assess pain
  - Client in the semi-Fowler's position
- Assess the client for complications
- Use medical and surgical asepsis
- Adrenalectomy preoperative care includes a dietary consultation
- Adrenalectomy postoperative care includes vital signs, monitoring intake and output

SUGGESTIONS FOR CLASSROOM ACTIVITIES	SUGGESTIONS FOR CLINICAL ACTIVITIES
• Develop care plans for both pre- and postoperative clients for adrenalectomy and subtotal thyroidectomy. Include nursing interventions and nursing diagnosis.	• Assign students to clients that have had a surgical intervention for an adrenalectomy and subtotal thyroidectomy.

LEARNING OUTCOME 5

Use the nursing process as a framework for providing individualized care to clients with disorders of the thyroid, parathyroid, adrenal, and pituitary glands.

CONCEPTS FOR LECTURE

1. Clients with disorders of the endocrine glands require nursing care for multiple problems.
2. Nursing care should be directed toward meeting physiological needs, providing education, and ensuring psychological support for the client and family.
3. Assessment should include a health history, physical assessment, and diagnostic testing.
4. Nursing diagnoses should include assessment of fluid volume deficit, anxiety, risk for injury, risk for infection, and body image disturbance.
5. Nursing Process and Frameworks of Care
   • Thyroid: hyperthyroid or hypothyroid goal is euthyroid function
   • Parathyroid
     ○ Hyperfunction: observe for renal calculi, muscle weakness, and polyuria
     ○ Hypofunction: observe for tetany, low serum calcium levels
   • Adrenal Gland
     ○ Cushing's syndrome: observe for pathologic fractures, hypertension, emotional disturbances
     ○ Addison's disease: observe for postural hypotension, syncope, Addisonian crisis
   • Anterior Pituitary Gland: observe for hypertension, voice changes, tongue enlargement, indicating acromegaly
   • Diabetes insipidus is manifested by polydipsia and polyuria
   • Posterior Pituitary: observe for signs of SIADH, which can occur as a result of water retention

POWERPOINT LECTURE SLIDES

Nursing Process and Frameworks of Care
   • Thyroid: hyperthyroid or hypothyroid goal is euthyroid function
   • Parathyroid
     ○ Hyperfunction: observe for renal calculi, muscle weakness, and polyuria
     ○ Hypofunction: observe for tetany, low serum calcium levels
   • Adrenal gland
     ○ Cushing's syndrome: observe for pathologic fractures, hypertension, emotional disturbances
     ○ Addison's disease: observe for postural hypotension, syncope, Addisonian crisis
   • Anterior pituitary gland: observe for hypertension, voice changes, tongue enlargement, indicating acromegaly
   • Diabetes insipidus is manifested by polydipsia and polyuria
   • Posterior pituitary: observe for signs of SIADH, which can occur as a result of water retention

SUGGESTIONS FOR CLASSROOM ACTIVITIES	SUGGESTIONS FOR CLINICAL ACTIVITIES
• Discuss the pathophysiology of syndrome of inappropriate ADH secretion (SIADH).	• Assign students to clients who are diagnosed with the endocrine disorders discussed in this chapter.

CHAPTER 20
NURSING CARE OF CLIENTS WITH DIABETES MELLITUS

RESOURCE LIBRARY

 PRENTICE HALL NURSING MEDIALINK DVD-ROM

Audio Glossary
NCLEX-RN© Review
Animations
  Diabetes Mellitus
  Glipizide

 COMPANION WEBSITE

Audio Glossary
NCLEX-RN© Review
Care Plan Activity: Diabetes Mellitus Type 2
Case Studies
  Compare and Contrast SIADH and DI
  Diabetes Mellitus Type 1
MediaLink Applications
  Diabetes and Nutrition
  Diabetes Foot Care
  Diabetic Neuropathy
Links to Resources

IMAGE LIBRARY

Figure 20.1 Regulation (homeostasis) of blood glucose levels by insulin and glucagon.

Figure 20.2 Pathophysiologic results of type 1 DM.

Figure 20.3 Determination of blood glucose levels by visual reading.

Figure 20.4 Sites of insulin injection.

Figure 20.5 In Type I diabetes mellitus, without adequate insulin, muscle (a) and fat (b) cells are

metabolized to provide sources of energy. Increased glucose (c) causes osmotic diuresis leading to dehydration and decreased circulatory volume.

Figure 20.6 Ulceration following trauma in the foot of the person with diabetes.

LEARNING OUTCOME 1

Apply knowledge of normal endocrine anatomy, physiology, and assessments when providing nursing care for clients with diabetes mellitus.

CONCEPTS FOR LECTURE

1. Diabetes mellitus (DM) is not a single disorder but a group of chronic disorders of the endocrine pancreas, all categorized under a broad diagnostic label. The condition is characterized by inappropriate hyperglycemia caused by a relative or absolute deficiency of insulin or by a cellular resistance to the action of insulin. Of the several classifications of diabetes, this chapter focuses on the two major types, type 1 and type 2. Type 1 DM is the result of pancreatic islet cell destruction and a total deficit of circulating insulin; type 2 DM results from insulin resistance with a defect in compensatory insulin secretion.

2. Clients with DM face lifelong changes in lifestyle and health status. Nursing care is provided in many settings for the diagnosis and care of the disease and treatment of complications. A major role of the nurse is that of educator in both hospital and community settings.

POWERPOINT LECTURE SLIDES

Nursing Care for DM
  • Clients face lifelong changes in lifestyle and health status
  • Major role of the nurse is that of educator in both hospital and community settings
  • Plan of care and content differ according to the type of diabetes
  • Nursing care focuses on teaching to manage the illness

3. Assessments, planning, and implementation differ for the person with newly-diagnosed diabetes, the person with long-term diabetes, and the person with acute complications of diabetes. The plan of care and content of teaching also differ according to the type of diabetes, the person's age and culture, and the person's intellectual, psychological, and social resources. However, nursing care often focuses on teaching the client to manage the illness.

4. The endocrine pancreas produces hormones necessary for the metabolism and cellular utilization of carbohydrates, proteins, and fats. The cells that produce these hormones are clustered in groups of cells called the islets of Langerhans. These islets have three different types of cells:
   - Alpha cells produce the hormone glucagon, which stimulates the breakdown of glycogen in the liver, the formation of carbohydrates in the liver, and the breakdown of lipids in both the liver and adipose tissue.
   - Beta cells secrete the hormone insulin, which facilitates the movement of glucose across cell membranes into cells, decreasing blood glucose levels.
   - Delta cells produce somatostatin, which is believed to be a eurotransmitter that inhibits the production of both glucagon and insulin.

5. All body tissues and organs require a constant supply of glucose; however, not all tissues require insulin for glucose uptake. The brain, liver, intestines, and renal tubules do not require insulin to transfer glucose into their cells. Skeletal muscle, cardiac muscle, and adipose tissue do require insulin for glucose movement into the cells.

6. Normal blood glucose is maintained in healthy people primarily through the actions of insulin and glucagon.

Suggestions for Classroom Activities

- Review anatomy and physiology of the pancreas in relationship to insulin production.

Learning Outcome 2

Describe the prevalence and incidence of diabetes mellitus.

Concepts for Lecture

1. Diabetes mellitus is a common chronic disease that requires continuing medical supervision and education.
2. Approximately 1.3 million new cases of DM are diagnosed each year in the United States. This chronic illness affects an estimated 18.2 million people; of that number, 13 million have been diagnosed and an estimated 5.2 million are undiagnosed.

PowerPoint Lecture Slides

Prevalence and Incidence of DM
- Approximately 1.3 million new cases of DM are diagnosed each year in the United States. This chronic illness affects an estimated 18.2 million people; of that number, 13 million have been diagnosed and an estimated 5.2 million are undiagnosed

3. Diabetes is a group of chronic disorders that result from insulin deficiency or a cellular resistance to the action of insulin.
4. Diabetes is the most frequent cause of nontraumatic amputations with an estimated 82,000 amputations in 2002 in people with diabetes.
5. The cost of illness and resulting loss of productivity for people with diabetes exceeds $132 billion per year, according to an estimate by the American Diabetes Association in 2002.
6. Diabetes is the sixth leading cause of death by disease in the United States.
7. 8.7% of all non-Hispanic whites aged 20 years or older have diabetes.
8. Millions of all non-Hispanic African Americans have diabetes, and those with type 2 diabetes have a higher rate of coronary heart disease, CVA, and end stage renal disease.
9. 2.5 million Hispanic/Latino Americans have diabetes and are 1.7 times as likely to have diabetes as non-Hispanic whites of similar age.
10. American Indians and Alaska Natives are 2.2 times more likely to have diabetes than non-Hispanic whites.

- Diabetes is the sixth leading cause of death by disease in the United States.
- 8.7% of all non-Hispanic whites aged 20 years or older have diabetes
  - Millions of all non-Hispanic African Americans have diabetes, and those with type 2 diabetes have a higher rate of coronary heart disease, CVA, and end stage renal disease
- 2.5 million Hispanic/Latino Americans have diabetes and are 1.7 times as likely to have diabetes as non-Hispanic whites of similar age
- American Indians and Alaska Natives are 2.2 times more likely to have diabetes than non-Hispanic whites

SUGGESTIONS FOR CLASSROOM ACTIVITIES

- Discuss the ethnic and socioeconomic implications of diabetes mellitus.
- Research new methods of treating diabetes mellitus.

SUGGESTIONS FOR CLINICAL ACTIVITIES

- Have each student determine if their client falls within one of the prevalences or incidents mentioned above.

LEARNING OUTCOME 3

Explain the pathophysiology, risk factors, manifestations, and complications of type 1 and type 2 diabetes mellitus.

CONCEPTS FOR LECTURE

1. DM is a group of metabolic diseases characterized by hyperglycemia resulting from defects in the secretion of insulin, the action of insulin, or both.
2. Type 1 diabetes was formerly called juvenile-onset, or insulin-dependent diabetes mellitus (IDDM).
3. Type 2 diabetes (90–95% of diagnosed cases) was formerly known as non-insulin-dependent diabetes mellitus (NIDDM).
4. Type 1 diabetes often occurs in childhood and adolescence and is characterized by hyperglycemia and the development of ketosis.
5. Risk factors for type 1 diabetes are genetic predisposition, and environmental factors such as exposure to viruses or chemical toxins in smoked meat.
6. Manifestations of type 1 diabetes are hyperglycemia and polyuria, polydipsia, and polyphagia.
7. Type 2 diabetes can occur at any age, but occurs most often in middle-age and older people.

POWERPOINT LECTURE SLIDES

Type 1 and Type 2 Diabetes
- Type 1
  - Occurs in childhood/adolescence
  - Genetic predisposition
  - Hyperglycemia
  - Polyuria, polyphagia, glucosuria, polydipsia
- Type 2
  - Occurs at any age
  - Heredity plays a role
  - Slow onset
  - Symptoms not as severe as type 1

8. Heredity is a factor in type 2, along with obesity, inactivity, hypertension, and hypercholesteremia.
9. Manifestations include hyperglycemia, although not as severe as in type 1. Polyphagia and weight loss are not often seen.
10. Complications of type 1 diabetes include cerebrovascular accident (CVA), coronary heart disease, neuropathies, slow wound healing, and retinopathies.

SUGGESTIONS FOR CLASSROOM ACTIVITIES

• Compare and contrast type 1 and type 2 diabetes.

SUGGESTIONS FOR CLINICAL ACTIVITIES

• Assign students to clients who have been diagnosed with diabetes mellitus.

LEARNING OUTCOME 4

Compare and contrast the manifestations and interdisciplinary care of hypoglycemia, diabetic ketoacidosis, and hyperosmolar hyperglycemic state.

CONCEPTS FOR LECTURE

1. Diabetic ketoacidosis (DKA) develops when there is an absolute deficiency of insulin and an increase in the insulin counterregulatory hormones.
2. Manifestations of diabetic ketoacidosis: Dehydration (from hyperglycemia)
   • Thirst
   • Weakness
   • Warm, dry skin with poor turgor
   • Malaise
   • Soft eyeballs
   • Rapid, weak pulse
   • Dry mucous membranes
   • Hypotension
   Metabolic acidosis (from ketosis)
   • Nausea and vomiting
   • Lethargy
   • Ketone (fruity, alcohol-like) breath odor
   • Coma
   Other manifestations
   • Abdominal pain (cause unknown)
   • Kussmaul's respirations (increased rate and depth of respirations, with a longer expiration; a compensatory response to prevent a further decrease in pH)
3. Hyperosmolar hyperglycemic state (HHS) occurs in clients who have type 2 diabetes and is characterized by a plasma osmolarity of 340 mOsm/L or greater, and blood glucose levels of over 600 mg/dL, which causes altered levels of consciousness.
4. Hypoglycemia usually occurs in clients with type 1 diabetes, although it may also occur in clients with type 2 diabetes.

POWERPOINT LECTURE SLIDES

Manifestations of Diabetic Ketoacidosis
• Dehydration (from hyperglycemia)
   ○ Thirst
   ○ Weakness
   ○ Warm, dry skin with poor turgor
   ○ Malaise
   ○ Soft eyeballs
   ○ Rapid, weak pulse
   ○ Dry mucous membranes
   ○ Hypotension
• Metabolic acidosis (from ketosis)
   ○ Nausea and vomiting
   ○ Lethargy
   ○ Ketone (fruity, alcohol-like) breath odor
   ○ Coma
• Other manifestations
   ○ Abdominal pain (cause unknown)
   ○ Kussmaul's respirations (increased rate and depth of respirations, with a longer expiration; a compensatory response to prevent a further decrease in pH)

Manifestations of Hyperosmolar Hyperglycemic State (HHS)
• Occurs in clients who have type 2 diabetes and is characterized by a plasma osmolarity of 340 mOsm/L or greater, and blood glucose levels of over 600 mg/dL, which causes altered levels of consciousness

5. Manifestations of hypoglycemia:
   - Manifestations caused by responses of the autonomic nervous system
     - Hunger
     - Shakiness
     - Nausea
     - Irritability
     - Anxiety
     - Rapid pulse
     - Pale, cool skin
     - Hypotension
     - Sweating
   - Manifestations caused by impaired cerebral function
     - Strange or unusual feelings
     - Slurred speech
     - Blurred vision
     - Headache
     - Decreasing levels of consciousness
     - Difficulty in thinking
     - Inability to concentrate
     - Seizures
     - Change in emotional behavior
     - Coma
6. Treatment of the client with diabetes focuses on maintaining blood glucose at levels as nearly normal as possible through medications, dietary management, and exercise.
7. Definitions of normal blood glucose levels vary in clinical practice, depending on the laboratory that performs the assay.
8. The pharmacologic treatment for diabetes mellitus depends on the type of diabetes.
9. The management of diabetes requires a careful balance between the intake of nutrients, the expenditure of energy, and the dose and timing of insulin or oral antidiabetic agents. Although everyone has the same need for basic nutrition, the person with diabetes must eat a more structured diet to prevent hyperglycemia. The goals for dietary management for adults with diabetes, based on guidelines established by the ADA.
10. People with diabetes should consult their primary healthcare provider before beginning or changing an exercise program. The ability to maintain an exercise program is affected by many different factors, including fatigue and glucose levels. It is as important to assess the person's usual lifestyle before establishing an exercise program as it is before planning a diet.

Manifestations of Hypoglycemia
- Manifestations of Hypoglycemia caused by responses of the autonomic nervous system
  - Hunger
  - Shakiness
  - Nausea
  - Irritability
  - Anxiety
  - Rapid pulse
  - Pale, cool skin
  - Hypotension
  - Sweating
- Manifestations caused by impaired cerebral function
  - Strange or unusual feelings
  - Slurred speech
  - Blurred vision
  - Headache
  - Decreasing levels of consciousness
  - Difficulty in thinking
  - Inability to concentrate
  - Seizures
  - Change in emotional behavior
  - Coma
- Interdisciplinary care
  - Maintaining blood glucose
  - Definitions of normal blood glucose levels vary in clinical practice, depending on the laboratory that performs the assay
  - Pharmacologic treatment for diabetes mellitus depends on the type of diabetes
  - Dietary management for adults with diabetes, based on guidelines established by the ADA.
  - The ability to maintain an exercise program is affected by many different factors

---

SUGGESTIONS FOR CLASSROOM ACTIVITIES

- Develop a nursing care plan for clients who are noncompliant. Include nursing diagnoses and nursing implications.

SUGGESTIONS FOR CLINICAL ACTIVITIES

- Assign students to care for clients with uncontrolled diabetes mellitus.

TABLE 20–5 DKA, HHS, and Hypoglycemia Comparison

		DKA	HHS	HYPOGLYCEMIA
Diabetes Type		Primary type 1	Type 2	Both
Onset		Slow	Slow	Rapid
Cause		↓ Insulin	↓ Insulin	↑ Insulin
		Infection	Older age	Omitted meal/snack
				Error in insulin dose
Risk Factors		Surgery	Surgery	Surgery
		Trauma	Trauma	Trauma
		Illness	Illness	Illness
		Omitted insulin	Dehydration	Exercise
		Stress	Medications	Medications
			Dialysis	Lipodystrophy
			Hyperalimentation	Renal failure
				Alcohol intake
Assessments	Skin	Flushed; dry; warm	Flushed; dry; warm	Pallor; moist; cool
	Perspiration	None	None	Profuse
	Thirst	Increased	Increased	Normal
	Breath	Fruity	Normal	Normal
	Vital signs	BP ↓	BP ↓	BP ↓
		P ↑	P ↑	P ↑
		R Kussmaul's	R normal	R normal
	Mental status	Confused	Lethargic	Anxious; restless
	Thirst	Increased	Increased	Normal
	Fluid intake	Increased	Increased	Normal
	Gastrointestinal effects	Nausea/vomiting; abdominal pain	Nausea/vomiting; abdominal pain	Hunger
	Fluid loss	Moderate	Profound	Normal
	Level of consciousness	Decreasing	Decreasing	Decreasing
	Energy level	Weak	Weak	Fatigue
	Other	Weight loss	Weight loss	Headache
		Blurred vision	Malaise	Altered vision
			Extreme thirst	Mood changes
			Seizures	Seizures
Laboratory Findings	Blood glucose	>300 mg/dL	>600 mg/dL	<50 mg/dL
	Plasma ketones	Increased	Normal	Normal
	Urine glucose	Increased	Increased	Normal
	Urine ketones	Increased	Normal	Normal
	Serum potassium	Abnormal	Abnormal	Normal
	Serum sodium	Abnormal	Abnormal	Normal
	Serum chloride	Abnormal	Abnormal	Normal
	Plasma pH	<7.3	Normal	Normal
	Osmolality	>340 mOsm/L	>340 mOsm/L	Normal
Treatment		Insulin	Insulin	Glucagon
		Treatment	Intravenous fluids	Rapid-acting carbohydrate
		Intravenous fluids	Electrolytes	Intravenous solution of 50% glucose
		Electrolytes		

LEARNING OUTCOME 5

Identify the diagnostic tests used for screening, diagnosis, and monitoring of diabetes mellitus.

CONCEPTS FOR LECTURE

1. Client should show symptoms of diabetes prior to testing.
2. Tests used for screening purposes include casual plasma glucose (PG) level, fasting plasma glucose (FPG), and 2 hour PG during an oral glucose tolerance test (OGTT).
3. Casual plasma glucose (PG): (>200 mg/dL) any time of day without regard to time since the last meal.
4. Fasting plasma glucose (FPG): (>126 mg/dL) no caloric intake in 8 hours.
5. Two-hour PG: (>200mg/dL) during an oral glucose tolerance test.
6. Each test must be confirmed on a following day using subsequent testing.
7. The following tests are used to measure diabetes management: FBG (fasting blood glucose), A1C (glycosylated hemoglobin (c), and urine glucose and ketone levels. Urine tests, serum cholesterol, and serum electrolytes are also used to assess diabetes management.
   - Fasting blood glucose (FBG). This test is often ordered, especially if the client is experiencing symptoms of hypoglycemia or hyperglycemia. In most people, the normal range is 70 to 110 mg/dL.
   - Glycosylated hemoglobin (c) (A1c). This test determines the average blood glucose level over approximately the previous 2 to 3 months. When glucose is elevated or control of glucose is erratic, glucose attaches to the hemoglobin molecule and remains attached for the life of the hemoglobin, which is about 120 days. The normal level depends on the type of assay done, but values above 7% to 9% are considered elevated. The ADA recommends that A1c be performed at the initial assessment, and then at regular intervals, individualized to the medical regimen used.
   - Urine glucose and ketone levels. These are not as accurate in monitoring changes in blood glucose as blood levels. The presence of glucose in the urine indicates hyperglycemia. Most people have a renal threshold for glucose of 180 mg/dL; that is, when the blood glucose exceeds 180 mg/dL, glucose is not reabsorbed by the kidney and spills over into the urine. This number varies highly, however. Ketonuria (the presence of ketones in the urine) occurs with the breakdown of fats and is an indicator of DKA; however, fat breakdown and ketonuria also occur in states of less than normal nutrition.
   - Urine test for the presence of protein as albumin (albuminuria). If albuminuria is present, a 24-hour urine test for creatinine clearance is used to detect the early onset of nephropathy.

POWERPOINT LECTURE SLIDES

DM Screening and Monitoring Tests
- DM Screening tests
  ○ Casual plasma glucose (PG): (>200 mg/dL) any time of day without regard to time since the last meal
  ○ Fasting plasma glucose (FPG): (>126 mg/dL) no caloric intake in 8 hours
  ○ Two-hour PG: (>200mg/dL) during an oral glucose tolerance test
- Management of diabetes
  ○ Fasting blood glucose (FBG): normal range 70–110 mg/dL
  ○ Glycosylated hemoglobin: used to determine the average glucose level over 2–3 months, values above 7%–9% considered elevated
  ○ Urine glucose and ketone levels: not as accurate as monitoring changes in blood glucose levels
  ○ Urine test: indicates presence of protein as albumin
  ○ Serum cholesterol and triglyceride levels: indicators of arthrosclerosis and increased cardiovascular impairment
  ○ Serum electrolytes: measure in clients who have DKA or HHS to determine imbalances

- Serum cholesterol and triglyceride levels. These are indicators of atherosclerosis and an increased risk of cardiovascular impairments. The ADA (2005) recommends treatment goals to lower LDL cholesterol to <100 mg/dL, raise HDL cholesterol to >45 mg/dL, and lower triglycerides to <150 mg/dL.
- Serum electrolytes. Levels are measured in clients who have DKA or hyperosmolar hyperglycemic state (HHS) to determine imbalances.

SUGGESTIONS FOR CLASSROOM ACTIVITIES

- Discuss the lab tests that are ordered to diagnose diabetes mellitus.

SUGGESTIONS FOR CLINICAL ACTIVITIES

- Review charts of clients who are diabetic. Note lab values.

LEARNING OUTCOME 6

Discuss the nursing implications for insulin and oral hypoglycemic agents used to treat clients with diabetes mellitus.

CONCEPTS FOR LECTURE

1. Insulin is used to treat clients with type 1 diabetes mellitus and is administered parenterally.
2. Oral hypoglycemics are used in the treatment of type 2 diabetes and are oral preparations.
3. Diabetic teaching and education is a very important component of medication management and will be discussed in depth in the next learning outcome.
4. Nursing implications for the insulin-dependent client include assessment of therapeutic response to the medication, teaching diet and exercise, and monitoring blood glucose levels. The nurse should also assess for signs of hypoglycemia or DKA.
5. Nursing implications for the clients using oral hypoglycemics includes assessing the client for therapeutic response to the medication, especially in the first seven days. Assess the client for signs of hypoglycemia or hyperglycemia.

POWERPOINT LECTURE SLIDES

Insulin and Oral Hypoglycemic Agents
- Insulin
  - Monitor storage and expiration of insulin
  - Monitor and maintain a record of blood glucose readings as prescribed
  - Monitor food intake
- Oral hypoglycemics
  - Administer with food
  - Assess diet and exercise
  - Monitor for hypoglycemia and hyperglycemia
  - Assess for side effects

SUGGESTIONS FOR CLASSROOM ACTIVITIES

- Develop a care plan that incorporates an educational component to teach the client about insulin administration and dietary control.

SUGGESTIONS FOR CLINICAL ACTIVITIES

- Practice administering insulin.
- Review the choice of insulin syringes.

LEARNING OUTCOME 7

Provide accurate information to clients with diabetes mellitus to facilitate self-management of medications, diet planning, exercise, and self-assessment, including foot care.

CONCEPTS FOR LECTURE

1. The client should be taught the proper method of medication administration including how to give themselves an injection, storage of medication, and

POWERPOINT LECTURE SLIDES

Self-Management of DM
- Maintain prescribed diet and exercise
- Insulin needs are increased if you have surgery, trauma, fever, or infection

how to read the blood glucose measurement as applied to a sliding scale.
2. Clients who have type 2 diabetes need to be taught safe medication practices concerning the self management of medications.
3. The family and the client should be taught to maintain a prescribed diet and exercise plan.
4. The management of diabetes requires a careful balance between the intake of nutrients, the expenditure of energy, and the dose and timing of insulin or oral antidiabetic agents. Although everyone has the same need for basic nutrition, the person with diabetes must eat a more structured diet to prevent hyperglycemia. The goals for dietary management for adults with diabetes, based on guidelines established by the ADA.
5. People with diabetes should consult their primary healthcare provider before beginning or changing an exercise program. The ability to maintain an exercise program is affected by many different factors, including fatigue and glucose levels. It is as important to assess the person's usual lifestyle before establishing an exercise program as it is before planning a diet.
6. The teaching plan should include self-assessment concerning skin integrity, especially foot care, and to be aware of the possible increased need for insulin in the case of severe illness or surgical intervention.
7. Use proper footwear, inspect the feet daily and after exercise, avoid exercise in extreme heat or cold, and avoid exercise during periods of poor glucose control.

- Monitor blood glucose
- Report any illness or side effects to healthcare provider
- Undergo periodic lab evaluations
- Avoid alcohol intake
- Take medications as prescribed
- Some medications (oral) may interfere with oral contraceptives

SUGGESTIONS FOR CLASSROOM ACTIVITIES

- Develop a teaching plan for a client who manages their DM by diet only.

SUGGESTIONS FOR CLINICAL ACTIVITIES

- Teach a diabetic foot care class to clients and their families.

LEARNING OUTCOME 8

Use the nursing process as a framework for providing individualized care to clients with diabetes mellitus.

CONCEPTS FOR LECTURE

1. All teaching plans need to be individualized and developed with the specific client.
2. The nursing process should address chronic complications of diabetes such as diabetic retinopathy, coronary artery disease, and hypertension.
3. Diabetic nephropathy is a disease of the kidneys characterized by the presence of albumin in the urine, hypertension, edema, and progressive renal insufficiency.
4. Coronary artery disease is a major risk factor in the development of myocardial infarction in people with diabetes, especially in the middle to older adult with type 2 DM. Coronary artery disease is the most common cause of death in people with diabetes.

POWERPOINT LECTURE SLIDES

Nursing Process Framework
- Health promotion
- Assessment
- Risk for impaired skin integrity
- Risk for infection
- Risk for injury
- Sexual dysfunction
- Ineffective coping

5. Hypertension (blood pressure ≥140/90 mmHg) is a common complication of DM. It affects 20% to 60% of all people with diabetes, and is a major risk factor for cardiovascular disease and microvascular complications such as retinopathy and nephropathy.

6. The plan of care should include risk for impaired skin integrity, risk for infection, and risk for injury.

7. The person with diabetes is at increased risk for altered skin integrity as a result of decreased or absent sensation from neuropathies, decreased tissue perfusion from cardiovascular complications, and infection. Injuries, lesions, and changes in skin hydration potentiate infections, delayed healing, and tissue loss in the person with diabetes mellitus.

8. The person with diabetes is at increased risk for infection. The risk of infection is believed to be due to vascular insufficiency that limits the inflammatory response, neurologic abnormalities that limit the awareness of trauma, and a predisposition to bacterial and fungal infections.

9. The person with diabetes is at risk for injury from multiple factors. Neuropathies may alter sensation, gait, and muscle control. Cataracts or retinopathy may cause visual deficits. Hyperglycemia often causes osmotic changes in the lenses of the eye, resulting in blurred vision. In addition, changes in blood glucose alter levels of consciousness and may cause seizures. The impaired mobility, sensory deficits, and neurologic effects of complications of diabetes increase the risk of accidents, burns, falls, and trauma.

10. Sexual dysfunction and ineffective coping should be addressed along with education for the family and the client.

11. Sexuality is a complex and inseparable part of every person. It involves not only physical sexual activities but also a person's self-perception as male or female, roles and relationships, and attractiveness and desirability. Changes in sexual function and in sexuality have been identified in both men and women with diabetes.

12. Coping is the process of responding to internal or environmental stressors or potential stressors. When coping responses are ineffective, the stressors exceed the individual's available resources for responding. The person diagnosed with diabetes is faced with lifelong changes in many parts of his or her life. Diet, exercise habits, and medications must be integrated into the person's lifestyle and be carefully controlled. Daily injections may be a reality. Fear of potential complications and of negative effects on the future is common.

SUGGESTIONS FOR CLASSROOM ACTIVITIES

• Develop a care plan that focuses on health maintenance and prevention of skin complications.

CHAPTER 21
ASSESSING CLIENTS WITH NUTRITIONAL AND GASTROINTESTINAL DISORDERS

RESOURCE LIBRARY

 PRENTICE HALL NURSING MEDIALINK DVD-ROM

Audio Glossary
NCLEX-RN® Review
Animation
   GI A&P

 COMPANION WEBSITE

Audio Glossary
NCLEX-RN® Review
Care Plan Activity: Gallstones
Case Studies
   Assessing Dietary Intake
   Counseling a College Student about Vitamins
Teaching Plan: Regular Dental Check-Ups and Older
   Adults
MediaLink Application: Nursing Tools for Assessing
   the Nutritional Status of Clients
Links to Resources

📖 IMAGE LIBRARY

Figure 21.1 Organs of the gastrointestinal tract and accessory digestive organs.

Figure 21.2 A schematic overview of nutrient use by body cells, including *A*, carbohydrates; *B*, proteins; *C*, fats; and *D*, ATP formation.

Figure 21.3 Structures of the mouth, the pharynx, and the esophagus.

Figure 21.4 The internal anatomic structures of the stomach, including the pancreatic, cystic, and hepatic ducts; the pancreas; and the gallbladder.

Figure 21.5 A barium x-ray of a healthy stomach.

Figure 21.6 Liver biopsy.

Figure 21.7 Measuring MAC with calipers.

Figure 21.8 Measuring MAC with a tape measure.

Figure 21.9 The four quadrants of the abdomen, with anatomic location of organs within each quadrant.

Figure 21.10 Auscultating the abdomen with the diaphragm of the stethoscope.

Figure 21.11 Location of placement of the stethoscope for auscultation of arteries of the abdomen.

Figure 21.12 Location of sites for systematic percussion of all four quadrants.

Figure 21.13 Anatomic location of the liver, with the midclavicular line (MCL) and midsternal line (MSL) superimposed.

Figure 21.14 Percussing the spleen.

Figure 21.15 Percussing for shifting dullness in ascites.

Figure 21.16 Light to moderate palpation of the abdomen.

Figure 21.17 Palpating the liver with the bimanual method.

LEARNING OUTCOME 1

Describe the sources of nutrients, and their functions in the human body.

CONCEPTS FOR LECTURE

1. The categories of nutrients are carbohydrates, proteins, fats, minerals, vitamins, and water.
2. The primary sources of carbohydrates are from plants. Carbohydrates are monosaccharides, disaccharides, and polysaccharides. Carbohydrates are converted to glucose to form adenosine triphosphate (ATP) in the cells.
3. Proteins are classified as complete or incomplete. Complete proteins are found in animal products.

POWERPOINT LECTURE SLIDES

Nutrient Sources
- Carbohydrates
  - Monosaccharides and disaccharides: milk, sugar cane, sugar beets, honey, fruits
  - Polysaccharide starch: grains, legumes, root vegetables
- Proteins
  - Complete proteins: eggs, milk, milk products, meat (contain high amounts of amino acids)

Proteins form amino acids which are necessary for tissue growth and maintenance. Incomplete proteins are found in nuts, grains, cereals, and vegetables. These sources lack one or more of the amino acids.

4. Neutral fats are the most abundant fat in the diet. They may be either saturated or unsaturated. Saturated fats are found in animal products; unsaturated fats are found in seeds, nuts, and most vegetable oils. Fats are a major source of energy, are used in cell membranes, and serve as protection in the form of adipose tissue.

5. Vitamins are organic compounds that facilitate the body's use of carbohydrates, proteins, and fats. Vitamins are categorized as fat-soluble or water-soluble. All vitamins may be found in foods except vitamins D and K.

6. Minerals work with other nutrients to maintain the structure and function of the body. The best sources of minerals are vegetables, legumes, milk, and some meats.

- ○ Incomplete proteins: legumes, nuts, cereal, grains, vegetables (contain low amounts or are lacking one or more amino acids)
- Fats
  - ○ Saturated: animal products (milk, meat) and some plant products (coconut)
  - ○ Unsaturated: seeds, nuts, most vegetable oils
  - ○ Cholesterol: meats, milk, egg yolks
- Vitamins
  - ○ Fat soluble
    - – A, D, E: fish liver oils, fortified milk, dark leafy green vegetables
    - – Vitamin D: synthesized by the skin from sunlight
    - – Vitamin K: synthesized by coliform bacteria in large intestine
  - ○ Water soluble
    - – B complex: leafy green vegetables, meats, fish
    - – Vitamin C: citrus fruits, tomatoes, potatoes

SUGGESTIONS FOR CLASSROOM ACTIVITIES

- Discuss sources of nutrients for each of the food groups.
- View a video of the Food Pyramid.

SUGGESTIONS FOR CLINICAL ACTIVITIES

- Have each student determine which diet the physician has ordered for the client he or she is taking care of.

LEARNING OUTCOME 2

Describe the anatomy, physiology, and functions of the gastrointestinal system.

CONCEPTS FOR LECTURE

1. The gastrointestinal tract is a hollow tube that extends from mouth to anus.
2. The digestive processes are: ingestion of food, movement of food and wastes; secretion of mucus, water, and enzymes; mechanical digestion of food; chemical digestion of food; and absorption of digested food.
3. The mouth (or oral or buccal cavity) is lined with mucous membranes and contains teeth, tongue, and salivary glands. It is enclosed by the cheeks and lips. The teeth masticate the food. The tongue mixes food with saliva and forms a bolus.
4. The oropharynx and laryngopharynx provide a passage for food to the esophagus.
5. The esophagus moves food into the stomach.
6. The stomach is an expandable pouch that can hold approximately 4 liters of food and liquid. Gastric juice is secreted and begins the second or gastric phase of digestion.
7. The small intestine begins at the pyloric sphincter and ends at the ileocecal junction at the entrance of the large intestine. Foods are chemically digested and most of it absorbed as it moves through the small intestine. Indigestible fibers, some water, and bacteria enter the large intestine and exit at the anus.
8. The accessory digestive organs are the liver, gallbladder, and exocrine pancreas.

POWERPOINT LECTURE SLIDES

Gastrointestinal System
- Mouth: mastication, forms food bolus
- Pharynx (oropharynx and laryngopharynx): moves food via peristalsis to the esophagus
- Esophagus: passageway for food to the stomach
- Stomach: storage reservoir, continues mechanical breakdown
- Small intestine: food is chemically digested and absorbed as it moves toward the large intestine
- Accessory organs: liver, gallbladder, exocrine, pancreas all produce enzymes necessary for digestion

SUGGESTIONS FOR CLASSROOM ACTIVITIES	**SUGGESTIONS FOR CLINICAL ACTIVITIES**
• Review anatomy and physiology of the gastrointestinal system. • Show students a model of the gastrointestinal system.	• Ask a gastroenterologist to speak to the class about gastrointestinal disorders.

LEARNING OUTCOME 3

Explain the processes of carbohydrate, fat, and protein metabolism.

CONCEPTS FOR LECTURE

1. After nutrients (carbohydrates, fats, and proteins) are ingested, digested, absorbed, and transported across cell membranes, they must be metabolized to produce and provide energy to maintain life.
2. Metabolism is the process of biochemical reaction that occurs in the body's cells.
3. Processes are either catabolic or anabolic.
4. Catabolism involves the breakdown of complex structures into simpler forms; for example, the breakdown of carbohydrates to produce adenosine triphosphate (ATP), an energy molecule that fuels cellular activity.
5. In the process of anabolism, simpler molecules combine to build more complex structures; for example, amino acids bond to form proteins.
6. The biochemical reactions of metabolism produce water, carbon dioxide, and ATP.

POWERPOINT LECTURE SLIDES

Metabolism
- Process of biochemical reaction occurring in cells
- Catabolism: breakdown of complex structures into simpler forms
- Anabolism: process of simpler molecules combining to build more complex structures
- Metabolism produce water, carbon dioxide, and ATP

SUGGESTIONS FOR CLASSROOM ACTIVITIES	**SUGGESTIONS FOR CLINICAL ACTIVITIES**
• Review the physiology of the cell and the metabolic process.	• Ask a nutritionist to speak to the class about the cell and the metabolic process.

LEARNING OUTCOME 4

Identify specific topics to consider during a health history assessment interview of the client with nutritional and gastrointestinal disorders.

CONCEPTS FOR LECTURE

1. The nurse should assess the client's perception of his or her health and health management.
2. Nutritional and metabolic assessment may be ascertained by asking questions about diet, fluid intake, vitamin/herbal medications weight gain or loss, and any gastrointestinal symptoms that have changed, including bowel habits.
3. Activity and exercise, along with sleep and rest patterns, must be assessed.
4. Self-perception, role relationships, and sexuality should be discussed in the health assessment interview.
5. Coping mechanisms and value belief systems are significant topics when obtaining a health history.

POWERPOINT LECTURE SLIDES

Topics to Consider for Health History Interview
- Health perception/health management
- Nutritional/metabolic
- Elimination
- Activity/exercise
- Sleep/rest
- Cognitive/perceptual
- Self-perception/self-concept
- Role relationships
- Sexuality
- Coping/stress tolerance
- Values/belief system

LEARNING OUTCOME 5

Explain techniques used for assessing nutritional and gastrointestinal status.

CONCEPTS FOR LECTURE

1. Diagnostic tests and physical assessment are used in assessment of nutritional and gastrointestinal status.
2. When conducting a health assessment interview, genetic history may be significant.
3. Physical assessment includes inspection, auscultation, percussion, and palpation.
4. Anthropometric data (height, weight, triceps skin folds, and midarm circumference) is collected as part of the physical assessment.

POWERPOINT LECTURE SLIDES

Diagnostic Tests
- Esophageal acidity and manometry
- Barium swallow or upper GI series
- Endoscopy (EGD)
- MRI
- Gastric analysis
- Gallbladder/pancreatic tests
- Ultrasound
- Liver biopsy
- Physical assessment
- Breath
- Abdomen
- Liver margins

LEARNING OUTCOME 6

Describe normal variations in assessment findings in the older adult.

CONCEPTS FOR LECTURE

1. Due to the possible decrease of adequate dentitia, nutritional deficits may occur, and there may be an increase in periodontal disease and tooth loss.
2. The older adult client may season food more highly due to tongue atrophy.
3. Swallowing may be more difficult in the older client due to a decrease in saliva production and a decrease in esophageal motility.
4. The increase in gastric irritation is due to the atrophy of the stomach and a decrease in the production of hydrochloric acid.
5. Gallstones may be more prevalent due to the liver's less efficient processing of fats.

POWERPOINT LECTURE SLIDES

Age-Related Gastrointestinal Changes
- Teeth
  - Increased number of root cavities
  - Cavities around existing dental work
  - Tooth enamel harder and more brittle
  - Dentin is more fibrous
  - Tooth cusps flatten
  - Root pulp shrinks
  - Increasing loss of bone supporting teeth
- Gums
  - Gingiva retracts
- Taste
  - Less acute as tongue atrophies (especially for sweet sensations)
- Saliva
  - Decreased amount is produced (1/3 of that produced in younger years)
- Esophageal motility
  - Decreased intensity of propulsive waves and slower emptying time
  - Weaker gag reflex

- Stomach
  - Mucosa atrophies
  - Decreased production of hydrochloric acid and pepsin leading to higher pH in stomach
- Liver
  - Less efficient handling of cholesterol and absorption

SUGGESTIONS FOR CLASSROOM ACTIVITIES

- Discuss the nutritional deficit in older adults and the causes.

SUGGESTIONS FOR CLINICAL ACTIVITIES

- Visit a gastroenterologist's office and assist in caring for clients with gastrointestinal disorders.

LEARNING OUTCOME 7

Identify abnormal findings that may indicate alterations in gastrointestinal function.

CONCEPTS FOR LECTURE

1. Diagnostic tests of the esophagus and stomach evaluate acid reflux, esophageal varices, any inflammation, hernia, and other alterations.
2. Gallbladder and pancreatic tissue can be assessed by ultrasound, x-ray, and direct visualization. These tests identify tumors, gallstones, obstructions, and other abnormalities.
3. A liver biopsy is used to rule out cancer, a cyst, or cirrhosis.
4. Blood tests used to rule out disease processes of the GI system are serum lipase and liver function testing.
5. Endoscopic exams are used to visualize gastrointestinal structures for strictures, cysts, polyps, and neoplasms.

POWERPOINT LECTURE SLIDES

Abnormal Findings Indicating Gastrointestinal Function
- Gallbladder and pancreatic tissue
  - Assessed by ultrasound, x-ray, and direct visualization
  - Identifies tumors, gallstones, obstructions, and other abnormalities
- Liver
  - Biopsy used to rule out cancer, cyst, or cirrhosis
- Blood tests
  - Rule out disease processes of the GI system

SUGGESTIONS FOR CLASSROOM ACTIVITIES

- Discuss the problems incurred with clients who have abnormal gallbladder and pancreatic studies.

SUGGESTIONS FOR CLINICAL ACTIVITIES

- Have each student assess their client's medical record for abnormal findings that may indicate alterations in gastrointestinal function.

CHAPTER 22
NURSING CARE OF CLIENTS WITH NUTRITIONAL DISORDERS

RESOURCE LIBRARY

 PRENTICE HALL NURSING MEDIALINK DVD-ROM

Audio Glossary
NCLEX-RN® Review

 COMPANION WEBSITE

Audio Glossary
NCLEX-RN® Review
Care Plan Activity: Malnutrition
Case Studies
   Enteral Feeding Complications
   Obesity
MediaLink Applications
   Anorexia Nervosa
   Establishing a Balanced Diet
   Adapting Diet Plans to Individualize Care
Links to Resources

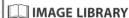 **IMAGE LIBRARY**

Figure 22.1 Types of surgical procedures to treat obesity.

Figure 22.2 A nasoduodenal tube and a jejunostomy tube.

Figure 22.3 The nurse secures the feeding tube of a client receiving a continuous enteral feeding.

Figure 22.4 Total parenteral nutrition through a catheter in the right subclavian vein.

LEARNING OUTCOME 1

Compare and contrast the pathophysiology and manifestations of nutritional disorders.

CONCEPTS FOR LECTURE

1. Obesity is one of the most prevalent diseases and preventable health problems in the United States. Obesity is defined as a body mass index (BMI) of over 30kg/m².
2. The incidence of obesity is higher in females, blacks, and in economically disadvantaged people of all races.
3. Obesity occurs when excess calories are stored as fat. The systems that regulate food intake and expenditure are not fully understood.
4. Malnutrition results from inadequate intake of nutrients, impaired absorption, and increased metabolic needs (due to infection or physiologic stressors).
5. The primary energy source for the body is carbohydrates. If inadequate carbohydrates are ingested, the body then relies on glycogen, body proteins, and lipids.
6. Eating disorders are characterized by severely disturbed eating behavior and weight management. Eating disorders are more common in affluent societies where food is plentiful. Women are much more commonly affected by eating disorders than men.

POWERPOINT LECTURE SLIDES

Nutritional Disorders
- Obesity-related problems
  ○ Cardiovascular
  ○ Respiratory
  ○ Gastrointestinal
  ○ Genitourinary
  ○ Musculoskeletal
  ○ Endocrine
  ○ Reproductive
- Malnutrition-related problems
  ○ Starvation
  ○ Hypermetabolism
  ○ Protein-calorie malnutrition
  ○ Abdominal edema
  ○ Diarrhea
  ○ Postural hypotension impaired immune function
- Eating disorders
  ○ Anorexia nervosa
  ○ Bulimia nervosa
  ○ Binge-eating disorder

SUGGESTIONS FOR CLASSROOM ACTIVITIES

- Divide the class into two groups. One group will research obesity, causes, pathophysiology, and morbidity. The other group will research malnutrition, and focus on eating disorders, pathophysiology, causes, morbidity. Both groups should cover the care, treatment, and nursing interventions.

SUGGESTIONS FOR CLINICAL ACTIVITIES

- Ask students to observe in a nutritionist's office.

LEARNING OUTCOME 2

Identify causes and predict effects of nutritional disorders on client health status.

CONCEPTS FOR LECTURE

1. Obesity occurs when excess calories are stored as fat; however, the complete process is not fully understood. Appetite may have little relationship to hunger.
2. Some studies suggest that leptin resistance is a cause of obesity.
3. Obesity is a significant risk factor for cardiovascular disease, including hypertension, coronary heart disease (CHD), and heart failure.
4. Malnutrition results from inadequate intake of nutrients. Malnutrition may be caused by inadequate nutrient intake; impaired absorption and use of nutrients; loss of nutrients due to diarrhea, hemorrhage, or renal failure; or increased metabolic needs (e.g., infection or physiologic stressors).
5. Malnourished clients have a much higher risk for infection than well-nourished people. Malnutrition affects many components of the immune system, including the skin, mucous membranes, and lymph tissue and cells.
6. Anorexia nervosa typically begins during adolescence. Clients with anorexia nervosa have a distorted body image and irrational fear of gaining weight.
7. Bulimia nervosa develops in late adolescence or early adulthood, and often follows failed attempts to lose weight through dieting.
8. While many of the characteristics of bulimia and binge-eating disorder (BED) are similar, clients with BED do not purge. BED commonly affects middle-aged adults and is slightly more common in women than in men. It affects blacks and whites equally. People with BED usually are overweight or obese, often morbidly obese. The cause of BED is unknown, although genetics may play a role in its development.

POWERPOINT LECTURE SLIDES

Cause and Effect of Nutritional Disorders
- Obesity
  - Caused by excess calories stored as fat
  - May also be due to leptin resistance
  - Significant risk factor for cardiovascular diseases
- Malnutrition
  - Possible causes
    - Inadequate nutrient intake
    - Impaired absorption and use of nutrients
    - Loss of nutrients due to diarrhea, hemorrhage, or renal failure
    - Increased metabolic needs
  - Higher risk for infection
  - Affects many components of the immune system
- Eating disorders
  - Anorexia nervosa: distorted body image and irrational fear of gaining weight
  - Bulimia nervosa: following failed attempts to lose weight through dieting
  - Binge-eating disorder: similar to bulimia but without purging

SUGGESTIONS FOR CLASSROOM ACTIVITIES

- Continue with the classroom activity for Learning Outcome 1.
- Research "leptin resistance."

SUGGESTIONS FOR CLINICAL ACTIVITIES

- Ask a nutritionist to speak to the class about nutritional disorders.

LEARNING OUTCOME 3

Explain interdisciplinary care for clients with nutritional disorders.

CONCEPTS FOR LECTURE

1. The treatment for obesity is far more complex than just reducing the amount of food intake.
2. Treatment for obesity is ongoing, and must be individualized for the obese client.
3. The treatment goal for malnutrition is to restore ideal body weight while replacing nutrients.
4. Age, severity of malnutrition, and any coexisting health problems help determine interventions.
5. Eating disorders, anorexia nervosa in particular, are difficult to effectively treat. Because of the intense fear of weight gain and the distorted body image of clients with anorexia, they strongly resist increasing food intake. While community-based care is appropriate for most clients with an eating disorder, complications of the disorder or resistance to treatment may necessitate hospitalization for some clients. In all cases, a comprehensive treatment plan for eating disorders includes medical care and monitoring, psychosocial interventions, and nutrition counseling.

POWERPOINT LECTURE SLIDES

Care for Clients with Nutritional Disorders
- Obesity
  - Medications (appetite suppressants)
  - A combination of diet, exercise, behavior modification
  - Successful treatment is rarely achieved
- Malnutrition
  - Medication-supplemental vitamins/minerals
  - Gradual refeeding
  - Nutritional supplements
  - Enteral nutrition, TPN
- Eating disorders
  - Difficult to effectively treat
  - Community-based care is appropriate for most clients
  - Hospitalization for some clients may be necessary
  - A comprehensive treatment plan for eating disorders includes medical care and monitoring, psychosocial interventions, and nutrition counseling

SUGGESTIONS FOR CLASSROOM ACTIVITIES

- Discuss multidisciplinary treatment of obesity and malnutrition.

SUGGESTIONS FOR CLINICAL ACTIVITIES

- Have each student develop a list of departments in a hospital setting that could be part of the interdisciplinary care for clients with nutritional disorders.

LEARNING OUTCOME 4

Develop strategies to promote nutrition for client populations.

CONCEPTS FOR LECTURE

1. Losing and maintaining weight are two separate issues. The client should be encouraged to continue to exercise and to self-monitor food intake. The client should be provided with treatment support.
2. The complex effects of malnutrition on multiple body systems place the client at high risk for a number of other problems. Clients should be closely monitored. The nurse should assess the client's knowledge. The client should have rest periods before and after meals.
3. Clients with eating disorders require extended treatment of the disorder. Involvement of the family and social support persons is vital to success. Encourage family members to participate in teaching and nutritional counseling sessions. Discuss the value of family therapy to address issues that have contributed to the disorder. Emphasize the need to provide consistent messages of support for healthy eating habits. Discuss using rewards for food and calorie intake rather than

POWERPOINT LECTURE SLIDES

Promoting Nutrition
- Obese client
  - Establish realistic weight goals
  - Identify factors that cause increased food intake
  - Behavior modification
  - Exercise
- Client with malnutrition
  - Hospitalized client requires an interdisciplinary approach
- Client with eating disorder
  - Anorexia nervosa, bulimia nervosa, binge eating disorder
  - Require hospitalization
  - Monitor weight
  - Observe client during and after meals
  - Multivitamin

weight gain. Provide referrals to a dietitian, nutritional support team, counseling, and support groups for people with eating disorders.

SUGGESTIONS FOR CLASSROOM ACTIVITIES	**SUGGESTIONS FOR CLINICAL ACTIVITIES**
• Create a nursing care plan for an obese client and a client with malnutrition. Include multidisciplinary methods for care.	• Make rounds with the nutritionist. Observe how the data is collected and strategies are developed.

CHAPTER 23
NURSING CARE OF CLIENTS WITH UPPER GASTROINTESTINAL DISORDERS

RESOURCE LIBRARY

💿 PRENTICE HALL NURSING MEDIALINK DVD-ROM

Audio Glossary
NCLEX-RN® Review
Animation
   Ranitidine

COMPANION WEBSITE

Audio Glossary
NCLEX-RN® Review
Care Plan Activity: Peptic Ulcer Disease and Pain
Case Studies
   GERD
   Peptic Ulcer Disease
MediaLink Applications
   Oral Cancer
   Reflux Dyspareunia
Links to Resources

📖 IMAGE LIBRARY

Figure 23.1 Oral cancer.
Figure 23.2 The esophagus.
Figure 23.3 Mechanisms of gastroesophageal reflux.
Figure 23.4 Nissen fundoplication.
Figure 23.5 Hiatal hernias.
Figure 23.6 Balloon dilation of the lower esophageal sphincter.
Figure 23.7 The client with a closed-system gastric lavage.

Figure 23.8 Common sites affected by peptic ulcer disease.
Figure 23.9 A superficial peptic ulcer.
Figure 23.10 The spread and forms (polypoid and ulcerating) of gastric cancer.
Figure 23.11 Partial and total gastrectomy procedures.
Figure 23.12 The pathogenesis and manifestations of dumping syndrome.
Figure 23.13 Gastrostomy.

LEARNING OUTCOME 1

Describe the pathophysiology of common disorders of the mouth, esophagus, and stomach.

CONCEPTS FOR LECTURE

1. Lesions of the mouth may have a variety of causes, including infection, mechanical trauma, irritants such as alcohol, and hypersensitivity. The lining of the mouth is very thin and fragile. Stomatitis is a very common disorder of the mouth. Oral cancer may develop on the lips, tongue, floor of the mouth, or other oral tissues.
2. A common disorder of the esophagus is reflux, or gastroesophageal reflux disease (GERD). In this condition, gastric contents reflux back into the esophagus from the stomach. Gastric juices contain acid, pepsin, and bile, which are corrosive. Prolonged exposure can cause esophagitis.
3. Hiatal hernia and esophageal cancer are also disease processes of the esophagus.
4. A hiatal hernia occurs when part of the stomach protrudes through the esophageal hiatus of the diaphragm into the thoracic cavity. Although hiatal hernia

POWERPOINT LECTURE SLIDES

Common Disorders of the Mouth, Esophagus, and Stomach
- Mouth
  - Stomatitis
    - Cold sore, fever blister (herpes simplex virus)
    - Aphthous ulcer (cause unknown)
    - Candidiasis/thrush (candida albicans)
    - Necrotizing ulcerative gingivitis (infection)
    - Oral mucositis (damage caused by chemotherapy or radiation therapy)
  - Oral cancer (usually squamous cell carcinoma)
- Esophagus
  - Gastroesophageal reflux disease (GERD): relaxation of lower sphincter, incompetent lower esophageal sphincter, and hiatal hernia

---

is thought to be a common problem, most affected individuals are asymptomatic. The incidence of hiatal hernia increases with age.

5. There are two types of esophageal tumors, adenocarcinoma and squamous cell carcinoma.

6. Cigarette smoking and chronic alcohol use are strong risk factors for squamous cell esophageal tumors, and also appear to contribute to the risk of developing adenocarcinoma.

7. Disorders of the stomach and duodenum include gastritis, peptic ulcer disease, and cancer of the stomach. Stomach disorders are often accompanied by nausea and vomiting.

8. Blood in the GI tract has several effects. It is irritating to the stomach, and typically leads to nausea and vomiting (hematemesis, vomiting blood). If the blood has been present in the stomach for a period of time and is partially digested, it may have a "coffee-grounds" appearance, rather than presenting as bright red blood. The accumulation of blood in the GI tract stimulates peristasis, leading to hyperactive bowel sounds and diarrhea. Stools may be black and tarry (melena) or frankly bloody (hematochezia); stool containing partially digested blood has a characteristic odor.

9. Nausea, an unpleasant subjective sensation, occurs when the vomiting center in the medulla of the brain is stimulated. Distention of the duodenum is a common stimulus for nausea. The vomiting center can be stimulated by input from several different sources.

- ○ Hiatal hernia: stomach protrudes through a defect in the diaphragm into the thoracic cavity
- ○ Esophageal cancer: uncommon in U.S., usually squamous cell, or adenocarcinoma
- Stomach
- ○ Gastritis: ingestion of gastric irritants
- ○ Peptic ulcer disease (PUD): use of ASA, NSAIDs, presence of *H. pylori*
- ○ Zollinger-Ellison syndrome: caused by gastrin-secreting tumor
- ○ Stomach cancer: *H. pylori*, genetic predisposition, carcinogenic factors in the diet

---

SUGGESTIONS FOR CLASSROOM ACTIVITIES

- Discuss how the conditions of the upper gastrointestinal tract affect nutritional status.

SUGGESTIONS FOR CLINICAL ACTIVITIES

- Ask a gastrointestinal nurse specialist to speak to the class about common disorders of the mouth, esophagus, and stomach.

LEARNING OUTCOME 2

Relate manifestations and diagnostic test results to the pathophysiologic processes involved in upper gastrointestinal disorders.

CONCEPTS FOR LECTURE

1. Nutritional status should be assessed due to either the inability of the client to eat or poor absorption due to disease process. Weight and general health status should also be assessed.

2. Diagnostic tests include electrolytes, liver, pancreatic, renal function studies, and radiographic studies if indicated.

3. Endoscopy is performed for direct visualization of problems with the esophagus and stomach.

4. Diagnostic tests for a client with gastritis may include gastric analysis to assess hydrochloric acid analysis, blood tests including CBC, and red blood cell indices.

5. GERD causes heartburn, usually after meals, with bending over, or when reclining. Regurgitation of sour

POWERPOINT LECTURE SLIDES

Diagnostic Tests
- Direct endoscopy
- Laboratory tests
- Radiologic exams: MRI, CT Scan
- Biopsy
- Assessment of nutritional status

material into the mouth, or difficulty and pain with swallowing may develop. Diagnostic tests that may be ordered for clients with manifestations of GERD include:

- Barium swallow to evaluate the esophagus, stomach, and upper small intestine.
- Upper endoscopy to permit direct visualization of the esophagus. Tissue may be obtained for biopsy to establish the diagnosis and rule out malignancy.
- 24-hour ambulatory pH monitoring may be performed to establish the diagnosis of GERD. For this test, a small tube with a pH electrode is inserted through the nose into the esophagus. The electrode is attached to a small box worn on the belt that records the data. The data are later analyzed by computer.
- Esophageal manometry measures pressures of the esophageal sphincters and esophageal peristalsis.

6. There are two types of esophageal tumors, adenocarcinoma and squamous cell carcinoma. Cigarette smoking and chronic alcohol use are strong risk factors for squamous cell esophageal tumors, and also appear to contribute to the risk of developing adenocarcinoma. Diagnostic and staging procedures for esophageal cancer may include esophagography, bronchoscopy, and scans to detect metastasis. The following diagnostic tests may be performed:

- Barium swallow to identify irregular mucosal patterns or narrowing of the lumen, which suggests esophageal cancer.
- Esophagoscopy to allow direct visualization of the tumor and obtain tissue for biopsy.
- Chest x-ray, CT scans, or MRI to identify possible tumor metastases to other organs or tissues.
- Complete blood count (CBC) may indicate anemia due to chronic blood loss. Serum albumin levels may be low due to malnutrition, and liver function tests (ALT, alkaline phosphatase, AST, and bilirubin) are elevated if liver metastases are present.

7. Blood in the GI tract has several effects. It is irritating to the stomach, and typically leads to nausea and vomiting (hematemesis, vomiting blood). Diagnostic testing focuses on determining the extent and effects of the bleed, as well as its cause. The following diagnostic tests may be performed:

- A complete blood count with hemoglobin and hematocrit are obtained. In an acute bleed, the CBC, hemoglobin, and hematocrit may not initially indicate the extent of blood loss because plasma is lost along with blood cells.
- Blood type and crossmatch are performed to prepare for transfusion as necessary.
- Serum electrolytes, osmolality, and BUN are obtained to determine the effects of the blood loss and protein digestion on blood chemistries.
- Liver function studies and a coagulation profile may be obtained to help determine the cause of the bleeding.

- An upper endoscopy is performed as soon as possible to identify and, if possible, treat the source of bleeding.

8. Chronic gastritis is often asymptomatic until atrophy is sufficiently advanced to interfere with digestion and gastric emptying. The client may complain of vague gastric distress, epigastric heaviness after meals, or ulcer-like symptoms. These symptoms typically are not relieved by antacids. Diagnostic tests that may be ordered for the client with gastritis include the following:

- Gastric analysis to assess hydrochloric acid secretion. A nasogastric tube is passed into the stomach, and pentagastrin is injected subcutaneously to stimulate gastric secretion of hydrochloric acid. Secretion may be decreased in clients with chronic gastritis.
- Hemoglobin, hematocrit, and red blood cell (RBC) indices are evaluated for evidence of anemia. The client with gastritis may develop pernicious anemia because of parietal cell destruction, or iron-deficiency anemia because of chronic blood loss.
- Serum vitamin B_{12} levels are measured to evaluate for possible pernicious anemia. Normal values for vitamin B_{12} are 200 to 1000 pg/mL, with lower levels seen in older adults.
- Upper endoscopy may be done to inspect the gastric mucosa for changes, identify areas of bleeding, and obtain tissue for biopsy. Bleeding sites may be treated with electro- or laser coagulation or injected with a sclerosing agent during the procedure.

SUGGESTIONS FOR CLASSROOM ACTIVITIES

- View diagnostic films of normal and abnormal upper gastrointestinal disease processes.
- Discuss normal and abnormal lab values for these disease processes.

SUGGESTIONS FOR CLINICAL ACTIVITIES

- Ask a gastroenterologist to speak to the class about the manifestations and diagnostic tests of the upper gastrointestinal disorders.

LEARNING OUTCOME 3

Explain interdisciplinary care for clients with upper gastrointestinal disorders.

CONCEPTS FOR LECTURE

1. Stomatitis is diagnosed by direct physical examination and, if indicated, cultures, smears, and evaluation for systemic illness. Treatment includes meticulous oral hygiene, topical medications, and oral antibiotics.

2. The first component of treating oral cancer is eliminating causative factors such as chewing tobacco, smoking, or drinking alcohol. Radiation, chemotherapy, and surgery are treatments of choice.

3. After the diagnosis of gastroesophageal reflux disease (GERD) is made, the treatment focuses on lifestyle changes, diet modification, and, in severe cases, surgery. Medications that neutralize stomach acid and increase motility and gastric emptying are prescribed.

POWERPOINT LECTURE SLIDES

Interdisciplinary Care for Upper Gastrointestinal Disorders
- Eliminate causative factors, foods, alcohol, lifestyle changes
- Medications
- Surgical interventions
- Radiation
- Chemotherapy
- Complementary and alternative medicines

4. Hiatal hernias may be treated with medications; however, severe cases may involve incarcerated herniation of the stomach. If incarceration occurs, surgical intervention is required.

5. Esophageal cancer usually requires surgical intervention, radiation, and chemotherapy.

6. Nausea and vomiting are common GI complaints. Nausea is caused by food poisoning, ingestion of toxins, gallbladder disease, or acute gastritis, and is usually relieved by vomiting. In most cases, nausea and vomiting are self-limited and require no treatment.

7. The treatment for gastrointestinal bleeding is dictated by the severity of the bleed. A client with a massive bleed must be treated aggressively in an intensive care setting.

8. Acute and chronic gastritis are generally handled in the community-based setting. Treatment usually includes medications, GI tract rest, and complementary therapies, such as herbal remedies or aromatherapy.

9. The treatment for the client with peptic ulcer disease (PUD) is the eradication of *H. pylori* infection, and treating and preventing ulcers related to the use of NSAIDs.

10. Cancer of the stomach is often diagnosed with an upper GI series, endoscopy, and a CBC. Surgical intervention is the treatment of choice. Radiation and chemotherapy are used in cases of metastasis.

SUGGESTIONS FOR CLASSROOM ACTIVITIES

- Ask students to select an upper gastrointestinal disorder and discuss the pathophysiology of the disease and the multidisciplinary treatment.

SUGGESTIONS FOR CLINICAL ACTIVITIES

- Assign students to clients with upper gastrointestinal disorders.

LEARNING OUTCOME 4

Describe the role of the nurse in interdisciplinary care of clients with upper gastrointestinal disorders.

CONCEPTS FOR LECTURE

1. Health promotion is foremost in clients with upper gastrointestinal disorders. Teach clients with stomatitis about good oral hygiene. Teach all clients about nutritious food choices, and to avoid chewing tobacco, alcohol, and carcinogenic meats.

2. Nursing assessment when completing a health history should collect both subjective and objective data.

3. The nurse should assess the effectiveness of the medication and whether the client is compliant in taking the prescribed medications.

POWERPOINT LECTURE SLIDES

Role of the Nurse in Interdisciplinary Care
- Health promotion: nutrition, lifestyle changes
- Assessment
- Medication assessment

SUGGESTIONS FOR CLASSROOM ACTIVITIES

- Develop a teaching plan for clients with upper gastrointestinal disorders that focuses on nutritional deficits.

SUGGESTIONS FOR CLINICAL ACTIVITIES

- Make rounds with the gastrointestinal nurse specialist. Observe how the data is collected.

CHAPTER 24
NURSING CARE OF CLIENTS WITH GALLBLADDER, LIVER, AND PANCREATIC DISORDERS

RESOURCE LIBRARY

 PRENTICE HALL NURSING MEDIALINK DVD-ROM

Audio Glossary
NCLEX-RN© Review
Animation
   Cirrhosis

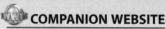 **COMPANION WEBSITE**

Audio Glossary
NCLEX-RN© Review
Care Plan Activity: A Client with Hepatitis A
Case Studies
   Hepatitis B
   Traditional Native American Diet and
    Gallbladder Disease
MediaLink Applications
   GI Disorders and Gallbladder Disease
   Treatment of Liver Cancer
Links to Resources

IMAGE LIBRARY

Figure 24.1 Common locations of gallstones.
Figure 24.2 T-tube placement in the common bile duct.
Figure 24.3 Asterixis.
Figure 24.4 Sites and position for paracentesis.
Figure 24.5 Triple-lumen nasogastric tube (Sengstaken-Blakemore) used to control bleeding esophageal varices.

Figure 24.6 Transjugular intrahepatic portosystemic shunt (TIPS).
Figure 24.7 Pancreatoduodenectomy (Whipple's procedure).

LEARNING OUTCOME 1

Describe the pathophysiology of commonly occurring disorders of the gallbladder, liver, and exocrine pancreas.

CONCEPTS FOR LECTURE

1. The gallbladder may have several disorders. Altered bile flow through the hepatic, cystic, or common bile duct is a common problem. Cholelithiasis (gallstones) and cholecystitis (inflammation of the gallbladder) are also common problems. Cancer of the gallbladder is very rare; however, it does carry a high mortality rate.
2. Gallstones form when several factors interact: abnormal bile composition, biliary stasis, and inflammation of the gallbladder. Most gallstones (80%) consist primarily of cholesterol; the rest contain a mixture of bile components. Excess cholesterol in bile is associated with obesity, a high-calorie, high-cholesterol diet, and drugs that lower serum cholesterol levels. When bile is supersaturated with cholesterol, it can precipitate out to form stones.
3. Gallbladder cancers spread by direct extension to the liver, and metastasize via the blood and lymph system.

POWERPOINT LECTURE SLIDES

Disorders of the Gallbladder, Liver, and Exocrine Pancreas
- Gallbladder
  - Cholelithiasis: cholesterol stones
  - Biliary colic: caused by obstructed cystic or common bile duct
  - Cholecystitis: may be acute or chronic
  - Cancer of the gallbladder: rare, very poor prognosis
- Liver
  - Hepatocellular failure: protein metabolism, glucose metabolism, impairs absorption of lipids, affects blood clotting
  - Jaundice (Icterus): caused by accumulation of bilirubin in tissue

4. The liver is a very complex organ with an extensive blood supply, which thereby exposes the organ to pathogens, toxins, drugs, and malignant cells. Liver dysfunction is manifested by disrupted liver cell function, impaired bilirubin conversion, and disrupted blood flow, which leads to portal hypertension.

5. The essential functions of the liver include the metabolism of proteins, carbohydrates, and fats. It also is responsible for the metabolism of steroid hormones and most drugs. It synthesizes essential blood proteins, including albumin and clotting factors in particular.

6. Common disorders of the pancreas include both acute and chronic pancreatitis and pancreatic cancer. Disorders of the exocrine pancreas also include diabetes mellitus, as discussed in Chapter 20. When there is an alteration in the normal function of the exocrine pancreas, the secretion of digestive enzymes is affected.

7. Acute pancreatitis is an inflammatory disorder that involves self-destruction of the pancreas by its own enzymes through autodigestion. The milder form of acute pancreatitis, interstitial edematous pancreatitis, leads to inflammation and edema of pancreatic tissue. It often is self-limiting. The more severe form, necrotizing pancreatitis, is characterized by inflammation, hemorrhage, and ultimately necrosis of pancreatic tissue.

8. Most cancers of the pancreas occur in the exocrine pancreas, are denocarcinomas, and cause death within 1 to 3 years after diagnosis. Cancer of the pancreas has a slow onset, with manifestations of anorexia, nausea, weight loss, flatulence, and dull epigastric pain. The pain increases in severity as the tumor grows. Other manifestations depend on the location of the tumor.

- ○ Portal hypertension: caused by impaired blood flow through liver causing increased venous pressure
- ○ Hepatitis: inflammation may be acute or chronic, may be caused by a virus, alcohol, drugs
- ○ Cirrhosis: end stage chronic disease, usual cause is alcohol, can be caused by viral hepatitis
- Pancreas
  - ○ Pancreatitis: acute or chronic
  - ○ Acute: self-destruction of the pancreas through autoingestion
  - ○ Chronic: primary cause is alcoholism
  - ○ Pancreatic cancer: very high mortality rate, 98% die

SUGGESTIONS FOR CLASSROOM ACTIVITIES

- Discuss the disorders of the gallbladder, liver, and pancreas.

SUGGESTIONS FOR CLINICAL ACTIVITIES

- Assign students to care for clients with these conditions.

LEARNING OUTCOME 2

Use knowledge of normal anatomy and physiology to understand the manifestations and effects of biliary, hepatic, and pancreatic disorders.

CONCEPTS FOR LECTURE

1. The gallbladder stores and secretes bile to aid in the digestion of fats and lipids. If a secretory duct is obstructed, the duct is distended, which leads to severe pain. Obstruction of the common duct will lead to bile reflux into the liver, which causes jaundice. Obstruction can also lead to cholecystitis, ischemia, and necrosis of the gallbladder. Stones do not form when the gallbladder empties completely in response to hormonal stimulation. Slowed or incomplete emptying allows cholesterol to concentrate and increases the risk of stone formation. Finally, inflammation of the gallbladder allows excess water and bile salt reabsorption, increasing the risk for lithiasis.

POWERPOINT LECTURE SLIDES

Effects of Biliary, Hepatic, and Pancreatic Disorders
- Gallbladder
  - ○ Stores and secretes bile to aid in the digestion of fats and lipids
  - ○ Obstructed secretory duct can lead to severe pain
  - ○ Obstructed common duct will lead to bile reflux into the liver, causing jaundice
  - ○ Obstruction can lead to cholecystitis, ischemia, and necrosis
- Liver
  - ○ Vital to digestion, metabolism, production of plasma proteins

2. The liver is vital to digestion and metabolism, production of plasma proteins, and excretion of many compounds including ammonia and toxins. If a client is in hepatocellular failure, all metabolic functions are greatly affected. Increased venous pressure in the liver causes dilation of the vessels in the gastrointestinal tract and abdominal wall. This will lead to esophageal varices, ascites, portal systemic encephalopathy, and renal failure.

3. The pancreas secretes digestive enzymes. When the organ becomes inflamed, self-destruction of the organ occurs through autodigestion, which leads to edema and possible necrosis of the pancreas. Pancreatitis can also be caused by a gallstone being lodged in the sphincter of Oddi. Other manifestations include nausea and vomiting; abdominal distention and rigidity; decreased bowel sounds; tachycardia; hypotension; elevated temperature; and cold, clammy skin. Within 24 hours, mild jaundice may appear. Retroperitoneal bleeding may occur 3 to 6 days after the onset of acute pancreatitis; signs of bleeding include bruising in the flanks (Turner's sign) or around the umbilicus (Cullen's sign).

- ○ Excretes many compounds, including ammonia and toxins
- ○ Hepatocellular failure affects all metabolism
- ○ Esophageal varices, ascites, and portal systemic encephalopathy, and renal failure
- Pancreas
  - ○ Secretes digestive enzymes
  - ○ Inflammation causes self-destruction of the organ occurs through autodigestion
  - ○ Pancreatitis also caused by a gallstone being lodged in the sphincter of Oddi

---

SUGGESTIONS FOR CLASSROOM ACTIVITIES

- Review the anatomy and physiology of the gallbladder, liver, and pancreas.
- Look at models of these structures and note the relationship of these organs.

SUGGESTIONS FOR CLINICAL ACTIVITIES

- Assign students to clients who are experiencing manifestations of biliary, hepatic, or pancreatic disorders.

LEARNING OUTCOME 3

Relate changes in normal assessment data to the pathophysiology and manifestations of gallbladder, liver, and exocrine pancreatic disorders.

CONCEPTS FOR LECTURE

1. The client with cholelithiasis or cholecystitis will require radiologic and laboratory diagnostic assessments. These assessments will differentiate gallbladder disease from other disorders.

2. Diagnostic tests are ordered to identify the presence and location of stones, identify possible complications, and help differentiate gallbladder disease from other disorders.
   - Serum bilirubin: elevated may indicate obstructed bile flow in the biliary duct system
   - Serum amylase and lipase: identifies possible pancreatitis due to common duct obstruction
   - WBC: elevated WBC is indicative of infection and inflammation of the gallbladder
   - Abdominal x-ray: shows gallstones with high calcium concentrate
   - Ultrasonography: accurately diagnosis cholelithiasis

POWERPOINT LECTURE SLIDES

Diagnostic Tests for Gallbladder, Liver, and Pancreatic Diseases
- Gallbladder disease
  - ○ Serum bilirubin
  - ○ Serum amylase and lipase
  - ○ WBC
  - ○ Abdominal x-ray
  - ○ Ultrasonography: accurately diagnose cholelithiasis
  - ○ Oral cystogram
  - ○ Gallbladder scan
- Liver disease
  - ○ Hepatitis
    - – Alanine aminotransferase (ALT)
    - – Aspartate aminotransferase (AST)
    - – Alakaline phosphotase (ALP)
    - – Gamma-glutamyltransferase (GGT)

- Oral cystogram[±]: assesses the gallbladder ability to concentrate and excrete bile
- Gallbladder scan: diagnose Biliary tree obstruction

3. The client with impaired liver function will have elevated liver function tests due to the enzymes that are released when liver cells are damaged. Endoscopy and liver biopsy may also be performed. Diagnostic tests may include the following:
   - Hepatitis
     ○ Alanine aminotransferase (ALT): damaged liver cells release this enzyme into blood.
     ○ Aspartate aminotransferase (AST): in severe damage, levels may be 20–100 X normal values
     ○ Alakaline phosphotase (ALP): elevated in hepatitis
     ○ Gamma-Glutamyltransferase (GGT): levels rise in hepatitis and obstructive biliary disease
     ○ Lactic dehydrogenase (LDH): LDH5 is specific indicator of liver damage
     ○ Serum bilirubin levels: elevated in viral hepatitis
   - Cirrhosis
     ○ ALT, AST, GGT: all elevated, but not as high as in acute hepatitis
     ○ CBC with platelets: low RBC indicates anemia due to bone marrow suppression, low platelets, and low WBC-spleenic involvement
     ○ Coagulation studies: prolonged PT indicates lack of vitamin K and impaired production of coagulation proteins
     ○ Bilirubin levels: elevated in severe cirrhosis
     ○ Serum ammonia: elevated as liver fails to convert ammonia into urea for excretion
     ○ Abdominal ultrasound: measures liver size
     ○ Esophagoscopy: determines presence of esophageal varices

4. Diagnostic assessments of the client with a pancreatic disease include laboratory and radiologic examinations. The following tests can be ordered to determine is a client has an exocrine pancrease:
   - Ultrasonography: identifies mass or pseudocyst
   - CT Scan: identifies enlargement, fluid collection, and perfusion deficits in areas or necrosis
   - Endoscopic Retrograde Cholangiopancreatography (ERCP): differentiates inflammation and fibrosis from carcinoma
   - Percutaneous Fine-Needle Aspiration Biopsy: differentiates between cancer and chronic pancreatitis

- – Lactic dehydrogenase (LDH)
- – Serum bilirubin levels
- ○ Cirrhosis
  - – ALT, AST, GGT
  - – CBC with platelets
  - – Coagulation studies
  - – Bilirubin levels
  - – Serum ammonia
  - – Abdominal ultrasound
  - – Esophagoscopy
- Exocrine pancreas
  ○ Ultrasonography
  ○ CT Scan
  ○ Endoscopic retrograde cholangiopancreatography (ERCP)
  ○ Percutaneous fine-needle aspiration biopsy

SUGGESTIONS FOR CLASSROOM ACTIVITIES

- Discuss the multidisciplinary approach for care of clients with disease conditions of the pancreas, gallbladder, and liver.

SUGGESTIONS FOR CLINICAL ACTIVITIES

- Assign students to clients who are undergoing diagnostic tests for gallbladder, liver, and pancreatic conditions.

CHAPTER 25
ASSESSING CLIENTS WITH BOWEL ELIMINATION DISORDERS

RESOURCE LIBRARY

 PRENTICE HALL NURSING MEDIALINK DVD-ROM

Audio Glossary
NCLEX-RN® Review

 COMPANION WEBSITE

Audio Glossary
NCLEX-RN® Review
Care Plan Activity: Bowel Elimination Disorder
Case Studies
  Abdominal Pain
  Post-Op Complications
MediaLink Application: Chronic Constipation
Links to Resources

📖 IMAGE LIBRARY

Figure 25.1 Anatomy of the large intestine.
Figure 25.2 Structure of the rectum and anus.

Figure 25.3 The four quadrants of the abdomen.
Figure 25.4 Digital examination of the *A*, anus; and *B*, rectum.

LEARNING OUTCOME 1
Describe the anatomy, physiology, and functions of the intestines.

CONCEPTS FOR LECTURE

1. The small intestine is about 20 feet long and about 1 inch in diameter. It is coiled around the abdominal cavity, suspended by mesentery, and surrounded by large intestine. Food is chemically digested and mostly absorbed as it moves through the small intestine. Enzymes in the small intestine break down carbohydrates, proteins, lipids, and nucleic acids.
2. The large intestine (colon) is about 5 feet long, begins at the ileocecal valve, and ends at the anus. It is divided into three parts: ascending, transverse, and descending colon. The main function of the large intestine is to eliminate indigestible food residue from the body and absorb water, salts, and vitamins formed by food residue and bacteria.

POWERPOINT LECTURE SLIDES

Basic Anatomy of Intestines
- Small intestine
  ○ 3 regions: duodenum, jejunum, ileum
- Large intestine
  ○ Cecum, appendix, colon, rectum, anal canal
  ○ Appendix is attached to the cecum

SUGGESTIONS FOR CLASSROOM ACTIVITIES

- Review the anatomy and physiology of the large and small intestine.
- Look at a model of the large and small intestine in relationship to other abdominal organs.

LEARNING OUTCOME 2

Explain the physiologic processes involved in bowel elimination.

CONCEPTS FOR LECTURE

1. Feces are moved along the intestine by peristalsis. The defecation reflex is initiated when feces enter the rectum and stretches the rectal wall.
2. The walls of the sigmoid colon contract and the anal sphincter relaxes.
3. The Valsalva maneuver facilitates the expulsion of feces.

POWERPOINT LECTURE SLIDES

Bowel Elimination
- Feces moved by peristalsis
- Defecation reflex
- Sigmoid colon contracts
- Anal sphincter relaxes
- Valsalva maneuver expels feces

SUGGESTIONS FOR CLASSROOM ACTIVITIES

- View a video about the process of bowel elimination.

LEARNING OUTCOME 3

Identify specific topics to consider during a health history assessment interview of the client with problems of bowel elimination.

CONCEPTS FOR LECTURE

1. Clients may feel embarrassed to talk about bowel elimination patterns. Begin the health history interview asking about less personal information such as inquiring about any medical conditions that may influence the client's bowel elimination pattern, such as a stroke or spinal cord impairment, inflammatory gastrointestinal diseases, endocrine disorders, and allergies. When rapport has been established, focus on the chief complaint.
2. Topics to consider for health history of client with a problem bowel:
   - Onset of problem
   - Characteristics and course
   - Severity
   - Precipitating and relieving factors
   - Cramping
   - Bleeding increased constipation
   - Recent travel outside the United States
   - Any changes in activities of daily living
   - Diarrhea
   - Constipation

POWERPOINT LECTURE SLIDES

Topics to Consider for Health History of Client with a Problem Bowel
- Onset of problem
- Characteristics and course
- Severity
- Precipitating and relieving factors
- Cramping
- Bleeding increased constipation
- Recent travel outside the United States
- Any changes in activities of daily living
- Diarrhea
- Constipation

SUGGESTIONS FOR CLASSROOM ACTIVITIES

- Discuss why travel outside the United States would impact bowel habits.

LEARNING OUTCOME 4

Describe techniques used to assess bowel integrity and function.

CONCEPTS FOR LECTURE

1. Physical assessment of the abdomen includes auscultation of bowel sounds, rectal exam, anal exam, and exam of client's stool sample.
   - Auscultate all four quadrants of the abdomen with the diaphragm of the stethoscope. Begin in the lower right quadrant, where bowel sounds are almost always present.
   - Auscultate the abdomen for vascular sounds with the bell of the stethoscope.
   - Ask the client to empty the bladder and have the client turn to the left lateral (Sims') position for the rectal examination.
   - Ask client to provide a fresh stool sample. A sterile container should be used to collect a stool sample for a culture. Ask women of childbearing age if they are having their menstrual period; if so, note this on the laboratory request.
   - Palpate the anus and rectum. Lubricate the gloved index finger and ask the client to bear down. Touch the tip of your finger to the client's anal opening. Flex the index finger, and slowly insert it into the anus, pointing the finger toward the umbilicus. Rotate the finger in both directions to palpate any lesions or masses.
2. Palpation should be used last when assessing the abdomen because pressure on the abdominal wall may cause pain and interfere with bowel sounds.

POWERPOINT LECTURE SLIDES

Physical Assessment of Bowel Integrity and Function
- Auscultation of bowel sounds
- Rectal exam
- Anal exam
- Exam of stool
- Palpation (do last)

SUGGESTIONS FOR CLASSROOM ACTIVITIES

- Discuss techniques and demonstrate the assessment of the abdomen including listening for bowel sounds in all quadrants.

SUGGESTIONS FOR CLINICAL ACTIVITIES

- Assign students to perform an abdominal assessment on their clients.

LEARNING OUTCOME 5

Describe normal variations in assessment findings for the older adult.

CONCEPTS FOR LECTURE

1. There are normal age-related intestinal changes.
2. In the small intestine there is a decreasing number of absorbing cells on the intestinal wall, slowed fat absorption, faulty absorption of vitamin B12, vitamin D, calcium, and iron.
3. In the large intestine there is decreasing mucous secretion and elasticity of the wall of the rectum, loss of tone in the internal sphincter with decreased awareness of the need to defecate.

POWERPOINT LECTURE SLIDES

Normal Age-Related Intestinal Changes
- Small intestine
  - Decreasing number of absorbing cells on the intestinal wall
  - Slowed fat absorption
  - Faulty absorption of vitamin B12, vitamin D, calcium, and iron
- Large intestine
  - Decreasing mucous secretion and elasticity of the wall of the rectum
  - Loss of tone in the internal sphincter with decreased awareness of the need to defecate

LEARNING OUTCOME 6

Identify manifestations of altered intestinal function.

CONCEPTS FOR LECTURE

1. Clients with altered intestinal function may display generalized abdominal distention and discomfort.
2. Generalized abdominal distention may be seen in gas retention or obesity.
3. Lower abdominal distention is seen in bladder distention, pregnancy, or ovarian mass.
4. Dilated veins are prominent in cirrhosis of the liver, ascites, portal hypertension, or venocaval obstruction.
5. Pulsation is increased in aortic aneurysm.
6. Bruits (blowing sound due to restriction of blood flow through vessels) may be heard over constricted arteries. A bruit over the liver may be heard in hepatic carcinoma.
7. A venous hum (continuous medium-pitched sound) may be heard over a cirrhotic liver.
8. Dullness is heard when the bowel is displaced with fluid or tumors or filled with a fecal mass.
9. Abnormal masses include aortic aneurysms, neoplastic tumors of the colon or uterus, and a distended bladder or distended bowel due to obstruction.
10. A rigid, boardlike abdomen may be palpated when the client has a perforated duodenal ulcer.
11. Hyperactive bowel sounds (borborygmus) is heard in diarrhea or the onset of bowel obstruction.
12. Frequent bouts of constipation may lead to external hemorrhoids at the area of the external hemorrhoidal plexus.
13. Rebound tenderness in the right lower quadrant occurs in acute appendicitis.
14. Left lower quadrant pain is seen in acute diverticulitis.
15. Bulges that appear in the inguinal area when the client bears down may indicate a hernia (a defect in the abdominal wall that allows abdominal contents to protrude outward).
16. Dilated anal veins in the perianal area appear with hemorrhoids. Fissures are caused by passing constipated stool.
17. Movable, soft masses may be polyps.
18. Hard, firm, irregular embedded masses may indicate carcinoma.
19. Stool should be tested for occult blood.

POWERPOINT LECTURE SLIDES

Altered Intestinal Function
- Abdominal assessment
- Inguinal assessment
- Perianal assessment
- Fecal assessment

SUGGESTIONS FOR CLASSROOM ACTIVITIES

- Disscuss the manifestation of altered bowel function including hyperactive bowel sounds, localized pain or tenderness, hemorrhoids, and generalized intestinal discomfort.

SUGGESTIONS FOR CLINICAL ACTIVITIES

- Assign students to clients with intestinal disease processes.

CHAPTER 26
NURSING CARE OF CLIENTS WITH BOWEL DISORDERS

RESOURCE LIBRARY

💿 PRENTICE HALL NURSING MEDIALINK DVD-ROM

Audio Glossary
NCLEX-RN® Review

COMPANION WEBSITE

Audio Glossary
NCLEX-RN® Review
Care Plan Activity: Irritable Bowel Syndrome
Case Studies
Enteral Tube Complications
Irritable Bowel Syndrome
Teaching Plan: Colon Cancer
MediaLink Applications
Crohn's Disease and Ulcerative Colitis
Crohn's Disease Teaching Sheet

📖 IMAGE LIBRARY

Figure 26.1 *A*, McBurney's point, located midway between the umbilicus and the anterior iliac crest in the right lower quadrant. *B*, In an appendectomy, the appendix and cecum are brought through the incision to the surface of the abdomen.

Figure 26.2 The weighted tip or inflated balloon at the end of an intestinal tube is drawn into the intestine by gravity and peristalsis.

Figure 26.3 *A*, Photomicrograph of the mucosa of the large intestine showing the entrances to the crypts of Lieberkühn. The crypts are the focal points for, *B*, ulcerative colitis and, *C*, Crohn's disease.

Figure 26.4 The progression of Crohn's disease.

Figure 26.5 Ileal pouch-anal anastomosis (IPAA).

Figure 26.6 A healthy-appearing stoma.

Figure 26.7 Continent (Kock's) ileostomy.

Figure 26.8 *A*, Tubular (or pedunculated) polyps; and *B*, villous (or sessile) polyps.

Figure 26.9 The distribution and frequency of cancer of the colon and rectum.

Figure 26.10 Various ostomy levels and sites.

Figure 26.11 A double-barrel colostomy.

Figure 26.12 An abdominal wall (ventral or incisional) hernia and an inguinal hernia.

Figure 26.13 Selected causes of mechanical obstruction.

Figure 26.14 Diverticula of the colon.

Figure 26.15 The location of internal and external hemorrhoids.

LEARNING OUTCOME 1

Compare and contrast the causes, pathophysiology, manifestations, interdisciplinary care and nursing care of clients with diarrhea, constipation, irritable bowel syndrome, and fecal incontinence.

CONCEPTS FOR LECTURE
DIARRHEA

1. Diarrhea is an increase in the frequency, volume, and fluid content of the stool. This increase may be caused by osmotic or secretory processes. Water and electrolytes can be lost in a large number of stools, which can lead to dehydration. Management focuses on identifying and treating the underlying cause. Nursing care of the client focuses on identifying the cause, relieving the manifestations, preventing complications, and preventing the potential spread to others.

POWERPOINT LECTURE SLIDES

Diarrhea, Constipation, IBS, and Fecal Incontinence
- Diarrhea
  - Increase in the frequency, volume, and fluid content of the stool
  - Water and electrolytes can be lost leading to dehydration
  - Management focuses on identifying and treating the underlying cause

2. Nursing interventions for diarrhea include:
   Risk for deficient fluid volume
   Risk for impaired skin integrity

CONSTIPATION

3. Constipation is defined as the infrequency or difficult passage of stools. It may be a primary problem or a manifestation of another disease or condition. Manifestations of constipation include having bowel movements less often than the usual pattern. Initial evaluation is based on the history and physical examination. Education can prevent constipation. Teach clients to eat a diet high in fiber.

4. Nursing interventions for the client with constipation focus chiefly on education.

IRRITABLE BOWEL SYNDROME

5. Irritable bowel syndrome (IBS) is also known as spastic bowel or functional colitis. It is a motility disorder of the GI tract, with no identifiable organic cause. IBS is characterized by abdominal pain that may be either colicky or dull and continuous. Diagnosis of IBS is based on the presence of abdominal pain that is relieved by defecation, and is associated with a change in frequency of elimination, or change in stool form. The primary nursing responsibility is education and referral.

6. The primary nursing responsibility is education; providing referrals and counseling are additional nursing responsibilities to clients who have irritable bowel syndrome.

FECAL INCONTINENCE

7. Fecal incontinence is the loss of voluntary control of defecation. Multiple factors may contribute to the condition, including both physiologic and psychologic factors. Diagnosis of fecal incontinence is based on client history and physical examination of the pelvic floor and anus to evaluate muscle tone.

8. Nurses are often responsible for instituting bowel training programs and other measures to manage fecal incontinence. Nursing interventions for fecal incontinence include:
   Risk for impaired skin integrity

- ○ Nursing care focuses on identifying the cause, relieving the manifestations, preventing complications, and prevention of the potential spread to others
- Constipation
  - ○ Infrequency or difficult passage of stools
  - ○ May be a primary problem or a manifestation of another disease or condition
  - ○ Evaluation based on the history and physical examination
  - ○ Nursing care focuses on education and modification of diet and exercise routines
- Irritable bowel syndrome (IBS)
  - ○ Motility disorder of the GI tract
  - ○ Diagnosis is based on presence of abdominal pain relieved by defecation and is associated with a change in frequency of elimination or change in stool form
  - ○ Nursing care is education and referral
- Fecal incontinence
  - ○ Loss of voluntary control of defecation
  - ○ Contributing factors included both physiologic and psychologic
  - ○ Diagnosis based on client history and physical examination of the pelvic floor and anus to evaluate muscle tone
  - ○ Nursing care includes bowel training programs and other measures to manage fecal incontinence

SUGGESTIONS FOR CLASSROOM ACTIVITIES

- Discuss irritable bowel syndrome, diarrhea, and constipation. What are the manifestations of these conditions and what are some of the causes?

LEARNING OUTCOME 2

Explain the pathophysiology, manifestations, complications, interdisciplinary care, and nursing care of clients with acute inflammatory and infectious bowel disorders, chronic inflammatory bowel disorders, malabsorption syndromes, neoplastic disorders, structural and obstructive bowel disorders, and anorectal disorders.

CONCEPTS FOR LECTURE

ACUTE INFLAMMATORY AND INFECTIOUS BOWEL DISORDERS

1. Most pathogens that affect the GI tract are ingested with food or water but also may be spread by direct contact and transmitted sexually.

2. Acute inflammatory disorders such as appendicitis and peritonitis result from contamination of damaged or normally sterile tissue by the client's own endogenous or resident bacteria. Appendicitis is the most common acute bowel disorder. Peritonitis is a serious complication of many acute abdominal disorders. It is caused by *E. coli, Klebsiella, Proteus,* or *Pseudomonas* bacteria.

3. Continuous mild generalized or upper abdominal pain is the initial characteristic manifestation of acute appendicitis. Over the next 4 hours, the pain intensifies and localizes in the right lower quadrant of the abdomen. It is aggravated by moving, walking, or coughing. On palpation, localized and rebound tenderness are noted at McBurney's point. Rebound tenderness is demonstrated by relief of pain with direct palpation of McBurney's point followed by pain on release of pressure. Extension or internal rotation of the right hip increases the pain. In addition to pain, a low-grade temperature, anorexia, nausea, and vomiting are often present.

4. Preoperative nursing care is directed toward preparing the client physically and psychologically for emergency surgery. Limited time is available for preoperative teaching. Nursing interventions for appendicitis include:

   Risk for infection
   Acute pain

5. Manifestations of peritonitis depend on the severity and extent of the infection, as well as the age and general health of the client. Both local and systemic manifestations are present. The client often presents with evidence of an acute abdomen, an abrupt onset of diffuse, severe abdominal pain. The pain may localize and intensify near the area of infection. Movement may intensify the pain. The entire abdomen is tender, with guarding or rigidity of abdominal muscles. The acute abdomen is often described as boardlike. Rebound tenderness may be present over the area of inflammation. Peritoneal inflammation inhibits peristalsis, resulting in a paralytic ileus. Nursing interventions for peritonitis include:

   Acute pain
   Deficient fluid volume
   Ineffective protection
   Anxiety

POWERPOINT LECTURE SLIDES

Bowel Disorders
- Acute bowel disorders
  - Appendicitis
    - Inflammation of the vermiform appendix
    - Pain localized in right lower quadrant with rebound tenderness
    - Danger of perforation if not treated within 24 hours of onset
  - Peritonitis
    - Inflammation of the peritoneum
    - Caused by many factors, including ruptured appendix, perforated diverticulum, perforated ulcer
    - Mortality rate can be as high as 40%
  - Paralytic ileus: peristalsis is slowed or stopped by inflammation
  - Gastroenteritis: inflammation of the stomach and small intestine caused by a viral or bacterial infection, producing inflammation and tissue damage
  - Exotoxins: bacteria produce and excrete exotoxins that enter the intestinal lumen causing inflammation and damage
  - Enterotoxins: staphylococcus, clostridium perfringens, clostridium botulinum, some strains of E. coli, and vibrio cholerae
- Specific types of gastrointestinal infections
  - Traveler's diarrhea
  - Staphylococcal food poisoning
  - Cholera
  - E. coli hemorrhagic colitis
  - C. difficile colitis
  - Shigellosis (bacillary dysentery)
- Parasites
  - Giardiasis (protozoa)
  - Amebiasis (amebic dysentery)
  - Cryptosporidiosis (coccidiosis)
  - Helminths (parasitic worms) round worms, flukes, tapeworms
- IBD
  - Ulcerative colitis
  - Crohn's disease
- Malabsorption syndrome
  - Celiac sprue: sensitive to gluten containing products
  - Tropical sprue: gluten intake has no effect
- Obstructive disorders
  - Hernias
  - Intestinal obstructions
  - Diverticular disease

6. Bacteria, parasites, viruses, or toxins also cause acute inflammatory bowel diseases. Manifestations of bacterial or viral infections of the GI tract are the result of two mechanisms: the production of exotoxins and invasion and ulceration of the mucosa. Anorexia, nausea, vomiting, and diarrhea are common manifestations of gastroenteritis. The severity of the manifestation is dependent upon the severity of the infection or inflammation.

7. Although the manifestations of bacterial and viral enteritis vary according to the organism involved, several features are common (i.e., nausea, vomiting, anorexia). Nursing diagnoses for bacterial and viral enteritis include:

    Deficient fluid volume

8. Protozoal bowel infection is caused by a parasite, giardiasis; and helminths, which are common in the United States. Other parasitic infections are caused by crytosporidiosis, which are found primarily in the tropics where sanitation is poor. Nursing interventions for the client with a protozoal GI infection are similar to those indicated for clients with bacterial or viral infections.

CHRONIC INFLAMMATORY BOWEL DISORDERS

9. Chronic inflammatory bowel disorder (IBD) includes two closely-related conditions: ulcerative colitis and Crohn's disease. Both are chronic and recurrent diseases. The cause is unknown; however, it appears to be regional (United States and Northern Europe) and tends to run in families.

10. Ulcerative colitis primarily affects the mucosa of the large bowel distally to proximally. Diarrhea is the predominant manifestation of ulcerative colitis, with stool that contains blood and mucous. Manifestations of toxic megacolon include fever, tachycardia, hypotension, dehydration, abdominal tenderness and cramping, and a change in the number of stools per day.

11. In Crohn's disease, patchy involvement is seen in the submucosal layers primarily in the small intestine. Crohn's disease can be so diverse that the manifestations are according to the location of the disease process. Certain complications of Crohn's disease (e.g., intestinal obstruction, abscess, and fistula) are so common that they are considered part of the disease process. Interdisciplinary care for inflammatory bowel disease begins by establishing the diagnosis and the extent and severity of the disease. Treatment is supportive, including medications and dietary measures to decrease inflammation, promote intestinal rest and healing, and reduce intestinal motility. Many clients with IBD require surgery at some point to manage the disease or its complications.

MALABSORPTION SYNDROME

12. Malabsorption syndrome is a condition in which the mucosa ineffectively absorbs nutrients. Diseases of the

- Anorectal disorders
  - Hemorrhoids
  - Anal fissures
  - Anorectal fistulas
  - Abscesses
  - Pilonidal disease

small intestine are often the cause of malabsorption syndromes, such as sprue. Manifestations of celiac sprue may develop at any age. Local manifestations include abdominal bloating and cramps, diarrhea, and steatorrhea. Systemic manifestations result from the effects of malabsorption and resulting deficiencies. Anemia is common. Manifestations of tropical sprue include sore tongue, diarrhea, and weight loss. Initially, diarrhea may be explosive and watery; as the disease progresses, stools become fewer in number and more solid with obvious steatorrhea. Folic acid deficiency is common. Vitamin B12 and iron deficiencies may occur, resulting in glossitis; stomatitis; dry, rough skin; and anemia. With any malabsorptive disorder, the initial focus of management is to identify the cause. Once this has been determined, specific therapy can be prescribed. Diarrhea and malnutrition are significant problems for the client with sprue and the priority foci for nursing intervention.

NEOPLASTIC DISORDERS

13. Malignant neoplasms of the lower bowel are the second leading cause of death in the United States. Bowel cancer may not present any manifestations until it is advanced. The primary focus of interdisciplinary care is prevention, early detection, and intervention. Most polyps are asymptomatic, found coincidentally during routine examination or diagnostic testing. Intermittent painless rectal bleeding, bright or dark red, is the most common presenting complaint. A large polyp may cause abdominal cramping, pain, or manifestations of obstruction. Diarrhea and mucous discharge may be associated with a large villous adenoma. The diagnosis of intestinal polyps is generally based on diagnostic studies such as sigmoidoscopy or colonoscopy. A rectal polyp may be palpable on digital examination, but further studies are necessary to determine its size and type and the extent of colon involvement, and to assess for malignancy. The incidence of intestinal polyps increases with age. They affect men and women equally. It is believed that an adenomatous polyp requires more than 5 years of growth to become significant in size and malignant potential. Advise all clients to have a screening for colorectal cancer (with a colonoscopy being the "gold standard" for diagnosis) at age 50 and as recommended thereafter for early detection of polyps (American Cancer Society).

STRUCTURAL AND OBSTRUCTIVE BOWEL DISORDERS

14. Any portion of the intestine may be affected by a structural or obstructive disorder. These disorders may be hernias, intestinal obstructions, or diverticular disease. Hernias are classified by location and may be congenital or acquired. Most hernias occur in the groin (inguinal or femoral hernias). Abdominal contents (peritoneum, bowel, and other abdominal organs) can

protrude through the abdominal wall to form a sac covered by skin and subcutaneous tissues. In most cases, abdominal contents move into the sac when intra-abdominal pressure increases, then return to the abdominal cavity when pressure returns to normal or when manual pressure is placed on the bulging sac. This is known as a reducible hernia. The risk for complications is low with a reducible hernia. If the contents of a hernia cannot be returned to the abdominal cavity, it is said to be incarcerated. Contents of an incarcerated hernia are trapped, usually by a narrow neck or opening to the hernia. Incarceration increases the risk of complications, including obstruction and strangulation. Obstruction occurs when the lumen of the bowel contained within the hernia becomes occluded, much like the crimping of a hose. A strangulated hernia develops when blood supply to bowel and other tissues in the hernia sac is compromised, leading to necrosis. The affected bowel can infarct, leading to perforation with contamination of the peritoneal cavity. Manifestations of a strangulated hernia include severe abdominal pain and distention, nausea, vomiting, tachycardia, and fever. The diagnosis of a hernia is made by a physical examination. The client is examined in a supine or standing position. A bulge may be seen or felt when the client coughs or bears down. No laboratory or diagnostic testing is usually required, unless bowel obstruction or strangulation is suspected.

ANORECTAL DISORDERS

15. Anorectal disorders include hemorrhoids, anal fissures, anorectal fistulas, abscesses, and pilonidal disease. Hemorrhoids develop when venous return from the anal canal is impaired. Straining to defecate increases venous pressure and is the most common cause of distended hemorrhoids. Pregnancy increases intra-abdominal pressure, raising venous pressure, and is another cause of hemorrhoids. Other factors that may contribute to symptomatic hemorrhoids include prolonged sitting, obesity, chronic constipation, and a low-fiber diet. Hemorrhoids may be internal or external. Lesions of the anorectal canal include fissures, abscesses, fistulas, and pilonidal disease. Pilonidal disease is an acute abscess or chronic draining sinus in the sacrococcygeal area. Because hemorrhoids are a normal condition, management is conservative unless complications such as permanent prolapsed or thrombosis occur.

SUGGESTIONS FOR CLASSROOM ACTIVITIES	**SUGGESTIONS FOR CLINICAL ACTIVITIES**
• Assign students to research one of the disease processes discussed in objective 2. Discuss the results of their findings with the class. • Discuss the effects of parasitic infections and treatments.	• Assign students to care for clients with one of the above disorders.

LEARNING OUTCOME 3

Discuss the purposes, nursing implications, and health education for the client and family of medications used to treat bowel disorders.

CONCEPTS FOR LECTURE

DIARRHEA

1. Antidiarrheal medications should be used sparingly or not at all until the cause of the diarrhea is known. Medications are usually absorbants and protectants. The medications bind substances that cause diarrhea. Most are available over-the-counter. The nurse should assess the contraindications of the therapy, and observe the client's response. Assess for contraindications to antidiarrheal or narcotic medications prior to giving these drugs. Administer paregoric undiluted with water. Do not administer difenoxin and diphenoxylate to clients receiving monoamine oxidase inhibitors (MAOIs); hypertensive crises may occur. Observe closely for increased effects of other CNS depressants, such as alcohol, narcotic analgesics, or barbiturate sedatives. Observe for abdominal distention; toxic megacolon may occur if these drugs are given to the client with ulcerative colitis.

CONSTIPATION

2. The only laxatives that are appropriate and safe for long-term use are bulking agents, such as psyllium seed, calcium polycarbophil, and methylcellulose. The agent softens the stool by drawing water into the feces. The nursing responsibilities for laxatives vary depending upon which type of laxative the client is using. Education can prevent constipation. Teach clients the importance of maintaining a diet high in natural fiber. Foods such as fresh fruits, vegetables, whole-grain products, and bran provide natural fiber. Encourage reducing consumption of meats and refined foods, which are low in fiber and can be constipating. Emphasize the need to maintain a high fluid intake every day, particularly during hot weather and exercise. Discuss the relationship between exercise and bowel regularity. Encourage clients to engage in some form of exercise, such as walking daily. Discuss normal bowel habits, and explain that a daily bowel movement is not the norm for all people. Encourage clients to respond to the urge to defecate when it occurs. Suggest setting aside a time, usually following a meal, for elimination.

IRRITABLE BOWEL SYNDROME

3. Irritable bowel syndrome is characterized by abdominal pain that often is relieved by defecation and a change in bowel habits. The pain may be either colicky, occurring in spasms, or dull and continuous. Although not curative, medications may be prescribed to manage the manifestations of IBS. The primary nursing responsibility is education; providing referrals and counseling are additional nursing responsibilities to clients who have irritable bowel syndrome.

POWERPOINT LECTURE SLIDES

Bowel Disorder Medications
- Antidiarrheal medications
  - Kaopectate, Donnagel, Pepto-Bismol
  - Nursing responsibilities
    - Administer on empty stomach
    - Assess for potential contraindications
  - Client and family teaching
    - Do not use for more than one week unless specified
    - Take in the morning
- Laxatives
  - Fibercon, Bran, Citrucel, Metamucil
  - Nursing responsibilities
    - Mix agent with at least 6 oz of water just prior to administering
    - Do not administer to clients with possible stool impaction or obstruction
  - Client and family teaching
    - Client should drink at least 6–8 glasses of fluid daily
    - Agents may be mixed with fruit juice, water or milk
    - Do not take at bedtime

See the previous sections on diarrhea and constipation for selected nursing interventions.

FECAL INCONTINENCE

4. Fecal incontinence, the loss of voluntary control of defecation, occurs less frequently than urinary incontinence but is no less distressing to the client. Multiple factors contribute to fecal incontinence, including both physiologic and psychologic conditions. The most common causes of fecal incontinence are those that interfere with either sensory or motor control of the rectum and anal sphincters. If the external sphincter is paralyzed as a result of spinal cord injury or disease, defecation occurs automatically when the internal sphincter relaxes with the defecation reflex. The diagnosis of fecal incontinence is based on the client's history. Physical examination of the pelvic floor and anus is performed to evaluate muscle tone and rule out a fecal impaction. Impaired sphincter muscle may be palpable on digital exam. Anorectal manometry or a rectal motility test may be used to evaluate the functional ability of the sphincter muscles. In this test, a small, flexible balloon catheter is introduced into the rectum, and pressures are measured in the rectum and internal and external sphincters. Normally, rectal dilation causes the internal sphincter to relax and the external sphincter to contract. Sigmoidoscopy also may be used to examine the rectum and anal canal. Management of fecal incontinence is directed toward the identified cause. Medications to relieve diarrhea or constipation may be prescribed. A high-fiber diet, ample fluids, and regular exercise are helpful for many clients. Exercises to improve sphincter and pelvic floor muscle tone (Kegel exercises) may be of long-term benefit.

SUGGESTIONS FOR CLASSROOM ACTIVITIES

- Create a teaching plan for clients and families with clients with bowel disorders. Incorporate over-the-counter (OTC) medications and diet.

SUGGESTIONS FOR CLINICAL ACTIVITIES

- Assign students to clients who are taking medication for a bowel disorder.

LEARNING OUTCOME 4

Explain the rationale for using selected diets, including those for diarrhea and constipation, low-residue, gluten-free, and high–fiber diets.

CONCEPTS FOR LECTURE

1. Fluid replacement is the primary concern for the client with diarrhea. Solid food should be withheld for 24 hours to rest the bowel. Lactose will aggravate the loose stools and should be added last.
2. The client with constipation should eat a diet high in fiber to increase stool bulk. The client should also

POWERPOINT LECTURE SLIDES

Selected Diets
- Diarrhea
  - Oral fluids, glucose electrolyte balanced (Gatorade, Pedialyte) for bowel rest
  - Soft foods after 24 hours
  - Add milk products and fat last

drink 6–8 ounces of fluid daily to assist bowel motility. The client should reduce the intake of refined foods and meats.

3. Low-residue diets are recommended for clients with ileostomies to avoid food blockage. Because food blockage is a potential problem, high-fiber foods are limited, and foods that may cause blockage, such as popcorn, corn, nuts, cucumbers, celery, fresh tomatoes, figs, strawberries, blackberries, and caraway seeds, are avoided. Symptoms of food blockage include abdominal cramping, swelling of the stoma, and absence of ileostomy output for over 4 to 6 hours.

4. Clients with sprue (celiac sprue) are placed on a gluten-free diet. Gliadin (a substance found in gluten) acts as an antigen in the intestinal mucosa, and causes inflammation.

- Constipation
  - High fiber (vegetable, raw fruits) to bulk up the stool mass
  - Reduce intake of refined foods and meats
- IBS
  - May benefit from high fiber diet
  - Adding bran and fluid reduces incidence of loose diarrheal stools and constipated stools
- Gluten free diet: prescribed for clients with sprue
- Low residue diet: for clients with ileostomies and colostomies to prevent blockage

SUGGESTIONS FOR CLASSROOM ACTIVITIES

- Ask a dietitian to speak to the students about special diets for clients with selected intestinal disease processes.

SUGGESTIONS FOR CLINICAL ACTIVITIES

- Have each student review a client's medical record and find the type of diet the physician has ordered for the client.

LEARNING OUTCOME 5

Describe the surgical procedures of the bowel, including colectomy, colostomy, ileostomy, and perianal surgery.

CONCEPTS FOR LECTURE

1. The treatment of choice for acute appendicitis is an appendectomy. The procedure may be through a laparoscopic approach, or an open incision at McBurney's point. If the appendix has not ruptured, the recovery is uneventful.

COLECTOMY AND ILEOSTOMY

2. Clients with extensive chronic ulcerative colitis may require a total colectomy. A colectomy is the surgical resection and removal of the colon. When the entire colon and rectum are removed, a pouch is formed at the terminal ileum (ileal pouch-anal anastomosis). A temporary ileostomy is performed at the same time to allow healing of the anal anastomosis. When the healing is complete, the ileostomy is closed and the client then has bowel movements through the anus. Assess the peristomal skin. Skin around the stoma should remain clean and pink and free of irritation, rashes, inflammation, or excoriation. Report abnormal assessment findings to the physician. Apply protective ointments to the perirectal area of clients with newly functioning ileoanal reservoirs and anastomoses.

3. The precise name of the ostomy depends on the location of the stoma. An ileostomy is made from the small intestine. A colostomy is formed from the large intestine.

POWERPOINT LECTURE SLIDES

Surgical Procedures of the Bowel
- Colectomy
- Colostomy
- Ileostomy
- Perianal surgery

Perianal Surgery

4. Perianal surgery involves hemorrhoidectomy, repair of anal fissures, and anal ulcers. Anal packing may be in place for the first 24 hours following the procedure. When removed, observe the client closely for bleeding. Pain is a common postoperative problem. Although the operative procedure is minor, postoperative discomfort can be significant because the anal region is richly innervated and muscle spasms may occur. In addition to systemic analgesics, sitz baths usually are ordered. These not only help promote relaxation and reduce discomfort but also clean the anal area. Use of a rubber ring or donut device minimizes pressure on the surgical site while the client sits in the bath. The primary nursing consideration is pain management.

5. Pilonidal disease is an acute abscess or chronic draining sinus in the sacrococcygeal area. The preferred treatment is to drain the cyst and excise the sinus tract. The incision may be closed or left open to secondary intention healing. Primary nursing care is to teach the client to keep the area clean and dry.

Suggestions for Classroom Activities

- Review the anatomy of the large and small intestine.
- Ask a surgeon to speak to the class about the procedures addressed in the objectives.

Suggestions for Clinical Activities

- Assign students to care for and develop a nursing care plan for clients with surgical interventions.

CHAPTER 27
ASSESSING CLIENTS WITH URINARY ELIMINATION DISORDERS

RESOURCE LIBRARY

 PRENTICE HALL NURSING MEDIALINK DVD-ROM

Audio Glossary
NCLEX-RN® Review
Animation
   The Kidney

 COMPANION WEBSITE

Audio Glossary
NCLEX-RN® Review
Care Plan Activity: Urinary System Disorder
Case Studies
   Urinary Calculi
   Urine Characteristics
MediaLink Applications
   Renal Function
   Urinary Diversions
Links to Resources

IMAGE LIBRARY

Figure 27.1 The urinary system.
Figure 27.2 Internal anatomy of the kidney.
Figure 27.3 The structure of a nephron, showing the glomerulus within the glomerular capsule.
Figure 27.4 Schematic view of the three major mechanisms by which the kidneys adjust to the composition of plasma.

Figure 27.5 The countercurrent exchange system is responsible for establishing and maintaining an osmotic gradient necessary to the composition, volume, and pH of urine.
Figure 27.6 Internal view of the urinary bladder and trigone.
Figure 27.7 Inspecting the urinary meatus of the male.

LEARNING OUTCOME 1

Describe the anatomy, physiology, and functions of the urinary system.

CONCEPTS FOR LECTURE

1. The organs of the urinary system include paired kidneys, paired ureters, the urinary bladder, and the urethra.
2. The kidneys are highly vascular and consist of three distinct regions, the cortex that contains the glomeruli, the medulla that contains the renal pyramids, and the pelvis that channels urine into the ureters.
3. The functions of the kidney are to: form urine; balance solute and water transport; and excrete metabolic waste products.
4. The functional units of each kidney are the approximately 1 million nephrons that process blood to make urine through glomerular filtration, tubular reabsorption, and tubular secretion.
5. The function of the ureters is transport of urine from the kidney pelvis to the urinary bladder.
6. The urinary bladder serves as a storage site for urine and its size varies with the amount of urine it contains.
7. The urethra channels urine to outside of the body.

POWERPOINT LECTURE SLIDES

Anatomy, Physiology, and Function of Urinary System
- Function of the urinary system
  - Kidneys
    - Urine formation
    - Water/solute balance
    - Excretion of metabolic waste products
    - Conserve nutrients
    - Regulate acid-base balance
    - Secrete hormones helping to regulate blood pressure, erythrocyte production, calcium metabolism
  - Ureters
    - Transport urine from the kidney to the bladder
  - Bladder
    - Stores urine until micturition
  - Urethra
    - Channels urine out of the body

LEARNING OUTCOME 2

Explain the role of the urinary system in maintaining homeostasis.

CONCEPTS FOR LECTURE

1. The healthy urinary system helps to maintain homeostasis by balancing fluid excretion, clearing waste products from the blood, and activating or synthesizing various hormones.
2. The dilution or concentration of urine is largely determined by the action of antidiuretic hormone (ADH), which is secreted by the posterior pituitary gland.
3. The kidneys excrete water-soluble waste products such as urea, creatinine, uric acid, ammonia, bacterial toxins, and water-soluble drugs.
4. Hormones either activated or synthesized by the kidneys include active vitamin D, erythropoietin, and natriuretic hormone.

POWERPOINT LECTURE SLIDES

The Urinary System and Homeostasis
- Regulates body fluids
- Filters metabolic wastes from bloodstream
- Reabsorbs needed substances and water into bloodstream
- Eliminates metabolic wastes and water

SUGGESTIONS FOR CLASSROOM ACTIVITIES

- Encourage classroom discussion of the implications of impaired kidney function.

SUGGESTIONS FOR CLINICAL ACTIVITIES

- Have students review medication records for medications that are cleared through the kidney and discuss implications of impaired kidney function in clients receiving those medications.

LEARNING OUTCOME 3

Identify specific topics for consideration during a health history assessment interview of the client with problems involving the urinary system.

CONCEPTS FOR LECTURE

1. Assessment of current urinary status should include: color, odor, and amount of urine; difficulty initiating a stream of urine; frequency of urination; painful urination; excessive urination at night; blood in the urine; voiding scant or excessive amounts of urine; discharge; flank pain; and changes in normal pattern of urination.
2. Assessment of history should include surgical procedures, previous urinary problems, and family occurrence of end-stage renal disease, renal calculi, or frequent urinary infections.
3. Lifestyle assessment should include diet, work history, exposure to toxic chemicals, usual fluid intake, type of fluid intake, and tobacco use.

POWERPOINT LECTURE SLIDES

Health History Assessment and the Urinary System
- Current urinary status assessment
  - Color, odor, amount of urine
  - Difficulty initiating stream
  - Frequency of urination
  - Dysuria
  - Nocturia
  - Hematuria
  - Oliguria
  - Polyuria
  - Discharge
  - Pain
- History
  - Previous surgical procedures
  - Previous urinary problems
  - Family history of renal disease, calculi, or infections

- Lifestyle
  - Diet
  - Work history, especially for exposure to toxic chemicals
  - Usual fluid intake including type of fluid
  - Tobacco use

Suggestions for Classroom Activities

- Have students review a case study history for findings that are significant to clients with urinary elimination disorder.
- Discuss interview methods that help to make the client more comfortable when discussing sensitive information.

Suggestions for Clinical Activities

- Have students review the client's history for indications of possible urinary dysfunction.

Learning Outcome 4

Describe techniques used to assess the integrity and function of the urinary system.

Concepts for Lecture

1. Urine may be tested for characteristics and components through routine analysis, urine culture, post-voiding residual urine amounts, and 24-hour collections for components such as creatinine.
2. The ability to empty the urinary bladder may be evaluated by ultrasonic bladder scan to evaluate for residual urine, uroflowmetry to measure the volume of urine voided per second, or cystometrogram (CMG) to evaluate bladder capacity, neuromuscular functions of the bladder, urethral pressures, and causes of bladder dysfunction.
3. Radiographic examinations include intravenous pyelogram, retrograde pyelogram, renal arteriogram, or angiogram.
4. Direct visualization of the bladder wall and urethra can be accomplished through cystoscopy which also allows for removal of small stones, tissue sampling, and contrast dye instillation.
5. Noninvasive tests include renal ultrasound, CT scan, MRI, and renal scan to determine kidney size and structure and presence of masses or obstruction. Renal scans can also evaluate kidney blood flow, perfusion, and urine production.
6. Kidney biopsy is done to obtain tissue to diagnose or monitor kidney disease.
7. Physical assessment of the urinary system should include: inspection of the skin and mucous membranes, inspection of the abdomen, inspection of the urinary meatus if indicated, auscultation of the renal arteries, percussion of kidneys for tenderness or pain, palpation of kidneys, percussion of the bladder for tone and position, and palpation of the bladder for distention.

PowerPoint Lecture Slides

Assessing Integrity and Function of Urinary System
- Laboratory studies
  - Routine urinalysis
  - Culture and sensitivity
  - Residual urine
  - 24-hour urine collections
- Testing ability to empty bladder
  - Ultrasound
  - Uroflowmetry
  - Cystometrogram
- Radiographic studies
  - Intravenous pyelogram
  - Retrograde pyelogram
  - Renal arteriogram/angiogram
  - CT/MRI/renal scans
- Invasive studies
  - Cystoscopy
  - Biopsy
- Physical assessment
  - Inspection of skin and mucous membranes
  - Inspection of the abdomen
  - Inspection of the urinary meatus (if indicated)
  - Auscultation of the renal arteries
  - Percussion of kidneys and bladder
  - Palpation of kidney and bladder

SUGGESTIONS FOR CLASSROOM ACTIVITIES

- Have students practice assessment techniques on mannequins.
- Discuss methods for ensuring accurate specimen collection for various urine studies.
- Have students manipulate urine collection devices.

SUGGESTIONS FOR CLINICAL ACTIVITIES

- Review client medical records for studies pertinent to the urinary system.
- Review laboratory study normal values.
- Have students perform urinary assessments on clients in the clinical area.

LEARNING OUTCOME 5

Describe normal variations in assessment findings for the older adult.

CONCEPTS FOR LECTURE

1. Atrophy of the kidneys may occur with aging.
2. Decrease in renal tubule function may result in less effective exchange of substances, water and sodium conservation. ADH secretion may be suppressed.
3. Bladder capacity decreases as muscles weaken. It becomes more difficult to empty the bladder and there is delay in the micturition reflex.

POWERPOINT LECTURE SLIDES

Normal Age-Related Changes
- Kidney atrophy
- Decrease in renal tubule function
- Decrease in bladder capacity

LEARNING OUTCOME 6

Identify manifestations of impairment of the urinary system.

CONCEPTS FOR LECTURE

1. Pallor, decreased turgor, edema, and uremic frost may be integumentary indicators of urinary dysfunction.
2. Abdominal assessment findings of asymmetry, masses, swelling, distention, glistening, or skin tightness may indicate urinary dysfunction.
3. Urinary dysfunction may manifest as increased redness, swelling, ulceration, displacement, or discharge from the urinary meatus.
4. Presence of systolic bruits over the renal arteries may indicate renal artery stenosis.
5. Percussion should reveal a bladder that is midline without dullness and no tenderness over the kidneys.
6. The bladder and kidneys are not normally palpable.

POWERPOINT LECTURE SLIDES

Manifestations of Impairment of the Urinary System
- Skin
  - Pallor, decreased turgor, edema, uremic frost
- Abdomen
  - Asymmetry, masses, swelling, distention, glistening, skin tightness
- Urinary Meatus
  - Redness, swelling, ulceration, displacement, discharge
- Kidneys
  - Arterial bruits, tenderness on percussion, enlargement, texture changes
- Bladder
  - Distention

SUGGESTIONS FOR CLASSROOM ACTIVITIES

- Discuss the case study on urine characteristics that is available on the Companion Website.

SUGGESTIONS FOR CLINICAL ACTIVITIES

- Help students identify manifestations of urinary dysfunction in clinical clients.

CHAPTER 28
NURSING CARE OF CLIENTS WITH URINARY TRACT DISORDERS

RESOURCE LIBRARY

PRENTICE HALL NURSING MEDIALINK DVD-ROM

Audio Glossary
NCLEX-RN® Review

COMPANION WEBSITE

Audio Glossary
NCLEX RN® Review
Care Plan Activity: Urinary Tract Infection
Case Studies
  Bladder Cancer
  Urinary Tract Infection
Concept Map: Bladder Cancer
MediaLink Applications
  Bladder Training
  Urinary Tract Disorders
Links to Resources

IMAGE LIBRARY

Figure 28.1 A competent vesicoureteral junction.
Figure 28.2 Appearance of the bladder wall affected by cystitis.
Figure 28.3 Development and location of calculi within the urinary tract.
Figure 28.4 Extracorporeal shock-wave lithotripsy.

Figure 28.5 Percutaneous ultrasonic lithotripsy.
Figure 28.6 Papillary transitional cell carcinoma of the urinary bladder.
Figure 28.7 Common urinary diversion procedures.
Figure 28.8 A sample voiding diary.

LEARNING OUTCOME 1

Explain the pathophysiology of common urinary tract disorders.

CONCEPTS FOR LECTURE
URINARY TRACT INFECTION

1. Urinary tract infections can be community acquired, but are often associated with instrumentation of the urinary tract in hospitalized clients.
2. Urinary tract infections can be categorized according to the organ involved: urethritis is inflammation of the urethra; prostatitis is inflammation of the prostate gland; cystitis is inflammation of the urinary bladder; and pyelonephritis is inflammation of the kidney and renal pelvis.
3. Risk factors for the development of urinary tract infection for women include: short, straight urethra, the proximity of the urinary meatus to the vagina and anus, being sexually active, use of diaphragm and spermicidal compounds for birth control, and pregnancy.
4. Risk factors for the development of urinary tract infection for males include being uncircumsized, presence of prostatic hypertrophy, and anal intercourse.

POWERPOINT LECTURE SLIDES

Pathophysiology of Common Urinary Tract Disorders
- Urinary tract infection
  ○ Bacteria colonized in the urethra, vagina, or perineal tissues
- Urinary calculi
  ○ Supersaturation
  ○ Nucleation
  ○ Lack of inhibitory substances
- Urinary tract tumor
  ○ Papillary lesions (papillomas)
  ○ Carcinoma in situ (CIS)
- Urinary retention
  ○ Benign prostatic hypertrophy (BPH)
  ○ Mechanical obstruction
  ○ Acute inflammation

5. Congenital or acquired factors such as urinary tract obstruction by tumors or calculi, structural abnormalities such as strictures, impaired bladder innervation, bowel incontinence, and chronic diseases such as diabetes mellitus increase risk of urinary tract infection for both sexes. Older clients also have greater risk.

6. Acute pyelonephritis is a bacterial infection of the kidney and usually results from an infection that ascends to the kidney from the lower urinary tract. Risk factors include any condition that results in status or backflow of urine.

7. Chronic pyelonephritis involves chronic inflammation of the kidney and is a common cause of renal failure. It may develop as a result of UTI, hypertension or other vascular conditions, severe reflux, or obstructions to the urinary tract.

URINARY CALCULI

8. Three factors contribute to urolithiasis: supersaturation, nucleation, and lack of inhibitory substances in the urine.

9. Types of kidney stones include calcium, uric acid, struvite, staghorn, and cystine.

10. The greatest risk factor for stone development is a prior personal or family history of urinary calculi. Other risk factors include dehydration, immobility, excess dietary intake of calcium, oxalate, or proteins, presence of gout or hyperparathyroidism, urinary stasis, or repeated urinary tract infection.

URINARY TRACT TUMOR

11. The most common site of urinary tract malignancy is the bladder.

12. Risk factors for tumor development include presence of carcinogens in the urine from smoking cigarettes, occupational exposure to dyes or solvents, and chronic urinary tract infections or bladder calculi.

URINARY RETENTION

13. Inability to completely empty the bladder can result from mechanical obstruction of the bladder outlet (commonly from benign prostatic hypertrophy) or from a functional problem that results from disrupted muscle function.

14. Risk factors for the development of urinary retention include abdominal or pelvic surgery and the use of anticholinergic medications or medications with anticholinergic side effects.

NEUROGENIC BLADDER

15. Disruption of the central or peripheral nervous system connections that influence bladder filling, the perception of fullness, the need to void, and bladder emptying may result in neurogenic bladder.

- Neurogenic bladder
  - Disruption at
    - Cerebral cortex
    - Micturition center of midbrain
    - Spinal cord tracts
    - Peripheral nerves of bladder
- Urinary incontinence
  - Pressure within urinary bladder exceeds urethral resistance

16. Spastic bladder dysfunction occurs when there is partial or total interruption of the sensory and voluntary control of urination, but when impulses to the detrusor muscle are intact. The most common cause of this interruption is spinal cord injury above the sacral segment.

17. Flaccid bladder dysfunction occurs when the perception of bladder fullness is lost, the bladder becomes overdistended, and there is weak and ineffective contraction of the detrusor muscle. This is commonly associated with myelomeningocele and during the spinal shock stage of a spinal cord injury above the sacral region.

URINARY INCONTINENCE

18. Urinary incontinence is the most common manifestation of impaired bladder control and is categorized as stress incontinence, urge incontinence, overflow incontinence, functional incontinence, mixed incontinence, and total incontinence.

19. Incontinence results when the pressure within the urinary bladder exceeds urethral resistance, which allows urine to escape. Relaxation of the pelvic musculature, disruption of cerebral and nervous system control, and disturbances of the bladder and its musculature are common contributing factors.

20. Causes of incontinence may be congenital (epispadias, meningomyelocele), acquired (CNS or spinal trauma, stroke, chronic neurologic disorders), or reversible (acute confusion, medication effects, prostatic enlargement, vaginal and uretheral atrophy, UTI, and fecal impaction).

SUGGESTIONS FOR CLASSROOM ACTIVITIES

- Review the anatomy and physiology of the urinary tract.
- Have students develop urinary tract health promotion teaching plans.

SUGGESTIONS FOR CLINICAL ACTIVITIES

- Have students review clinical client health histories for evidence of risk factors for development of urinary disorders.

LEARNING OUTCOME 2

Describe the manifestations of urinary tract disorders, relating manifestations to the pathophysiology of the disorder.

CONCEPTS FOR LECTURE
URINARY TRACT INFECTION (UTI)

1. Cystitis is the most common UTI and tends to remain superficial, and involve bladder mucosa. Hemorrhage of the bladder wall and presence of pus from the inflammatory response is common. Classic manifestations of cystitis are dysuria, frequency, urgency, and nocturia. The urine may be cloudy with a foul odor or hematuria may be present. This is a result of mucus and excess white cells in the urine, and bleeding of the inflamed bladder wall. Suprapubic pain and tenderness may also be present.

POWERPOINT LECTURE SLIDES

Manifestations of Common Urinary Tract Disorders
- Urinary tract infection
  ○ Cystitis
    – Dysuria
    – Frequency
    – Urgency
    – Nocturia
    – Pyuria
    – Hematuria
    – Suprapubic discomfort

2. Classic symptoms of cystitis may be absent in the older individual. Nonspecific manifestations such as nocturia, incontinence, confusion, behavioral changes, lethargy, anorexia, or "not feeling right" may occur. Fever may be present, but hypothermia may also occur.

3. Catheter-associated UTIs are often asymptomatic, but can result in gram-negative bacteremia.

4. Acute pyelonephritis manifests rapidly, with chills and fever, malaise, vomiting, flank pain, costovertebral tenderness, urinary frequency, and dysuria. Symptoms of cystitis may also be present. Older adults may manifest behavior changes, confusion, incontinence, or general deterioration in condition.

5. Chronic pyelonephritis may be asymptomatic or have mild manifestations.

URINARY CALCULI

6. Manifestations may be mild or acute and develop as a result of urine flow obstruction, distention, and tissue trauma. Renal colic is acute, severe flank pain caused by ureteral spasm. Other manifestations may mimic UTI. Gross or microscopic hematuria may be present, with gross hematuria often being the only sign of bladder stones.

7. A major complication of urinary calculi is obstruction, which can lead to urinary stasis with infection or hydronephrosis.

URINARY TRACT TUMOR

8. Manifestations of urinary tract tumor include painless hematuria and signs of urinary tract infection. If the tumor obstructs outflow, colicky pain may occur.

URINARY RETENTION

9. The client with urinary retention is unable to empty the bladder completely and may have overflow voiding or incontinence. Assessment reveals a firm, distended bladder that may be displaced to one side of midline. Percussion reveals a dull tone.

NEUROGENIC BLADDER

10. Manifestations include incontinence, overfilling of the bladder, or incomplete emptying of the bladder.

INCONTINENCE

11. Manifestations include inability to control micturation.

- ○ Acute pyelonephritis
  - – Urinary
    - · Urinary frequency
    - · Dysuria
    - · Pyuria
    - · Hematuria
    - · Flank pain
    - · Costovertebral tenderness
  - – Systemic
    - · Vomiting
    - · Diarrhea
    - · Acute fever
    - · Shaking chills
    - · Malaise
- • Urinary calculi
  - ○ Kidney stones
  - ○ Ureteral stones
  - ○ Bladder stones
- • Urinary tract tumor
  - ○ Painless hematuria
  - ○ Frequency
  - ○ Urgency
  - ○ Dysuria
  - ○ Colicky pain
- • Urinary retention
  - ○ Inability to empty bladder completely
  - ○ Overflow voiding or incontinence
- • Neurogenic bladder
  - ○ Incontinence, overfilling or incomplete emptying of bladder
- • Urinary incontinence
  - ○ Inability to control micturition

LEARNING OUTCOME 3

Discuss tests used to diagnose disorders affecting the urinary tract with their nursing implications.

CONCEPTS FOR LECTURE

URINARY TRACT INFECTION

1. Laboratory testing includes: urinalysis, gram stain of urine, urine culture and sensitivity, and WBC with differential.
2. Additional diagnostic testing may include: intravenous pyelography, voiding cystourethrography, cystoscopy, and manual pelvic or prostate examinations.

URINARY CALCULI

3. Laboratory testing includes urinalysis, chemical analysis of any stones passed, measurement of urine calcium, uric acid, and oxalate levels, and measurement of serum calcium, phosphorus, and uric acid levels.
4. Diagnostic testing includes KUB (flat plate x-ray of the kidney, ureters, and bladder), renal ultrasonography, CT scan, IVP, and cystoscopy.

URINARY TRACT TUMOR

5. Laboratory testing includes urinalysis for hematuria and urine cytology.
6. Diagnostic testing includes ultrasound of the bladder, IVP, cystoscopy, ureteroscopy, CT scan, and MRI.

URINARY RETENTION

7. Diagnostic testing includes bladder scan and catheterization for residual urine.

NEUROGENIC BLADDER

8. Laboratory testing includes urine culture, urinalysis, serum BUN, and serum creatinine.
9. Diagnostic testing includes post-void catheterization for residual urine and cystometrography.

INCONTINENCE

10. Laboratory testing includes urinalysis and urine culture.
11. Diagnostic testing includes catheterization for post-voiding residual volume, cystometrography, uroflowmetry, IVP, cystoscopy, and ultrasonography.

POWERPOINT LECTURE SLIDES

Diagnostic Testing for Urinary Disorders
- Urinary tract infection
  - Urinalysis, gram stain of urine, urine culture and sensitivity, WBC with differential
  - Intravenous pyelography, voiding cystourethrography, cystoscopy, and manual pelvic or prostate examinations
- Urinary calculi
  - Urinalysis, chemical analysis of any stones passed, measurement of urine calcium, uric acid, and oxalate levels, and measurement of serum calcium, phosphorus, and uric acid levels
  - KUB (flat plate x-ray of the kidney, ureters, and bladder), renal ultrasonography, CT scan, IVP, and cystoscopy
- Urinary tract tumor
  - Urinalysis for hematuria and urine cytology
  - Ultrasound of the bladder, IVP, cystoscopy, ureteroscopy, CT scan, and MRI
- Urinary retention
  - Bladder scan and catheterization for residual urine
- Neurogenic bladder
  - Urine culture, urinalysis, serum BUN, and serum creatinine
  - Post-void catheterization for residual urine and cystometrography
- Incontinence
  - Urinalysis and urine culture
  - Catheterization for post-voiding residual volume, cystometrography, uroflowmetry, IVP, cystoscopy, and ultrasonography

LEARNING OUTCOME 4

Discuss the nursing implications of medications and treatments prescribed for clients with urinary tract disorders.

CONCEPTS FOR LECTURE
URINARY TRACT INFECTIONS

1. Uncomplicated lower urinary tract infections may be treated with short course antibiotics which reduces treatment costs, increases compliance, and has a lower rate of side effects. A 3-day course of treatment is generally preferred over a 1-day course. Commonly prescribed drugs are trimethoprim-sulfamethoxazole (TMP-SMZ), TMP, or a quinalone antibiotic such as ciprofloxacin (Cipro). Phenazophyridine (Pyridium) is a urinary analgesic and is also often prescribed.

2. Clients with pyelonephritis, urinary tract abnormalities or stones, or a history of previous antibiotic-resistant infections require 7–10 days of therapy. Commonly prescribed drugs are TMP-SMZ, ciprofloxacin (Cipro), or ofloxacin (Floxin).

3. Severely ill clients may require hospitalization with administration of intravenous medications such as ciprofloxacin (Cipro), gentamicin (Garamycin), ceftriaxone (Rocephin), or ampicillin (Polycillin).

4. Follow-up urine culture is scheduled 10 days to 2 weeks after treatment completion to ensure eradication of bacteria from the urinary tract.

5. Clients with frequent symptomatic UTI may be treated with TMP-SMZ, TMP, or nitrofurantoin (Furadantin).

6. Common nursing diagnoses include: Pain, Impaired Urinary Elimination, and Ineffective Health Maintenance. Community-based care education should include information on risk factors for development of UTI, early manifestations, how to maintain an optimal immune system, the importance of completing prescribed treatments and keeping follow-up appointments, and minimizing the risk of UTI if an indwelling urinary catheter is necessary.

POWERPOINT LECTURE SLIDES

Medication and Treatments for Urinary Tract Disorders
- Urinary tract infections
  - Medications: short or long course antibiotics, urinary analgesics, hospitalization for IV antibiotics may be required
  - Follow-up urine culture 10 days to 2 weeks after treatment completion
- Urinary calculi
  - Medications: pain relief, often with IV morphine sulfate
  - Hydration with oral or intravenous fluids
  - Analysis of stone composition
    - Medications to inhibit further stone formation
  - Diet modification
- Urinary tract tumor
  - Intravesical instillation of immunologic or chemotherapeutic agents
- Urine retention
  - Indwelling catheter or intermittent catheterization
  - Cholinergic medications
- Neurogenic bladder
  - Medications
    - Increase or decrease contractility of the detrusor muscle
    - Increase or decrease tone of the internal sphincter
    - Relax the external urethral sphincter
  - Nutritional measures
  - Bladder retraining or intermittent catheterization

URINARY CALCULI

7. Focus of immediate care is pain relief, often with intravenous morphine sulfate or indomethacin (Indocin) by suppository, and hydration with oral or intravenous fluids.

8. After analysis of stone composition, various medications may be ordered to inhibit or prevent further stone development.

9. Diet modification may be necessary to change the composition of the urine for prevention of further stone development. Increase fluid intake is often prescribed regardless of stone composition.

10. Common nursing diagnoses include: Acute Pain, Impaired Urinary Elimination, and Deficient Knowledge. Community-based care education should include the importance of maintaining fluid intake; information about medication; dietary recommendations; prevention, recognition, and management of UTI; how to change dressings if indicated; assessment of wound for healing if indicated; and how to manage drainage systems if present.

URINARY TRACT TUMOR

11. The primary treatment of bladder cancer includes the intravesical instillation of immunologic or chemotherapeutic agents.

12. Common nursing diagnoses include: Impaired Urinary Elimination, Disturbed Body Image, and Risk for Infection. Community-based care education should include teaching about signs of tumor recurrence, care of stoma if indicated, prevention of urine reflux and infection, indications of possible UTI and renal calculi, and use of clean technique in self-catheterization if indicated.

URINE RETENTION

13. Clients with urinary retention may be treated with an indwelling urinary catheter or with intermittent straight catheterization.

14. Close review of medications is necessary. A medication with no anticholinergic side effects may be substituted when retention is a problem.

15. Cholinergic medications such as bethanechol chloride (Urotone) may be used to promote detrusor muscle contraction and bladder emptying.

16. The primary nursing diagnosis is Impaired Urinary Elimination. Community-based care education includes intermittent catheterization if indicated, avoidance of over-the-counter medications with an anticholinergic effect, bladder training information, and information regarding care of an indwelling urinary catheter if indicated.

- Incontinence
  - ○ Medications: dependent upon type of incontinence
  - ○ Complementary therapies: biofeedback, relaxation techniques

NEUROGENIC BLADDER

17. Medications may be prescribed to increase or decrease contractility of the detrusor muscle, increase or decrease tone of the internal sphincter, or to relax the external urethral sphincter.

18. Nutritional measures to reduce risk for UTI and urinary calculi are often suggested.

19. Clients with spastic neurogenic bladder may require bladder retraining to stimulate reflex voiding, allowing for scheduled toileting. The client with a flaccid bladder may require intermittent catheterization on a routine schedule.

20. Common nursing diagnoses include: Impaired Urinary Elimination, Self-Care Deficit: Toileting, Risk for Impaired Skin Integrity, and Risk for Infection. Community-based care education includes measures to stimulate reflex voiding and promote bladder emptying, use of prescribed medication, and manifestations of UTI or calculi with measures to reduce the risk of those complications.

INCONTINENCE

21. Phenylpropanolamine administration may reduce episodes of mild stress incontinence. Estrogen therapy may improve incontinence associated with postmenopausal atrophic vaginitis, and preparations that increase bladder capacity are useful in the treatment of urge incontinence.

22. Complementary therapies include biofeedback and relaxation techniques.

23. Common nursing diagnoses include: Urinary Incontinence: Stress and/or Urge, Self-Care Deficit: Toileting, and Social Isolation. Community-based education includes causes of incontinence and their treatment, fluid intake management, perineal care, and products for clothing protection.

SUGGESTIONS FOR CLASSROOM ACTIVITIES

- Have students research complementary therapies for prevention and treatment of urinary tract infection.
- Using the case study "Urinary Tract Infection" provided on the textbook Companion Website, lead students through the development of a nursing care plan for this client's care.
- Have students develop a teaching plan to assist clients in compliance with diet modifications necessary for various stone compositions.
- Have students develop a nursing plan of care for clients experiencing urinary calculi.

SUGGESTIONS FOR CLINICAL ACTIVITIES

- Have students review clinical client medication records for medications used to treat urinary disorders. Require medication information cards that list nursing implications of therapy with those medications.
- Have students review clinical client medication records for medications that may have side effects that affect the urinary tract. Discuss alternative medications or treatments.

LEARNING OUTCOME 5

Describe surgical procedures used in treating urinary tract disorders.

CONCEPTS FOR LECTURE

URINARY TRACT INFECTION

1. Surgery such as ureteroplasty with stent placement may be indicated in cases of recurrent UTI if stones, structural abnormalities, or strictures are present.

URINARY CALCULI

2. The preferred treatment for urinary calculi is lithotripsy. Extracorporeal shock wave lithotripsy is the noninvasive technique. Other forms of lithotripsy include percutaneous ultrasonic lithotripsy and laser lithotripsy. Stent placement often follows lithotripsy procedures.
3. Surgical procedures may be necessary to remove calculi. Variations of this procedure include ureterolithotomy (incision into the ureter), pyelolithotomy (incision into the kidney pelvis), and nephrolithotomy (incision into the body of the kidney).
4. Bladder stones may be removed through cystoscopy.

URINARY TRACT TUMOR

5. Surgical treatment ranges from simple resection of noninvasive tumors to removal of the bladder. If tumors are located in sites other than the bladder, other surgical procedures may be necessary.
6. Invasive cancer of the bladder results in cystectomy (bladder removal); removal of prostate and seminal vessels in males that results in impotence; and removal of uterus, uterine tubes, and ovaries that results in sterility in females. At the time of surgery a urinary diversion, either an ileal conduit or continent urinary diversion, is created.
7. Radiation is another adjunctive treatment of urinary tract tumor.

URINARY RETENTION

8. Surgical procedures such as resection of the prostate gland and stricture removal may be necessary in the client with urinary retention.

NEUROGENIC BLADDER

9. Surgery may be required when urination cannot be controlled using more conservative measures. Surgical procedures include rhizotomy to destroy the nerve supply to the detrusor muscle or external sphincter, urinary diversion, or implantation of an artificial sphincter.

INCONTINENCE

10. Surgery may be used to treat stress incontinence associated with cystocele or urethrocele and overflow incontinence associated with enlargement of the prostate gland.

POWERPOINT LECTURE SLIDES

Surgical Procedures Used in Treating Urinary Tract Disorders
- Urinary tract infection
  - Ureteroplasty with stent placement
- Urinary calculi
  - Lithotripsy with stent placement
  - Ureterolithotomy, pyelolithotomy, nephrolithotomy
  - Cystoscopy
- Urinary tract tumor
  - Simple resection to removal of bladder
  - Cystectomy
  - Urinary diversion
  - Radiation
- Urinary retention
  - Resection of prostate and/or stricture removal
- Neurogenic bladder
  - Rhizotomy, urinary diversion, implantation of artificial sphincter
- Incontinence
  - Surgery to correct cystocele or urethrocele

SUGGESTIONS FOR CLASSROOM ACTIVITIES

- Arrange a guest lecture by a registered nurse who works in a lithotripsy unit.
- Discuss the nursing care implications of cystectomy.
- Arrange a guest lecture by a client who has undergone cystectomy.
- Discuss the possible results of prostate gland resection.

SUGGESTIONS FOR CLINICAL ACTIVITIES

- Arrange for students to observe in a lithotripsy unit.
- Arrange for students to attend a meeting of a support group for clients who have undergone cystectomy.

CHAPTER 29
NURSING CARE OF CLIENTS WITH KIDNEY DISORDERS

RESOURCE LIBRARY

 PRENTICE HALL NURSING MEDIALINK DVD-ROM

Audio Glossary
NCLEX-RN® Review
Animation/Video
  Furosemide
  The Kidney

🌐 COMPANION WEBSITE

Audio Glossary
NCLEX-RN® Review
Care Plan Activity: Acute Glomerulonephritis
Case Studies
  Acute Glomerulonephritis
  Kidney Transplant
MediaLink Applications
  Kidney Disorders
  Renal Insufficiency
Links to Resources

📖 IMAGE LIBRARY

Figure 29.1 A polycystic kidney.
Figure 29.2 The pathogenesis of glomerulonephritis.
Figure 29.3 Severe edema characteristic of nephrotic syndrome.
Figure 29.4 Incisions used for kidney surgery.
Figure 29.5 Acute tubular necrosis.
Figure 29.6 *A*, The components of a hemodialysis system. *B*, A woman receiving kidney dialysis.
Figure 29.7 Continuous arteriovenous hemofiltration (CAVH).
Figure 29.8 An arteriovenous fistula.

Figure 29.9 *A*, Peritoneal dialysis. *B*, Woman receiving peritoneal dialysis.
Figure 29.10 The most common causes of chronic renal failure.
Figure 29.11 The relationship of renal function to BUN and serum creatinine values through the course of chronic renal failure.
Figure 29.12 Placement of a transplanted kidney in the iliac fossa with anastomosis to the hypogastric artery, iliac vein, and bladder.

LEARNING OUTCOME 1

Describe the pathophysiology of common kidney disorders, relating pathophysiology to normal physiology and manifestations of the disorder.

CONCEPTS FOR LECTURE
CONGENITAL KIDNEY MALFORMATION

1. Developmental malformations such as agenesis (absence of kidney) and hypoplasia (underdevelopment of kidney) typically affect only one of the paired organs, so renal function remains normal unless the unaffected kidney is compromised.
2. Abnormal position of the kidneys affects urine flow and increases risk for urinary tract infection and stone formation.
3. Horseshoe kidney is a condition where the two kidneys are fused at either the upper or lower pole. Kidney function is not typically affected, but there is an increased risk for hydronephrosis, UTI, and renal calculi.

POWERPOINT LECTURE SLIDES

Pathophysiology of Common Kidney Disorders
- Congenital kidney malformation
  - Agenesis—absence of kidney
  - Hypoplasia—underdevelopment of kidney
  - Alterations in kidney position—affects ureters and urine flow
  - Horseshoe kidney—increased risk for hydronephrosis
- Polycystic kidney disease
  - Autosomal dominant—common form affecting adults
  - Cyst formation and massive kidney enlargement

POLYCYSTIC KIDNEY DISEASE

4. Polycystic kidney disease is characterized by cyst formation and massive kidney enlargement. The two forms include the more common autosomal dominant form that affects adults, and the rarer autosomal recessive form that is present at birth.

5. As the renal cysts develop, fill, and enlarge, renal blood vessels and tissues are compressed and compromised.

6. Persons with polycystic kidney disease often develop cysts in other areas of the body such as the liver, spleen, pancreas, and other organs. Diverticular disease of the colon is common.

7. Manifestations of polycystic kidney disease include flank pain, hematuria, proteinuria, polyuria, nocturia, UTI, renal calculi, hypertension, and presence of palpable kidneys that feel large and knobby.

GLOMERULAR DISORDER

8. Glomerular disorder may be primary (often immunologic or idiopathic in origin) or secondary to a multisystem disease or hereditary condition.

9. Glomerular disease affects the structure and function of the glomerulus and disrupts glomerular filtration. The capillary membrane becomes more permeable which results in hematuria, proteinuria, and edema.

10. Acute glomerulonephritis is inflammation of the glomerular capillary membrane. The most common form is acute poststreptococcal glomerulonephritis, also known as acute proliferative glomerulonephritis, which occurs subsequent to an infection of the pharynx or skin with group A beta-hemolytic streptococcus. Staphylococcal or viral infections can lead to a similar postinfectious acute glomerulonephritis.

11. Manifestations of acute proliferative glomerulonephritis include abrupt onset of hematuria, proteinuria, salt and water retention, azotemia, brown or cola-colored urine, periorbital and dependent edema, hypertension, fatigue, anorexia, nausea, vomiting, and headache.

12. Rapidly progressive glomerulonephritis (RPGN) is characterized by manifestations of severe glomerular injury without a specific, identifiable cause. RPGN may be idiopathic or secondary to systemic disorder. Glomerular cells proliferate and form lesions that obliterate Bowman's space. RPGN leads to rapid, progressive decline in renal function with rapid decline to irreversible renal failure.

13. Manifestations of RPGN are weakness, nausea, vomiting, history of flu-like illness, oliguria, abdominal pain, moderate hypertension, hematuria, and massive proteinuria.

14. Goodpasture's syndrome is a rare autoimmune disorder of unknown etiology and is characterized by formation of antibodies to the glomerular and alveolar basement membranes. These antibodies interfere with normal glomerular and alveolar function.

- ○ Cysts in other areas
- ○ Diverticular disease
- ○ Congential intracranial aneurysm
- ○ Heart valve defects
- Glomerular disorder
  - ○ Primary
    - – Acute glomerulonephritis
    - – Rapidly progressive glomerulonephritis
    - – Chronic glomerulonephritis
    - – Nephritic syndrome
  - ○ Secondary
    - – Diabetic nephropathy
    - – Lupus nephritis
- Vascular kidney disorder
  - ○ Renal function is dependent upon adequate blood supply
  - ○ Hypertension can result from or cause kidney disease
  - ○ Renal artery or venous occlusion
  - ○ Renal artery stenosis
- Kidney trauma
  - ○ Blunt trauma most common
  - ○ Penetrating injuries
    - – Hematuria, flank or abdominal pain, oliguria, anuria
- Renal tumor
  - ○ Benign are infrequent, malignant can be primary or secondary
  - ○ Often silent with few manifestations
  - ○ Often result in paraneoplastic syndrome
    - – Hypercalcemia, hypertension, and hyperglycemia
- Acute renal failure
  - ○ Prerenal, intrinsic or intrarenal, and postrenal
  - ○ Most common cause: ischemia, nephrotoxins
- Chronic renal failure
  - ○ Progressive renal tissue destruction with loss of function
  - ○ Eventually progresses to end stage renal disease (ESRD)
  - ○ Chronic renal failure stages
    - – Decreased renal reserve
    - – Renal insufficiency
    - – Renal failure
    - – ESRD

15. Renal manifestations of Goodpasture's syndrome include hematuria, proteinuria, and edema with rapid progression to renal failure. Respiratory manifestations include cough, SOB, and hemoptysis that can lead to life-threatening pulmonary hemorrhage.

16. Nephrotic syndrome is a group of clinical findings, not a specific disorder and is associated with minimal change disease (MCD), membranous glomerulonephropathy, focal sclerosis, and membranoproliferative glomerulonephritis. Nephrotic syndrome is characterized by massive proteinuria, hypoalbuminemia, hyperlipidemia, edema, and disruption of the coagulation system.

17. Chronic glomerulonephritis is typically the end stage of other glomerular disorders, but can also occur when no previous glomerular disease is present. The disorder is characterized by slow, progressive destruction of glomeruli and gradual decline in renal function.

18. Diabetic nephropathy is common in the later stages of DM and results in glomerulosclerosis.

19. Lupus nephritis develops in clients with SLE and may have an insidious or fulminant onset.

VASCULAR KIDNEY DISORDER

20. Renal function is dependent upon adequate blood supply.

21. Hypertension can result from or cause kidney disease.

22. Renal artery or venous occlusion can occur from a primary process that affects renal vessels or by emboli, clots, or other foreign material. Manifestations depend upon how rapidly the occlusion occurs.

23. Renal artery stenosis is generally the result of atherosclerosis in men, but may be caused by fibromuscular dysplasia in young women. This disorder is suspected when hypertension develops before age 30 or after age 50 with no previous history of high blood pressure.

KIDNEY TRAUMA

24. Blunt trauma is the most common cause of kidney damage. Injury ranges from small contusions or hematomas, to fragmentation or shattering of the kidney that causes significant blood loss and urine extravasation. Tearing of the renal vessels may cause rapid hemorrhage and death.

25. Penetrating injuries range from minor capsule or cortex lacerations to destruction of renal parenchyma or vascular supply. Renal vessel and renal pelvis lacerations are critical injuries.

26. Primary manifestations of kidney trauma are hematuria, flank or abdominal pain, and oliguria or anuria. Localized swelling, tenderness, or ecchymoses in the flank region may occur.

RENAL TUMOR

27. Benign renal tumors are infrequent; malignant renal tumors can be primary or secondary.

28. Renal tumors are often silent with few manifestations, but the classic triad is gross hematuria, flank pain, and a palpable abdominal mass. Systemic manifestations include fever without infection, fatigue, and weight loss.

29. Renal tumors often result in paraneoplastic syndrome with such manifestations as hypercalcemia, hypertension, and hyperglycemia.

ACUTE RENAL FAILURE

30. Acute renal failure (ARF) is a rapid decline in renal function with azotemia and fluid and electrolyte imbalance. The most common causes are ischemia and nephrotoxins.

31. The causes and pathophysiology of ARF are commonly categorized as prerenal, intrinsic or intrarenal, and postrenal.

32. Acute tubular necrosis (ATN) causes abrupt and progressive decline of renal function. Prolonged ischemia is the primary cause of ATN, but it can occur from ingestion of nephrotoxic substances, hemolysis of red blood cells, and rhabdomyolysis.

33. The course of ARF that is caused by ATN has three phases: initiation, maintenance, and recovery.

CHRONIC RENAL FAILURE

34. Chronic renal failure is the progressive destruction of renal tissue with loss of function. Eventually the kidneys are unable to excrete metabolic wastes and regulate fluid and electrolyte balance adequate. This condition is known as end stage renal disease (ESRD).

35. Chronic renal failure develops through stages identified as: decreased renal reserve, renal insufficiency, renal failure, and ESRD.

36. Manifestations of CRF affect all body systems.

SUGGESTIONS FOR CLASSROOM ACTIVITIES

- Review the kidney animation provided on the textbook DVD-ROM.
- Use anatomical models to help students visualize the interrelationships of urinary tract organs and how damage in one area can affect another area.

SUGGESTIONS FOR CLINICAL ACTIVITIES

- Review clinical client medical records, health histories, and assessments for indications of kidney disorder. Help students relate those manifestations to the specific disorder.

LEARNING OUTCOME 2

Discuss risk factors for kidney disorders and nursing care to reduce these risks.

CONCEPTS FOR LECTURE
GLOMERULAR DISORDERS

1. Risk factors for development of primary glomerular disorders such as acute proliferative glomerulonephritis include infection with a group A beta-hemolytic streptococcus. Staphylococcal and viral infections are also implicated. Nursing support of early and effective

POWERPOINT LECTURE SLIDES

Risk Factors for Kidney Disorders
- Glomerular disorder
  - Primary glomerular disorders: infection with a group A beta-hemolytic streptococcus, staphylococcus and viruses

---

treatment of these infections can lessen their severity and the possibility of renal involvement.

2. Secondary glomerular disorders can be related to the presence of chronic systemic diseases. Nursing management of those conditions should include measures to reduce the risk of associated nephritis, such as effectively managing the diseases, treating hypertension, and avoiding drugs and substances that are potentially toxic to the kidneys.

VASCULAR KIDNEY DISORDER

3. Since vascular kidney disorder is often a result of vessel damage from hypertension or the presence of emboli, management of such disorders as atrial fibrillation and hypertension are essential. Nursing management includes education about the disease process, medications, and treatments.

KIDNEY TRAUMA

4. The most common causes of kidney trauma are blunt force and penetrating injuries. Educating clients about routine personal safety and good health practices may help to prevent these injuries.

RENAL TUMOR

5. Major risk factors for the development of renal cancers are smoking and obesity. Chronic irritation from renal calculi may also contribute. Nursing management includes education about smoking cessation and a healthy diet. Specific dietary and medication education may be required to reduce the risk of calculi development.

ACUTE RENAL FAILURE

6. Risk factors for the development of acute renal failure can be divided into prerenal, intrarenal, and postrenal factors. Nursing education for risk factor management can include support of hydration, control of systemic diseases, and careful management of obstructive disorders such as renal calculi and benign prostatic hypertrophy.

CHRONIC RENAL FAILURE

7. Since chronic renal failure often results from acute renal failure, nursing management of risk factors includes astute care of clients with any kidney disorder.

- Need early and effective treatment of these infections
- Secondary glomerular disorders: related to presence of chronic systemic diseases
  - Need measures to reduce the risk of associated nephritis
- Vascular kidney disorder
  - Often a result of vessel damage from hypertension or presence of emboli
  - Need management of such disorders as atrial fibrillation and hypertension
- Kidney trauma
  - Often result of blunt force and penetrating injuries
  - Routine personal safety and good health practices
- Renal tumor
  - Major risk factors: smoking and obesity
  - Contributing factor: chronic irritation from renal calculi
  - Need education about smoking cessation and healthy diet
  - Need specific dietary and medication education to reduce risk of calculi
- Acute renal failure
  - Risk factors: prerenal, intrarenal, and post-renal
  - Education include support of hydration, control of systemic diseases, and management of obstructive disorders
- Chronic renal failure
  - Often results from acute renal failure
  - Astute care of clients with any kidney disorder

SUGGESTIONS FOR CLASSROOM ACTIVITIES

- Have students develop a "life plan" for the maintenance of healthy kidney function.

SUGGESTIONS FOR CLINICAL ACTIVITIES

- Help students identify clinical clients with kidney disorders. Have students develop a teaching plan for clients that will help the client manage risk factors for kidney disorders.
- Discuss the difference between activities designed to improve kidney health and those designed to reduce progression to ESRD.

LEARNING OUTCOME 3

Explain diagnostic studies used to identify disorders of the kidneys and their effects.

CONCEPTS FOR LECTURE

CONGENITAL KIDNEY MALFORMATION

1. Renal ultrasonography and IVP are used to diagnose malformations.

POLYCYSTIC KIDNEY DISEASE

2. Renal ultrasonography, IVP, and CT scans are used to diagnose polycystic kidney disease.

GLOMERULAR DISORDER

3. Laboratory tests include: throat or skin cultures, anti-streptolysin O (ASO) titers, erythrocyte sedimentation rate (ESR), BUN, serum creatinine, urine creatinine, creatinine clearance, serum electrolytes, and urinalysis.
4. Diagnostic tests include: KUB abdominal x-ray, kidney scans, and biopsy.

VASCULAR KIDNEY DISORDER

5. Laboratory tests include: blood chemistry and renal enzyme levels.
6. Diagnostic tests include renal ultrasound and renal angiography.
7. Renal artery stenosis diagnosis may include a captopril test for renin activity.

KIDNEY TRAUMA

8. Laboratory tests include: hemoglobin and hematocrit, urinalysis, and AST levels.
9. Diagnostic tests include: renal ultrasonography, CT scan, IVP, and renal arteriography.

RENAL TUMOR

10. Diagnostic tests include: renal ultrasonography, CT scan, IVP, MRI, renal angiography, orthography, inferior venacavography, chest x-ray, bone scan, and liver function studies.

ACUTE RENAL FAILURE

11. Laboratory testing includes: urinalysis, serum creatinine, BUN, serum electrolytes, arterial blood gases, and CBC.
12. Diagnostic testing includes: renal ultrasonography, CT scan, IVP, and renal biopsy.

CHRONIC RENAL FAILURE

13. Laboratory testing includes: urinalysis, urine culture, BUN and serum creatinine, creatinine clearance, serum electrolytes, and CBC.
14. Diagnostic testing includes: renal ultrasonography and kidney biopsy.

POWERPOINT LECTURE SLIDES

Diagnostic Studies to Identify Kidney Disorders
- Congenital kidney malformation
  - Diagnostic tests: renal ultrasound and IVP
- Polycystic kidney disease
  - Diagnostic tests: renal ultrasound, IVP, CT
- Glomerular disease
  - Laboratory: throat or skin cultures, antistreptolysin O (ASO) titers, and erythrocyte sedimentation rate (ESR), BUN, serum creatinine, urine creatinine, creatinine clearance, serum electrolytes, and urinalysis
  - Diagnostic: KUB abdominal x-ray, kidney scans, biopsy
- Vascular kidney disorder
  - Laboratory: blood chemistry and renal enzyme levels
  - Diagnostic: renal ultrasound and renal angiography
  - Renal artery stenosis diagnosis: captopril test for renin activity
- Kidney trauma
  - Laboratory: H&H, urinalysis, AST levels
  - Diagnostic: renal ultrasonography, CT scan, IVP, renal arteriography
- Renal tumor
  - Diagnostic: ultrasound, CT, MRI, IVP, angiography, aortography, inferior venacavography, chest x-ray, bone scan, liver function testing
- Acute renal failure
  - Laboratory: urinalysis, serum creatinine, BUN, serum electrolytes, ABGs, CBC
  - Diagnostic: renal ultrasonography, CT scan, IVP, renal biopsy
- Chronic renal failure
  - Laboratory: urinalysis, urine culture, BUN and serum creatinine, creatinine clearance, serum electrolytes, and CBC.
  - Diagnostic: renal ultrasonography and kidney biopsy

LEARNING OUTCOME 4

Discuss the effects and nursing implications for medications and treatments used for clients with kidney disorders.

CONCEPTS FOR LECTURE

CONGENITAL KIDNEY MALFORMATION

1. Nursing care is primarily educational and is focused on health promotion.
2. Clients with horseshoe kidney may require surgical resection of the connection between kidneys.

POLYCYSTIC KIDNEY DISEASE

3. Hypertension associated with polycystic kidney disease is generally controlled using angiotensin-converting enzyme inhibitors or other antihypertensive medications.
4. Ultimately clients will experience end-stage renal failure that requires dialysis or renal transplantation. Genetic counseling and screening of family members is important.
5. Common nursing diagnoses are Excess Fluid Volume, Anticipatory Grieving, Deficient Knowledge, and Risk for Ineffective Coping.

GLOMERULAR DISORDER

6. No medications are available to cure glomerular disease, so medication use is focused on treating underlying disorders, reducing inflammation, and managing symptoms.
7. Treatments may include bed rest, limitation of sodium intake, dietary protein restriction, plasmapheresis, and dialysis.
8. Common nursing diagnoses include: Excessive Fluid Volume, Fatigue, and Ineffective Role Performance.

VASCULAR KIDNEY DISORDER

9. Clients who are experiencing vascular kidney disorder may undergo surgery or anticoagulant therapy. Hypertension control is essential.

KIDNEY TRAUMA

10. Treatment for minor kidney trauma is conservative, and includes bed rest and monitoring. More major trauma treatment focuses on controlling hemorrhage

POWERPOINT LECTURE SLIDES

Effects and Implications for Kidney Disorder Medications and Treatments
- Congenital kidney malformation
  - Nursing care is primarily educational
  - Focus on health promotion
  - Clients with horseshoe kidneys may require surgery
- Polycystic kidney disease
  - ACE inhibitors or other anti-hypertensives
  - Clients will ultimately require dialysis or transplant
  - Genetic testing important
- Glomerular disease
  - No medications available for cure
  - Focus on treating underlying disorders, reducing inflammation, managing symptoms
  - Treatments: bedrest, sodium/protein restriction, plasmapheresis, dialysis
- Vascular kidney disorder
  - Surgery, anticoagulant therapy, hypertension control
- Kidney trauma
  - Treatment for minor kidney trauma is conservative
  - More major trauma treatment focuses on controlling hemorrhage and treating or preventing shock
  - Nursing care focus: assessment and timely intervention to prevent complications
- Renal tumor
  - Treatment: radical nephrectomy; chemotherapy generally not effective
- Acute renal failure
  - Treatment focus: restoration/maintenance of renal perfusion, elimination of nephrotoxic substances
  - Common treatments: IV fluids, Dopamine infusion, diuretics, aggressive hypertension management, antacids, histamine H2-receptor antagonists or proton-pump inhibitors, and

and treating or preventing shock. Removal of damaged kidney tissue may be required. Nursing care focuses on assessment and timely intervention to prevent complications.

RENAL TUMOR

11. Treatment includes radical nephrectomy. Chemotherapy is generally not effective.
12. Nursing diagnoses include: Pain, Risk for Impaired Urinary Elimination, and Anticipatory Grieving. Teaching includes measures to protect the remaining kidney.

ACUTE RENAL FAILURE

13. Focus of treatment is restoration and maintenance of renal perfusion and elimination of nephrotoxic substances.
14. Common treatments include IV fluids, dopamine infusion, diuretics, aggressive hypertension management, antacids, histamine H2-receptor antagonists or proton-pump inhibitors, and methods to control hyperkalemia and hyperphosphatemia. Dialysis may be required.
15. Nursing diagnoses include: Excess Fluid Volume, Imbalanced Nutrition: Less than Body Requirements, and Deficient Knowledge. Teaching includes avoiding exposure to nephrotoxins; preventing infection; monitoring weight, blood pressure, and pulse; manifestations of relapse; and dietary restrictions.

CHRONIC RENAL FAILURE

16. Chronic renal failure affects both the pharmacokinetic and pharmacodynamic effects of drug therapy.
17. Commonly administered medications include drugs to manage fluid balance, electrolyte imbalance, and anemia.
18. Nutrition and fluid management is necessary as renal function declines.
19. When fluid and electrolyte balances can no longer be managed by pharmacologic and dietary changes, renal replacement therapies such as dialysis or kidney transplantation are considered.
20. Common nursing diagnoses include: Impaired Tissue Perfusion: Renal, Imbalanced Nutrition: Less than Body Requirements, Risk for Infection, and Disturbed Body Image.
21. Education needs include topics necessary for the day-to-day care of a seriously ill client at home.

methods to control hyperkalemia and hyperphosphatemia
  ○ Dialysis may be required
• Chronic renal failure
  ○ Affects pharmacokinetics and pharmacodynamics of drug therapy
  ○ Medications include drugs to manage fluid balance, electrolyte imbalance, and anemia
  ○ Nutrition and fluid management as renal function declines
  ○ Dialysis or kidney transplant becomes necessary when medication/dietary treatments are no longer effective

---

SUGGESTIONS FOR CLASSROOM ACTIVITIES

• Review the case study and care plan activity about acute glomerulonephritis that are provided on the textbook Companion Website.

SUGGESTIONS FOR CLINICAL ACTIVITIES

• Have students investigate methods for individualizing standard "textbook" interventions to the care of the specific client with kidney disorder.

LEARNING OUTCOME 5

Compare and contrast dialysis procedures used to manage acute and chronic renal failure.

CONCEPTS FOR LECTURE

1. The most common therapies for ESRD in the United States are hemodialysis, peritoneal dialysis, and kidney transplant.
2. Hemodialysis is most commonly performed in a dialysis center and is typically done three times a week for a total of 9–12 hours.
3. The most common type of peritoneal dialysis is continuous ambulatory peritoneal dialysis (CAPD). Another type of peritoneal dialysis is continuous cyclic peritoneal dialysis (CCPD).
4. Each type of dialysis has advantages and disadvantages.
5. Kidney transplant is the treatment of choice for many clients with ESRD. The transplanted organ may come from a living donor or may be from a cadaver.

POWERPOINT LECTURE SLIDES

Dialysis Procedures to Manage Renal Failure
- Renal replacement therapies
  - Hemodialysis
  - Peritoneal dialysis
  - Kidney transplant
- Hemodialysis
  - Dialysis center
  - Three times/week, 9–12 total hours
- Peritoneal dialysis
  - Continuous ambulatory peritoneal dialysis
  - Continuous cyclic peritoneal dialysis
- Kidney transplant
  - May be living donor or cavaderic

SUGGESTIONS FOR CLASSROOM ACTIVITIES

- Arrange for a registered nurse who works in a dialysis unit to speak to the class.
- Arrange for a hemodialysis client to speak to the class.
- Have students plan a 1-month traveling vacation for a client who is on hemodialysis and for a client who is on peritoneal dialysis. Compare and contrast issues for each client.

SUGGESTIONS FOR CLINICAL ACTIVITIES

- Arrange for clinical students to visit a dialysis unit.
- Have students develop an assessment documentation flow sheet for clients undergoing routine hemodialysis.

CHAPTER 30

ASSESSING CLIENTS WITH CARDIAC DISORDERS

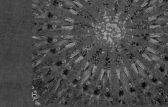

RESOURCE LIBRARY

 PRENTICE HALL NURSING MEDIALINK DVD-ROM

Audio Glossary
NCLEX-RN® Review
Animation/Videos
   Cardiac A&P
   Dysrhythmias
   Heart Sounds
   Hemodynamics
   Oxygen Transport

 COMPANION WEBSITE

Audio Glossary
NCLEX-RN® Review
Care Plan Activity: Cardiac Catheterization
Case Study: Chest Pain
MediaLink Application: Heart Sounds
Links to Resources

📖 **IMAGE LIBRARY**

Figure 30.1 Location of the heart in the mediastinum of the thorax.
Figure 30.2 Coverings and layers of the heart.
Figure 30.3 The internal anatomy of the heart, frontal section.
Figure 30.4 Pulmonary and systemic circulation.
Figure 30.5 Coronary circulation.
Figure 30.6 The cardiac cycle has three events: (1) ventricular filling in mid-to-late diastole,

(2) ventricular systole, and (3) isovolumetric relaxation in early diastole.
Figure 30.7 The intrinsic conduction system of the heart.
Figure 30.8 Action potential of a cardiac muscle cell.
Figure 30.9 Pericardiocentesis.
Figure 30.10 Areas for inspection and palpation of the precordium, indicating the sequence for palpation.
Figure 30.11 Areas for auscultation of the heart.

LEARNING OUTCOME 1

Describe the anatomy, physiology, and functions of the heart.

CONCEPTS FOR LECTURE

1. The heart is a muscular pump and its purpose is to move blood through the body to nourish tissue cells and remove wastes.
2. The pericardium is a double-layered fibroserous membrane that surrounds the heart and anchors it to surrounding structures. The small space between the two layers of this membrane is filled with lubricating pericardial fluid, which helps to cushion the heart.
3. The heart wall consists of three layers. The outermost epicardium covers the heart and the great vessels. The myocardium is the middle layer and consists of specialized cardiac muscle cells that provide the bulk of the contractile heart muscle. The endocardium is the innermost layer and lines the inside of the heart's chambers and great vessels.
4. The heart is divided into two upper atria and two lower ventricles that are separated longitudinally by the interventricular septum. The chambers are separated by valves that allow unidirectional blood flow to the next chamber or great vessel.

POWERPOINT LECTURE SLIDES

Anatomy, Physiology, and Functions of the Heart
- The heart
  - Muscular pump that moves blood through the body
    - Nourishes tissues cells
    - Removes wastes
- The pericardium
  - Double-layered fibroserous membrane surrounding the heart
    - Anchors the heart to surrounding structures
  - Space between layers is filled with pericardial fluid
    - Lubricates heart muscle
    - Helps to cushion the heart
- The heart wall
  - Consists of three layers
    - Epicardium
    - Myocardium
    - Endocardium

---

5. The cardiac cycle is based upon electrical activity. Each cardiac muscle cell possesses the ability for self-excitation, which would result in electrical chaos if not under the control of specialized cells. These areas are the sinoatrial (SA) node and the atrioventricular (AV) node.
6. The SA node is located at the junction of the superior vena cava and the right atrium and acts as the normal "pacemaker" of the heart. Impulses from the SA node travel across the atria via internodal pathways to the AV node.
7. The AV node is located in the floor of the interatrial septum and acts to slightly delay the transmission of impulses to the ventricles. The impulse then travels down the bundle of His, down the interventricular septum, and out to the Purkinje fibers in the ventricular muscle walls.
8. Movement of ions across cell membranes causes the electrical impulse that stimulates muscle contraction. This electrical action potential depolarizes cells, which contract and then rest (repolarization). The period in which cells resist stimulation (the refractory period) protects cardiac muscle from spasm and tetany.

- Chambers
  - Two upper atria
  - Two lower ventricles
  - Chambers separated by valves
- The cardiac cycle
  - Each cardiac cell possesses ability for self-excitation which would result in chaos if not controlled
  - Control is exercised by SA and AV nodes
- The SA (Sinoatrial) node
  - Located at junction of superior vena cava and right atrium
  - Acts as "pacemaker" of the heart
  - Impulses move via internodal pathways to AV node
- The AV (Atrioventricular) node
  - Located in the floor of the interatrial septum
  - Slows the transmission of impulses to the ventricle
  - Impulse then travels through bundle of His and across Purkinje fibers
- Electrical action potential
  - Depolarizes cells, causing contraction
  - Repolarization is phase of cell rest
  - Refractory period is protective of heart cells

SUGGESTIONS FOR CLASSROOM ACTIVITIES

- Bring anatomical models to the classroom to demonstrate the size and structure of the heart and great vessels.
- Use anatomical models to trace electrical activity through the heart.
- View the animation about cardiac anatomy and physiology provided on the textbook DVD-ROM.

LEARNING OUTCOME 2

Trace the circulation of blood through the heart and coronary vessels.

CONCEPTS FOR LECTURE

1. Deoxygenated blood returns from the body to the right atria via the superior vena cava, the inferior vena cava, and the coronary sinus. Blood then moves through the tricuspid valve to the right ventricle.
2. The right ventricle pumps the blood through the pulmonic valve to the pulmonary artery and into the pulmonary capillary bed for oxygenation.
3. Oxygenated blood returns to the left atria via the pulmonary veins. It then travels through the mitral valve to the left ventricle.
4. The blood is pumped through the aortic valve and into the aorta and the arterial circulation.
5. Since the heart is a muscle, it must have a blood supply to its tissues. The left and right coronary arteries originate at the base of the aorta and branch out to encircle the myocardium. After moving through the coronary arteries, the cardiac veins drain the blood into the coronary sinus, which then empties into the right atrium.

POWERPOINT LECTURE SLIDES

Circulation of Blood
- Deoxygenated blood returns to the heart to right atrium
- Blood moves to right ventricle
- Blood moves to the lungs
- Oxygenated blood returns to the heart
- Blood moves to left ventricle
- Blood is pumped to the body
- Coronary circulation

LEARNING OUTCOME 3

Identify normal heart sounds and relate them to the corresponding events in the cardiac cycle.

CONCEPTS FOR LECTURE

1. Heart sounds are caused by mechanical events that occur in the heart. The typical "lub-dub" associated with the heart is produced by closure of the heart valves.
2. The first heart sound, "lub," is termed S1 and is the result of closure of the atrioventricular (AV) valves. This sound occurs at the onset of contraction or systole.
3. The second heart sound, "dub," is termed S2 and is the result of closure of the semilunar valves. This sound occurs at the onset of relaxation or diastole.

POWERPOINT LECTURE SLIDES

Normal heart sounds
- Etiology of heart sounds
  ○ Caused by mechanical events occurring in the heart
  ○ Typical "lub-dub" is produced by closure of heart valves
- First heart sound
  ○ "lub"
  ○ S1
  ○ Closure of the AV valves
  ○ Occurs at onset of systole (contraction)
- Second heart sound
  ○ "dub"
  ○ S2
  ○ Closure of the semilunar valves
  ○ Occurs at onset of diastole (relaxation)

SUGGESTIONS FOR CLASSROOM ACTIVITIES	SUGGESTIONS FOR CLINICAL ACTIVITIES
• Review the animation about heart sounds provided on the textbook DVD-ROM.	• Have students practice identifying heart sounds during assessment of clinical clients.

LEARNING OUTCOME 4

Explain cardiac output and explain the influence of various factors in its regulation.

CONCEPTS FOR LECTURE

1. Cardiac output (CO) is the amount of blood pumped by the ventricles into the pulmonary and systemic circulation in one minute.
2. Cardiac output is determined by multiplying the amount of blood pumped each minute (stroke volume) times the heart rate: CO = HR x SV. Average adult cardiac output ranges from 4 to 8 L/min.
3. Four major factors in determining cardiac output are heart rate, contractility, preload, and afterload.
4. If heart rate increases, cardiac output increases (up to a point) even if there is no change in stroke volume. If heart rate increases to the point that there is inadequate relaxation time for ventricular filling, the cardiac output will decrease because stroke volume decreases. Cardiac output will decrease if the client experiences bradycardia because the number of cardiac cycles are decreased.

POWERPOINT LECTURE SLIDES

Factors Influencing Cardiac Output
- Heart rate
  ○ Increase HR increases CO even without increased SV
  ○ However, there must be time for ventricles to fill
    – Too rapid heart rate does not allow for ventricular filling, so CO may decrease
  ○ Bradycardia will result in decreased CO if heart rate is too slow
- Contractility
  ○ Inherent capability of cardiac muscle fibers to shorten
  ○ Poor contractility reduce blood
  ○ Increased contractility m heart

5. Contractility is the inherent capability of the cardiac muscle fibers to shorten. Poor contractility reduces forward flow of blood and increases ventricular pressures from the accumulation of blood volume. These two factors work together to reduce cardiac output. Increased contractility may stress the heart, which results in eventual decrease in cardiac output.

6. Preload is the amount of cardiac muscle stretch existing just before contraction of the ventricles. This stretch is related to the amount of blood present in the ventricle and the compliance of the ventricular tissues. The greater the stretch of the cardiac muscle, the more forceful the contraction of the fibers (Starling's law of the heart). Eventually, this relationship reaches its physiologic limit; overstretching the muscle fibers results in ineffective contraction and decreased cardiac output. Decreased venous return to the heart also results in decreased preload.

7. Afterload is the force the ventricles must overcome to eject their blood volume. Since the pulmonary system is lower pressure than the systemic circulation, the right ventricular afterload (pulmonary vascular resistance) is lower than the left ventricular afterload (systemic vascular resistance). Afterload increases when resistance increases. As this workload increases, consumption of myocardial oxygen increases and the compromised heart cannot meet the demand.

8. Cardiac index is the cardiac output adjusted to the client's body surface area. Because body size is taken into consideration, the cardiac index is a more meaningful indicator of the heart's ability to perfuse tissues. Cardiac index is determined by dividing CO by BSA. An adequate range is 2.5 to 4.2 L/min/m2.

9. Ejection fraction is the stroke volume divided by volume of blood that is held in the ventricles just before contraction (end-diastolic volume). This value represents the fraction or percent of blood that is ejected by each contraction. Normal ejection fraction ranges from 50% to 70%.

- Pre-load
  - Amount of stretch in cardiac muscle fibers just before ventricular contraction
    - Related to amount of blood in ventricles
    - Related to ventricular compliance
  - Starling's law of the heart
    - The greater the stretch on the cardiac muscle fibers, the more forceful the contraction
    - Overstretching the muscle fibers results in ineffective contraction
  - Decreased venous return to the heart also results in decreased preload
- Afterload
  - The force the ventricles must overcome to eject their blood volume
  - Right side of the heart has a lower afterload (pulmonary vascular resistance) because it pumps to the lower pulmonary circulation
  - Left side of the heart has a higher afterload (systemic vascular resistance) because it pumps to the higher systemic circulation
  - Afterload increases as resistance increases
  - As workload increases, myocardial oxygen consumption increases

---

SUGGESTIONS FOR CLASSROOM ACTIVITIES

- Present various values for cardiac output, cardiac index, and ejection fraction and have students identify normal values.
- Discuss implications of abnormal values.

SUGGESTIONS FOR CLINICAL ACTIVITIES

- Have students identify abnormal cardiac output, cardiac index, and ejection fraction values in clinical clients and help them identify clinical findings associated with those values.

LEARNING OUTCOME 5

Describe normal variations in assessment findings for the older adult.

CONCEPTS FOR LECTURE

1. Aging may cause decreased myocardial efficiency and contractility resulting in decreased cardiac output when under physiologic stress.

POWERPOINT LECTURE SLIDES

Age-Related Changes
- Decreased myocardial efficiency and contractility
  - Decreased cardiac output

2. Aging may cause changes in the left ventricle resulting in increased stroke volume and increased blood pressure.
3. There are age-related changes in valves and blood vessels that results in blood pressure.

- Left ventricular changes
  ○ Increased stroke volume
    – Increased blood pressure
- Valve and blood vessels changes
  ○ Increased blood pressure

SUGGESTIONS FOR CLINICAL ACTIVITIES

- Have students review the assessment of an older adult to identify normal age-related changes.

LEARNING OUTCOME 6

Identify manifestations of impaired cardiac structure and functions.

CONCEPTS FOR LECTURE

1. Apical impulse assessment may reveal changes in placement, strength of impulse, or change in duration of impulse.
2. Heart rate assessment may reveal changes in rate (tachycardia or bradycardia) or rhythm (dysrhythmia).
3. Heart sound assessment may reveal the presence of abnormal heart sounds such as splitting, presence of S3 or S4, or murmur.

POWERPOINT LECTURE SLIDES

Manifestations of Impaired Cardiac Structure and Functions
- Apical impulse assessment
  ○ Changes in placement
  ○ Changes in strength of impulse
  ○ Change in duration of impulse
- Heart rate assessment
  ○ Changes in rate (tachycardia or bradycardia)
  ○ Changes in rhythm (dysrhythmia)
- Heart sound assessment
  ○ Presence of abnormal heart sounds
    – Splitting
    – S3
    – S4
    – Murmur

SUGGESTIONS FOR CLASSROOM ACTIVITIES

- Have students practice assessment activities on mannequins or volunteers.
- Discuss the implication of abnormal assessment findings.

SUGGESTIONS FOR CLINICAL ACTIVITIES

- Have students perform cardiac assessments on clinical clients.
- Discuss the relationship between cardiac assessments and client physical manifestations.

CHAPTER 31
NURSING CARE OF CLIENTS WITH CORONARY HEART DISEASE

RESOURCE LIBRARY

💿 PRENTICE HALL NURSING MEDIALINK DVD-ROM

Audio Glossary
NCLEX-RN® Review
Animation/Video
  Automated External Defibrillation
  Coronary Heart Disease
  Dysrhythmias
  Nifedipine
  Propranolol

📖 IMAGE LIBRARY

Figure 31.1 ECG changes during an episode of angina.
Figure 31.2 Percutaneous coronary revascularization.
Figure 31.3 Coronary artery bypass grafting using the internal mammary artery and a saphenous vein graft.
Figure 31.4 A diagrammatic representation of cardiopulmonary bypass.
Figure 31.5 ECG changes characteristic of MI.
Figure 31.6 The intra-aortic balloon pump.

🌐 COMPANION WEBSITE

Audio Glossary
NCLEX-RN® Review
Care Plan Activity: Perioperative Pacemaker Care
Case Study: Myocardial Infarction
Exercise: Match the Rhythm
MediaLink Applications
Links to Resources

Figure 31.7 Toursades de pointes.
Figure 31.8 Placement of paddles for defibrillation.
Figure 31.10 A permanent epicardial pacemaker.
Figure 31.11 A permanent transvenous (endocardial) pacemaker with the lead placed in the right ventricle via the subclavian vein.
Figure 31.12 Pacing artifacts.
Figure 31.13 Schematic of an automated external defibrillator (AED) attached to a client.

LEARNING OUTCOME 1

Discuss the coronary circulation and electrical properties of the heart.

CONCEPTS FOR LECTURE

1. The two main coronary arteries supply blood, oxygen, and nutrients to the myocardium.
2. The left main coronary artery divides to form the anterior descending and circumflex arteries.
3. The anterior descending artery supplies the anterior interventricular septum and left ventricle.
4. The circumflex branch supplies the lateral wall of the left ventricle.
5. The right coronary artery supplies the right ventricle.
6. The posterior descending artery supplies the posterior portion of the heart.
7. Collateral channels develop between small arteries. If larger vessels are gradually occluded, these channels enlarge, which provides alternative routes for blood flow.
8. Five unique properties of cardiac cells allow effective heart function: automaticity, excitability, conductivity, refractoriness, and contractility.
9. Automaticity is the ability of pacemaker cells to spontaneously initiate an electrical impulse.

POWERPOINT LECTURE SLIDES

Coronary Circulation and Electrical Properties of the Heart
- Left main coronary artery
  - Anterior descending
    - Supplies anterior interventricular septum and left ventricle
  - Circumflex branch
    - Supplies lateral wall of left ventricle
- Right coronary artery
  - Supplies the right ventricle
  - Posterior descending artery supplies posterior portion of heart
- Collateral channels
  - Develop between small arteries
  - Providing alternative routes for blood flow
- Five unique properties of cardiac cells
  - Automaticity
  - Excitability
  - Conductivity

10. Excitability is the ability of myocardial cells to respond to stimuli generated by pacemaker cells.
11. Conductivity is the ability of cardiac cells to transmit an impulse from one cell to another cell.
12. Refractoriness is the inability of cardiac cells to respond to additional stimuli immediately following depolarization.
13. Contractility is the ability of myocardial fibers to shorten in response to a stimulus.
14. The electrical activity of the heart is normally controlled by the cardiac conduction system.

- ○ Refractoriness
- ○ Contractility
- ○ Controlled by the cardiac conduction system

SUGGESTIONS FOR CLASSROOM ACTIVITIES

- Using anatomic models, review the structure and blood flow through the heart.
- Using anatomic models, review the electrical pathways of the heart.

LEARNING OUTCOME 2

Compare and contrast the pathophysiology and manifestations of coronary heart disease and common cardiac dysrhythmias.

CONCEPTS FOR LECTURE
ATHEROSCLEROSIS

1. Atherosclerosis is a progressive disease characterized by atheroma formation. The keys to its development appear to be abnormal lipid metabolism and injury to, or inflammation of, the endothelial cells that line the arteries. In addition to obstructing blood flow, atherosclerosis weakens arterial walls and is a major cause of aneurysm.

MYOCARDIAL ISCHEMIA

2. Myocardial cells become ischemic when oxygen supply is inadequate to meet metabolic demands.
3. Coronary heart disease is divided into chronic ischemic heart disease and acute coronary syndromes.
4. Chronic ischemic heart disease includes stable and vasospastic angina, and silent myocardial ischemia.
5. Acute coronary syndromes range from unstable angina to myocardial infarction.

ANGINA PECTORIS

6. Angina is chest pain that results from reduced coronary blood flow or ischemia. Three types of angina have been identified: stable angina, Prinzmetal's (variant) angina, and unstable angina.
7. Silent myocardial ischemia is asymptomatic ischemia and is thought to be common in people with CHD. It is associated with an increased chance of myocardial infarction and death.
8. The cardinal manifestation of angina is chest pain, which is typically precipitated by an identifiable event. The classic sequence is activity—pain, rest—relief.

POWERPOINT LECTURE SLIDES

Coronary Heart Disease and Common Cardiac Dysrhythmias
- Coronary heart disease (CHD)
  - ○ Affects 13.2 million people in the United States
  - ○ Caused by impaired blood flow to myocardium
  - ○ May be asymptomatic, or may lead to
    - Angina pectoris
    - Acute coronary syndrome
    - Myocardial infarction
    - Dysrhythmias
    - Heart failure
    - Sudden death
- Cardiac dysrhythmias
  - ○ Disturbance or irregularity in electrical system of heart
    - Automaticity
    - Excitability
    - Conductivity
    - Refractoriness
  - ○ May be benign or lethal
  - ○ Can significantly affect cardiac performance

9. Client may describe pain as tight, squeezing, heavy, or constricting substernal pain that radiates to the jaw, epigastric area, or back. Additional manifestations include dyspnea, pallor, tachycardia, and great anxiety or fear.

10. Women frequently present with atypical symptoms: indigestion, nausea, vomiting, and upper back pain.

11. Angina is graded I–IV by the degree to which it limits the client's activities.

ACUTE CORONARY SYNDROME

12. Acute coronary syndrome (ACS) is a condition of unstable cardiac ischemia, including unstable angina and acute myocardial ischemia with or without significant injury of myocardial tissue.

13. ACS is a state in which coronary blood flow is acutely reduced, but not fully occluded. Myocardial cells are injured by the resulting acute ischemia.

14. ACS is precipitated by one or more reasons: 1) rupture or erosion of atherosclerotic plaque with formation of blood clot that does not fully occlude the vessel; 2) coronary artery spasm; 3) progressive vessel obstruction by plaque or by restenosis after treatment; 4) inflammation of a coronary artery; and 5) increased myocardial oxygen demand and/or decreased supply.

15. Manifestations are substernal or epigastric chest pain that often radiates to the neck, left shoulder, and/or left arm. Dyspnea, diaphoresis, pallor, and cool skin may be present. Tachycardia and hypotension may occur. There may be a feeling of nausea or light-headedness.

MYOCARDIAL INFARCTION

16. Acute myocardial infarction (AMI) is death of myocardial cells and is a life-threatening event. It occurs when blood flow to a portion of cardiac muscle is completely blocked, which results in prolonged tissue ischemia and irreversible cell damage.

17. AMI can be classified as subendocardial or non-Q wave infarction, or as transmural or Q-wave infarction.

18. Tissue effects of AMI may include tissue death, stunning or hibernation of tissue, or myocardial remodeling. Rapid restoration of blood flow limits these changes.

19. AMI can also be described by the damaged area of the heart.

20. AMI may develop due to cocaine ingestion. Clients who present with cocaine-induced MI may manifest an altered level of consciousness, confusion, restlessness, seizure activity, tachycardia, hypotension, increased respiratory rate, and respiratory crackles.

21. Manifestations of AMI include pain of sudden onset that is not linked to activity and is described as crushing, severe, squeezing, tightness, or burning. Pain often begins in the center of the chest and may radiate to shoulders, neck, jaw, or arms. Women and older adults often experience indigestion, heartburn, nausea, and vomiting.

22. Other frequent manifestations of AMI include anxiety, tachycardia or bradycardia, cool, clammy, mottled skin, blood pressure changes, nausea, and vomiting.

CARDIAC DYSRHYTHMIAS

23. Cardiac dysrhythmia is a disturbance or irregularity in the electrical system of the heart. These dysrhythmias may be benign or lethal.
24. Dysrhythmias arise through disruption of the heart's automaticity, excitability, conductivity, and refractoriness. They are classified as tachydysrhythmias, bradydysrhythmias, and ectopic rhythms.
25. Sick sinus syndrome results from sinus node disease or dysfunction that causes problems with impulse formation, transmission, and conduction.

SUDDEN CARDIAC DEATH

26. Sudden cardiac death (SCD) is defined as unexpected death that occurs within one hour of the onset of cardiovascular symptoms. It is usually caused by ventricular fibrillation and cardiac arrest.
27. SCD may be preceded by typical manifestations of acute coronary syndrome or myocardial infarction. The event itself is abrupt, with complete loss of consciousness and death within minutes.

SUGGESTIONS FOR CLASSROOM ACTIVITIES

- View the animations/videos about coronary heart disease and dysrhythmia that are provided on the textbook DVD-ROM.
- Present dysrhythmia recognition techniques, and focus on common dysrhythmias.
- Use the MediaLink Application: Match the Rhythm to help students identify common dysrhythmias.

SUGGESTIONS FOR CLINICAL ACTIVITIES

- Assign students to the care of clients with different cardiac disorders. Have students relate the manifestations seen in these clients to the pathophysiology that occurs. In conference, have students compare and contrast manifestations and pathophysiology from different disorders.
- Assign students to a cardiac monitor unit where they can observe monitor strip interpretation.

LEARNING OUTCOME 3

Describe interdisciplinary and nursing care for clients with coronary heart disease and cardiac dysrhythmias.

CONCEPTS FOR LECTURE
CORONARY HEART DISEASE

1. Care of coronary heart disease (CHD) focuses on aggressive risk factor management to slow atherosclerotic process and maintain myocardial perfusion.
2. Conservative management of CHD focuses on risk factor modifications, including smoking, diet, exercise, and management of contributing conditions.
3. Common nursing diagnoses include: Imbalanced Nutrition: More than Body Requirements and Ineffective Health Maintenance.
4. Education includes techniques for maintaining the lifestyle changes necessary to reduce risk of CHD.

POWERPOINT LECTURE SLIDES

Care for Clients with Coronary Heart Disease and/or Cardiac Dysrhythmias
- Coronary heart disease
  - Care focuses on aggressive risk factor management
- Angina
  - Management focuses on maintaining coronary blood flow and cardiac function
- Acute coronary syndrome
  - Clients generally admitted to acute care unit
  - Nursing care is similar to that for clients with angina and AMI

ANGINA

5. Management focuses on maintaining coronary blood flow and cardiac function.
6. Common nursing diagnoses include: Ineffective Tissue Perfusion: Cardiac and Risk for Ineffective Therapeutic Regimen Management.
7. Education should include: information about CHD, use of medications including nitroglycerin (NTG), and the importance of seeking medical care for unrelieved chest pain. If the client has undergone cardiac surgery, then education should include information about respiratory care, activity, pain management, the importance of participation in rehabilitation, and manifestations of infection or other potential complications and their management.

ACUTE CORONARY SYNDROME

8. The pain of acute coronary syndrome (ACS) may be unrelieved by nitroglycerin (NTG) or may be more severe and of longer duration than the client's normal angina.
9. Clients are generally admitted to the acute care unit. Coronary revascularization may be performed within 48 hours.
10. Coronary revascularization procedures include: percutaneous coronary revascularization; percutaneous transluminal coronary angioplasty; intracoronary stents placement; coronary artery bypass grafting; minimally invasive coronary artery surgery; and transmyocardial laser revascularization.
11. Nursing care is similar to that for clients with angina and acute myocardial infarction (AMI).

ACUTE MYOCARDIAL INFARCTION

12. Immediate treatment goals for acute myocardial infarction (AMI) are to relieve chest pain, reduce the extent of myocardial damage, maintain cardiovascular stability, decrease cardiac workload, and to prevent complications.
13. Many AMI clients are treated with immediate or early percutaneous coronary revascularization such as angioplasty and stent placement.
14. Other invasive procedures include intra-aortic balloon pump placement and ventricular assist device placement.
15. Cardiac rehabilitation is a long-term program of medical evaluation, exercise, risk factor modification, education, and counseling designed to limit the physical and psychological effects of cardiac illness and to improve the client's quality of life.
16. Nursing diagnoses include: Acute Pain; Ineffective Tissue Perfusion; Ineffective Coping; and Fear.
17. Education includes normal anatomy and physiology of the heart, the specific area of heart damage, the process of CHD and implications of MI, purposes and

- Acute myocardial infarction
  - Immediate treatment goals
    - Relieve chest pain
    - Reduce the extent of myocardial damage
    - Maintain cardiovascular stability
    - Decrease cardiac workload
    - Prevent complications.
  - Other invasive procedures
    - Intra-aortic balloon pump placement
    - Ventricular assist device placement
  - Cardiac rehabilitation
- Cardiac rhythm disorders
  - Major goals of care
    - Identifying the dysrhythmias
    - Evaluating its effects on the physical and psychosocial well-being
    - Treating underlying causes
  - Countershock
    - Synchronized cardioversion
    - Defibrillation
- Sudden cardiac death
  - Goal of care: to restore cardiac output and tissue perfusion
  - Basic and advanced cardiac life support measures
  - Important concepts of emergency cardiac care are
    - Treat the client, not the monitor
    - Activate emergency medical system
    - Begin and continue basic cardiac life support
    - Continually assessing effectiveness of intervention
    - Defibrillating pulseless VT or VF as soon as possible
    - Initiate ALS protocols early

side effects of prescribed medications, the importance of complying with the medical regimen and cardiac rehabilitation program and keeping follow-up appointments; and information about community resources.

CARDIAC RHYTHM DISORDERS

18. Recognizing lethal dysrhythmias is a matter of life and death. Major goals of care include identifying the dysrhythmias, evaluating its effects on the physical and psychosocial well-being, and treating underlying causes.

19. Countershock is used to interrupt cardiac rhythms that compromise cardiac output and the client's welfare.

20. Nursing responsibilities for cardioversion include preparing the client before the procedure; obtaining any laboratory tests ordered; obtaining and documenting ECG strips prior to, during, and after treatment; setting up the equipment; and monitoring the client's response.

21. Defibrillation can be delivered internally (done only by physicians) or externally (provided by any trained healthcare provider).

22. A pacemaker is a pulse generator used to provide an electrical stimulus to the heart when the heart fails to generate or conduct its own at a rate that maintains the cardiac output. Pacemakers can be temporary or permanent.

23. The implantable cardioverter-defibrillator detects life-threatening changes in the cardiac rhythm and automatically delivers an electric shock to convert the dysrhythmia back into a normal rhythm.

24. Cardiac mapping and catheter ablation are used to locate and destroy an ectopic focus.

25. Nursing diagnoses include Decreased Cardiac Output; Ineffective Tissue Perfusion; Activity Intolerance; and Fear or Anxiety.

26. Major teaching efforts focus on coping strategies and lifestyle changes, as well as specific management of prescribed therapies.

SUDDEN CARDIAC DEATH

27. The goal of care is to restore cardiac output and tissue perfusion. Basic and advanced cardiac life support measures must be instituted within 2–4 minutes of cardiac arrest.

28. Important concepts of emergency cardiac care are: treat the client, not the monitor; activate emergency medical system; begin and continue basic cardiac life support, continually assessing effectiveness of intervention; defibrillate pulseless VT or VF as soon as possible; and initiate ALS protocols early.

29. Common nursing diagnoses include: Ineffective Tissue Perfusion; Impaired Spontaneous Ventilation; Spiritual Distress; Disturbed Thought Processes; and Fear.

30. Postresuscitation care should also include the risk for future episodes.

LEARNING OUTCOME 4

Relate the outcomes of diagnostic tests and procedures to the pathophysiology of cardiac disorders and implications for client responses to the disorder.

CONCEPTS FOR LECTURE
CORONARY HEART DISEASE

1. Lipid profiles are used to assess total serum cholesterols, HDL levels, LDL levels, and triglyceride levels.
2. C-reactive protein is a protein associated with the inflammatory process. High levels may be predictive of CHD.
3. Ankle-brachial blood pressure index may be predictive of CHD.
4. Exercise ECG testing is considered "positive" if myocardial ischemia is detected on ECG, the client develops chest pain, or the test is stopped due to excess fatigue, dysrhythmias, or other symptoms.
5. Electron beam computed tomography is a noninvasive test that requires no preparation and can identify clients at risk for developing myocardial infarction.
6. Myocardial perfusion imaging may be used to evaluate myocardial blood flow and perfusion.

ANGINA

7. Diagnosis is based on past medical history and family history, a comprehensive description of the chest pain, and physical assessment findings.
8. Electrocardiography may reveal changes such as nonspecific ST and T wave changes. During periods of ischemia, the ST segment is depressed or downsloping, and the T wave may flatten or invert.
9. Other diagnostic testing includes ECG stress testing, radionuclide testing, echocardiography, and coronary angiography.

ACUTE CORONARY SYNDROME

10. The ECG is used in conjunction with blood levels of cardiac markers to differentiate between unstable angina and acute myocardial infarction.
11. Serum cardiac markers including cardiac muscle troponins, creatine kinase, and CK-MB are often used to diagnose ACS.
12. Several procedures may be used to restore blood flow and oxygen to ischemic tissue: transluminal coronary angioplasty, laser angioplasty, coronary atherectomy, intracoronary stents, and coronary artery bypass grafting.

POWERPOINT LECTURE SLIDES

Outcomes of Diagnostic Tests and Procedures
- General diagnostic testing
  - Lipid profiles
  - C-reactive protein
  - Ankle-brachial blood pressure index
  - Exercise ECG testing
  - Electron beam computed tomography
  - Myocardial perfusion imaging
- Angina
  - Diagnosis
    - Past medical history and family history
    - Comprehensive description of the chest pain
    - Physical assessment findings
  - Electrocardiography
    - Nonspecific ST and T wave changes
    - ST segment is depressed or downsloping
    - T wave may flatten or invert
  - Other diagnostic testing
    - ECG stress testing
    - Radionuclide testing
    - Echocardiography
    - Coronary angiography
- Acute coronary syndrome
  - Diagnostic testing
    - ECG
    - Serum cardiac markers
  - Procedures
    - Transluminal coronary angioplasty
    - Laser angioplasty
    - Coronary atherectomy
    - Intracoronary stents
    - Coronary artery bypass grafting
- Acute myocardial infarction
  - Laboratory testing
    - Creatine kinase
    - CK-MB
    - Cardiac-specific troponin
    - Cardiac-specific troponin I
    - Myoglobin
    - CBC
    - ABGs
  - Diagnostic testing
    - Electrocardiography

ACUTE MYOCARDIAL INFARCTION

13. Laboratory testing includes measurement of creatine kinase, CK-MB, cardiac-specific troponin, cardiac-specific troponin I, myoglobin, CBC, and ABGs.
14. Electrocardiography, echocardiography, and myocardial nuclear scans are the most common diagnostic tests performed when AMI is suspected. Hemodynamic monitoring may be initiated when AMI significantly affects cardiac output and hemodynamic status.

CARDIAC RHYTHM DISORDER

15. Diagnostic tests include the ECG, cardiac monitoring, and electrophysiology studies.
16. Laboratory tests include serum electrolytes, drug levels, and arterial blood gases.

- – Echocardiography
- – Myocardial nuclear scans
- – Hemodynamic monitoring
- Cardiac rhythm disorder
  - ○ Diagnostic tests
    - – ECG
    - – Cardiac monitoring
    - – Electrophysiology studies
  - ○ Laboratory tests
    - – Serum electrolytes
    - – Drug levels
    - – Arterial blood gases

SUGGESTIONS FOR CLASSROOM ACTIVITIES

- Present laboratory and diagnostic test results. Have students identify normal and abnormal results. Discuss nursing implications of those results.
- Divide students into small groups. Assign each group a common diagnostic procedure and have them develop a guideline for nursing care for that procedure.

SUGGESTIONS FOR CLINICAL ACTIVITIES

- Have students review cardiac client medical records for laboratory and diagnostic testing results. Help students relate the results of these tests to the manifestations and goals of care for specific clients.

LEARNING OUTCOME 5

Discuss nursing implications for medications and treatments used to prevent and treat coronary heart disease and dysrhythmias.

CONCEPTS FOR LECTURE
CORONARY HEART DISEASE

1. Drug therapy to lower total serum cholesterol and LDL levels and to raise HDL levels now is an integral part of CHD management.
2. Four classes of cholesterol-lowering drugs are statins, bile acid sequestrants, nicotinic acid, and fibrates.

ANGINA

3. The goal of medication treatment is to reduce oxygen demand and increase oxygen supply to cardiac muscle. The three major classes of medications used are nitrates, beta blockers, and calcium channel blockers. Low-dose aspirin is also recommended.

ACUTE CORONARY SYNDROME

4. Medications include drugs to reduce myocardial ischemia (nitrates and beta blockers) and those to reduce the risk for blood clotting (aspirin, other antiplatelet drugs, and heparin).

POWERPOINT LECTURE SLIDES

Medications and Treatments to Prevent and Treat Coronary Heart Disease and Dysrhythmias
- Coronary heart disease
  - ○ Drug therapy to lower total serum cholesterol and LDL levels and to raise HDL levels
  - ○ Four classes of cholesterol-lowering drugs
    - – Statins
    - – Bile acid dequestrants
    - – Nicotinic acid
    - – Fibrates
- Angina
  - ○ Goal is to reduce oxygen demand and increase oxygen supply
  - ○ Three major classes of medications
    - – Nitrates
    - – Beta blockers
    - – Calcium channel blockers
  - ○ Low dose aspirin
- Acute coronary syndrome
  - ○ Medications include drugs
    - – To reduce myocardial ischemia (nitrates and beta blockers)

ACUTE MYOCARDIAL INFARCTION

5. Aspirin is now considered an essential part of treating AMI. Fibrinolytic agents, analgesics, and antidysrhythmic agents are among the principal classes of drugs used in treating AMI.

CARDIAC RHYTHM DISORDERS

6. The goal of drug therapy is to suppress dysrhythmia formation. Antidysrhythmic drugs are primarily used for acute treatment of dysrhythmias, although they may also be used to manage chronic conditions.

- To reduce the risk for blood clotting (aspirin, other antiplatelet drugs, and heparin)
- Acute myocardial infarction
  - Aspirin is now considered an essential part of treating AMI
  - Fibrinolytic agents
  - Analgesics
  - Antidysrhythmic agents
- Cardiac rhythm disorders
  - Goal of drug therapy: to suppress dysrhythmia formation
  - Antidysrhythmic drugs
    - Used for acute management
    - Used for chronic management

SUGGESTIONS FOR CLASSROOM ACTIVITIES

- Discuss the expected therapeutic effects of common cardiac medications.
- Discuss nursing implications of adverse effects of common cardiac medications.
- Have students identify medication-related changes in cardiac output. Discuss the concept of polypharmacy as it applies to the cardiac client.

SUGGESTIONS FOR CLINICAL ACTIVITIES

- Require students to develop medication information sheets for common cardiac medications.
- Have students review client medication administration records for cardiac medications and relate those medications to changes in client clinical findings.
- Investigate the costs associated with cardiac maintenance drugs.

LEARNING OUTCOME 6

Describe nursing care for the client undergoing diagnostic testing, an interventional procedure, or surgery for coronary heart disease or a dysrhythmia.

CONCEPTS FOR LECTURE

1. Preoperative or preprocedure nursing responsibilities include: comprehensive physical assessment and education regarding the procedure or surgery being performed.
2. Postoperative or postprocedure nursing responsibilities include: close monitoring of vital signs, cardiac rhythm, output, respiratory status, and general physical assessment. The nurse must also monitor and manage IV medication administration, and monitor and treat pain.
3. Common postoperative or postprocedure nursing diagnoses include: Hypothermia; Acute Pain; Ineffective Airway Clearance/Impaired Gas Exchange; Risk for Infection; Disturbed Thought Processes; and Activity Intolerance.

POWERPOINT LECTURE SLIDES

Nursing Care
- Pre-operative or pre-procedure nursing responsibilities include
  - Comprehensive physical assessment
  - Education regarding the procedure or surgery being performed
- Post-operative or post-procedure nursing responsibilities include
  - Close monitoring of VS, cardiac rhythm, output, respiratory status, and general physical assessment
  - Monitor and manage IV medication administration
  - Monitor and treat pain
- Nursing diagnoses
  - Hypothermia
  - Acute pain
  - Ineffective airway clearance/impaired gas exchange
  - Risk for infection
  - Disturbed thought processes
  - Activity intolerance

SUGGESTIONS FOR CLASSROOM ACTIVITIES

- Review the animation/video about automated external defibrillation that is provided on the textbook DVD-ROM.
- Access the care plan activity about perioperative pacemaker care that is provided on the textbook Companion Website. Have students develop individualized nursing interventions using the information provided.

SUGGESTIONS FOR CLINICAL ACTIVITIES

- Assign students to units where clients are prepared for, or recovered from, cardiac procedures.
- Have students develop case studies of clients who have undergone cardiac procedures. Have students present those case studies to other students who have not cared for similar clients.

CHAPTER 32
NURSING CARE OF CLIENTS WITH CARDIAC DISORDERS

RESOURCE LIBRARY

PRENTICE HALL NURSING MEDIALINK DVD-ROM

Audio Glossary
NCLEX-RN® Review
Animations
   Digoxin
   Hemodynamics

COMPANION WEBSITE

Audio Glossary
NCLEX-RN® Review
Care Plan Activity: Acute Pulmonary Edema
Case Study: Rheumatic Fever
MediaLink Applications
   Beta Blockers
   Heart Failure
Links to Resources

IMAGE LIBRARY

Figure 32.1 The hemodynamic effects of left-sided heart failure.
Figure 32.2 The hemodynamic effects of right-sided heart failure.
Figure 32.3 A hemodynamic monitoring setup.
Figure 32.4 Inflation of the balloon on the flow-directed catheter allows it to be carried through the pulmonic valve into the pulmonary artery.
Figure 32.5 Typical waveforms seen when measuring (*A*) pulmonary artery pressure and (*B*) pulmonary wedge pressure.
Figure 32.6 Cardiac transplantation.

Figure 32.7 A vegetative lesion of bacterial endocarditis.
Figure 32.8 Cardiac tamponade.
Figure 32.9 Constrictive pericarditis.
Figure 32.10 Valvular heart disorders.
Figure 32.11 Mitral stenosis.
Figure 32.12 Mitral regurgitation.
Figure 32.13 Mitral valve prolapse.
Figure 32.14 Aortic stenosis.
Figure 32.15 Aortic regurgitation.
Figure 32.16 Balloon valvuloplasty.

LEARNING OUTCOME 1

Compare and contrast the etiology, pathophysiology, and manifestations of common cardiac disorders, including heart failure, structural disorders, and inflammatory disorders.

CONCEPTS FOR LECTURE
HEART FAILURE

1. Heart failure is a complex syndrome in which the heart is unable to pump enough blood to meet the metabolic demands of the body. As a result of this inability, cardiac output falls and tissue perfusion decreases.
2. It is often the result of structural and inflammatory disorders, but can also result from excessive demands on a normal heart.
3. As the heart begins to fail, compensatory mechanisms are activated. Primary compensatory mechanisms are the Frank-Starling mechanism, neuroendocrine responses, and myocardial hypertrophy.
4. As heart failure progresses, the compensatory mechanisms begin to be detrimental to muscle function. Heart function continues to deteriorate.
5. The client with heart failure has little or no cardiac reserve and does not tolerate physical or psychologic stress.

POWERPOINT LECTURE SLIDES

Etiology, Pathophysiology, and Manifestations of Common Cardiac Disorders
- Heart failure
- Pulmonary edema
- Rheumatic fever/rheumatic heart disease
- Infective endocarditis
- Myocarditis
- Pericarditis
- Valvular heart disease
- Mitral stenosis
- Mitral regurgitation
- Mitral valve prolapse
- Aortic stenosis
- Aortic regurgitation
- Tricuspid stenosis
- Tricuspid regurgitation
- Pulmonic stenosis

- Pulmonic regurgitation
- Cardiomyopathy

6. Systolic failure occurs when the ventricle does not contract adequately and manifests as weakness, fatigue, and decreased exercise tolerance. Diastolic failure occurs when the heart does not relax completely, which impairs its filling ability. It manifests as shortness of breath, tachypnea, respiratory crackles, distended neck veins, liver enlargement, anorexia, and nausea. Many clients have components of both systolic and diastolic failure.

7. Left-sided failure is often caused by coronary heart disease and manifests as fatigue and activity intolerance, dizziness, syncope, dyspnea, shortness of breath, cough, orthopnea, cyanosis, presence of inspiratory crackles and wheezes, and presence of an S3 gallop.

8. Right-sided failure is often caused by factors that restrict blood flow to the lungs. It manifests as congestion of abdominal organs and development of peripheral edema, especially in dependent tissues.

9. Low-output failure occurs when the cardiac output drops due to structural or inflammatory disorders of the heart muscle. In this case, supply is low.

10. High-output failure occurs when demand is increased as when the client is in a hypermetabolic state. In this case, demand is high.

11. Acute failure is abrupt in onset, which results in suddenly decreased cardiac function and output. Chronic failure is a progressive deterioration of the heart muscle.

PULMONARY EDEMA

12. Pulmonary edema is an abnormal accumulation of fluid in the interstitial tissue and alveoli of the lung, caused by both cardiac and noncardiac disorders. Cardiogenic pulmonary edema is a sign of severe cardiac decompensation.

13. This is a true medical emergency because the client is literally drowning in the fluid in the lungs. Immediate treatment is necessary.

14. As contractility of the left ventricle decreases, pulmonary hydrostatic pressure increases, which forces fluid into interstitial tissues. Eventually this increase in pressure causes fluid to enter the alveoli. Ventilation and gas exchange are severely disrupted.

15. Manifestations include dyspnea; shortness of breath; orthopnea; cyanosis, cool, clammy, diaphoretic skin; productive cough with pink, frothy sputum; crackles in lung fields; restlessness; and confusion.

RHEUMATIC FEVER AND RHEUMATIC HEART DISEASE

16. Rheumatic fever is a systemic inflammatory disease that is caused by an abnormal immune response to pharyngeal infection by group A beta-hemolytic streptococci.

17. It is thought that antigens from an abnormal immune response bind to cells in the heart, muscles, brain, and synovial joints, which causes inflammation. Carditis and Aschoff bodies may develop. Damage to valve structures may occur.

18. Rheumatic heart disease is a slowly progressive valvular deformity that results in stenosis or regurgitation of the heart valves.

19. Manifestations of rheumatic fever include chest pain, friction rub, heart murmur, migratory polyarthritis, erythema marginatum, subcutaneous nodules over joint extensors, and Sydenham's chorea.

INFECTIVE ENDOCARDITIS

20. Endocarditis is inflammation of the endocardium. It is generally infectious in nature and results in colonization of the cardiac structures by a pathogen.

21. Prosthetic valve endocarditis (PVE) occurs in clients who have undergone valve replacement. PVE may develop early in the postoperative course due to contamination of the prosthetic valve during surgery or perioperative bacteriemia and usually has a rapid course with high mortality. Late PVE has a course more like subacute endocarditis.

22. Development of endocarditis requires entry of pathogens into the bloodstream. Vegetations of pathogens form on the cardiac structures, most commonly the valve leaflets. As these vegetations grow, they interfere with the normal movement of blood through the heart. The vegetations may also fracture and embolize.

23. Classifications of endocarditis are: acute infectious endocarditis which has an abrupt onset and a rapidly progressive course; and subacute infective endocarditis which has a more gradual onset.

24. Manifestations of endocarditis can be nonspecific and flu-like with presence of chills, fever, general malaise, fatigue, cough, dyspnea, and joint pain. There is also often presence of a heart murmur. Anorexia and abdominal pain may develop with splenomegaly. Peripheral manifestations occur from microemboli or circulating immune complexes and include petechiae, splinter hemorrhages of the nails, Osler's nodes on finger and toe pads, Janeway lesions on the palms and soles of the feet, and Roth's spots on the retina.

25. Common complications of endocarditis are embolization of vegetative fragments, heart failure, abscess, and aneurysm. Without treatment, endocarditis is almost universally fatal. Antibiotic therapy is generally effective in treating the disease.

MYOCARDITIS

26. Myocarditis is inflammation of the heart muscle, and usually results from infection, most commonly viral in nature.

27. The extent of muscle damage ultimately determines the long-term outcome of the disease. Severe myocarditis may result in cardiomyopathy and heart failure.

28. Myocarditis is often preceded by a nonspecific febrile illness or upper respiratory illness and manifestations often appear similar to those illnesses. Muffling of S1,

presence of S3, murmur, or pericardial friction rub may be heard. Chest pain may also be present.

PERICARDITIS

29. Pericarditis is inflammation of the pericardium and may be a primary disorder or develop secondary to another disorder. It is usually viral, but affects 40–50% of clients with ESRD and uremia. MI and cardiac surgery are also common causes.
30. Inflammation of the pericardium may result in pericardial effusion, fibrosis, or scarring. These changes restrict cardiac function.
31. Classic manifestations include chest pain, a pericardial friction rub, and fever. Dyspnea and tachycardia are common.
32. Common complications are pericardial effusion, cardiac tamponade, and constrictive pericarditis.

VALVULAR HEART DISEASE

33. Valvular heart disease interferes with blood flow to and from the heart. Acquired valvular disease may be a result of an acute condition such as infective endocarditis or from a chronic condition such as rheumatic heart disease or MI. Congenital heart defects may also affect heart valve function.
34. Two major types of heart disease are stenosis and regurgitation. Stenosis is when the valve opening narrows and becomes rigid. Regurgitation occurs when valves are insufficient or incompetent and do not close.

MITRAL STENOSIS

35. Mitral stenosis is a narrowing of the mitral valve and obstructs blood flow from the left atrium into the left ventricle. It is usually caused by rheumatic heart disease or bacterial endocarditis.
36. Manifestations depend upon cardiac output and pulmonary vascular pressures. Dyspnea on exertion is typically the earliest symptom. Other manifestations are cough, hemoptysis, frequent pulmonary infections, paroxysmal nocturnal dyspnea, orthopnea, weakness, fatigue, and palpitations. As stenosis worsens, manifestations of right heart failure, jugular venous distension, hepatomegaly, ascites, and peripheral edema develop. Cyanosis of the face and extremities may occur with severe mitral stenosis. Heart sounds may reveal a loud S1, split S2, a mitral opening snap, and a low-pitched, rumbling, crescendo-decrescendo murmur.
37. Complications include atrial dysrhythmias with resulting thrombi and emboli production.

MITRAL REGURGITATION

38. Mitral regurgitation allows blood to flow back into the left atrium during systole and results in left atrial enlargement. This regurgitation can result from bacterial endocarditis vegetations, scarring from MI, or cardiac dilation.

39. Manifestations may include fatigue, weakness, exertional dyspnea, and orthopnea. Pulmonary congestion and edema may occur with severe or acute regurgitation. The murmur of mitral regurgitation is loud, high-pitched, rumbling, and holosystolic and may be accompanied by a palpable thrill. It is heard best at the cardiac apex.

MITRAL VALVE PROLAPSE

40. Mitral valve prolapse is a condition in which one or both mitral valve cusps billow into the atrium during ventricular systole. It can result from acute or chronic rheumatic damage, ischemic heart disease, or other cardiac disorders. It commonly affects people with Marfan syndrome.

41. Mitral valve prolapse is often asymptomatic. There may be a midsystolic ejection click or murmur. This murmur is high-pitched and occurs late in systole. Atypical chest pain related to fatigue may be present along with tachyarrhythmias.

AORTIC STENOSIS

42. Aortic stenosis obstructs blood flow from the left ventricle into the aorta. It may be idiopathic or may result from a congenital defect, rheumatic damage, or degenerative changes.

43. Aortic stenosis may be asymptomatic for years. Classic manifestations include dyspnea on exertion, angina pectoris, and exertional syncope. Aortic stenosis produces a harsh systolic murmur with a palpable thrill. This murmur is heard best in the second intercostal space to the right of the sterum.

AORTIC REGURGITATION

44. Aortic regurgitation or insufficiency allows blood to flow back into the left ventricle from the aorta. The most common cause is rheumatic heart disease. It is also caused by congenital disorders, infective endocarditis, blunt chest trauma, aortic aneurysm, syphilis, Marfan syndrome, and chronic hypertension.

45. Aortic regurgitation may be asymptomatic for years, even when severe. Manifestations include persistent palpitations with a characteristic head bob (Musset's sign), dizziness, fatigue, exertional dyspnea, orthopnea, and paroxysmal nocturnal dyspnea, and murmur. The murmur is a blowing, high-pitched sound and is associated with a palpable thrill and ventricular heave. It is heard best at the third left intercostal space.

TRICUSPID STENOSIS

46. Tricuspid stenosis obstructs blood flow from the right atrium to the right ventricle. The most common cause is rheumatic heart disease.

47. Manifestations include increased central venous pressure, jugular venous distention, ascites, hepatomegaly, peripheral edema, fatigue, and weakness. The associated murmur is low-pitched and rumbling and is heard over the fourth intercostal space at the left sternal border or over the xiphoid.

TRICUSPID REGURGITATION

48. Tricuspid regurgitation allows blood flow back into the right atrium during systole. The major cause is right ventricular dilation that results from left ventricular failure or pulmonary hypertension. The valve may also be damaged by rheumatic heart disease, infective endocarditis, inferior MI, and trauma.

49. Manifestations include systemic venous congestion and atrial fibrillation. The associated murmur is high-pitched and blowing is heard over the xiphoid.

PULMONIC STENOSIS

50. Pulmonic stenosis obstructs blood flow from the right ventricle into the pulmonary system and is usually congenital.

51. Pulmonary stenosis is generally asymptomatic unless severe. Manifestations may include dyspnea on exertion, fatigue, peripheral edema, ascites, hepatomegaly, and increased venous pressure. The murmur of pulmonic stenosis is a harsh, systolic crescendo-decrescendo murmur heard best at the second left intercostal space.

PULMONIC REGURGITATION

52. Incomplete valve closure allows blood to flow back into the right ventricle during diastole, which decreases blood flow to the lungs. Pulmonary regurgitation is often a complication of pulmonary hypertension, but it can also be a result of infective endocarditis, pulmonary artery aneurysm, or syphilis.

53. Pulmonary regurgitation manifests as right-sided heart failure. The associated murmur is high-pitched, decrescendo, and blowing and is heard along the left sternal border during diastole.

CARDIOMYOPATHY

54. Cardiomyopathies affect the heart muscle and can be either primary or secondary in origin. Primary cardiomyopathies are idiopathic. Secondary cardiomyopathies occur as a result of ischemia, infection, exposure to toxins, connective tissue disorders, metabolic disorders, or nutritional deficiencies.

55. Dilated cardiomyopathy is the most common type and is often idiopathic. Reversible dilated cardiomyopathy may develop as a result of alcohol and cocaine abuse, chemotherapeutic drugs, pregnancy, and systemic hypertension. Basic physiology is the dilation of the heart chambers with resulting impairment of ventricular contraction.

56. Manifestations of dilated cardiomyopathy develop gradually. Right- and left-sided failure develops with dyspnea on exertion. Orthopnea, paroxysmal nocturnal dyspnea, weakness, fatigue, peripheral edema, and ascites occur. Heart sounds include S3 and S4 along with an AV regurgitation murmur. Dysrhythmias are common and mural thrombi may form in the left ventricular apex and embolize to other parts of the body.

57. Hypertrophic cardiomyopathy is characterized by decreased compliance of the left ventricle and hypertrophy of the ventricular muscle mass.

58. Usual manifestations of hypertrophic cardiomyopathy are dyspnea, angina, and syncope. Ventricular dysrhythmias and atrial fibrillation are common. Heart sounds include a harsh, crescendo-decrescendo systolic murmur that is heard best at the lower left sternal border and apex. An S4 may be present.

59. Restrictive cardiomyopathy is the least common type of cardiomyopathy and is characterized by rigid ventricular walls. Causes include myocardial fibrosis and infiltrative processes, such as amyloidosis. Manifestations include heart failure and decreased tissue perfusion. Dyspnea on exertion, exercise intolerance, JVD, and presence of S3 and S4 are common.

SUGGESTIONS FOR CLASSROOM ACTIVITIES

- Have students develop a chart that outlines the etiology, pathophysiology, and manifestations of common cardiac disorders. Using these student-developed charts, compare and contrast the manifestations to the pathophysiology of the disorders.

SUGGESTIONS FOR CLINICAL ACTIVITIES

- Assign students to care for clients with various cardiac disorders. Have students review client physical assessments and health history for manifestations of cardiac disorders.

LEARNING OUTCOME 2

Explain risk factors and preventive measures for cardiac disorders such as heart failure, inflammatory disorders, and valve disorders.

CONCEPTS FOR LECTURE
HEART FAILURE

1. Risk factors for the development of heart failure include any condition that decreases cardiac output below the level of metabolic need. Such conditions include coronary artery disease, cardiomyopathies, hypertension, and congenital and valvular heart disease.

2. Health promotion activities to reduce the risk for heart failure include teaching the client about how to reduce the risk factors for coronary heart disease. Controllable factors include hypertension and diabetes mellitus.

POWERPOINT LECTURE SLIDES

Risk Factors and Preventive Measures for Cardiac Disorders
- Heart failure
  - Risk factors
    - Coronary artery disease
    - Cardiomyopathies
    - Hypertension
- Congenital and valvular heart disease prevention
  - Education regarding coronary artery disease and diabetes mellitus
- Rheumatic fever and rheumatic heart disease
  - Risk factors
    - Crowded living conditions
    - Malnutrition

RHEUMATIC FEVER AND RHEUMATIC HEART DISEASE

3. Risk factors for streptococcal infections of the pharynx include environmental and economic factors such as crowded living conditions, malnutrition, immunodeficiency, and poor access to health care.
4. There may also be a genetic factor in susceptibility to rheumatic fever.
5. Prompt identification and treatment of streptococcal throat infections helps decrease spread of the pathogen and the risk of rheumatic fever. The importance of finishing the complete course of medications should be emphasized.

INFECTIVE ENDOCARDITIS

6. Risk factors for infective endocarditis include the presence of congenital deformities of the heart, tissue damage due to ischemic disease, valve prosthesis, intravenous drug use, invasive catheters, dental procedures or poor dental health, and recent heart surgery.
7. Education of susceptible people is a key part of prevention. Clients with preexisting heart valve damage or replacement may require prophylactic antibiotic administration prior to invasive procedures, including routine dental work.

MYOCARDITIS

8. Any factor that alters immune response, such as advanced age, malnutrition, alcohol use, immunosuppression, exposure to radiation, and stress increase the risk for myocarditis.

VALVULAR HEART DISEASE

9. Since valvular heart disease is often a consequence of rheumatic heart disease, measures to prevent rheumatic fever are essential. The registered nurse should emphasize early and effective treatment of strep throat, including the importance of completing the full prescription of antibiotics. Prophylactic antibiotic therapy before invasive procedures is also important.

- – Immunodeficiency
- – Poor access to health care
- – Genetic factor may be present
  - ○ Prevention
    - – Prompt identification, treatment
    - – Importance of finishing medications
- • Infective endocarditis
  - ○ Risk factors
    - – Congenital deformities
    - – Tissue damage due to ischemic disease
    - – Valve prosthesis
    - – Intravenous drug use
    - – Invasive catheters
    - – Dental procedures or poor dental health
    - – Recent heart surgery
  - ○ Prevention
    - – Education is key
    - – Prophylactic antibiotics
- • Myocarditis
  - ○ Risk factors are anything that alters immune response
    - – Advanced age
    - – Malnutrition
    - – Alcohol use
    - – Immunosuppression
    - – Exposure to radiation
    - – Stress
- • Valvular heart disease
  - ○ Measures to prevent rheumatic fever
    - – Emphasis on early and effective treatment of strep throat
    - – Importance of completing the full rescription of antibiotic
- • Prophylactic antibiotic therapy before invasive procedures

---

SUGGESTIONS FOR CLASSROOM ACTIVITIES

- • Have students develop a community outreach teaching plan regarding strep infections of the throat, including common manifestations, the need for health care intervention, and the importance of taking the entire prescription of antibiotics.

SUGGESTIONS FOR CLINICAL ACTIVITIES

- • Have students teach discharged at-risk clients about manifestations that indicate the need for reassessment by a healthcare professional.
- • Have students teach discharged at-risk clients about measures to prevent the development of cardiac disorders.

LEARNING OUTCOME 3

Discuss indications for and management of clients undergoing hemodynamic monitoring.

CONCEPTS FOR LECTURE

1. Hemodynamics is the study of forces involved in blood circulation. The main goals are to evaluate cardiac and circulatory function and responses to interventions.
2. Hemodynamic parameters include heart rate, arterial blood pressure, central venous or right atrial pressure, pulmonary pressure, and cardiac output.
3. These parameters can be measured directly (straight from the monitor) or indirectly (calculated using direct data.)
4. Nursing care of clients with hemodynamic monitoring includes interventions focused on safety, infection control, and accuracy of measurement. Knowledge of hemodynamic equipment being used is paramount.

POWERPOINT LECTURE SLIDES

Hemodynamic Monitoring
- Hemodynamics
  - Study of forces involved in blood circulation
  - Main goals
    - Evaluation of cardiac and circulatory function
    - Evaluation of responses to interventions
- Hemodynamic parameters
  - Heart rate
  - Arterial blood pressure
  - Central venous or right atrial pressure
  - Pulmonary pressure
  - Cardiac output
- How parameters are measured
  - Directly (straight from the monitor)
  - Indirectly (calculated using direct data)
- Nursing Care Focus
  - Safety
  - Infection control
  - Accuracy of measurement
  - Knowledge of equipment being used

SUGGESTIONS FOR CLASSROOM ACTIVITIES

- Arrange for a registered nurse who has extensive hemodynamic monitoring experience to discuss the use of this equipment in practice.
- Have students search the internet for types of hemodynamic monitoring equipment. In class, discuss the similarities and differences of this equipment.

SUGGESTIONS FOR CLINICAL ACTIVITIES

- Arrange for students to observe registered nurses caring for clients who are being hemodynamically monitored.

LEARNING OUTCOME 4

Discuss the effects and nursing implications for medications commonly prescribed for clients with cardiac disorders.

CONCEPTS FOR LECTURE

HEART FAILURE

1. Clients receive multiple medications for heart failure. The main classes are ACE inhibitors, angiotension II receptor blockers, beta-blockers, diuretics, inotropic medications, direct vasodilators, and antidysrhythmic drugs.
2. Nursing diagnoses include: Decreased Cardiac Output; Excess Fluid Volume; Activity Intolerance; and Deficient Knowledge: Low-Sodium Diet.

PULMONARY EDEMA

3. This medical emergency requires astute assessment and rapid intervention. Medications commonly administered include morphine sulfate; potent loop diuretics such as furosemide (Lasix); vasodilators such as nitroprusside (Nipride); dopamine (Dopastat)

POWERPOINT LECTURE SLIDES

Medications for Cardiac Disorders
- Heart failure
  - ACE inhibitors
  - Angiotensin II receptor blockers
  - Beta-blockers
  - Diuretics
  - Inotropic medications
  - Direct vasodilators
  - Antidysrhythmic drugs
- Pulmonary edema
  - Morphine sulfate
  - Potent loop diuretics such as furosemide
  - Vasodilators such as nitroprusside; dopamine or dobutamine
  - Aminophylline to reduce bronchospasm

or dobutamine (Dobutrex) to improve myocardial contractility; and aminophylline (Corophyllin) to reduce bronchospasm.

4. Nursing diagnoses include: Impaired Gas Exchange; Decreased Cardiac Output; and Fear.

RHEUMATIC FEVER

5. As soon as diagnosis is made, antibiotic therapy is initiated. Penicillin (PCN) is the drug of choice with erythromycin (Erythrocin) or clindamycin (Cleocin) used for those who are allergic to PCN. Antibiotic therapy may continue for 5 to 10 years to prevent recurrence.

6. Joint pain and fever are managed with antiinflammatory medications.

7. Nursing diagnoses include: Acute Pain and Activity Intolerance.

INFECTIVE ENDOCARDITIS

8. Antibiotic therapy effectively treats infective endocarditis in most cases. The fibrin covering over the vegetative lesions protects them from antibiotics, so a prolonged course of therapy is generally necessary.

9. Nursing diagnoses include: Risk for Imbalanced Body Temperature; Risk for Ineffective Tissue Perfusion; and Ineffective Health Maintenance.

MYOCARDITIS

10. Medications administered for myocarditis depend upon the likely causative factor. Common medications include antibiotics and antiviral therapy if infection is the cause. Immunosuppressives may be used to minimize the inflammatory response if inflammation is a factor. Heart failure is treated with ACE inhibitors and other drugs, but digitalis preparations should be used with caution. Other medications include antidysrhythmic agents and anticoagulants.

11. Nursing diagnoses include: Activity Intolerance; Decreased Cardiac Output; Fatigue; Anxiety; and Excess Fluid Volume.

PERICARDITIS

12. Medication is administered according to manifestations. Aspirin (ASA) and acetaminophen are used for fever. NSAIDs are used to decrease inflammation and for comfort. Corticosteroids may be used.

13. Pericardiocentesis may be indicated to remove pericardial fluid.

14. Nursing diagnoses include: Acute Pain; Ineffective Breathing Pattern; Risk for Decreased Cardiac Output; and Activity Intolerance.

VALVULAR HEART DISEASE

15. If heart failure is present, the client is treated with diuretics, ACE inhibitors, vasodilators, and possibly digitalis. If atrial fibrillation is present, digitalis, small doses of

- Rheumatic fever
  - Antibiotics
    - Penicillin
    - Erythromycin, Clindamycin
  - Anti-inflammatory drugs
- Infective endocarditis
  - Prolonged course of antibiotics
- Myocarditis
  - Antibiotics and antiviral therapy if infection
  - Immunosuppressives to minimize the inflammatory response
  - ACE inhibitors and other drugs
    - Digitalis preparations should be used with caution
  - Antidysrhythmic agents
  - Anticoagulants
- Pericarditis
  - According to manifestations
    - ASA and acetaminophen
    - NSAIDs
    - Corticosteroids
- Valvular heart disease
  - Diuretics, ACE inhibitors, vasodilators, and possibly digitalis if heart failure
  - Digitalis, small doses of beta-blockers, and anticoagulant therapy if atrial fibrillation
  - Prophylactic antibiotics prior to any dental work, invasive procedures, or surgery
  - Surgery and invasive procedures
  - Percutaneous balloon valvuloplasty
  - Valvuloplasty
  - Open commissurotomy
  - Annuloplasty
  - Valve replacement
- Cardiomyopathies
  - Dilated and restrictive cardiomyopathies
    - ACE inhibitors, vasodilators, and digitalis
    - Beta-blockers with caution in dilated cardiomyopathy
    - Anticoagulants and antidysrhythmics
  - Hypertrophic cardiomyopathy
    - Beta-blockers
    - Vasodilators, digitalis, nitrates, and diuretics are contraindicated
  - Surgery and invasive treatments
  - Cardiac transplant
  - Ventricular assist devices
  - Removal of excess muscle
  - Dual-chamber pacemakers
  - Implantable cardioverter-defibrillators

beta-blockers, and anticoagulant therapy is prescribed. Antibiotics are prescribed prophylactically prior to any dental work, invasive procedures, or surgery.

16. Surgical and invasive procedures include percutaneous balloon valvuloplasty; valvuloplasty; open commissurotomy; annuloplasty; and valve replacement.

17. Nursing diagnoses include: Decreased Cardiac Output; Activity Intolerance; Risk for Infection; and Ineffective Protection.

CARDIOMYOPATHIES

18. Dilated and restrictive cardiomyopathies are treated with ACE inhibitors, vasodilators, and digitalis. Beta-blockers may be used with caution in dilated cardiomyopathy. Anticoagulants and antidysrhythmics are also administered.

19. Hypertrophic cardiomyopathy is treated with beta-blockers. Vasodilators, digitalis, nitrates, and diuretics are contraindicated.

20. Definitive treatment is cardiac transplant. Ventricular assist devices may be used until a donor heart is available. Removal of excess muscle may be indicated in severely symptomatic clients with obstructive hypertrophic cardiomyopathy. Dual-chamber pacemakers and implantable cardioverter-defibrillators may be inserted.

21. Nursing diagnoses include: Decreased Cardiac Output; Fatigue; Ineffective Breathing Pattern; Fear; Ineffective Role Performance; and Anticipatory Grieving.

SUGGESTIONS FOR CLASSROOM ACTIVITIES

- Have students review the case studies about rheumatic fever and acute pulmonary edema that are provided on the textbook Companion Website.

SUGGESTIONS FOR CLINICAL ACTIVITIES

- Have students obtain standard plans of care or clinical pathways for various cardiac disorders from clinical sites. Compare and contrast the care to be provided. Discuss the RN role in ensuring quality care for these clients.

LEARNING OUTCOME 5

Describe nursing care for the client undergoing cardiac surgery or cardiac transplant.

CONCEPTS FOR LECTURE

1. Placement of a circulatory assistance device such as an intra-aortic balloon pump or left-ventricular assist device may be used to allow the myocardium to rest or as a bridge to transplant.

2. Heart transplant is the treatment of choice for end-stage heart disease.

3. Nursing care of the heart transplant client is similar to care of any cardiac surgery client. Particularly important are monitoring chest tube drainage, cardiac rate and rhythm, cardiac output, pulmonary artery pressures, and CVP.

4. The nurse manages rewarming procedures and administration of intravenous medications.

POWERPOINT LECTURE SLIDES

Nursing Care
- Placement of a circulatory assistance device
  - Intra-aortic balloon pump
  - Left-ventricular assist device
- Heart transplant
- Nursing care of the heart transplant client
  - Similar to care of any cardiac surgery client
  - Monitoring chest tube drainage
  - Monitoring cardiac rate and rhythm
  - Monitoring cardiac output, pulmonary artery pressures and CVP
- Manage
  - Rewarming procedures
  - Administration of intravenous medications

5. Infection and rejection are major postoperative concerns. Aggressive nursing care is directed at prevention of infection. Limit visitors with communicable disease, pulmonary hygiene measures, early ambulation, and strict aseptic technique.

- Aggressive nursing care to prevent infection
  - Limit visitors with communicable diseases
  - Pulmonary hygiene
  - Early ambulation
  - Strict aseptic technique

SUGGESTIONS FOR CLASSROOM ACTIVITIES

- Have students search the internet for pictures of circulatory assistance devices and methods of cardiac transplant. Review these pictures in class, and compare and contrast the equipment and methods available.
- Arrange for a registered nurse who works in an organ procurement organization to discuss management of the donor and recipient of heart transplant.
- Arrange for a heart transplant recipient to speak to the class.

SUGGESTIONS FOR CLINICAL ACTIVITIES

- Arrange for students to observe during cardiac surgery.
- Have students talk to a registered nurse who routinely cares for postoperative cardiac clients.
- Assign students to a 1-day observation experience in a postcardiac surgery intensive care unit.

CHAPTER 33
ASSESSING CLIENTS WITH HEMATOLOGIC, PERIPHERAL VASCULAR, AND LYMPHATIC DISORDERS

RESOURCE LIBRARY

 PRENTICE HALL NURSING MEDIALINK DVD-ROM

Audio Glossary
NCLEX-RN® Review
Animation
  Oxygen Transport

 COMPANION WEBSITE

Audio Glossary
NCLEX-RN® Review
Care Plan Activity: Peripheral Vascular System
Case Study: Arterial Blood Pressure
MediaLink Application: Blood Pressure
Links to Resources

📖 IMAGE LIBRARY

Figure 33.1 Blood cell formation from stem cells.

Figure 33.2 Top and side view of a red blood cell (erythrocyte).

Figure 33.3 The hemoglobin molecule includes globin (a protein) and heme, which contains iron.

Figure 33.4 Erythropoiesis.

Figure 33.5 Platelet plug formation and blood clotting.

Figure 33.7 Clot formation.

Figure 33.8 Major arteries of the systemic circulation.

Figure 33.9 Major veins of the systemic circulation.

Figure 33.10 Structure of arteries, veins, and capillaries.

Figure 33.11 The lymphatic system.

Figure 33.12 Body sites at which peripheral pulses are most easily palpated.

Figure 33.13 Evaluation of edema.

Figure 33.14 Auscultation sites of the abdominal aorta and its branches.

Figure 33.15 Percussing the spleen.

LEARNING OUTCOME 1

Describe the anatomy, physiology, and functions of the hematologic, peripheral vascular, and lymphatic systems.

CONCEPTS FOR LECTURE
HEMATOLOGIC SYSTEM

1. The hematologic system is the blood components of the circulation. Blood consists of plasma, solutes, red blood cells, white blood cells, and platelets.

2. The hematopoietic, or blood-forming, system includes bone marrow and lymphoid tissues. All blood cells originate from stem cells (hemocytoblasts).

3. The functions of blood include transporting oxygen, nutrients, hormones, and metabolic wastes; protecting against invasion of pathogens; maintaining blood coagulation; and regulating fluids, electrolytes, acids, bases, and body temperature.

4. Red blood cells carry hemoglobin that transports oxygen to body tissues and are the most common type of blood cells. Red blood cell production (erythropoiesis) begins in red bone marrow and is completed in the blood or spleen.

POWERPOINT LECTURE SLIDES

Hematologic, Peripheral Vascular, and Lymphatic Systems
- Hematologic system
  - Consists of the blood components of the circulation
    - Plasma
    - Solutes
    - Red blood cells
    - White blood cells
    - Platelets
- Hematopoietic system
  - The blood forming system
    - Bone marrow
    - Lymphoid tissues
  - All blood cells originate from stem cells (hemocytoblasts)

5. White blood cells are a part of the body's defense against microorganisms. WBCs originate from hemopoietic stem cells in the bone marrow and are classified as granular leukocytes and nongranular leukocytes.

6. Platelets are necessary for hemostasis and are produced in the bone marrow. The five stages of hemostasis are (1) vessel spasm, (2) formation of the platelet plug, (3) development of an insoluble fibrin clot, (4) clot retraction, and (5) clot dissolution.

PERIPHERAL VASCULAR SYSTEM

7. The two main components of the peripheral vascular system are the arterial network and the venous network. The arterial network includes major artery branches from the aorta that branch into successively smaller arteries and then into arterioles and finally into the capillary bed. The venous system begins with exchange areas in the capillary bed that grow into venules, which in turn join into larger and larger veins. These veins empty into the inferior and superior vena cavae and then into the right atrium.

8. Arteries have an elastic inner layer that allow them to alternately expand and recoil as the heart contracts and relaxes with each beat. This produces a pressure wave that can be felt as a pulse over an artery.

9. Venous blood travels at lower pressure than does arterial blood. Veins have thinner walls, a larger lumen, and greater capacity than do arteries and many are equipped with valves that help blood flow against gravity back to the heart.

10. The capillaries connect arterioles and venules and are permeable to the gases and molecules exchanged between blood and tissue cells. The capillaries are typically found in interwoven networks.

11. Factors that affect arterial circulation are blood flow, peripheral vascular resistance, and blood pressure.

LYMPHATIC SYSTEM

12. The lymphatic system consists of lymphoid organs (lymph nodes, spleen, thymus, tonsils, and Peyer's patches of the small intestine) and lymphatic vessels.

13. Lymph nodes are distributed along the lymphatic vessels and assist the immune system by removing foreign material, infectious organisms, and tumor cells from lymph.

14. The main function of the spleen is to filter the blood by breaking down old red blood cells, to synthesize lymphocytes, store platelets for blood clotting, and to serve as a reservoir for blood.

15. The thymus gland is most active during childhood and facilitates the immune action of lymphocytes.

16. Tonsils and Peyer's patches protect the upper respiratory and digestive tracts from foreign pathogens.

17. Lymphatic vessels form a network around the arterial and venous channels and serve to collect and drain excess tissue fluid called lymph.

- Functions of the blood
  - Transporting oxygen, nutrients, hormones, and metabolic wastes
  - Protecting against invasion of pathogens
  - Maintaining blood coagulation
  - Regulating fluids, electrolytes, acids, bases, and body temperature
- Peripheral vascular system: two main components
  - Arterial network
    - Major artery branches from aorta
    - Successively small arteries
    - Arterioles
    - Capillary bed
  - Venous system
    - Capillary bed
    - Venules
    - Veins
    - Inferior and superior vena cavae
    - Right atrium
- Lymphatic system components
  - Lymphoid organs
    - Lymph nodes
    - Spleen
    - Thymus
    - Tonsils
    - Peyer's patches of small intestine
  - Lymphatic vessels

LEARNING OUTCOME 2

Explain the physiologic dynamics of blood flow, peripheral resistance, and blood pressure.

CONCEPTS FOR LECTURE

1. Blood flow refers to the volume of blood transported in a vessel, in an organ, or throughout the entire circulation over a given period of time and is commonly expressed as liters or milliliters per minute or cubic centimeters per second.
2. Peripheral vascular resistance refers to the opposing forces or impedance to blood flow as arterial channels become more distant from the heart. It is determined by blood viscosity, length of the vessel, and diameter of the vessel.
3. Blood pressure is the force exerted against the walls of the arteries by the blood as it is pumped from the heart. Mean arterial pressure (MAP) is regulated by cardiac output (CO) and peripheral vascular resistance (PVR): MAP = CO x PVR.
4. Systolic blood pressure is the highest pressure that occurs at the peak of ventricular contraction (systole).
5. Diastolic blood pressure is the lowest pressure that is exerted during ventricular relaxation (diastole).

POWERPOINT LECTURE SLIDES

Blood Flow, Peripheral Resistance, and Blood Pressure
- Blood flow
  - The volume of blood transported in a vessel, in an organ, or throughout the circulation over a given period of time
  - Commonly expressed as liters or milliliters per minute or cubic centimeters per second
- Peripheral vascular resistance
  - The opposing forces or impedance to blood flow as arterial channels become more distant from the heart
  - Determined by blood viscosity, length of vessel, and diameter of vessel
- Blood pressure
  - Force exerted against walls of arteries by blood as it is pumped from the heart
  - Mean arterial pressure is regulated by cardiac output and peripheral vascular resistance
    - MAP = CO x PVR
- Systolic blood pressure
  - Highest pressure that occurs at peak of ventricular contraction (systole)
- Diastolic blood pressure
  - Lowest pressure that occurs during ventricular relaxation (diastole)

LEARNING OUTCOME 3

Compare and contrast the major factors influencing arterial blood pressure.

CONCEPTS FOR LECTURE

1. The sympathetic and parasympathetic nervous systems are the primary mechanisms that regulate blood pressure. Sympathetic nervous system stimulation causes vasoconstriction of the arterioles, which thereby increases blood pressure. Parasympathetic stimulation causes vasodilation of the arterioles, which lowers blood pressure.
2. Baroreceptors and chemoreceptors in the aortic arch, carotid sinus, and other large vessels are sensitive to

POWERPOINT LECTURE SLIDES

Arterial Blood Pressure
- Sympathetic nervous system
  - Causes vasoconstriction of arterioles, increasing BP
- Parasympathetic nervous system
  - Causes vasodilation of arterioles, lowering BP
- Baroreceptors and chemoreceptors
  - Located in the aortic arch, carotid sinus, and other large vessels

pressure and chemical changes and cause sympathetic stimulation.

3. The kidneys help maintain blood pressure by excreting or conserving sodium and water by initiating the renin-angiotensin mechanism and responding to pituitary release of antidiuretic hormone.

4. Environmental temperatures may affect peripheral resistance: cold causes vasoconstriction and heat causing vasodilation.

5. Chemicals, hormones, and drugs can influence blood pressure by affecting cardiac output and/or peripheral vascular resistance.

6. Dietary factors such as intake of salt, saturated fats, and cholesterol elevate blood pressure by affecting blood volume and vessel diameter.

7. Race, gender, age, weight, time of day, position, exercise, and emotional state may also affect arterial blood pressure.

8. Systemic venous pressure can also be influenced by blood volume, venous tone, and right atrial pressure.

- ○ Sensitive to pressure and chemical changes and cause sympathetic stimulation
- Kidneys
  - ○ Excrete or conserve sodium and water
  - ○ Renin-angiotensin mechanism
  - ○ Antidiuretic hormone released by pituitary
- Environmental temperatures
  - ○ Cold causes vasoconstriction; heat causes vasodilation
- Chemicals, hormones, drugs
  - ○ Influence blood pressure by affecting cardiac output and/or peripheral vascular resistance
- Dietary factors
  - ○ Salt, saturated fats, and cholesterol elevate blood pressure by affecting blood volume and vessel diameter
- Personal factors
  - ○ Arterial blood pressure can be affected by race, gender, age, weight, time of day, position, exercise and emotional state
  - ○ Systemic venous pressure can be influenced by blood volume, venous tone, and right atrial pressure

---

SUGGESTIONS FOR CLASSROOM ACTIVITIES

- Review the case study about arterial blood pressure that is provided on the textbook DVD-ROM. Develop a nursing plan of care using information from the case study.

SUGGESTIONS FOR CLINICAL ACTIVITIES

- Assign students to clinical clients with hypertension. Lead post-clinical conference discussion of factors that affect individual client blood pressure.

LEARNING OUTCOME 4

Describe normal variations in assessment findings for the older adult.

CONCEPTS FOR LECTURE

1. Aging may result in a decrease in the ability of the bone marrow to respond to the need for increased RBCs, WBCs, and platelets. This change makes the older adult more prone to the development of anemia.

2. Aging may result in changes in the tunica intima and tunica media layers of the blood vessel structure. These changes result in a systolic blood pressure rise and vascular changes in the heart, kidneys, and pituitary gland. The older adult may manifest postural hypotension, reduction of ability to respond to cold temperatures, edema, inflammation, pressure ulcers, and changes in the effects of medications.

3. Changes in the immune system make the older adult at risk for infection with decreased manifestations of acute infection. There is an increased incidence of cancers, an altered response to antigens such as PPD, and a possible reactivation of TB.

POWERPOINT LECTURE SLIDES

Results of Aging
- Decrease bone marrow activity
  - ○ Risk for anemia
- Blood vessel changes
  - ○ Postural hypotension
  - ○ Cold intolerance
  - ○ Edema
  - ○ Inflammation
  - ○ Pressure ulcers
  - ○ Changes in effects of medications
- Immune system
  - ○ Increased risk of infection
  - ○ Increased risk of cancers
  - ○ Altered response to antigens
  - ○ Possible reactivation of TB

SUGGESTIONS FOR CLASSROOM ACTIVITIES

- Discuss the implications of age-related changes to risk factor management in the older adult.

SUGGESTIONS FOR CLINICAL ACTIVITIES

- Have students review the assessment of an older adult and identify those assessment findings that are a result of the aging process.

LEARNING OUTCOME 5

Identify manifestations of impairment in the function of the hematologic, peripheral vascular, and lymphatic systems.

CONCEPTS FOR LECTURE

1. Assessment of blood pressure may reveal hypotension, hypertension, orthostatic hypotension, or widening or narrowing of pulse pressure.
2. Skin assessment findings of pallor or cyanosis may result from circulatory abnormalities. Edema, redness, induration, or lesions over regional lymph nodes may be the result of lymphangitis, lymphedema, infection, or malignancy.
3. Assessment of arteries and veins may reveal redness, swelling, nodules, or the presence of a thrill or bruit. Assessment of pulses may reveal alterations in symmetry, rate, rhythm, or variations in pulse amplitude.
4. Assessment of the extremities may reveal edema, color changes, temperature variations, inadequate capillary refill, arterial insufficiency, lesions, skin thickening, or varicose veins.
5. Abdominal assessment may reveal pulsations, bulging, or presence of bruits. Presence of a palpable spleen may indicate splenomegaly.

POWERPOINT LECTURE SLIDES

Hematologic, Peripheral Vascular, and Lymphatic Systems
- Assessment of blood pressure may reveal
  - Hypotension
  - Hypertension
  - Orthostatic hypotension
  - Narrowing or widening of pulse pressure
- Skin assessment may reveal
  - Pallor or cyanosis from circulatory abnormalities
  - Edema, redness, induration, lesions resulting from lymphangitis, lymphedema, infection, or malignancy
- Artery and vein assessment may reveal
  - Redness, swelling, nodules, or presence of thrill or bruit
  - Pulses may be asymmetrical or have changes in rate, rhythm, or amplitude
- Extremity assessment may reveal
  - Edema, color changes, temperature variations, inadequate capillary refill, arterial insufficiency, lesions, skin thickening, or varicose veins
- Abdominal assessment may reveal
  - Pulsations, bulging, bruits
  - Presence of palpable spleen (splenomegaly)

SUGGESTIONS FOR CLASSROOM ACTIVITIES

- Discuss the pathophysiologic basis of the changes listed.

SUGGESTIONS FOR CLINICAL ACTIVITIES

- Have students complete assessment of the hematologic, peripheral pulses, and lymphatic systems of clinical clients.
- Help students relate manifestations of disorders to their physiologic basis.

Chapter 34
Nursing Care of Clients with Hematologic Disorders

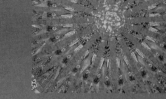

Resource Library

 PRENTICE HALL NURSING MEDIALINK DVD-ROM

Audio Glossary
NCLEX-RN® Review
Animation/Video
   Sickle Cell Anemia

 COMPANION WEBSITE

Audio Glossary
NCLEX-RN® Review
Care Plan Activity: Acute Myelocytic Leukemia
Case Studies
   Disseminated Intravascular Coagulation
   Immune Thrombocytopenic Purpura
MediaLink Applications
   Blood Alternatives
   Sickle Cell Anemia
   Stem Cell Transplant
   Synthetic Blood Products
Links to Resources

IMAGE LIBRARY

Figure 34.1 The skin of the client with anemia appears pale beside that of a person with a normal hemoglobin and hematocrit.

Figure 34.2 A blood smear showing RBCs characteristically seen in iron deficiency anemia.

Figure 34.3 Inheritance pattern for sickle cell anemia.

Figure 34.4 Blood smear containing normal red blood cells and sickle cells.

Figure 34.5 A blood smear from the bone marrow of a client with acute myeloid leukemia.

Figure 34.6 The Philadelphia chromosome.

Figure 34.7 A blood smear from the bone marrow of a client with acute lymphocytic leukemia.

Figure 34.8 Allogeneic bone marrow transplant.

Figure 34.9 Cervical lymphadenopathy in a client with lymphoma of the neck.

Figure 34.10 Patterns of radiation therapy used to treat lymphoma based on the location and extent of the disease.

Figure 34.11 An illustration of the progress of multiple myeloma in an African American male.

Figure 34.12 Significant ecchymosis of the eyelid associated with minor trauma in a client with thrombocytopenia.

Figure 34.13 The inheritance pattern of hemophilia A and B. Both are transmitted as X-linked recessive disorders.

Figure 34.14 Disseminated intravascular coagulation (DIC).

Learning Outcome 1

Relate the physiology and assessment of the hematologic system and related systems to commonly occurring hematologic disorders.

Concepts for Lecture
Anemia

1. Slowly-developing anemia may be asymptomatic as long as compensatory mechanisms are adequate. If the oxygen demands of the body increase due to exercise or infection, manifestations develop.
2. Pallor of the skin, mucous membranes, conjunctiva, and nail beds develops as a result of blood redistribution to vital organs and lack of hemoglobin.
3. Heart and respiratory rates rise in an attempt to increase cardiac output and tissue perfusion.

PowerPoint Lecture Slides

Commonly Occurring Hematologic Disorders
- Anemia
- Iron deficiency anemia
- Vitamin B$_{12}$ deficiency anemia
- Folic acid deficiency anemia
- Sickle cell anemia
- Thalassemia
- Acquired hemolytic anemia
- Glucose 6-phosphate dehydrogenase anemia

4. Tissue hypoxia may cause angina, fatigue, dyspnea of exertion, and night cramps.
5. Increased erythropoietin release stimulates RBC production in the bone marrow, which leads to bone pain.
6. Cerebral hypoxia can lead to headache, dizziness, and dim vision.
7. With rapidly-developing anemia, initial manifestations include tachycardia and tachypnea and pale, cool, clammy skin. Signs of circulatory shock include hypotension, tachycardia, decreased level of consciousness, and oliguria.

IRON DEFICIENCY ANEMIA

8. Chronic iron deficiency may also lead to brittle, spoon-shaped nails; cheilosis; a smooth, sore tongue; and pica.

VITAMIN B$_{12}$ DEFICIENCY ANEMIA

9. Manifestations develop gradually as bodily stores of B$_{12}$ are depleted. Specific manifestations include paresthesias and problems with proprioception.
10. Pernicious anemia may result in a smooth, sore, beefy tongue and diarrhea.

FOLIC ACID DEFICIENCY ANEMIA

11. Manifestations include pallor, progressive weakness and fatigue, shortness of breath, and heart palpitations. Glossitis, cheilosis, and diarrhea are common. There are no neurologic symptoms with folic acid deficiency anemia.
12. Folic acid deficiency anemia is strongly associated with neural tube defects such as meningomyelocele.

SICKLE CELL ANEMIA

13. Red blood cell sickling causes general manifestations of hemolytic anemia, including pallor, fatigue, jaundice, and irritability. Extensive sickling can precipitate a sickle cell crisis in which the microcirculation occludes. This occlusion leads to issue ischemia, infarction, and severe pain.
14. Sickling affects all body systems. Common findings are painful swelling of the hands, feet, and joints; abdominal pain; stroke; priapism; ulceration of the skin; enlargement of the spleen and liver; renal insufficiency; and gallstone development. Acute chest syndrome and sequestration crisis may also develop.

THALASSEMIA

15. People with thalassemia minor often are asymptomatic. When manifestations do occur they include mild to moderate anemia, mild splenomegaly, bronze skin coloring, and bone marrow hyperplasia.
16. Thalassemia major causes severe anemia; heart failure; fractures of long bones, ribs, and vertebrae; jaundice; liver failure; and failure of the pancreas.

- Aplastic anemia
- Myelodysplastic syndrome
- Polycythemia
- Multiple myeloma
- Neutropenia
- Infectious mononucleosis

ACQUIRED HEMOLYTIC ANEMIA

17. Manifestations depend upon the extent of hemolysis and the body's ability to replace destroyed RBCs. Findings may include mild to moderate anemia, splenic enlargement, jaundice, and in severe cases, deformity and pathologic fractures of the bones.

GLUCOSE 6-PHOSPHATE DEHYDROGENASE ANEMIA

18. Manifestations develop within days of exposure to the stressor drugs. Findings may include pallor, jaundice, hemoglobinuria, and an elevated reticulocyte count.

APLASTIC ANEMIA

19. Manifestations vary with the severity of the pancytopenia and may be sudden or insidious. Manifestations include fatigue, pallor, progressive weakness, exertional dyspnea, headache, tachycardia, bleeding tendencies, fever, and heart failure.

MYELODYSPLASTIC SYNDROME

20. Anemia is the predominant early manifestation and in many cases the client is asymptomatic, and learns about the anemia only as a result of routine blood count.
21. Manifestations include fatigue, weakness, dyspnea, pallor, splenomegaly, and hepatomegaly with resulting upper abdominal pain, abnormal bleeding, and increased infection.

POLYCYTHEMIA

22. Polycythemia vera (PV) is initially asymptomatic. Manifestations include hypertension, headache, dizziness, vision and hearing disruptions, plethora, mental status changes, weight loss, and night sweats.
23. Complications of PV include thrombosis and hemorrhage.
24. Secondary polycythemia manifestations are similar to those of primary polycythemia.

MULTIPLE MYELOMA

25. Multiple myeloma develops slowly. Manifestations are due to its effects on the bone and the impaired immune system. Bone pain is the most common presenting symptom. Rapid bone destruction leads to hypercalcemia and manifestations of neurologic dysfunction.

NEUTROPENIA

26. The manifestations of neutropenia include opportunistic bacterial, fungal, and protozoal infections that commonly affect the respiratory tract and mucosa of the mouth, GI tract, and vagina. Malaise, chills, and fever with extreme weakness are common.

INFECTIOUS MONONUCLEOSIS

27. The onset of mononucleosis is insidious with headache, malaise, and fatigue. Other manifestations may include fever, sore throat, cervical lymphadenopathy, and splenomegaly.

SUGGESTIONS FOR CLASSROOM ACTIVITIES

• Assign each major hematologic disorder to a small group of students. Have the students explain how the disorder relates to the pathophysiology of the hematological system as if they were explaining it to a lay audience.

LEARNING OUTCOME 2

Describe the pathophysiology of common hematologic disorders.

CONCEPTS FOR LECTURE

1. A number of factors can lead to anemia, but they all reduce the oxygen-carrying capacity of the blood, which leads to tissue hypoxia. Basic factors include decreased RBC production and increased RBC loss or destruction.

2. In acute blood loss anemia, the RBCs are normocytic and the RBC count, hemoglobin, and hematocrit may be normal. As blood loss continues, fluid shifts into the vascular space to maintain circulating volume and the RBC count, hemoglobin, and hematocrit fall.

NUTRITIONAL ANEMIAS

3. Nutritional anemias result from nutrient deficits that affect RBC formation or hemoglobin synthesis. The deficit may occur from inadequate diet, malabsorption of the nutrient, or an increased need for the nutrient.

4. Iron deficiency anemia is the most common type of anemia and develops when the supply of iron is inadequate for optimal RBC formation and hemoglobin synthesis.

5. Vitamin B_{12} deficiency occurs when inadequate vitamin B_{12} is consumed, or, more commonly, when it is poorly absorbed from the GI tract.

6. Folic acid is necessary for DNA synthesis and normal maturation of red blood cells. Folic acid deficiency anemia is characterized by fragile, large, immature cells. Those at risk of developing folic acid deficiency are those with chronic malnutrition and those with impaired folic acid absorption.

HEMOLYTIC ANEMIA

7. Hemolytic anemias are characterized by premature lysis of RBCs. In response to this lysis the hematopoietic activity of bone marrow increases, which leads to immature RBCs in circulating blood.

SICKLE CELL ANEMIA

8. Sickle cell anemia is a hereditary, chronic hemolytic anemia characterized by episodes when RBCs become

POWERPOINT LECTURE SLIDES

Pathophysiology of Common Hematologic Disorders
- Anemia
  - Decreased RBC production
  - Increased RBC loss
  - Increased RBC destruction
- Nutritional anemias
  - Nutrient deficits affect RBC formation or hemoglobin synthesis
  - Inadequate diet
  - Malabsorption of the nutrient
  - Increased need for the nutrient
- Hemolytic anemia
  - Premature lysis of RBCs
  - Hematopoietic activity increases
  - Causes immature RBCs
- Sickle cell anemia
  - Hereditary, chronic hemolytic anemia
  - RBCs become abnormally crescent shaped or sickled
  - Causes synthesis of an abnormal form of hemoglobin
  - Autosomal recessively transmitted
  - Sickle cell crisis
- Thalassemia
  - Inherited disorders of hemoglobin synthesis
    - Mediterranean, Asian, or African American
  - Results in RBCs called target cells
    - Distinctive bull's-eye appearance
- Acquired hemolytic anemia
  - Hemolysis due to factors outside the RBC
    - Mechanical trauma to the RBC
    - Autoimmune disorders
    - Bacterial or protozoal infection
    - Immune system-mediated response
    - Response to drugs, toxins, chemical agents, or venoms
- Glucose-6-phosphate dehydrogenase anemia (G6PD)
  - Hereditary defect in RBC metabolism

abnormally crescent-shaped or sickled. This defect causes synthesis of an abnormal form of hemoglobin and is autosomal recessively transmitted.

THALASSEMIA

9. Thalassemia is an inherited disorder of hemoglobin synthesis that generally affects people of Mediterranean, Asian, or African American descent. The disorder results in RBCs called target cells because of their distinctive bull's-eye appearance.

10. The disorder results from missing or defective alpha or beta chains of the hemoglobin. Severity of symptoms depends upon which chains and genes are affected.

ACQUIRED HEMOLYTIC ANEMIA

11. Acquired hemolytic anemia results from hemolysis due to factors outside the RBC. Some factors include mechanical trauma to the RBC, autoimmune disorders, bacterial or protozoal infection, immune system-mediated response, and response to drugs, toxins, chemical agents, or venoms.

GLUCOSE-6-PHOSPHATE DEHYDROGENASE ANEMIA

12. Glucose-6-phosphate dehydrogenase (G6PD) anemia is caused by a hereditary defect in RBC metabolism and is relatively common in people of African or Mediterranean descent. The defect has many variations, but generally causes direct oxidation of hemoglobin, which damages the RBC. It is often triggered by exposure to drugs such as aspirin, sulfonamides, or vitamin K derivatives.

APLASTIC ANEMIA

13. In aplastic anemia, the bone marrow fails to produce all three types of blood cells, which leads to pancytopenia. The cause of about 50% of aplastic anemia is idiopathic; other cases are caused by exposure to radiation, certain chemicals such as benzene, some antibiotics, and chemotherapeutic drugs.

14. Faconi anemia is a rare aplastic anemia caused by defects of DNA repair.

MYELODYSPLASTIC SYNDROME

15. Myelodysplastic syndrome (MDS) is a group of blood disorders characterized by abnormal-appearing bone marrow and cytopenia.

16. Anemia that does not respond to treatment (refractory anemia) is a characteristic of most forms of MDS.

17. Primary MDS is idiopathic. Secondary MDS may be related to exposure to environmental toxins such as cigarette smoke, benzene and radiation, radiation therapy, or chemotherapy.

- ○ Generally causes direct oxidation of hemoglobin
- ○ Triggered by exposure to drugs
  - – Aspirin
  - – Sulfonamides
  - – Vitamin K derivatives
- Aplastic anemia
  - ○ Bone marrow fails to produce all three types of blood cells
  - ○ Leading to pancytopenia
- Myelodysplastic syndrome
  - ○ Abnormal appearing bone marrow and cytopenia
  - ○ Causes refractory anemia
  - ○ Stem cells fail to reproduce and differentiate
  - ○ Genetic components of stem cells altered
  - ○ Ability to produce normal cells is lost
- Polycythemia
  - ○ Excess of RBCs (hematocrit higher than 55%)
  - ○ Types: primary, secondary, and relative
- Multiple myeloma
  - ○ Malignancy in which plasma cells multiply uncontrollably
  - ○ Cells infiltrate bone marrow, lymph nodes, spleen
  - ○ Affected bones are weakened
  - ○ Pathologic fractures
- Neutropenia
  - ○ Development/maturation of granulocytes in the bone marrow suppressed
  - ○ Number of circulating neutrophils falls rapidly
  - ○ Immunity is significantly reduced
- Infectious mononucleosis
  - ○ Epstein-Barr viral invasion of oropharyngeal lymphoid tissues
  - ○ Usually benign and self-limiting
  - ○ Incubation period: 4 to 8 weeks

18. MDS occurs when stem cells fail to reproduce and differentiate into the various types of blood cells. Genetic components of stem cells are altered and the ability to produce normal cells is lost. In severe cases, people with MDS may develop leukemia.

POLYCYTHEMIA

19. Polycythemia is an excess of RBCs characterized by a hematocrit higher than 55%.
20. Primary polycythemia (polycythemia vera) is caused by an increase of RBC production. PV uncommon and most commonly affects men of European Jewish ancestry. It is considered a myeloproliferative disorder and is of idiopathic origin.
21. Secondary polycythemia (erythrocytosis) occurs when erythropoietin levels are elevated and may affect clients of any age or origin. It is most commonly a response to hypoxia.
22. Relative polycythemia occurs due to fluid deficit, not excess RBCs. The hematocrit is elevated because of cell concentration.

MULTIPLE MYELOMA

23. Multiple myeloma is a malignancy in which plasma cells multiply uncontrollably and infiltrate the bone marrow, lymph nodes, spleen, and other tissues. Affected bones are weakened and may break without trauma.

NEUTROPENIA

24. Leukopenia is a decrease in the total circulating white blood cell count. Neutropenia is a decrease in circulating neutrophils. Agranulocytosis is severe neutropenia.
25. When the development and maturation of granulocytes in the bone marrow is suppressed, the number of circulating neutrophils falls rapidly. As a result, immunity is significantly reduced.

INFECTIOUS MONONUCLEOSIS

26. Infectious mononucleosis is characterized by the invasion of the Epstein-Barr virus into oropharyngeal lymphoid tissues. The disease is usually benign and self-limiting. The incubation period for infectious mononucleosis is 4 to 8 weeks.

SUGGESTIONS FOR CLASSROOM ACTIVITIES

- Using the same small group approach as in the previous suggestion for classroom activities, have the student groups explain the pathophysiology of their assigned disorders. Be certain that students explain the pathophysiology as if they were speaking to a lay audience.
- Review the animation about sickle cell anemia provided on the textbook DVD-ROM.

LEARNING OUTCOME 3

Explain nursing implications for medications and other treatments prescribed for hematologic disorders.

CONCEPTS FOR LECTURE

ANEMIA

1. Medications to treat anemia depend on its cause. Common medications include: iron replacement therapy for iron deficiency anemia; parenteral vitamin B_{12} for vitamin B_{12} deficiency anemia; folic acid supplementation for all women of childbearing age and clients with folic acid deficiency or sickle cell anemia; hydroxyurea for clients with sickle cell anemia; erythropoietin; and immunosuppressive therapy for aplastic anemia.

2. Blood transfusions may be indicated to treat anemia.

3. Nursing diagnoses include: Activity Intolerance; Impaired Oral Mucous Membranes; Risk for Decreased Cardiac Output; and Self-Care Deficit.

MYELODYSPLASTIC SYNDROME

4. Management of MDS is based on the severity of the disease. Therapy is guided by classification of the disease according to severity using the French-American-British system, the International Prognostic Scoring System, or the World Health Organization classification system.

5. Treatments include frequent red blood cell transfusion, iron chelation therapy to remove excess iron; administration of blood cell growth factors, platelet transfusion, and antibiotic therapy. Chemotherapy regimens similar to those used to treat leukemia may be administered. Stem cell transplant is the only hope for a cure.

6. Nursing diagnoses include: Activity Intolerance and Risk for Ineffective Health Maintenance.

POLYCYTHEMIA

7. Treatment of PV may include use of chemotherapeutic agents that may increase the client's risk for leukemia.

8. Secondary polycythemia clients may require no treatment if asymptomatic. Smokers are urged to quit.

9. Periodic phlebotomy, which removes 300 to 500 mL of blood, may benefit clients with both primary and secondary polycythemia.

10. Other medications may include antihistamines to treat itching and aspirin (ASA) to control thrombosis.

11. Nursing diagnoses include: Decisional Conflict Regarding Smoking Cessation; Pain; and Risk for Ineffective Tissue Perfusion.

MULTIPLE MYELOMA

12. There is no cure for multiple myeloma. The disease may have a very slow course for many years. When indicated, standard treatment includes induction

POWERPOINT LECTURE SLIDES

Nursing Implications
- Anemia
  - Medications
    - Iron replacement therapy for iron deficiency anemia
    - Parenteral vitamin B_{12} for vitamin B_{12} deficiency anemia
    - Folic acid supplementation
    - Hydroxyurea for sickle cell anemia
    - Erythropoietin
    - Immunosuppressive therapy to treat aplastic anemia
  - Treatments
    - Blood transfusion
  - Nursing diagnoses
    - Activity Intolerance
    - Impaired Oral Mucous Membranes
    - Risk for Decreased Cardiac Output
    - Self-Care Deficit
- Myelodysplastic syndrome
  - Treatments
    - Frequent red blood cell transfusion
    - Iron chelation therapy
    - Administration of blood cell growth factors
    - Platelet transfusion
    - Antibiotic therapy
    - Chemotherapy regimens
    - Stem cell transplant is the only hope for a cure
  - Nursing diagnoses
    - Activity Intolerance
    - Risk for Ineffective Health Maintenance
- Polycythemia
  - Treatment
    - Chemotherapeutic agents
    - Smoking cessations
    - Periodic phlebotomy
  - Medications
    - Antihistamines
    - ASA
  - Nursing diagnoses
    - Decisional Conflict Regarding Smoking Cessation
    - Pain
    - Risk for Ineffective Tissue Perfusion
- Multiple myeloma
  - Treatment
    - No cure
    - Induction chemotherapy
    - Stem cell transplant
    - Maintenance chemotherapy
  - Nursing diagnoses
    - Chronic Pain

chemotherapy followed by stem cell transplant and maintenance chemotherapy.

13. Nursing diagnoses include: Chronic Pain; Impaired Physical Ability; and Risk for Injury.

NEUTROPENIA

14. Hematopoietic growth factor may be administered to stimulate granulocyte maturation and differentiation. Antibiotics and isolation may be used to treat infection.

15. The primary nursing diagnosis is Risk for Infection.

INFECTIOUS MONONUCLEOSIS

16. Treatment includes bed rest and analgesic agents to alleviate symptoms.

17. Nursing care is primarily educational to prevent further spread of the disease.

- – Impaired Physical Ability
- – Risk for Injury
- Neutropenia
  - ○ Treatments
    - – Hematopoietic growth factor
    - – Antibiotics
    - – Isolation
  - ○ Primary nursing diagnosis
    - – Risk for Infection
- Infectious mononucleosis
  - ○ Treatment
    - – Bedrest
    - – Analgesic agents
  - ○ Nursing care
    - – Primarily educational

SUGGESTIONS FOR CLASSROOM ACTIVITIES

- Have each small group outlined in Outcome 1 and 2 create a nursing plan of care for clients with the disorder they are investigating.

SUGGESTIONS FOR CLINICAL ACTIVITIES

- Assign students to the care of clients with a hematologic disorder. Have students review the client's health assessment and diagnostic test results for indications of a hematologic disorder. Have students present findings in a clinical post-conference.

LEARNING OUTCOME 4

Discuss indications for and complications of bone marrow or stem cell transplantation, as well as related nursing care.

CONCEPTS FOR LECTURE

1. Bone marrow transplant (BMT) is the treatment of choice for some types of leukemia. Two major categories of BMT are used.

2. Allogeneic BMT uses bone marrow cells from a donor. Prior to cell transfusion, high doses of chemotherapy and/or total body irradiation are used to destroy leukemic cells in the bone marrow.

3. Autologous BMT uses the client's own bone marrow and is often called bone marrow rescue. About 1 L of bone marrow is aspirated from the client during a period of disease remission. The marrow is frozen and stored for future use. If relapse occurs, lethal doses of chemotherapy or radiation are given to destroy the immune system and malignant cells, and the thawed marrow is administered.

4. In both allogeneic and autologous BMT, the client is critically ill during the period of bone marrow destruction. Potential complications include malnutrition, infection, and bleeding.

5. Allogeneic stem cell transplant (SCT) is an alternative to BMT. SCT results in complete and sustained replacement of the recipient's blood cell lines with cells derived from donor stem cells. The risks for infection and other complications are similar to those of BMT.

POWERPOINT LECTURE SLIDES

Bone Marrow or Stem Cell Transplantation
- Bone marrow transplant
  - ○ Allogeneic BMT
    - – Donor bone marrow
    - – Prior to transfusion leukemic cells are destroyed
  - ○ Autologous BMT (bone marrow rescue)
    - – Uses the client's own remission bone marrow
    - – Administered in case relapse occurs
    - – Lethal doses of chemotherapy or radiation are given
    - – Thawed marrow is administered
  - ○ Nursing care
    - – In both, client is critically ill
    - – Bone marrow is destroyed
    - – Potential complications include malnutrition, infection, and bleeding
- Allogeneic stem cell transplant (SCT)
  - ○ Alternative to BMT
  - ○ Complete/sustained replacement of blood cell lines
- Nursing care
  - ○ Complications is similar to those of BMT

6. Graft-versus-host disease (GVHD) develops in up to 60% of clients who receive an allogeneic BMT or SCT. It results when the immune cells of the donated bone marrow (graft) identify the recipient's body (host) as foreign.
7. Acute GVHD develops within days or weeks of the transplant. Manifestations are a pruritic, maculopapular rash that begins on the palms and soles of the feet and jaundice.
8. Chronic GVHD develops 100 or more days after the transplant and may follow acute GVHD or may develop in clients with no prior symptoms.
9. Priority nursing diagnoses include: Risk for Infection; Imbalanced Nutrition; and Impaired Protection (Bleeding).

SUGGESTIONS FOR CLASSROOM ACTIVITIES

- Have students list the possible sources of nosocomial infection that are of danger to a client undergoing bone marrow or stem cell transplantation. Help students relate common nursing interventions to the development of those infections, focusing on prevention.
- Have students outline the typical sequence of procedures performed when clients undergo bone marrow or stem cell transplantation. Focus students on the ability of the nurse to decrease the client's risk for injury secondary to those procedures.
- Arrange for a post-bone marrow or stem cell transplant client to speak to the class.

SUGGESTIONS FOR CLINICAL ACTIVITIES

- Have students research the isolation capabilities of the nursing unit on which they have clinical. Lead a post-conference discussion about what would be necessary for a bone marrow or stem cell transplant client.

LEARNING OUTCOME 5

Compare and contrast the pathophysiology, manifestations, and management of bleeding disorders.

CONCEPTS FOR LECTURE

1. Bleeding disorders may result from deficient platelets, disruption of the clotting cascade, or a combination of factors.

THROMBOCYTOPENIA

2. Thrombocytopenia is a platelet count less than 100,000 per milliliter of blood and can lead to abnormal bleeding.
3. Thrombocytopenia results from one of three mechanisms: decreased production, increased sequestration in the spleen, or accelerated destruction.
4. Two types of primary thrombocytopenia are immune thrombocytopenic purpura (ITP) and thrombotic thrombocytopenic purpura (TTP).
5. ITP is also known as idiopathic thrombocytopenic purpura. It is an autoimmune disorder in which platelet destruction is accelerated.
6. Manifestations of ITP are due to bleeding from small vessels and mucous membranes. Common findings are petechiae, purpura, bruising, epistaxis, hematuria, excess

POWERPOINT LECTURE SLIDES

Bleeding Disorders
- Thrombocytopenia
  - Immune thrombocytopenic purpura (ITP)
    - Manifestations—petechiae, purpura, bruising, epistaxis, hematuria, excess menstrual bleeding, bleeding gums
  - Thrombotic thrombocytopenic purpura (TTP)
    - Manifestations—purpura, petechiae, headache, seizures, altered consciousness
  - Heparin induced thrombocytopenia (HIT)
    - Manifestations—bleeding, arterial thrombosis, venous thrombosis
- Hemophilia
  - Manifestations—hemarthrosis, easy bruising, bleeding, hematuria, epistaxis, pain
- Disseminated intravascular coagulation (DIC)
  - Manifestations—oozing to frank hemorrhage

menstrual bleeding, and bleeding gums. Spontaneous intracranial bleeding is rare but does occur.

7. TTP is a rare disorder in which thrombi occlude arterioles and capillaries of the microcirculation. This occlusion affects the heart, kidneys, and brain. Platelet aggregation is a key feature of the disorder.

8. TTP may be acute or chronic. The acute form may be fatal within months if not effectively treated. Manifestations include purpura, petechiae, headache, seizures, and altered consciousness.

9. Heparin-induced thrombocytopenia (HIT) develops as a result of an abnormal response to heparin therapy.

10. Bleeding is a common manifestation of HIT. Manifestations of an arterial thrombosis, or of venous thrombosis, may develop.

11. Interdisciplinary care of thrombocytopenia focuses on treating or removing any causative factors and treating the platelet deficiency.

12. Medications include oral glucocorticoids. Prompt withdrawal of heparin therapy is vital.

13. Platelet transfusions may be required. Plasmapheresis or plasma exchange therapy is the primary treatment for acute TTP.

14. Splenectomy may be required.

15. Nursing diagnoses may include: Ineffective Protection and Impaired Oral Mucous Membranes.

HEMOPHILIA

16. Hemophilia is a group of hereditary clotting disorders associated with deficiencies of clotting factors VII, IX, and XI.

17. Hemophilia A (classic hemophilia) is the most common type of hemophilia and is caused by deficiency of dysfunction of clotting factor VIII. It is transmitted as an X-linked recessive disorder from mothers to sons.

18. Severity of disease is related to the amount of clotting factor present. Mild and moderate hemophilia (concentrations of 1% of normal or above) results in infrequent bleeding that is usually associated with trauma. Severe hemophilia (less than 1% of normal concentration) results in frequent bleeding, often in the absence of any trauma.

19. Hemophilia B is also known as Christmas disease and is caused by deficiency of factor IX.

20. Despite the differences in etiology of hemophilia A and hemophilia B, they are clinically identical.

21. Von Willebrand's disease is considered a type of hemophilia and is caused by a deficit of, or defect in, von Willebrand (vW) factor. Reduced levels of factor VIII are also present, because vW factor carries factor VIII.

22. Hemophilia C is caused by factor XI deficiency and is usually a mild disorder.

23. Manifestations include hemarthrosis, easy bruising, bleeding from gums, prolonged bleeding, GI bleeding, hematuria, epistaxis, and pain. Intracranial hemorrhage can be life-threatening.

24. Interdisciplinary care includes preventing or treating bleeding episodes. Deficient clotting factors and fresh frozen plasma are replaced on an individual basis. Aspirin (ASA) is avoided in all types of hemophilia.
25. Nursing diagnoses include: Ineffective Protection and Risk for Ineffective Health Maintenance.

DISSEMINATED INTRAVASCULAR COAGULATION

26. DIC is a clinical syndrome characterized by widespread intravascular clotting and bleeding. It may be severe and life-threatening or very mild. The most common etiology is sepsis.
27. DIC begins with endothelial damage, which initiates the clotting cascade. Normal anticoagulants in the blood become overwhelmed and widespread clotting occurs in the microvasculature. Clotting factors are depleted, the ability to form clots is lost, and hemorrhage occurs.
28. Manifestations of DIC range from oozing to frank hemorrhage.
29. Interdisciplinary care is directed toward treating the underlying disorder and preventing further bleeding or massive thrombosis.
30. Treatments include administration of fresh frozen plasma and platelets. Heparin may be administered to interfere with the clotting cascade, which thereby prevents further clotting factor consumption.
31. Nursing diagnoses include: Ineffective Tissue Perfusion; Impaired Gas Exchange; Pain; Alteration in Safety; and Fear.

SUGGESTIONS FOR CLASSROOM ACTIVITIES

- Review the case study about immune thrombocytopenia purpura that is provided on the textbook Companion Website. Have students develop a nursing plan of care based upon the information presented.
- Have students problem-solve the nursing actions that are necessary for emergency treatment of a client who develops DIC.
- Pain is a common nursing diagnosis for bleeding disorders. Have students research the pathophysiology of this pain and plan nursing interventions to prevent or treat the pain.

SUGGESTIONS FOR CLINICAL ACTIVITIES

- Have students identify clinical clients who are at risk for developing bleeding disorders. Discuss assessment findings that would indicate developing of the disorder and interventions to prevent or minimize health impact.
- Discuss the risks of bloodborne pathogen transmission in clients with hemophilia. Plan nursing care to protect the client and care providers from these disorders.

LEARNING OUTCOME 6

Describe the major types of leukemia and the most common treatment modalities and nursing interventions.

CONCEPTS FOR LECTURE

1. Leukemic cells proliferate slowly and do not differentiate normally. They accumulate in the bone marrow and compete with the proliferation of normal cells. Leukemic cells do not function as mature WBCs and are ineffective in the inflammatory and immune

POWERPOINT LECTURE SLIDES

Major Types of Leukemia
- Acute lymphocytic (lymphoblastic) leukemia (ALL)
- Chronic lymphocytic leukemia (CLL)
- Acute myeloid (myeloblastic) leukemia (AML)
- Chronic myeloid (myelogenous) leukemia (CML)

processes. As these cells leave the bone marrow, they infiltrate other body tissues.

2. Leukemia results in severe anemia, splenomegaly, and bleeding disorders. Death is usually secondary to internal hemorrhage and infections.

3. Manifestations of leukemia include pain and tissue swelling, headache, alteration of the level of consciousness, cranial nerve impairment, nausea, vomiting, renal failure, heat intolerance, weight loss, dyspnea on exertion, and tachycardia.

4. Leukemias are classified by their acuity and the predominant cell type involved. General types of leukemia include: acute lymphocytic (lymphoblastic) leukemia (ALL); chronic lymphocytic leukemia (CLL); acute myeloid (myeloblastic) leukemia (AML); and chronic myeloid (myelogenous) leukemia (CML).

5. ALL is characterized by uncontrolled proliferation of myeloblasts and hyperplasia of the bone marrow and spleen. Manifestations include severe infections, petechiae, purpura, ecchymoses, epistaxis, hematosis, hematuria, GI bleeding, bone pain, and anemia. Death usually results from infections or hemorrhage.

6. CML is characterized by abnormal proliferation of all bone marrow elements. CML is usually associated with a chromosome abnormality called the Philadelphia chromosome. Initially, clients are often asymptomatic, and then the disease progresses to a more aggressive phase in 3 to 4 years. Manifestations during this stage include fatigue, weight loss, sweating, heat intolerance, splenic enlargement, bleeding, and increased bruising. The final stage of the disease, the terminal blast phase, is characterized by significant illness. Death often occurs within 2–4 months of this stage.

7. AML is the most common leukemia in children and young adults. It most often results from malignant transformation of B cells. Onset is generally rapid. Manifestations include bleeding, anemia, bone pain, lymphadenopathy, liver enlargement, frequent infections, headaches, visual disturbances, vomiting, and seizures.

8. CLL is characterized by proliferation and accumulation of small, abnormal, mature lymphocytes in the bone marrow, peripheral blood, and body tissues. These lymphocytes are unable to maintain immunity. Manifestations are vague and may include anemia, infection, enlarged lymph nodes, splenomegaly, and hepatomegaly. Years may elapse before treatment is necessary.

9. Treatment for leukemia generally includes single or combination chemotherapy. During the induction phase, high doses of drug are given to eradicate leukemic cells from the bone marrow. Colony-stimulating factors are often administered to rescue the bone marrow following induction chemotherapy. Post-remission chemotherapy is administered to continue to eradicate any additional leukemic cells, prevent relapse, and prolong survival.

10. Radiation therapy may also be administered.
11. Bone marrow transplant is the treatment of choice for some types of leukemia and is often used in conjunction with, or following, chemotherapy or radiation.
12. Biologic therapies such as interferons and interleukins may be used to treat some leukemias.
13. Common nursing diagnoses include: Risk for Infection; Imbalanced Nutrition: Less than Body Requirements; Impaired Oral Mucous Membranes; Ineffective Protection; and Anticipatory Grieving.
14. Client and family teaching focuses on encouraging self-care, providing information, preventing infection, and promoting nutrition.

SUGGESTIONS FOR CLASSROOM ACTIVITIES

- Assign the different classifications of leukemia to small groups of students. Have each group explain the pathophysiology of the disease and the nursing care required.
- Have students access internet sources for current statistics and treatments associated with leukemia.
- Discuss the statement, "Leukemia is a death sentence." Have students support their opinions on the statement with facts gathered from internet research.
- Complete the care plan activity about acute myelocytic leukemia that is provided on the textbook Companion Website.

SUGGESTIONS FOR CLINICAL ACTIVITIES

- If possible, assign the care of a client with leukemia to clinical students. If not possible, have students discuss how care would be planned and provided.
- Many clients with CLL live years after initial diagnosis and may be hospitalized with disorders that are not related to CLL. Have students discuss how caring for these clients differs from caring for similar clients without CLL.

LEARNING OUTCOME 7

Differentiate Hodgkin's disease from non-Hodgkin's lymphomas.

CONCEPTS FOR LECTURE

1. Lymphomas are malignancies of lymphoid tissue. The most common types are Hodgkin's disease and non-Hodgkin's lymphoma.
2. Hodgkin's disease develops in a single lymph node or chain of nodes, and spreads to adjoining nodes. Involved lymph nodes contain Reed-Steinberg cells. These cells invade the spleen, liver, lungs, digestive tract, and CNS. The immune system is impaired by rapid proliferation of these malignant cells. Both Epstein-Barr virus and genetic factors appear to play a role in its development.
3. The most common symptom of Hodgkin's disease is one or more painlessly enlarged lymph nodes that are generally in the cervical or subclavicular regions. Symptoms may also include persistent fever, night sweats, fatigue, weight loss, malaise, pruritus, and anemia.
4. Non-Hodgkin's lymphoma is a group of lymphoid tissue malignancies that do not contain Reed-Steinberg cells. The cause is unknown, but viral infections such as EBV, HTLV-1 and HTLV-2, and HIV, are thought to play a role. Extranodal spread may involve

POWERPOINT LECTURE SLIDES

Hodgkin's Disease and Non-Hodgkin's Lymphomas
- Hodgkin's disease
  - Develops in a single lymph node or chain of nodes
  - Spreads to adjoining cells
  - Reed-Steinberg cells
  - Immune system impairment
  - Etiology
    - Epstein-Barr virus
    - Genetic factors
- Manifestations
  - Painlessly enlarged lymph nodes
    - Generally cervical or subclavicular
    - Persistent fever, night sweats
    - Fatigue, malaise
    - Weight loss
    - Pruritus
    - Anemia
- Non-Hodgkin's lymphoma
  - Do not contain Reed-Steinberg cells
  - Etiology
    - Often unknown
    - Viral infections may play a role

the nasopharynx, gastrointestinal tract, bone, CNS, thyroid, testes, and soft tissue.

5. Early manifestations are similar to those of Hodgkin's disease. Systemic manifestations such as fever, night sweats, fatigue, and weight loss are less common than in Hodgkin's disease.

6. Interdisciplinary care includes chemotherapy and radiation therapy, either alone or in combination. Stem cell transplant can also be a treatment option.

7. Staging, using the Ann Arbor Staging System, is done to determine the extent of the disease and appropriate treatment.

8. Nursing diagnoses include: Fatigue; Nausea, Disturbed Body Image; Sexual Dysfunction; and Risk for Impaired Skin Integrity.

- Manifestations
  - Early similar to Hodgkin's disease
  - Fever, night sweats, fatigue, and weight loss are less common

SUGGESTIONS FOR CLASSROOM ACTIVITIES

- Have students explain why staging is an important part of the care of clients with lymphoma. Discuss the Ann Arbor Staging system.
- The textbook lists common nursing diagnoses for clients experiencing lymphoma. Have students explain how these nursing diagnoses are appropriate and the assessment data that indicates the appropriate nursing diagnoses.

SUGGESTIONS FOR CLINICAL ACTIVITIES

- Help students learn to assess cervical and subclavicular lymph nodes. Discuss conditions other than lymphomas that could cause lymph node enlargement.

CHAPTER 35
NURSING CARE OF CLIENTS WITH PERIPHERAL VASCULAR DISORDERS

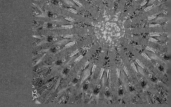

RESOURCE LIBRARY

 PRENTICE HALL NURSING MEDIALINK DVD-ROM

Audio Glossary
NCLEX-RN® Review

 COMPANION WEBSITE

Audio Glossary
NCLEX-RN® Review
Care Plan Activity: Lymphedema
Case Study: Abdominal Aortic Aneurysm
MediaLink Applications
  Calcium Channel Overdose
  Peripheral Vascular Disease
Links to Resources

📖 IMAGE LIBRARY

Figure 35.1 Factors affecting blood pressure.
Figure 35.2 Algorithm for treating hypertension.
Figure 35.3 Sites of antihypertensive drug action.
Figure 35.4 A magnetic resonance angiogram (MRA) showing a circumferential aneurysm of the lower abdominal aorta.
Figure 35.5 An angiogram showing a saccular (berry) aneurysm in the carotid artery of a 50-year-old man.
Figure 35.6 An angiogram showing a large aneurysm of the ascending aorta and aortic arch.

Figure 35.7 An angiogram showing several popliteal aneurysms.
Figure 35.8 Repair of an abdominal aortic aneurysm.
Figure 35.9 Hands of a client with Raynaud's phenomenon.
Figure 35.10 Common locations of venous thrombosis.
Figure 35.11 Venal caval filters.
Figure 35.12 Chronic venous insufficiency.

LEARNING OUTCOME 1

Describe the etiology, pathophysiology, and manifestations of common peripheral vascular and lymphatic disorders.

CONCEPTS FOR LECTURE
BLOOD PRESSURE DISORDERS

1. Cardiac output and systemic (or peripheral) vascular resistance are the primary factors that determine blood pressure.
2. A decrease in cardiac output or decreased peripheral vascular resistance causes the blood pressure to fall.
3. Increased cardiac output or increased peripheral vascular resistance causes the blood pressure to rise.
4. Sympathetic nervous system stimulation, epinephrine and norepinephrine, and the hormones angiotensin II and vasopressin are vasoconstrictors that increase the blood pressure.
5. Parasympathetic nervous system stimulation and the hormones atrial natriuretic peptide and adrenomedulin are vasodilators that decrease the blood pressure.
6. The hormones aldosterone and ADH promote sodium and water retention, which increases the blood pressure.

POWERPOINT LECTURE SLIDES

Common Peripheral Vascular and Lymphatic Disorders
- Primary hypertension
  - Pathophysiologic causes
    - Sympathetic nervous system overstimulation
    - Alterations of the renin-angiotensin-aldosterone system
    - Chemical mediators of vasomotor tone and blood volume
    - Interaction between insulin resistance, hyperinsulinemia, and endothelial function
  - Manifestations
    - Initially asymptomatic
    - Headache, confusion
    - Nocturia
    - Nausea and vomiting
    - Visual disturbances
  - Complications
    - Cardiovascular
    - Neurologic
    - Renal systems

PRIMARY HYPERTENSION

7. Primary hypertension is also known as essential hypertension and has no identified cause. Hypertension is defined as a systolic blood pressure of 140 mm Hg or higher, or diastolic blood pressure of 90 mm Hg or higher, based on the average of three or more readings taken on separate occasions.

8. Pathophysiologic causes of hypertension include: sympathetic nervous system overstimulation; alterations of the renin-angiotensin-aldosterone system; chemical mediators of vasomotor tone and blood volume; and the interaction between insulin resistance, hyperinsulinemia, and endothelial function.

9. Initially, primary hypertension may be asymptomatic. Manifestations include headache, nocturia, confusion, nausea and vomiting, and visual disturbances.

10. Complications of sustained hypertension affect the cardiovascular, neurologic, and renal systems.

SECONDARY HYPERTENSION

11. Secondary hypertension is elevation of the blood pressure that can be related to a specific underlying cause. Common causes are kidney disease, coarctation of the aorta, endocrine disorders, neurologic disorders, drug use, and pregnancy.

HYPERTENSIVE CRISIS

12. Hypertensive emergency or malignant hypertension is rapid elevation of the blood pressure to greater than 180 mm Hg systolic and 120 mm Hg diastolic. Treatment is initiated within 1 hour to prevent cardiac, renal, and vascular damage.

13. Manifestations of hypertensive crisis include headache, confusion, papilledema, blurred vision, restlessness, and motor and sensory defects.

LYMPHADENOPATHY

14. Lymphadenopathy, which is enlarged lymph nodes, can be localized or generalized.

15. Localized lymphadenopathy generally results from an inflammatory process.

16. Lymphangitis is inflammation of the lymph vessels that drain an infected area of the body and is characterized by a red streak along inflamed vessels.

LYMPHEDEMA

17. Primary lymphedema is uncommon and may be associated with genetic disorders.

18. Secondary lymphedema results from damage, obstruction, or removal of lymphatic vessels.

- Secondary hypertension
  - Related to a specific underlying cause
    - Kidney disease
    - Coarctation of the aorta
    - Endocrine disorders
    - Neurologic disorders
    - Drug use
    - Pregnancy
- Hypertensive crisis
  - Malignant hypertension
  - Rapid elevation of the blood pressure
  - Treatment is initiated within 1 hour
  - Manifestations
    - Headache, confusion
    - Papilledema, blurred vision
    - Restlessness
    - Motor and sensory defects
- Lymphadenopathy
  - Enlarged lymph nodes
  - Can be localized or generalized
- Localized lymphadenopathy
  - Generally results from an inflammatory process
- Lymphangitis
  - Inflammation of the lymph vessels
  - Characterized by a red streak
- Lymphedema
  - Primary lymphedema
  - Secondary lymphedema

LEARNING OUTCOME 2

Compare and contrast the manifestations and effects of disorders affecting large and small vessels, arteries, and veins.

CONCEPTS FOR LECTURE

ANEURYSM

1. An aneurysm is an abnormal dilation of a blood vessel. Aneurysms commonly affect the aorta and peripheral arteries and may also develop in the ventricles.
2. Aneurysms form due to weakness of the arterial wall. Hypertension is a major contributing factor.
3. Types of aneurysms include true aneurysms, fusiform aneurysms, circumferential aneurysms, false aneurysms, and berry aneurysms.
4. Aneurysms may dissect if a break or tear in the tunica intima and media allows blood to invade or dissect the layers of the vessel wall.
5. Thoracic aneurysms are frequently asymptomatic. When manifestations do occur they vary according to the location, size, and growth rate of the aneurysm.
6. Abdominal aortic aneurysms are associated with arteriosclerosis and hypertension. These aneurysms may be asymptomatic, but the client may present with a pulsating abdominal mass with pain in the midabdominal region or back.
7. Thrombi often develop within aneurysms and can embolize. Rupture of aneurysms causes hemorrhage, hypovolemic shock, and can lead to death.
8. Popliteal and femoral aneurysms may be asymptomatic, but may result in intermittent claudication, pain, and numbness. Thrombus and emboli may lead to gangrene and the need for amputation.

AORTIC DISSECTION

9. Dissection is a life-threatening condition in which a tear in the inner layer of the artery allows blood to dissect or split the vessel wall.
10. Type A dissection (proximal dissection) affects the ascending aorta.
11. Type B dissection (distal dissection) affects the descending aorta.
12. Manifestations include sudden, excruciating pain over the area of the dissection, syncope, dyspnea, weakness, and absence of peripheral pulses.

POWERPOINT LECTURE SLIDES

Disorders Affecting Large and Small Vessels, Arteries, and Veins
- Aneurysm
  - Abnormal dilation of a blood vessel
  - Commonly affect aorta and peripheral arteries
  - May also develop in the ventricles
  - Form due to weakness of the arterial wall
  - Hypertension is major contributing factor
- Aortic dissection
  - A life-threatening condition
  - Tear in artery inner layer allows blood to dissect or split the vessel wall
- Peripheral vascular disease
  - Hardening and narrowing of peripheral arteries
  - Impairing blood supply to peripheral tissues
  - Collateral circulation usually inadequate
- Thromboangitis obliterans
  - Also called Buerger's disease
  - Occlusive vascular disease
  - Inflammation and spasm cause clots to form in peripheral arteries
- Raynaud's disease and phenomenon
  - Episodes of intense vasospasm in the small arteries and arterioles
  - Raynaud's disease
    - No identifiable cause
    - Blue-white disease
  - Raynaud's phenomenon
    - Secondary to another disease or condition
- Acute arterial occlusion
  - May occur acutely by thrombus or by embolism
- Venous thrombosis
  - Also known as thrombophlebitis
  - Condition in which a blood clot forms on the wall of a vein
  - Causes inflammation of the vein
  - Some degree of venous blood flow obstruction
- Chronic venous insufficiency
  - Disorder of inadequate venous return over a prolonged period

13. Complications such as obstruction of the carotid artery, infarction of the myocardium, kidney, or bowel, and aortic regurgitation may develop.

PERIPHERAL VASCULAR DISEASE

14. Peripheral vascular disease (PVD) occurs when atherosclerosis hardens and narrows the peripheral arteries, which impairs blood supply to peripheral tissues.
15. Intermittent claudication is a cramping or aching pain in the calves of the legs, the thighs, and the buttocks that occurs with a predictable level of activity and is characteristic of PVD.
16. Rest pain occurs during periods of inactivity and increases with elevation of the legs. Pain decreases when legs are dependent.
17. The skin is often thin, shiny, and hairless, with discolored areas. Toenails may be thickened. Areas of skin breakdown may be present, along with edema.
18. Complications include gangrene, rupture of abdominal aortic aneurysms, infection, and sepsis.

THROMBOANGITIS OBLITERANS

19. Thromboangitis obliterans is also called Buerger's disease. It is an occlusive vascular disease in which inflammation and spasm cause clots to form in small and mid-sized peripheral arteries.
20. Pain is the primary manifestation and occurs in the form of claudication and rest pain.
21. Assessment reveals thin, shiny skin with thickened and malformed nails. Involved digits and/or extremities are pale, cyanotic, or ruddy, and cool or cold to touch. Peripheral pulses are weak or absent. Painful ulcers and gangrene may develop.

RAYNAUD'S DISEASE

22. Raynaud's disease and phenomenon are characterized by episodes of intense vasospasm in the small arteries and arterioles of the fingers and sometimes the toes.
23. Raynaud's disease has no identifiable cause and Raynaud's phenomenon is secondary to another disease or condition.
24. Raynaud's disease is also known as "blue-white-red disease."

ACUTE ARTERIAL OCCLUSION

25. Arterial occlusion may occur acutely by thrombus or by embolism.
26. Manifestations include painful, pale, and cold tissues, absence of distal pulses, paresthesias, cyanosis, mottling, and paralysis. A line of demarcation between normal and ischemic tissue may be visible.

- ○ Most common cause is deep vein thrombosis
- ○ Venous status occurs, impairing arterial circulation
- Varicose veins
  - ○ Irregular, tortuous veins with incompetent valves
  - ○ Commonly found in the lower extremities

VENOUS THROMBOSIS

27. Venous thrombosis is also known as thrombophlebitis and is a condition in which a blood clot forms on the wall of a vein, which causes inflammation of the vein, along with some degree of venous blood flow obstruction.
28. Deep vein thrombosis (DVT) is a common complication of hospitalization, surgery, and immobilization.
29. The three pathological factors (Virchow's triad) associated with thrombophlebitis are stasis of blood, vessel damage, and increased blood viscosity.
30. Manifestations are calf pain, tenderness, swelling, warmth, and erythema of the affected extremity. The extremity may be cyanotic and is often edematous.

CHRONIC VENOUS INSUFFICIENCY

31. Chronic venous insufficiency is a disorder of inadequate venous return over a prolonged period.
32. The most common cause is deep vein thrombosis which occludes a large vein, increasing the pressure in other veins of the extremity. This results in impaired unidirectional blood flow and deep vein emptying.
33. Brown skin pigmentation is a result of breakdown of red blood cells in the congested tissues. Venous ulcers develop.
34. Manifestations include lower leg edema; itching; discomfort that increases with prolonged standing; cyanosis; and shiny, atrophic skin that has a brown pigmentation.

VARICOSE VEINS

35. Varicose veins are irregular, tortuous veins with incompetent valves and are commonly found in the lower extremities.
36. Primary varicose veins are those with no deep vein involvement and secondary varicose veins that are caused by obstruction of deep veins.
37. Manifestations are severe aching leg pain, leg fatigue, leg heaviness, itching, or feelings of heat in the legs. Assessment reveals obviously dilated, tortuous veins.

SUGGESTIONS FOR CLASSROOM ACTIVITIES

• Using the case study provided on the textbook Companion Website, have students identify manifestations and effects of abdominal aortic aneurysm. Include pertinent nursing assessment and emergency nursing interventions.
• Discuss the nursing implications of manifestations of disorders of large and small vessel disease.

SUGGESTIONS FOR CLINICAL ACTIVITIES

• Have students identify clinical clients who are at risk for development, or who have already developed, disorders of large and small vessel disease. In post-conference, have students compare and contrast the manifestations seen and interventions for care of these clients.

LEARNING OUTCOME 3

Explain risk factors for and measures to prevent peripheral vascular disorders and their complications.

CONCEPTS FOR LECTURE

PRIMARY HYPERTENSION

1. Risk factors for development of primary hypertension include aging; race (prevalence of hypertension is highest among African-American females); family history of hypertension; high sodium intake; low potassium, calcium, and magnesium intake; obesity; insulin resistance; excess alcohol consumption; and stress.
2. Education focuses on modifiable risk factors for hypertension development.

HYPERTENSIVE CRISIS

3. Most hypertensive emergencies occur when clients suddenly stop taking their medications or when their hypertension is poorly controlled.

ANEURYSM

4. Risk factors for the development of aortic dissection include hypertension, cystic medial necrosis, male gender, advancing age, pregnancy, congenital defects of the aortic valve, coarctation of the aorta, and inflammatory aortitis.

PERIPHERAL VASCULAR DISEASE

5. Risk factors are diabetes mellitus, hypercholesterolemia, hypertension, cigarette smoking, and high homocysteine levels.

THROMBOANGITIS OBLITERANS

6. Cigarette smoking is the single most significant cause of the disease.
7. If gangrene develops, amputation may be necessary.

RAYNAUD'S DISEASE

8. There may be a genetic predisposition to Raynaud's disease.
9. With repeated attacks, the fingertips thicken and the nails become brittle.
10. Ulceration and gangrene are serious complications, but they seldom occur.

ACUTE ARTERIAL OCCLUSION

11. Clients with arteriosclerosis, sepsis, cancer, who are pregnant, have broken long bones, myocardial infarction, valvular heart disease, and atrial fibrillation are at risk for embolism. Embolism may also occur from foreign objects such as air bubbles.
12. Arterial occlusion can result in permanent vessel and limb damage such as tissue necrosis and gangrene.

POWERPOINT LECTURE SLIDES

Risk Factors for Peripheral Vascular Disorders
- Primary hypertension
  - Aging
  - Race
  - Family history of hypertension
  - High sodium intake
  - Low potassium, calcium, and magnesium intake
  - Obesity
  - Insulin resistance
  - Excess alcohol consumption
  - Stress
- Hypertensive crisis
  - Sudden discontinuance of medications
  - Poorly controlled hypertension
- Aneurysm
  - Hypertension
  - Cystic medial necrosis
  - Male gender
  - Advancing age
  - Pregnancy
  - Congenital defects of the aortic valve
  - Coarctation of the aorta
  - Inflammatory aortitis
- Peripheral vascular disease
  - Diabetes mellitus
  - Hypercholesterolemia
  - Hypertension
  - Cigarette smoking
  - High homocysteine levels
- Thromboangitis obliterans
  - Cigarette smoking
- Raynaud's disease
  - Genetic predisposition
- Acute arterial occlusion
  - Arteriosclerosis (or atherosclerosis)
  - Sepsis
  - Cancer
  - Pregnancy
  - Long bone fracture
  - Myocardial infarction
  - Valvular heart disease
  - Atrial fibrillation
  - Foreign body embolism
- Venous thrombosis
  - Hospitalization
  - Immobility
  - Abdominal or thoracic surgery
  - Certain cancers
  - Trauma
  - Pregnancy
  - Use of oral contraceptives
  - Hormone replacement therapy

13. Visceral arterial occlusion may result in compartment syndrome, acute respiratory failure, stroke, or renal failure.

VENOUS THROMBOSIS

14. Risk factors for venous thrombosis include hospitalization, immobility, abdominal or thoracic surgery, certain cancers, trauma, pregnancy, and use of oral contraceptives or hormone replacement therapy.
15. The major complications of deep vein thrombosis are chronic venous insufficiency and pulmonary embolism.

CHRONIC VENOUS INSUFFICIENCY

16. The most frequent cause of chronic venous insufficiency is deep vein thrombosis, but varicose veins and leg trauma may also contribute. Risk factor management focuses on measures to increase venous return and to prevent trauma.

VARICOSE VEINS

17. Risk factors for the development of varicose veins are aging, prolonged standing, obesity, venous thrombosis, congenital arteriovenous malformations, and sustained pressure on abdominal veins.
18. Complications of varicose veins are venous insufficiency, stasis ulcers, development of chronic stasis dermatitis, and superficial venous thrombosis.

- Chronic venous insufficiency
  - Deep vein thrombosis
  - Varicose veins
  - Leg trauma
- Varicose veins
  - Aging
  - Prolonged standing
  - Obesity
  - Venous thrombosis
  - Congenital arteriovenous malformations
  - Sustained pressure on abdominal veins

SUGGESTIONS FOR CLASSROOM ACTIVITIES

- Have students identify risk factors for development of common peripheral vascular disorders. Group these disorders according to methods of prevention. Using these groupings, have students identify teaching interventions to prevent the development of the disorder.

SUGGESTIONS FOR CLINICAL ACTIVITIES

- Have students review clinical client medical records for risk factors for developing peripheral vascular disease. Have students develop a teaching plan for clients at risk. In post-conference, have students compare and contrast their findings and their teaching plans.

LEARNING OUTCOME 4

Explain the nursing implications for medications and other interdisciplinary treatments used for clients with peripheral vascular disorders.

CONCEPTS FOR LECTURE
PRIMARY HYPERTENSION

1. Hypertension management focuses on reducing the blood pressure to less than 140 mm Hg systolic and 90 mm Hg diastolic. The ultimate goal is to reduce cardiovascular and renal morbidity and mortality.
2. Lifestyle modifications recommended for clients with hypertension or pre-hypertension include weight loss, dietary changes, restricted alcohol use and cigarette smoking, increased physical activity, and stress reduction.

POWERPOINT LECTURE SLIDES

- Primary hypertension
  - Medications
    - Diuretics
    - Beta-adrenergic blockers
    - Central acting sympatholytics
    - Vasodilators
    - ACE inhibitors
    - Angiotensin II receptor blockers
    - Calcium channel blockers
  - Nursing diagnoses
    - Ineffective Health Maintenance
    - Risk for Noncompliance

3. Medications include one or more of the following: diuretics, beta-adrenergic blockers, central acting sympatholytics, vasodilators, ACE inhibitors, angiotensin II receptor blockers, and calcium channel blockers.
4. Nursing diagnoses include: Ineffective Health Maintenance; Risk for Noncompliance; Imbalanced Nutrition: More than Body Requirements; and Excess Fluid Volume.

HYPERTENSIVE CRISIS

5. The goal of care in hypertensive crisis is to reduce the blood pressure by no more than 25% within minutes to 1 hour, then toward 160/100 within 2 to 6 hours.
6. Drug treatment includes IV antihypertensives, such as sodium nitroprusside.
7. Nursing care includes: continuous blood pressure monitoring, titrating medications to blood pressure readings, avoiding rapid blood pressure changes, and providing calm reassurance to the client and family.

ANEURYSM

8. Thoracic aortic aneurysms may be treated with long-term beta-blockers and other antihypertensive medications.
9. Clients with aortic dissection are treated with IV beta-blockers, sodium nitroprusside, and calcium channel blockers. Direct vasodilators are avoided. Postoperative anticoagulant therapy is initiated.
10. Treatment depends upon the size of the aneurysm. Small, asymptomatic aneurysms are medically managed. Large aneurysms are at risk for rupture and require surgery.
11. Treatments include constant monitoring of vital signs, hemodynamics, and urine output.
12. Surgical treatment of aneurysm may include endovascular stent grafts (EVSG) or surgical excision and replacement of the area with a synthetic graft.
13. Nursing diagnoses include: Risk for Ineffective Tissue Perfusion; Risk for Injury; and Anxiety.

PERIPHERAL VASCULAR DISEASE

14. Management of PVD focuses on slowing the atherosclerotic process and maintaining tissue perfusion.
15. Medications include drugs to inhibit platelet aggregation, platelet inhibitors, drugs to decrease blood viscosity, and parenteral vasodilator prostaglandins.
16. Smoking cessation and meticulous foot care are essential. Regular, progressively strenuous exercise is important. It is also important to control diabetes, hypertension, cholesterol levels, and weight.
17. Revascularization procedures such as percutaneous transluminal angioplasty, stent placement, or atherectomy may be used. Surgical options include endarterectomy and bypass grafts.

- – Imbalanced Nutrition: More than Body Requirements
- – Excess Fluid Volume
- Hypertensive crisis
  - Medications
    - – IV antihypertensives
  - Nursing care
    - – Continuous blood pressure monitoring
    - – Titrating medications to blood pressure readings
    - – Avoiding rapid blood pressure changes
    - – Providing calm reassurance to the client and family
- Aneurysm
  - Thoracic aortic aneurysms
    - – Long-term beta-blockers
    - – Other antihypertensive medications
  - Aortic dissection
    - – IV beta-blockers
    - – Sodium nitroprusside
    - – Calcium channel blockers
    - – Direct vasodilators are avoided
    - – Post-operative anticoagulant therapy
  - Nursing diagnoses
    - – Risk for ineffective tissue perfusion
    - – Risk for injury
    - – Anxiety
- Peripheral vascular disease
  - Medications
    - – Drugs to inhibit platelet aggregation
    - – Platelet inhibitors
    - – Drugs to decrease blood viscosity
    - – Parenteral vasodilator prostaglandins
  - Nursing diagnoses
    - – Ineffective Tissue Perfusion: Peripheral
    - – Pain
    - – Impaired Skin Integrity
    - – Activity Intolerance
- Thromboangitis obliterans
  - Surgical treatment
    - – Sympathectomy
    - – Arterial bypass graft
  - Nursing care
    - – Promotion of arterial circulation
    - – Prevention of prolonged tissue hypoxia
    - – Smoking cessation support
    - – Relief of acute manifestations
- Raynaud's disease
  - Medications
    - – Vasodilators
    - – Sustained release calcium channel blockers
    - – Alpha-adrenergic blockers
    - – Transdermal nitroglycerine
    - – Longer-acting oral nitrates
  - Nursing care
    - – Education
    - – Support

18. Nursing diagnoses include Ineffective Tissue Perfusion: Peripheral; Pain; Impaired Skin Integrity; and Activity Intolerance.

THROMBOANGITIS OBLITERANS

19. Smoking cessation is the single most important component of disease management. Keeping extremities warm, managing stress, keeping the affected extremities in a dependent position, preventing injury, and regular exercise are also important components of treatment.
20. Surgical treatment may include sympathectomy or arterial bypass graft.
21. Nursing care focuses on promoting arterial circulation and preventing prolonged tissue hypoxia. Smoking cessation and relieving acute manifestations are also important.

RAYNAUD'S DISEASE

22. Medications to treat Raynaud's may include vasodilators, sustained release calcium channel blockers, alpha-adrenergic blockers, and transdermal nitroglycerine or longer-acting oral nitrates.
23. Treatments are conservative and include keeping hands warm, avoiding injury to the hands, smoking cessation, stress reduction, reducing dietary fats, increasing activity level, and maintaining normal body weight.
24. Nursing care is primarily educative and supportive.

ACUTE ARTERIAL OCCLUSION

25. Emergency embolectomy or thromboendarterectomy may be necessary.
26. Anticoagulation or thrombolytic therapy is often used to open the vessel or to keep it open.
27. Nursing diagnoses include Ineffective Tissue Perfusion: Peripheral; Anxiety; and Altered Protection.

VENOUS THROMBOSIS

28. Prevention of venous thrombosis includes use of low-molecular-weight heparins and oral anticoagulation.
29. Anticoagulants, thrombolytics, and NSAIDs may be used to treat venous thrombosis.
30. Venous thrombectomy and insertion of filters to capture emboli may be used.
31. Nursing diagnoses are Pain; Ineffective Tissue Perfusion: Peripheral; Ineffective Protection; Impaired Physical Mobility, and Risk for Ineffective Tissue Perfusion: Cardiopulmonary.

CHRONIC VENOUS INSUFFICIENCY

32. Collaborative care focuses on relieving symptoms, promoting adequate circulation, and healing and preventing tissue damage.

- Acute arterial occlusion
  ○ Medications
    – Anticoagulation
    – Thrombolytic therapy
  ○ Nursing diagnoses
    – Ineffective Tissue Perfusion: Peripheral
    – Anxiety
    – Altered Protection
- Venous thrombosis
  ○ Medications
    – Anticoagulants
    – Thrombolytics
    – NSAIDs
  ○ Nursing diagnoses
    – Pain
    – Ineffective Tissue Perfusion: Peripheral
    – Ineffective Protection
    – Impaired Physical Mobility
    – Risk for Ineffective Tissue Perfusion: Cardiopulmonary
- Chronic venous insufficiency
  ○ Medications
    – Corticosteroids
    – Zinc oxide
    – Clotrimazole
    – Miconazole
    – Burrow's solution
  ○ Nursing diagnoses
    – Disturbed Body Image
    – Ineffective Health Maintenance
    – Risk for Infection
    – Impaired Physical Mobility
    – Impaired Skin Integrity
    – Ineffective Tissue Perfusion: Peripheral
- Varicose veins
  ○ Treatments
    – Compression stockings
    – Regular, daily walking
    – Discouraging prolonged sitting or standing
    – Regular periods of leg elevation
  ○ Nursing diagnoses
    – Chronic Pain
    – Ineffective Tissue Perfusion: Peripheral
    – Risk for Impaired Skin Integrity
    – Risk for Peripheral Neurovascular Dysfunction
- Lymphedema
  ○ Treatments
    – Generally conservative
    – Positioning
    – Avoidance of infection
    – Diuretic therapy
  ○ Nursing diagnoses
    – Impaired Tissue Integrity
    – Excess Fluid Volume
    – Disturbed Body Image

33. Conservative management focuses on reducing edema and treating ulcerations.
34. Medications include topical treatments for ulcerations including corticosteroids, zinc oxide, clotrimazole (Canesten), miconazole (Monistat-Derm), and Burrow's solution.
35. Large, chronic ulcers may require surgery to excise ulcerated tissue and skin grafts.
36. Nursing care is educative with common nursing diagnoses of Disturbed Body Image; Ineffective Health Maintenance; Risk for Infection; Impaired Physical Mobility; Impaired Skin Integrity; and Ineffective Tissue Perfusion: Peripheral.

VARICOSE VEINS

37. Management is generally conservative; however, surgery may be required for severe symptoms or if complications arise.
38. Treatments include compression stockings, regular, daily walking, discouraging prolonged sitting or standing, and regular periods of leg elevation.
39. Compression sclerotherapy is a treatment in which a sclerosing solution is injected into the vein and a compression bandage is applied. This results in obliteration of the vein.
40. Surgical stripping of the varicosed vein is generally reserved for the most serious cases.
41. Nursing diagnoses include: Chronic Pain; Ineffective Tissue Perfusion: Peripheral; Risk for Impaired Skin Integrity; and Risk for Peripheral Neurovascular Dysfunction.

LYMPHEDEMA

42. Interdisciplinary care focuses on relieving edema and preventing or treating infection.
43. Treatment is generally conservative and includes positioning, avoidance of infection, and diuretic therapy when indicated.
44. Nursing diagnoses include: Impaired Tissue Integrity; Excess Fluid Volume, and Disturbed Body Image.

SUGGESTIONS FOR CLASSROOM ACTIVITIES

- Have students list the common medications used to treat peripheral vascular diseases. Review these medications and list nursing implications. Compare these nursing implications and look for similarities and differences among and between medications.

SUGGESTIONS FOR CLINICAL ACTIVITIES

- Have students review clinical client medication administration records for medications identified in the classroom activity listed in the previous paragraph. Have students complete medication information sheets that list the common dosages, nursing implications and warnings, and client education for each drug.

LEARNING OUTCOME 5

Describe preoperative and postoperative nursing care of clients having vascular surgery.

CONCEPTS FOR LECTURE

1. Preoperative care should include teaching and routine preoperative care. Implement measures to reduce anxiety and fear.
2. Careful management of medications to control blood pressure may be important to the preoperative safety of clients scheduled for vascular surgery.
3. Postoperative care includes close adherence to specific measures according to the surgical procedure performed.

POWERPOINT LECTURE SLIDES

Preoperative and Postoperative Nursing Care
- Preoperative care
  - Teaching
  - Routine preoperative care
  - Reduction of anxiety and fear
  - Medications to control blood pressure
- Postoperative care
  - According to surgical procedure performed

SUGGESTIONS FOR CLASSROOM ACTIVITIES

- Have students prepare a plan of care for a client scheduled to undergo vascular surgery.
- Discuss the postoperative care of clients who have undergone vascular surgery.
- List critical findings that would indicate postoperative emergencies and the nursing interventions associated with those findings.

SUGGESTIONS FOR CLINICAL ACTIVITIES

- Assign students to the care of a client who is scheduled to undergo vascular surgery.
- Assign students to the care of a client who has undergone vascular surgery.
- Ask an RN who regularly cares for clients who are scheduled for or who have undergone vascular surgery to speak to the post-conference group.

CHAPTER 36
ASSESSING CLIENTS WITH RESPIRATORY DISORDERS

RESOURCE LIBRARY

PRENTICE HALL NURSING MEDIALINK DVD-ROM

Audio Glossary
NCLEX-RN® Review
Animation/Video
   Carbon Dioxide Transport
   Oxygen Transport

COMPANION WEBSITE

Audio Glossary
NCLEX-RN® Review
Case Study: Respiratory Assessment
MediaLink Applications
   Pulmonary Function Testing
   Wheezes and Crackles
Links to Resources

IMAGE LIBRARY

Figure 36.1 The upper respiratory system.
Figure 36.2 Sinuses, frontal and lateral views.
Figure 36.3 The lower respiratory system, showing the location of the lungs, the mediastinum, and layers of visceral and parietal pleura.
Figure 36.4 Respiratory bronchi, bronchioles, alveolar ducts, and alveoli.
Figure 36.5 *A*, Anterior rib cage, showing intercostal spaces. *B*, Posterior rib cage.
Figure 36.6 Respiratory inspiration: lateral and anterior views.

Figure 36.7 Respiratory expiration: lateral and anterior views.
Figure 36.8 Oxygen-hemoglobin dissociation curve.
Figure 36.9 Fiberoptic bronchoscopy.
Figure 36.10 Palpating for chest expansion.
Figure 36.11 Sequence for lung percussion.
Figure 36.12 Measuring diaphragmatic excursion.
Figure 36.13 Sequence for lung auscultation.

LEARNING OUTCOME 1

Describe the anatomy, physiology, and functions of the respiratory system.

CONCEPTS FOR LECTURE

1. The upper respiratory system serves as a passageway for air moving into the lungs and carbon dioxide moving out into the external environment. As air moves through these structures, it is cleaned, humidified, and warmed. Major structures of the upper respiratory system are the nose, sinuses, pharynx, larynx, and trachea.
2. The lower respiratory system includes the lungs. Within the lungs are the bronchi and alveoli which contain the respiratory membrane where gas exchange takes place.

POWERPOINT LECTURE SLIDES

The Respiratory System
   - Upper respiratory system
     ○ Nose, sinuses, pharynx, larynx, trachea
     ○ Passageway for air, cleanses, humidifies, warms
   - Lower respiratory system
     ○ Lungs, bronchi, alveoli
     ○ Respiratory membrane for gas exchange

SUGGESTIONS FOR CLASSROOM ACTIVITIES

- Using anatomic models, demonstrate the anatomy of the respiratory system.

LEARNING OUTCOME 2

Explain the mechanics of ventilation.

CONCEPTS FOR LECTURE

1. There are two phases of pulmonary ventilation: inspiration and expiration. These phases occur as the result of changes in the position of the diaphragm and rib cage which change the intrapleural pressures. Since gases follow their pressure gradients, these changes in pressure result in gases flowing into or out of the lung to equalize the pressure.

2. Inspiration occurs when diaphragmatic and rib cage position changes decrease intrapleural pressures. During inspiration, air enters the lungs through the primary bronchus and then moves through the increasingly smaller passageways of the lungs to the alveoli.

3. Oxygen and carbon dioxide are exchanged at the respiratory membrane of the alveoli by simple diffusion.

4. Expiration occurs when those inspiratory muscles relax, which increases intrapleural pressures. Expiration is primarily a passive process. Carbon dioxide is expelled through expiration.

POWERPOINT LECTURE SLIDES

Mechanics of Ventilation
- Ventilation
  - Inspiration
    - Occurs when changes decrease interpleural pressures
    - Air enters the lungs through the primary bronchus
    - Oxygen and carbon dioxide are exchanged at the alveolar respiratory membrane
    - Simple diffusion
  - Expiration
    - Occurs when changes increase interpleural pressures
    - Primarily passive
    - Carbon dioxide is expelled through expiration

SUGGESTIONS FOR CLASSROOM ACTIVITIES

- View the animations/videos about carbon dioxide transport, gas exchange, and oxygen transport that are provided on the textbook DVD-ROM.

LEARNING OUTCOME 3

Compare and contrast factors affecting respiration.

CONCEPTS FOR LECTURE

1. Factors that affect respiration include: changes in volume and capacity; air pressures; oxygen, carbon dioxide, and hydrogen ion concentration in the blood; airway resistance; lung compliance and elasticity; and alveolar surface tension.

2. Respiratory volume and capacity are affected by gender, age, weight, and health status. The volumes can be measured by pulmonary function tests.

3. Pulmonary ventilation depends on volume changes in the thoracic cavity.

4. Oxygen, carbon dioxide, and hydrogen ion concentrations affect the respiratory centers in the medulla oblongata and pons of the brain, and the chemoreceptors located in the medulla and in the carotid and aortic bodies.

5. Airway resistance, lung compliance, and elasticity also affect respiration. Increased airway resistance results in a decrease in gas flow. Lung compliance is the distensibility of the lungs and can be decreased by factors that decrease the elasticity of the lungs, block the respiratory passages, or interfere with rib cage movement. Lung elasticity is essential for lung expansion and recoil and can be decreased from disease such as emphysema.

POWERPOINT LECTURE SLIDES

Factors that Affect Respiration
- Changes in volume and capacity
  - Affected by gender, age, weight, and health status
  - Measured by pulmonary function tests
- Air pressure
  - Pressure changes in the thoracic cavity drive inspiration/expiration
- Oxygen, carbon dioxide, hydrogen ion Concentrations
  - Affect respiratory centers in medulla oblongata, pons, medulla, carotid and aortic bodies
- Airway resistance, lung compliance, and elasticity
  - Increase airway resistance, decreased lung compliance or decreased elasticity decrease gas flow
- Alveolar surface tension
  - Along with presence of surfactant, prevent alveolar collapse between breaths

6. Alveolar surface tension and presence of surfactant helps to prevent alveolar collapse between breaths.

SUGGESTIONS FOR CLASSROOM ACTIVITIES	SUGGESTIONS FOR CLINICAL ACTIVITIES
• Discuss how gender, age, and weight can affect respiration.	• Have students identify factors that impact respiration in their clinical clients.

LEARNING OUTCOME 4

Identify specific topics for consideration during a health history interview of the client with health problems involving the respiratory system.

CONCEPTS FOR LECTURE

1. If the client has a problem with respiratory function, analyze its onset, characteristics, course, severity, precipitating and relieving factors, and associated symptoms, noting timing and circumstances.
2. Observe client for difficulty breathing, sustaining normal conversation, hoarseness, changes in voice quality, or cough.
3. Ask about present health status, medical history, family health history, and risk factors for illness. Include questions about allergies, asthma, respiratory illnesses, surgery, trauma, other chronic illnesses, and medication usage.
4. Lifestyle questions should include asking about smoking history, exposure to environmental substances that might affect respiratory health, exercise patterns, and use of alcohol and recreational drugs.

POWERPOINT LECTURE SLIDES

Health History
- Current illness
- Observe for respiratory compromise
- Present health status, medical history, family history, risk factors
- Lifestyle questions
  - Smoking history
  - Exposure to environmental substances
  - Exercise
  - Use of recreational drugs

SUGGESTIONS FOR CLASSROOM ACTIVITIES	SUGGESTIONS FOR CLINICAL ACTIVITIES
• Review the case study about respiratory assessment that is provided on the textbook Companion Website. Use the material provided to discuss materials to include in assessment and assessment techniques.	• Have students complete respiratory assessments on clinical clients.

LEARNING OUTCOME 5

Describe normal variations in assessment findings for the older adult.

CONCEPTS FOR LECTURE

1. Aging may cause a decrease in the elastic recoil of the lung, a loss of skeletal muscle strength in the thorax and diaphragm, more fibrosis in the alveoli, and fewer functional capillaries. These changes result in an increase in anterior-posterior chest diameter, a reduction in vital capacity, and an increase in residual volume.
2. The cough may become less effective with aging, increasing risk of respiratory infections such as pneumonia.
3. PO_2 reduces as much as 15% by age 80.

POWERPOINT LECTURE SLIDES

Age-Related Changes
- Decrease in elastic recoil of the lung
- Loss of skeletal muscle strength in thorax and diaphragm
- Fibrosis in the alveoli
- Fewer functional capillaries
- Less effective cough
- Decrease in PO_2

LEARNING OUTCOME 6

Identify manifestations of impairment of the respiratory system.

CONCEPTS FOR LECTURE

1. Nasal assessment findings of asymmetry, redness, swelling, septum abnormalities, purulent drainage, or changes in ability to smell may indicate a respiratory disorder.
2. Tender frontal or maxillary sinuses may indicate allergies or infection.
3. Thoracic assessment findings of markedly increased or decreased respiratory rate, abnormal AP diameter, intercostal retraction or bulging, asymmetric chest expansion, malposition of the trachea, changes in tactile fremitus, dullness or hyperresonance on percussion, or asymmetric diaphragmatic excursion are indicative of a respiratory disorder.
4. Breath sound assessment that reveals adventitious sounds, absence of breath sounds, or malposition of normal quality breath sounds require further investigation.

POWERPOINT LECTURE SLIDES

Manifestations of Possible Respiratory Disorder
- Nasal assessment
  - Asymmetry, redness, swelling, septum abnormalities, purulent drainage, changes in ability to smell
- Frontal or maxillary sinus assessment
  - Tenderness
- Thoracic assessment
  - Markedly increased or decreased respiratory rate, abnormal AP diameter, intercostal retraction or bulging, asymmetric chest expansion, malposition of the trachea, changes in tactile fremitus, dullness or hyperresonance on percussion or asymmetric diaphragmatic excursion
- Breath sound assessment
  - Adventitious sounds, absence of breath sounds, or malposition of normal quality breath sounds

Chapter 37

Nursing Care of Clients with Upper Respiratory Disorders

Resource Library

 PRENTICE HALL NURSING MEDIALINK DVD-ROM

Audio Glossary
NCLEX-RN® Review

 COMPANION WEBSITE

Audio Glossary
NCLEX-RN® Review
Care Plan Activity: Epistaxis
Case Study: Sleep Apnea
MediaLink Applications
  Laryngectomy
  Pulse Oximetry
Links to Resources

📖 IMAGE LIBRARY

Figure 37.1 Incision to access ethmoid and frontal sinuses.

Figure 37.2 The appearance of the oral pharynx and tonsils in acute pharyngitis and tonsillitis.

Figure 37.3 Posterior nasal packing.

Figure 37.4 Administering abdominal thrusts (the Heimlich maneuver) to *A*, a conscious victim, and *B*, an unconscious victim.

Figure 37.5 A client using a nasal mask and CPAP to treat sleep apnea.

Figure 37.6 Laryngoscopy showing a polyp on the left vocal cord.

Figure 37.7 Cancer of the larynx and epiglottis.

Figure 37.8 Following a total laryngectomy, the client has a permanent tracheostomy.

Figure 37.9 The tracheoesophageal prosthesis allows diversion of air from the trachea through a one-way valve into the esophagus and oropharynx, producing speech when the tracheostomy stoma is occluded.

Figure 37.10 Speech generators.

LEARNING OUTCOME 1

Relate anatomy and physiology of the upper respiratory tract to commonly occurring disorders and risk factors for these disorders.

CONCEPTS FOR LECTURE

INFECTIOUS OR INFLAMMATORY DISORDERS

1. Rhinitis is inflammation of the nasal cavities and is the most common upper respiratory disorder.
2. Acute viral rhinitis is the common cold.
3. Allergic rhinitis is a sensitivity reaction to allergens such as plant pollen.
4. Vasomotor rhinitis has manifestations much like allergic rhinitis, but is not linked to allergic reaction. Its etiology is unknown.
5. Atrophic rhinitis is characterized by changes in the mucous membrane of the nasal cavities.

VIRAL UPPER RESPIRATORY INFECTION

6. Viral upper respiratory infections or URI are also known as the common cold and are the most common respiratory tract infections. These infections are

POWERPOINT LECTURE SLIDES

Upper Respiratory Tract Disorders and Risk Factors
- Infectious or inflammatory disorders
  ○ Rhinitis
  ○ Acute viral rhinitis
  ○ Allergic rhinitis
  ○ Vasomotor rhinitis
  ○ Atrophic rhinitis
- Respiratory syncytial virus
  ○ Respiratory syncytial virus (RSV)
  ○ In older children and adults manifests as a common cold
  ○ May cause severe illness or death in immunocompromised
- Influenza
  ○ Highly contagious viral respiratory disease
  ○ Usually occurs in epidemics or pandemics
  ○ Avian influenza: possible pandemic

highly contagious, with peak incidence in September, late January, and late April.

RESPIRATORY SYNCYTIAL VIRUS

7. Respiratory syncytial virus (RSV) is a common virus that is the primary cause of respiratory illness in children and the majority of lower respiratory disease in infants.
8. Older children and adults are commonly infected with RSV, which usually manifests as a common cold.

INFLUENZA

9. Influenza is a highly contagious viral respiratory disease that usually occurs in epidemics or pandemics.

SINUSITIS

10. The sinuses are normally sterile air-filled cavities in the facial bones that open into the turbinates of the nasal cavity.
11. Sinusitis is inflammation of the mucous membranes of one or more of these sinuses and commonly follows a URI. The risk for sinusitis is higher in clients with impaired immunity.

PHARYNGITIS OR TONSILLITIS

12. Pharyngitis is acute inflammation of the pharynx. It is one of the most commonly identified clinical problems and is generally viral, but may also be caused by one of a variety of bacteria.
13. Tonsillitis is acute inflammation of the palatine tonsils. It is sometimes viral in nature, but is generally due to streptococcal infection.

EPIGLOTTITIS

14. Epiglottitis is a rapidly progressive cellulitis that begins between the base of the tongue and the epiglottis. It is a medical emergency, as the airway may be threatened.

LARYNGITIS

15. Laryngitis is inflammation of the larynx. It is a common disorder and may occur alone or along with another URI.
16. Laryngitis may occur secondary to overuse of the voice, sudden changes in temperature, or exposure to environmental irritants. Laryngitis may be acute or chronic.

DIPHTHERIA

17. Diphtheria is an acute, contagious disease caused by *Corynebacterium diptheriae*. The disease has been uncommon in the United States because of adequate immunization.
18. Asymptomatic carriers of the disease can be a factor in spreading this infection.

- Sinusitis
  - Sterile air-filled cavities in the facial bones
  - Sinusitis
- Pharyngitis or tonsillitis
  - Pharyngitis
    - Acute inflammation of pharynx
    - Generally viral
    - May be bacterial
  - Tonsillitis
    - Acute inflammation of palatine tonsils
    - Generally due to streptococcal infection
    - May be viral
- Epiglottitis
  - Rapidly progressive cellulitis
  - Begins between base of tongue and epiglottis
  - Medical emergency, as airway may be threatened
- Laryngitis
  - Inflammation of the larynx
  - Occurs alone or with other URI
  - May be acute or chronic
- Diphtheria
  - Acute, contagious disease
  - Caused by *Corynebacterium diphtheriae*
  - Uncommon in U.S.
- Pertussis
  - Whooping cough
  - Highly contagious
- Epistaxis
  - Nosebleed
  - May indicate a bleeding disorder
- Nasal trauma or surgery
  - Nose is most commonly broken facial bone
  - Can result in
    - Deviation of the septum
    - Soft tissue trauma
- Laryngeal obstruction or trauma
  - Narrowest portion of upper airway
  - At risk for obstruction
- Sleep apnea
  - Obstructive sleep apnea
  - Central sleep apnea
- Nasal polyps
  - Benign grapelike growths of lining of nose
  - Interfere with air movement
  - May obstruct openings, leading to sinusitis
- Laryngeal tumor
  - Benign
    - Papillomas
    - Nodules
    - Polyps
- Malignant
  - Fairly uncommon
  - Often curable if detected early

PERTUSSIS

19. Pertussis is also known as whooping cough and is highly contagious.
20. Adults are thought to be an important reservoir for this disease.

EPISTAXIS

21. The nose is richly supplied with blood. Epistaxis may be precipitated by trauma, drying of nasal mucous membranes, infection, substance abuse, arteriosclerosis, or hypertension.
22. Epistaxis may also indicate a bleeding disorder secondary to acute leukemia, thrombocytopenia, aplastic anemia, or severe liver disease. Treatment with anticoagulant or antiplatelet drugs may also cause epistaxis.

NASAL TRAUMA OR SURGERY

23. The nose is the most commonly broken bone of the face, usually as a result of sports injury, trauma related to violence, or motor vehicle crashes. Deviation of the septum and soft tissue trauma can result from nasal fracture.

LARYNGEAL OBSTRUCTION OR TRAUMA

24. The larynx is the narrowest portion of the upper airway and is at risk for obstruction.

OBSTRUCTIVE SLEEP APNEA

25. Sleep apnea is intermittent absence of airflow through the mouth and nose during sleep. It is a serious and life-threatening disorder.
26. Obstructive sleep apnea is the most common type. The respiratory drive remains intact, but airflow ceases due to occlusion of the oropharyngeal airway.
27. Central sleep apnea is a rare neurological disorder that involves transient impairment of the neurologic drive to respiratory muscles.

NASAL POLYPS

28. Nasal polyps are benign grapelike growths of the mucous membrane that lines the nose. These are benign tumors that may interfere with air movement through the nasal passages or that may obstruct openings, which leads to sinusitis.

LARYNGEAL TUMOR

29. Laryngeal tumors may be either benign or malignant.
30. Benign tumors of the larynx include papillomas, nodules, and polyps.
31. Cancer of the larynx is uncommon and is often curable if detected early.

LEARNING OUTCOME 2

Describe the pathophysiology of common upper respiratory tract disorders, relating their manifestations to the pathophysiologic process.

CONCEPTS FOR LECTURE

VIRAL UPPER RESPIRATORY INFECTION

1. The most common cause of viral URI is rhinovirus, but they are also caused by parainfluenza viruses, respiratory syncytial viruses, coronaviruses, and adenoviruses.
2. These viruses are spread by aerosolized droplet nuclei during sneezing or coughing or by direct contact. Viruses are then picked up by the hands and fingers and carried to the eyes or mucous membranes of the susceptible host.
3. Local response to the virus includes a local inflammatory response and swelling of the mucous membranes of the nasal passages that results in hyperemia, engorgement, and hyperactivity of the mucus-secreting glands. This response is an attempt to trap the invading organism in the upper-respiratory tract and prevent spread to more vulnerable areas.
4. Manifestations of acute upper respiratory infection are nasal congestion, profuse nasal discharge (coryza), sneezing, coughing, sore throat, low-grade fever, headache, malaise, and muscle aches.
5. Acute viral upper respiratory infection is generally mild and self-limited, but complications such as sinusitis or otitis media can occur.

RESPIRATORY SYNCYTIAL VIRUS

6. Transmission of RSV occurs much the same as other URIs. The incubation period is 4–6 days.
7. Adult manifestations of RSV are those of other commonly occurring URIs.
8. In older adults, RSV may present as a lower respiratory infection with fever or pneumonia.
9. In infants, RSV may manifest as a URI, but is more likely to progress to pneumonia, bronchiolitis, and tracheobronchiolitis.

INFLUENZA

10. Influenza virus is spread by airborne droplet and direct contact. The three major strains of flu are influenza A virus, influenza B virus, and influenza C virus.
11. The incubation period for flu is 18–72 hours. The virus invades the respiratory epithelium and rapidly replicates, and spreads to neighboring cells. Inflammation leads to necrosis and shedding of serous and ciliated cells of the respiratory tract.

POWERPOINT LECTURE SLIDES

Viral Upper Respiratory Infection
- Pathophysiology
  - Local inflammatory response
  - Swelling of mucous membranes of nasal passages
  - Hyperactivity of mucus-secreting glands
  - Immunity produced only to individual virus
- Manifestations
  - Nasal congestion
  - Profuse nasal discharge (coryza)
  - Sneezing
  - Coughing
  - Sore throat
  - Low-grade fever
  - Headache
  - Malaise
  - Muscle aches

Sinusitis
- Pathophysiology
  - Sinus opening obstruction, impaired drainage
- Manifestations
  - Pain and tenderness
  - Headache, fever, and malaise
  - Nasal congestion
  - Purulent nasal discharge
  - Bad breath

Epiglottitis
- Pathophysiology
  - Inflammation/swelling pushes the epiglottis posteriorly
  - Possible airway obstruction
- Manifestations in adults
  - 1–2 day history of sore throat
  - Painful swallowing
  - Dyspnea
  - Drooling
  - Stridor

Laryngitis
- Pathophysiology
  - Mucous membrane lining of larynx becomes inflamed
  - Vocal cords edema
- Manifestations
  - Change in voice quality
  - Sore, scratchy throat
  - Dry, harsh cough

12. Infection produces one of three syndromes: uncomplicated nasopharyngeal inflammation, viral upper respiratory infection followed by bacterial infection, or viral pneumonia. Onset is rapid, with profound malaise that may develop in a matter of minutes.

13. Manifestations include: abrupt onset of chills and fever, malaise, muscle aches, and headache. Respiratory manifestations include dry, nonproductive cough, sore throat, substernal burning, and coryza. Acute symptoms subside within 2–3 days. Fever may last as long as a week. Cough may be severe and productive and can persist for days or several weeks.

14. Complications of influenza include secondary bacterial infections such as sinusitis or otitis media. Tracheobronchitis may develop and last for weeks.

15. Influenza is clearly linked to increased risk for development of pneumonia. Primary influenza viral pneumonia is uncommon, but may be fatal. Bacterial pneumonia is more likely to occur in older at-risk adults and presents as a relapse of influenza.

16. Reye's syndrome is a rare but potentially fatal complication of influenza and is often associated with influenza B. These clients may experience rapid development of hepatic failure and encephalopathy.

17. Other complications include myositis, myocarditis, and central nervous system disorders.

SINUSITIS

18. Sinusitis develops when the sinus openings are obstructed, which impairs drainage. The mucus secretion that collects in the sinuses is a medium for bacterial growth. Blockage of the sinus openings also causes swelling and pressure.

19. Chronic sinusitis can develop when acute sinusitis is inadequately treated. Isolation of bacteria, thickening of mucous membranes and fungal infections may occur.

20. Manifestations are pain and tenderness across the infected sinuses, headache, fever, and malaise. Symptoms worsen for 3–4 hours after awakening, and become less severe in the afternoon and evening as sinuses drain. Other symptoms may include nasal congestion, purulent nasal discharge, and bad breath.

21. Complications include periorbital abscess, cellulitis, cavernous sinus thrombosis, hearing loss, meningitis, brain abscess, or sepsis.

PHARYNGITIS OR TONSILLITIS

22. Pharyngitis and tonsillitis are spread by droplet nuclei and have incubation periods of a few hours to several days, depending upon the causative organism. Symptoms typically resolve 3–10 days after onset.

23. Streptococcal pharyngitis manifests abruptly with high fever, severe sore throat, dysphagia, malaise, arthralgias, myalgias, and enlargement of the anterior lymph nodes.

Diphtheria
- Pathophysiology
  - Tonsils and pharynx are common site of infection
  - Thick, grayish, rubbery pseudomembrane forms over posterior pharynx/trachea
- Manifestations
  - Fever
  - Malaise
  - Sore throat
  - Malodorous breath
  - Lymphadenopathy
  - Stridor
  - Cyanosis

Pertussis
- Pathophysiology
  - Damage/effects caused by bacterial toxins
- Manifestations
  - Follow predictable pattern
  - Begin with typical URI symptoms
  - 1–2 weeks cough becomes more frequent
  - Paroxysms of coughing occur frequently
  - Vomiting commonly follows coughing episode

Laryngeal Trauma
- Manifestations
  - Subcutaneous emphysema or crepitus
  - Voice changes
  - Dysphagia
  - Pain with swallowing
  - Inspiratory stridor
  - Hemoptysis
  - Cough

Obstructive Sleep Apnea
- Pathophysiology
  - Loss of normal pharyngeal muscle tone
  - Pharynx to collapse during inspiration
  - Tongue is pulled against posterior pharyngeal wall
  - Obstruction causes O_2 sat, PO_2, and pH to fall, and P_{CO_2} to rise
  - Asphyxia causes brief arousal from sleep
  - Restores airway patency and airflow
  - Episodes may occur hundreds of times a night
- Manifestations
  - Loud snoring during sleep
  - Excessive daytime drowsiness
  - Headache
  - Irritability
  - Restless sleep

24. Viral pharyngitis manifests more slowly, with low-grade fever, sore throat, mild hoarseness, headache, and rhinorrhea.
25. Tonsillitis manifests as a sore throat, difficulty swallowing, general malaise, fever, and pain referred to the ear. White exudate is present on the tonsil and pressing on the tonsil may produce purulent discharge. Cervical lymph nodes are usually tender and enlarged.
26. Bacterial pharyngitis can lead to complications such as abscess, scarlet fever, toxic shock syndrome, rheumatic fever, or acute poststreptococcal glomerulonephritis.

EPIGLOTTITIS

27. As the tissues between the tongue and the epiglottis become inflamed, swelling pushes the epiglottis posteriorly, which threatens the airway.
28. Manifestations of epiglottitis in adults include a 1–2 day history of sore throat, painful swallowing, dyspnea, and possible drooling and stridor.

LARYNGITIS

29. In laryngitis, the mucous membrane that lines the larynx becomes inflamed; the vocal cords also may become edematous.
30. The primary manifestation of laryngitis is a change in the quality of the voice; however, a sore, scratchy throat and dry, harsh cough may also be present.

DIPHTHERIA

31. Diphtheria is spread through droplet nuclei and is easily spread in areas with poor sanitation, crowded living conditions, and limited access to health care.
32. Common sites of infection with diphtheria are the tonsils and pharynx. Exudate from inflamed tissues produces a thick, grayish, rubbery pseudomembrane over the posterior pharynx and sometimes into the trachea that may interfere with eating, drinking, and breathing.
33. Manifestations are fever, malaise, sore throat, malodorous breath, lymphadenopathy, and presence of a gray or white exudate that extends to form the classic membrane. Dislodging the membrane may cause bleeding.

PERTUSSIS

34. Pertussis is spread by respiratory droplets. The damage and effects of pertussis are due to the toxins produced by the bacteria. These toxins damage the nasopharyngeal mucosa and paralyze the cilia, which impairs the clearance of respiratory secretions and increases risk for pneumonia. This prompts the inflammatory response and inhibits immunity.
35. Manifestations follow a predictable pattern and begin with typical URI symptoms. After 1–2 weeks cough becomes more frequent and is characterized by paroxysms of rapid cough, followed by an audible whooping sound caused by rapid inspiration.

The paroxysms of coughing may occur from several times an hour to 5–10 per day and interfere with eating and sleeping. Vomiting commonly follows an episode of coughing.

36. Complications include development of pneumonia, neurologic complications secondary to hypoxia, pneumothorax, weight loss, inguinal hernia, rib fracture, and cough syncope.

EPISTAXIS

37. Ninety percent of nosebleeds arise from Kiesselbach's area in the anterior nasal septum. This area is very susceptible to trauma, drying, and infection.
38. Posterior nosebleeds occur from the terminal branches of the sphenopalatine and internal maxillary arteries. They are more commonly associated with disorders such as blood dyscrasias, hypertension, or diabetes. Posterior nosebleeds are more severe and more commonly occur in adults.
39. Manifestations of anterior nosebleeds include obvious bleeding from the nares, as well as bleeding into the posterior nasal and oral pharynx. Posterior bleeding may be less apparent with most of the blood draining into the posterior nasopharynx. Nausea and vomiting may occur from swallowing blood.

NASAL TRAUMA OR SURGERY

40. Unilateral nasal fracture involves only one side of the nose. It causes little displacement or cosmetic deformity.
41. Bilateral fractures are more common, with depression or displacement of both nasal bones to one side.
42. Complex fractures may involve the septum, ascending processes of the maxilla, and frontal bones of the face.
43. Manifestations include epistaxis, hematomas, periorbital edema and ecchymoses, and bony crepitus. Bilateral fractures may result in a flattened appearance to the nose or an S or C configuration from deviation.
44. Complications of nasal fracture include septal hematomas and abscess formation, septal perforation or deviation, and cerebrospinal fluid leakage. Obstruction can occur.
45. Fractures in the nasoethmoidal or frontal region can disrupt the dura, causing CSF leakage or rhinorrhea. CSF rhinorrhea is suspected by watery nasal drainage that tests positive for glucose.

LARYNGEAL OBSTRUCTION OR TRAUMA

46. Complete or partial obstruction may occur from aspiration, laryngospasm, or edema.
47. A *café coronary* or food aspiration is the most common cause of obstruction in adults.
48. Presence of a foreign body in the airway causes pain, laryngospasm, dyspnea, and inspiratory stridor. Infection may develop if the foreign body lodges in the trachea or lungs.

49. Laryngospasm occurs due to trauma, chemical irritation, or hypocalcemia. Acute hypersensitivity reactions may lead to angioedema of the upper airways and severe laryngeal edema, which results in obstruction.

50. Manifestations of obstruction are coughing, choking, gagging, obvious difficulty breathing, inspiratory stridor, cyanosis, respiratory distress, or death.

51. Laryngeal trauma can occur with motor vehicle and other accidents, assaults, or traumatic intubation attempts. The thyroid and/or cricoid cartilage may be fractured. Soft-tissue injuries cause swelling and obstruction.

52. Manifestations of laryngeal trauma may include subcutaneous emphysema or crepitus, voice changes, dysphagia, and pain with swallowing, inspiratory stridor, hemoptysis, and cough.

OBSTRUCTIVE SLEEP APNEA

53. Loss of normal pharyngeal muscle tone permits the pharynx to collapse during inspiration as pressure within the airways becomes negative in relation to atmospheric pressure. The tongue is pulled against the posterior pharyngeal wall, which increases obstruction.

54. Airway obstruction causes the oxygen saturation, PO_2, and pH to fall, and the PCO_2 to rise. This progressive asphyxia causes brief arousal from sleep, which restores airway patency and airflow.

55. Sleep can be severely fragmented as these episodes may occur hundreds of times a night.

56. Manifestations are loud snoring during sleep, excessive daytime drowsiness, headache, irritability, and restless sleep.

57. Complications include secondary physiologic effects. Neurologic effects include excessive daytime drowsiness, impaired intellect, memory loss, and personality changes. Cardiac effects include myocardial ischemia and angina, dysrhythmias, heart failure, and systemic and pulmonary hypertension.

58. Sudden cardiac death is believed to be a potential fatal complication of obstructive sleep apnea.

59. Clients with sleep apnea who undergo gastric bypass surgery to treat obesity are at significant risk for postoperative respiratory complications.

60. Risk factors for developing sleep apnea include increasing age, obesity, and large neck circumference. Use of alcohol and other CNS depressants may also contribute to sleep apnea.

NASAL POLYPS

61. Chronic irritation and swelling of the mucous membranes from allergic rhinitis may cause slow polyp formation.

62. Polyps are pale, edematous masses covered with mucous membrane and generally develop in dependent areas. They are usually bilateral and have a stem-like base, which makes them movable.

63. Polyps can continue to enlarge and reach the size of a grape. Large polyps may cause nasal obstruction, rhinorrhea, and loss of the sense of smell.

LARYNGEAL TUMOR

64. Papillomas are small, wart-like growths that are believed to be viral in origin.
65. Nodules occur as paired lesions on the free edge of the vocal cords.
66. Manifestations of benign vocal cord tumors include hoarseness and a breathy voice quality.
67. The most common malignancy of the larynx is squamous cell carcinoma. Leukoplakia are white, patchy, precancerous lesions. Red, velvety patches, called erythroplakia, are thought to represent a later stage of carcinoma development. Initial cancerous lesion, carcinoma in situ (CIS), is superficial and if untreated will develop into squamous cell cancer.
68. Laryngeal cancer spreads by both direct invasion of surrounding tissues and by metastasis.
69. Laryngeal cancer may develop in the glottis, the supraglottis, and the subglottis.
70. Cancers of the true vocal cords or glottis tend to be well-differentiated and slow-growing. Metastasis occurs late in the illness. Manifestations are hoarseness or a change in voice quality.
71. Cancer of the supraglottis (the epiglottis, aryepiglottic folds, arytenoid muscles and cartilage, and false vocal cords) often invade locally and metastasize early. Manifestations are painful swallowing, sore throat, or a feeling of a lump in the throat. Dyspnea, foul breath, and pain that radiates to the ear are later manifestations.
72. Subglottic tumors (below the vocal cords) are often asymptomatic until the enlarging tumor obstructs the airway.
73. Risk factors for laryngeal cancer development include tobacco use, alcohol consumption, poor nutrition, human papillomavirus infection, exposure to asbestos, and race.

SUGGESTIONS FOR CLASSROOM ACTIVITIES

- Have the students develop a chart that lists common upper respiratory tract disorders and their manifestations. Using the chart, look for commonalities and differences among these disorders.
- List common manifestations of upper respiratory tract disorders. Discuss the pathophysiology of these manifestations.

SUGGESTIONS FOR CLINICAL ACTIVITIES

- Have students assess clinical clients for manifestation of common respiratory disorders. Review the medical records for risk factors that lead to the development of the disorder. Relate how the pathophysiology is expressed in manifestations.

LEARNING OUTCOME 3

Discuss nursing implications for medications and other interdisciplinary care measures to treat upper respiratory disorders.

CONCEPTS FOR LECTURE
VIRAL UPPER RESPIRATORY INFECTION

1. Treatment is symptomatic and may include rest and fluids. Mild decongestants and OTC antihistamines may relieve coryza and nasal congestion. Warm salt-water gargles, throat lozenges, and mild analgesics may be used for sore throat.

2. Complementary therapies include echinacea and garlic which may have antiviral and antibiotic effects. Aromatherapy may reduce congestion and promote comfort and recovery. Acupuncture and acupressure may also be effective in treating adult URI.

RESPIRATORY SYNCYTIAL VIRUS

3. Treatment for adults with RSV is symptomatic, and includes hydration and mobilization of respiratory secretions. Aerosolized ribavirin (Virazole) may be prescribed for older adults and immunocompromised clients with RSV pneumonia.

INFLUENZA

4. The primary focus of interdisciplinary care is preventing community outbreaks and protecting vulnerable populations. Immunization is an important aspect of preventing influenza and is recommended for those over 65, residents of nursing homes, those with chronic cardiopulmonary disorders or chronic metabolic diseases, and for healthcare workers who have frequent contact with high-risk clients.

5. Amantadine (Symmetrel) or rimantadine (Flumadine) may be used as prophylaxis in unvaccinated people who are exposed to the virus. The drug should be given within 48 hours of exposure and, if possible, unvaccinated persons should receive the vaccine along with the antiviral drug.

6. Amantadine (Symmetrel), rimantadine (Flumadine), zanamivir (Relenza), oseltamivir (Tamiflu), and ribavirin (Virazole) may also be used to reduce the severity and duration of flu symptoms. OTC drugs such as ASA, acetaminophen, and NSAIDs may provide symptomatic relief of fever and muscle aches. Antitussives may decrease cough, which promotes rest. Antibiotics are not indicated.

7. Nursing diagnoses include: Ineffective Breathing Pattern, Disturbed Sleep Pattern, and Risk for Infection.

SINUSITIS

8. Interdisciplinary care of sinusitis focuses on draining obstructed sinuses, controlling infection, relieving pain, and preventing complications.

POWERPOINT LECTURE SLIDES

Influenza
- Medications
  ○ Prophylaxis
  ○ Treatment to reduce severity
    – Amantadine
    – Rimantadine
    – Zanamivir
    – Oseltamivir
    – Ribavirin
  ○ Symptom relief also include
    – ASA
    – Acetaminophen
    – NSAIDs
    – Antitussives
    – Antibiotics are not indicated

Sinusitis
- Medication therapy
  ○ Antibiotics
  ○ Oral or topical decongestants
  ○ Antihistamines
  ○ Saline nose drops or sprays
  ○ Systemic mucolytic agents

Pharyngitis or Tonsillitis
- Medications
  ○ Antibiotics for bacterial infections
  ○ Antipyretics
  ○ Mild analgesics

Epiglottitis
- Medications
  ○ Antibiotics for infection
  ○ Corticosteroids

Pertussis
- Medications
  ○ Erythromycin
  ○ Prophylactically to all household/close contacts

Epistaxis
- Medications
  ○ Topical vasoconstrictors
  ○ Chemical agents for cauterization
  ○ Topical anesthetics if packing is required
  ○ Prophylactic antibiotic therapy

Nasal Polyps
- Medications
  ○ Topical corticosteroid nasal sprays
  ○ Low-dose corticosteroids

9. Medication therapy includes antibiotics, oral or topical decongestants, antihistamines, saline nose drops or sprays, and systemic mucolytic agents.

10. Complementary therapies include aromatherapy, herbal teas, hot or cold compresses, steam inhalation, and acupuncture.

11. Nursing diagnoses include: Pain and Imbalanced Nutrition: Less than Body Requirements.

PHARYNGITIS OR TONSILLITIS

12. Both viral and bacterial pharyngitis are usually self-limited diseases, but because of the potential complications of streptococcal infections, an effort is usually made to establish an accurate diagnosis and to treat bacterial pharyngitis.

13. Medications for treatment of pharyngitis and tonsillitis include antibiotics for bacterial infections, as well as antipyretics and mild analgesics for symptomatic relief.

14. Home care is generally appropriate for uncomplicated pharyngitis and tonsillitis. Nursing care focuses on education regarding medications, symptom control, and potential complications.

EPIGLOTTITIS

15. Using a tongue blade to view the oropharynx may cause laryngospasm and airway obstruction. When epiglottis is suspected, a flexible fiberoptic laryngoscope is used to visualize the area and to establish a diagnosis. Nasotracheal intubation may be necessary to ensure airway patency.

16. Medications include antibiotics for infection and corticosteroids to suppress the inflammatory response and rapidly reduce swelling.

17. The focus of nursing care is maintenance of airway patency.

LARYNGITIS

18. There is no specific treatment for laryngitis other than reducing exposure to precipitating factors. Voice rest is encouraged. Inhalation of steam and spraying the throat with antiseptic solution may offer some relief.

19. The primary nursing diagnoses is: Impaired Verbal Communication.

DIPHTHERIA

20. Collaborative care goals for diphtheria are to prevent its transmission, treat the infection, neutralize toxins, and provide respiratory support.

21. Strict isolation procedures are instituted. All contacts are screened and immunized.

22. Medications include antitoxin for which a skin test for sensitivity must be administered. Antibiotics are also administered.

23. Intensive nursing care is required and includes monitoring for airway obstruction, cardiac manifestations, and CNS complications. Nutrition and fluid balance are closely managed.
24. Diphtheria is immediately reported to the local health department and the Centers for Disease Control and Prevention.

Pertussis

25. Active immunization with pertussis vaccine is the primary preventive strategy.
26. Erythromycin (Akne-Mycin) is the antibiotic of choice and is given prophylactically to all household and close contacts of the infected client.
27. Respiratory isolation is maintained until 5 days after antibiotic therapy is initiated.
28. Nursing care is primarily educative, including immunizations, control of respiratory secretions, maintenance of nutrition and fluid balance, and medication administration.
29. Pertussis is a reportable communicable disease.

Epistaxis

30. Interdisciplinary care includes management of bleeding. Anterior bleeding can usually be managed by simple first-aid measures. Posterior bleeding may require nasal packing.
31. Medications include topical vasoconstrictors, chemical agents for cauterization, topical anesthetics if packing is required, and prophylactic antibiotic therapy.
32. Priority nursing diagnoses are: Anxiety and Risk for Aspiration.

Nasal Trauma or Surgery

33. Major treatment goals of nasal fractures are to maintain a patent airway and prevent deformity.
34. Treatments include simple reduction and external splint application. Ice is often used to control edema and bleeding. Nasal packing may be necessary to control epistaxis.
35. Nursing diagnoses include: Ineffective Airway Clearance and Risk for Infection.

Laryngeal Obstruction or Trauma

36. The treatment goal is to maintain an open airway. Rapidity of intervention depends upon extent of obstruction.
37. For anaphylaxis, epinephrine may be administered to reduce laryngeal edema and relieve obstruction.
38. For complete foreign body airway obstruction, the Heimlich maneuver is performed immediately. Endotracheal intubation, cricothyrotomy, or tracheostomy may become necessary.
39. The priority of nursing care in laryngeal obstruction or trauma is restoring a patent airway to prevent cerebral anoxia and death.

OBSTRUCTIVE SLEEP APNEA

40. The goal of care for obstructive sleep apnea is to restore airflow and prevent adverse effects of the disorder.
41. Treatments of mild to moderate sleep apnea include weight reduction, alcohol abstinence, improving nasal patency, and avoiding the prone sleeping position.
42. Nasal continuous positive airway pressure (CPAP) is the treatment of choice for sleep apnea.
43. A newer device, the BiPAP ventilator, delivers higher pressures than CPAP during inhalation and lower pressures during expiration, which provides less resistance to exhaling.
44. Nursing diagnoses include: Disturbed Sleep Pattern; Fatigue; Ineffective Breathing Pattern; Impaired Gas Exchange; Risk for Injury; and Risk for Sexual Dysfunction.

NASAL POLYPS

45. If polyps are secondary to an acute URI, they may regress spontaneously with resolution of the infection.
46. Medications prescribed include topical corticosteroid nasal sprays or low-dose corticosteroids. Polyps will continue to enlarge when corticosteroid therapy is discontinued.
47. Nursing care generally focuses on education, as well as preoperative and postoperative care of the polypectomy client.

LARYNGEAL TUMOR

48. Benign tumors may resolve with correction of the underlying cause.
49. Treatment of laryngeal cancers varies with extent of the disease.
50. Nursing diagnoses include: Risk for Impaired Airway Clearance; Impaired Verbal Communication; Impaired Swallowing, Imbalanced Nutrition: Less than Body Requirements; and Anticipatory Grieving.

SUGGESTIONS FOR CLASSROOM ACTIVITIES

- Have students list medications commonly prescribed for clients with an upper respiratory disorder. List the nursing implications of each of those medications. Have students relate the action of the medication to the pathophysiology of the disorder.
- Review the case study on sleep apnea and the care plan activity on epistaxis provided on the textbook Companion Website. Use the information provided to create a nursing care plan for clients who have these disorders.

SUGGESTIONS FOR CLINICAL ACTIVITIES

- Have students review clinical client medication administration records for medications that are commonly prescribed for upper respiratory disorders. Have students relate the use of this medication to manifestations assessed in the client. Require students to create medication information sheets listing appropriate dose ranges, nursing implications, and client/family teaching information for the medications identified.

Describe surgical procedures used to treat upper respiratory disorders and their implications for client care and recovery.

CONCEPTS FOR LECTURE

SINUSITIS

1. Clients who do not respond to pharmacologic measures and who experience persistent facial pain, headache, or nasal congestion may require endoscopic sinus surgery. This surgery is most effective for local disease, recurrent acute sinusitis, or for removing anatomic obstructions.

2. Antral irrigation can be done in the physician's office under local anesthetic. Saline solution is instilled through a needle inserted into the maxillary sinus, irrigating the area.

3. If endoscopic sinus surgery is unsuccessful, the Caldwell-Luc procedure may be indicated. An opening between the maxillary sinus and lateral nasal wall is created to increase aeration of the sinus and to promote drainage into the nasal cavity. Diseased mucous membrane and periosteum tissue is removed.

4. In external sphenoethmoidectomy, an incision along the side of the nose from the middle of the eyebrow is used to open and remove diseased tissue from the sphenoid or ethmoid sinuses.

PHARYNGITIS AND TONSILLITIS

5. Peritonsillar abscess may be treated with needle aspiration or by incision and drainage.

6. Tonsillectomy is indicated for recurrent or nonresponsive chronic infections, tonsillar hypertrophy with possible airway obstruction, repeated episodes of purulent otitis media, and tonsil malignancy. Adenoid tissue is usually removed at the same time.

7. Following tonsillectomy, nursing care focuses on ensuring a patent airway, monitoring for and controlling hemorrhage, and control of pain and swelling.

EPISTAXIS

8. Chemical or surgical cautery procedures may be used to sclerose involved vessels.

9. In some cases occlusion of the internal maxillary artery is necessary. This procedure is done by ligating or embolizing the artery and may result in facial paralysis, paresthesia, facial pain, or dental injury.

NASAL TRAUMA OR SURGERY

10. Complex nasal fractures, nasal septal deviation, or persistent CSF leakage may require surgical repair.

11. Rhinoplasty is surgical reconstruction of the nose.

12. Septoplasty and submucous resection are procedures done to correct a deviated septum.

13. Endoscopic repair may be necessary to correct defects in the cribriform plate, fovia ethmoidalis, or sphenoid sinus associated with persistent CSF leakage. Large defects may require craniotomy for repair.

POWERPOINT LECTURE SLIDES

Sinusitis
- Endoscopic sinus surgery
- Antral irrigation
- Caldwell-Luc procedure
- External sphenoethmoidectomy

Pharyngitis and Tonsillitis
- Peritonsillar abscess
- Tonsillectomy

Epistaxis
- Chemical or surgical cautery to sclerose involved vessels
- Ligation or embolization of internal maxillary artery

Nasal Trauma or Surgery
- Surgical repair
  ○ Complex nasal fractures
  ○ Nasal septal deviation
  ○ Persistent CSF leakage
  ○ Rhinoplasty is surgical reconstruction of the nose
  ○ Deviation of the septum repair
  ○ Endoscopic repair

Obstructive Sleep Apnea
- Tonsillectomy
- Adenoidectomy
- Uvulopalatopharyngoplasty (UPPP)
- Tracheostomy

Nasal Polyps
- Polypectomy
- Laser surgery
- Repeat surgeries may be necessary

OBSTRUCTIVE SLEEP APNEA

14. Tonsillectomy and adenoidectomy may relieve upper airway obstruction in some clients. Uvulopalatopharyngoplasty (UPPP) is the removal of obstructive tissue from the soft palate, uvula, and posterior lateral pharyngeal wall. In severe cases, tracheostomy may be required.

NASAL POLYPS

15. Polypectomy or laser surgery may be necessary if polyps obstruct normal breathing.
16. Repeat surgeries may be necessary, as polyps have a tendency to recur.

SUGGESTIONS FOR CLASSROOM ACTIVITIES

- Lead a discussion of the surgical procedures used to ensure an open airway.
- Discuss why surgery might be an appropriate treatment for someone with a sinus infection.

SUGGESTIONS FOR CLINICAL ACTIVITIES

- Assign students to the care of a client who is scheduled to undergo surgery for an upper respiratory disorder. Have students prepare a teaching plan for the postoperative care of this client.
- Review the medical record of a client who has undergone surgery of the upper respiratory tract. Review the nursing and medical orders for this client and have students identify the pathophysiologic or psychosocial rationale for that order.

LEARNING OUTCOME 5

Identify health promotion activities related to reducing the incidence of upper respiratory disorders, describing the appropriate population and setting for implementing identified measures.

CONCEPTS FOR LECTURE
VIRAL UPPER RESPIRATORY INFECTION

1. Maintaining good general health and stress-reducing activities support the immune system and help to prevent URI. Limiting exposure to crowds and using good hand washing techniques can also reduce incidence of URI.
2. Teaching should include hygiene, hand washing, and prevention of rebound effect from nasal decongestants.

RESPIRATORY SYNCYTIAL VIRUS

3. The focus of nursing care for the adult with URI manifestations of RSV is on teaching for self-care, identification of complications, and prevention of viral spread.

INFLUENZA

4. Health promotion activities should include immunization education and information to reduce risk of contracting influenza, such as avoiding crowds and people who are ill.

POWERPOINT LECTURE SLIDES

Health Promotion Activities
Viral Upper Respiratory Infection
- Maintaining good general health
- Stress-reducing activities
- Limiting exposure to crowds
- Good hand washing

Influenza
- Immunization education
- Risk reduction activities
  - Avoiding crowds
  - Avoiding those who are ill

Sinusitis
- Promote nasal drainage
- Encouraging liberal fluid intake
- Judicious use of nasal decongestants
- Treating any obstructive process

Pharyngitis or Tonsillitis
- Education regarding need to seek treatment

SINUSITIS

5. Measures to prevent sinusitis are those to promote nasal drainage; encouraging liberal fluid intake, judicious use of nasal decongestants; and treating any obstructive process.

PHARYNGITIS OR TONSILLITIS

6. Because of the risk of significant complications associated with streptococcal pharyngitis, all clients with symptoms that persist for several days or that include fever, lymphadenopathy, and myalgias should be encouraged to seek evaluation and treatment.

DIPHTHERIA AND PERTUSSIS

7. Nurses are instrumental in promoting effective immunizations of all infants and young children.

OBSTRUCTIVE SLEEP APNEA

8. The nurse should provide teaching regarding the relationship between sleep apnea and obesity, alcohol use, and sedative use. Referral to programs for weight loss and alcohol use cessation may be appropriate. If the client is to use CPAP, information on proper use of the equipment and the importance of its continuous use at night should be included. Referral to support groups of persons with sleep apnea syndrome may be helpful.

NASAL TRAUMA OR SURGERY

9. All people should be taught about the importance of wearing helmets and facial protection when participating in high-risk sports such as football, hockey, and baseball catching. Promote the use of seatbelts with shoulder harness and airbags in vehicles to reduce the risk of facial injury in motor vehicle crashes.

LARYNGEAL OBSTRUCTION OR TRAUMA

10. Health promotion activities include measures to prevent food aspiration, teaching about CPR and Heimlich maneuver, and measures to identify and provide rapid intervention to those with anaphylactic responses.

NASAL POLYPS

11. People who have asthma and nasal polyps may have an associated aspirin allergy of which they are unaware.

LARYNGEAL TUMOR

12. Health promotion activities to prevent laryngeal cancer focus on preventing smoking among children, adolescents, and young adults; and promoting smoking cessation in people who do smoke. Activities to promote abstinence or moderate alcohol use are also beneficial.

Diptheria and Pertussis
- Immunizations

Obstructive Sleep Apnea
- General teaching about process and treatments

Nasal Trauma or Surgery
- Safety measures
  - Helmets
  - Facial protection
  - Seatbelts with shoulder harnesses
  - Airbags

Laryngeal Obstruction or Trauma
- Measures to prevent food aspiration
- CPR teaching
- Measures to identify/provide rapid intervention for anaphylaxis

Nasal Polyps
- Possibility of aspirin allergy for those with asthma and nasal polyps

Laryngeal Tumor
- Smoking prevention and cessation activities
- Activities to promote abstinence or moderate alcohol use

LEARNING OUTCOME 6

Discuss treatment options for oral and laryngeal cancers with their implications for the client's body image and functional health.

CONCEPTS FOR LECTURE

1. Laryngeal cancer treatment is determined by staging the cancer, combining T (tumor size and location), N (number of involved lymph nodes), and M (presence of metastasis) to assign a stage.
2. Radiation therapy is often the treatment of choice in early laryngeal cancer.
3. Chemoradiotherapy is radiation therapy combined with chemotherapy and is used to treat more advanced laryngeal cancers.
4. Chemotherapy is used to treat distant metastasis and for palliation when the tumor is unresectable.
5. The goals of surgery for laryngeal cancer are to remove the malignancy, maintain airway patency, and achieve optimal cosmetic appearance.
6. Carcinoma in situ, vocal cord polyps, and early vocal cord cancers may be removed by laser during laryngoscopy procedure. Normal eating, speaking, and breathing are restored.
7. Laryngectomy is removal of the larynx. Partial laryngectomy may be used for tumors localized to a portion of the larynx with limited extension beyond the larynx. Normal speaking, breathing, and swallowing are restored.
8. Total laryngectomy is required for cancers that extend beyond the vocal cords. The entire larynx, epiglottis, thyroid cartilage, several tracheal rings, and the hyoid bone are removed. Normal speech is lost and a permanent tracheostomy is created.
9. Radical or modified neck dissection may be performed if cervical lymph nodes are involved but there is no evidence of distal metastasis.
10. In radical neck dissection, all soft tissues from the lower edge of the mandible down to the clavicle is removed, including cervical lymph nodes, the sternocleidomastoid muscle, internal jugular vein, cranial nerve XI, and submaxillary salivary gland. Significant deformity results from this procedure.
11. Modified neck dissection surgery results in removal of all of the neck contents, but leaves the sternocleidomastoid muscle, internal jugular vein, and spinal accessory nerve.

POWERPOINT LECTURE SLIDES

Treatment of Laryngeal Cancer
- Determined by staging the cancer
- Radiation therapy
- Chemoradiotherapy
- Chemotherapy

Goals of Surgery
- Remove the malignancy
- Maintain airway patency
- Achieve optimal cosmetic appearance

Procedures
- Laser laryngoscopy
- Laryngectomy
- Radical neck dissection
- Modified neck dissection

Speech Rehabilitation
- Necessary if entire larynx is removed
- Techniques
  ○ Tracheoesophageal puncture with placement of a one-way shunt valve
  ○ Esophageal speech
  ○ Use of speech generators

12. Speech rehabilitation is necessary after total laryngectomy. Techniques include tracheoesophageal puncture with placement of a one-way shunt valve, esophageal speech, and use of speech generators.

SUGGESTIONS FOR CLASSROOM ACTIVITIES	**SUGGESTIONS FOR CLINICAL ACTIVITIES**
• Have student access the MediaLink application about laryngectomy that is provided on the textbook Companion Website. Assign each student to the investigation of a treatment option for these clients. Compare and contrast these treatments in class. • Arrange for a client who has undergone radical neck dissection to come to the classroom.	• Assign clinical students to the care of clients who are preparing to undergo or who have undergone surgery for an oral or laryngeal cancer. • Have other students investigate the nursing care for clients who are undergoing treatments other than surgery for oral or laryngeal cancer. • Compare and contrast these treatment modalities with emphasis on the nursing implications.

CHAPTER 38
NURSING CARE OF CLIENTS WITH VENTILATION DISORDERS

RESOURCE LIBRARY

 PRENTICE HALL NURSING MEDIALINK DVD-ROM

Audio Glossary
NCLEX-RN® Review
Animation
  Tuberculosis

 COMPANION WEBSITE

Audio Glossary
NCLEX-RN® Review
Care Plan Activity: Pneumonia
Case Study: TB Medication and Compliance
MediaLink Applications
  Health Promotion Among Vulnerable Populations
  SARS
Links to Resources

IMAGE LIBRARY

Figure 38.1 In pneumonia, the inflammatory response causes fluid to accumulate in the alveoli and edema to form as alveolar capillaries dilate and allow fluid to leak into interstitial tissues.

Figure 38.2 The pathogenesis of pneumococcal pneumonia.

Figure 38.3 Low-flow oxygen delivery devices.

Figure 38.4 Venturi mask, a high-flow oxygen delivery system.

Figure 38.5 *A*, Percussing (clapping) the upper posterior chest. *B*, Vibrating the upper posterior chest.

Figure 38.6 Positions for postural drainage.

Figure 38.7 *A*, Intradermal injection for tuberculin testing. *B*, The injection causes a local inflammatory response (wheal). *C*, Measurement of induration following tuberculin testing.

Figure 38.8 Thoracentesis.

Figure 38.9 The Heimlich one-way valve allows air to escape from the pleural space, helping to reestablish negative pressure and allowing the lung to reexpand.

Figure 38.10 A closed-chest drainage system.

Figure 38.11 Flail chest with paradoxic movement.

Figure 38.12 The pathogenesis of near-drowning, freshwater and saltwater.

LEARNING OUTCOME 1

Relate the pathophysiology and manifestations of lower respiratory infections and inflammation, lung cancer, chest wall disorders, and trauma to the ability to maintain effective ventilation and respiration (gas exchange).

CONCEPTS FOR LECTURE
ACUTE BRONCHITIS

1. Infectious bronchitis can be viral, bacterial, or inflammatory.
2. The response of the bronchial tissue to viral or bacterial invasion or the presence of irritating substances causes increased mucus production and mucosal irritation.
3. Acute bronchitis generally begins with a nonproductive cough that later becomes productive. The cough is paroxysmal and is aggravated by cold, dry, or dusty air. Chest pain, moderate fever, and general malaise may also be present.

PNEUMONIA

4. Pneumonia is inflammation of the lung parenchyma. It may be infectious or noninfectious.

POWERPOINT LECTURE SLIDES

Pathophysiology and Manifestations of Lower Respiratory Infections
Acute Bronchitis
- Manifestations
  - Non-productive cough
    - Later becomes productive
  - Cough is paroxysmal
  - Cough aggravated by cold, dry, or dusty air
  - Chest pain
  - Moderate fever
  - General malaise

Pneumonia
- Pathophysiology
  - Inflammation of lung parenchyma
  - Infectious
  - Noninfectious

5. Bacteria, viruses, fungal protozoa, and other microbes can lead to infectious pneumonia.
6. Noninfectious causes of pneumonia include aspiration of gastric contents and inhalation of toxic or irritating gases.
7. Pneumonias can be classified as community-acquired, nosocomial, or opportunistic.
8. Pathogens may enter the lungs by aspiration of oropharyngeal secretions, inhalation of contaminated air or water, or through the bloodstream from infection elsewhere in the body.
9. Pneumonia may develop in four distinct patterns: lobar pneumonia, bronchopneumonia, interstitial pneumonia, and miliary pneumonia.

ACUTE BACTERIAL PNEUMONIA

10. The inflammatory response initiated by the causative organism results in alveolar edema and the formation of exudate. Consolidation of lung tissue occurs when serous exudate, blood cells, fibrin, and bacteria fill the alveoli and respiratory bronchioles. The lower lobes of the lungs are usually affected because of gravity.
11. Lobar pneumonia is consolidation of a large portion of an entire lung lobe.
12. Bronchopneumonia is a patchy consolidation that involves several lobules.
13. Manifestations of bacterial pneumonia are acute, rapid onset, shaking chills, fever, and cough productive of rust-colored or purulent sputum. Pleuritic pain is common. Limited breath sounds, fine crackles, rales, or pleural friction rubs may be heard over the affected area of the lung. Dyspnea and cyanosis may be noted.
14. Bronchopneumonia has a more insidious onset with low-grade fever, cough, and scattered crackles.
15. Atypical presentation including fever, tachypnea, and altered mentation or agitation may be seen in the older adult or debilitated client.

LEGIONNAIRE'S DISEASE

16. Legionnaire's disease is a form of bronchopneumonia caused by *Legionella pneumophila* that occurs in warm standing water. The disease was first recognized in 1976 when an outbreak occurred at an American Legion convention.
17. Manifestations are dry cough, dyspnea, general malaise, chills and fever, headache, confusion, anorexia and diarrhea, myalgias, and arthralgias.

PRIMARY ATYPICAL PNEUMONIA

18. Pneumonia caused by *Mycoplasma pneumoniae* is generally classified as primary atypical pneumonia, because its presentation and course significantly differ from other bacterial pneumonias.
19. Manifestations are fever, headache, myalgias, and arthralgias. The associated cough is dry, hacking, and

- ○ Can be classified as community acquired, nosocomial, or opportunistic
- ○ Pathogens enter the lungs
  - – Aspiration of oropharyngeal secretions
  - – Inhalation of contaminated air or water
  - – Through the bloodstream
- ○ Pneumonia may develop in four distinct patterns
  - – Lobar pneumonia
  - – Bronchopneumonia
  - – Interstitial pneumonia
  - – Miliary pneumonia

Legionnaire's Disease
- • Manifestations
  - ○ Dry cough
  - ○ Dyspnea
  - ○ General malaise
  - ○ Chills and fever
  - ○ Headache confusion
  - ○ Anorexia
  - ○ Diarrhea
  - ○ Myalgia
  - ○ Arthralgias

Primary Atypical Pneumonia
- • Manifestations
  - ○ Fever
  - ○ Headache
  - ○ Myalgias
  - ○ Arthralgias
  - ○ Dry, hacking, nonproductive cough

Viral Pneumonia
- • Manifestations
  - ○ Flu-like symptoms
  - ○ Headache
  - ○ Fever
  - ○ Fatigue
  - ○ Malaise
  - ○ Muscle aches

Pneumocystis Pneumonia
- • Manifestations
  - ○ Abrupt onset
  - ○ Fever
  - ○ Tachypnea
  - ○ Shortness of breath
  - ○ Dry, nonproductive cough
  - ○ Respiratory distress can be significant
    - – Intercostal retractions
    - – Cyanosis

Severe Acute Respiratory Syndrome (SARS)
- • Manifestations
  - ○ High fever
  - ○ Chills
  - ○ Headache
  - ○ Malaise
  - ○ Muscle aches

nonproductive. Alveolar exudate and consolidation of lung tissue are not features of atypical pneumonia.

VIRAL PNEUMONIA

20. Influenza and adenovirus are primary causative agents of viral pneumonia. Cytomegalovirus pneumonia is increasing in immunocompromised people.
21. Manifestations are flulike symptoms of headache, fever, fatigue, malaise, and muscle aches.

PNEUMOCYSTIS PNEUMONIA

22. Infection with *Pneumocystis* produces patchy involvement throughout the lungs, which causes affected alveoli to thicken, become edematous, and fill with foamy, protein-rich fluid. Gas exchange is severely impaired as the disease progresses.
23. Manifestations include abrupt onset with fever, tachypnea and shortness of breath, and a dry, nonproductive cough. Respiratory distress can be significant, with intercostal retractions and cyanosis.

ASPIRATION PNEUMONIA

24. Aspiration of gastric contents into the lungs results in a chemical and bacterial pneumonia known as aspiration pneumonia.
25. The low pH of gastric contents causes a severe inflammatory response when aspirated into the respiratory tract. Pulmonary edema and respiratory failure may result.
26. Complications include abscesses, bronchiectasis, and gangrene of pulmonary tissue.

SEVERE ACUTE RESPIRATORY SYNDROME

27. Severe acute respiratory syndrome (SARS) is a lower respiratory illness of unknown etiology. The infective agent is a coronavirus not previously identified in humans.
28. The virus spreads primarily by contact with respiratory secretions or by direct contact with an infected person or contaminated objects.
29. The primary pathophysiologic process is the development of a hyaline membrane that interferes with gas exchange within the alveoli.
30. Manifestations include high fever, chills, headache, malaise, muscle aches, nonproductive cough, shortness of breath, dyspnea, and hypoxemia.
31. Complications include acute respiratory failure or multiorgan dysfunction.

LUNG ABSCESS

32. A lung abscess is a localized area of lung destruction or necrosis and pus formation.
33. A lung abscess forms when a consolidated area becomes necrotic and fills with purulent material.

- ○ Nonproductive cough
- ○ Shortness of breath
- ○ Dyspnea
- ○ Hypoxemia

Lung Abscess
- • Manifestations
  - ○ Productive cough
  - ○ Chills and fever
  - ○ Pleuritic chest pain
  - ○ Malaise
  - ○ Anorexia
  - ○ Temperature elevation
  - ○ Foul-smelling, purulent, blood-streaked sputum

Tuberculosis (TB)
- • Manifestations
  - ○ Fatigue
  - ○ Weight loss
  - ○ Anorexia
  - ○ Low-grade afternoon fever
  - ○ Dry cough
    - – May become productive of purulent or bloody sputum
  - ○ Night sweats

Inhalation Anthrax
- • Manifestations
  - ○ Flulike
  - ○ Malaise
  - ○ Dry cough
  - ○ Fever
  - ○ Abrupt onset of severe dyspnea
  - ○ Stridor
  - ○ Cyanosis
  - ○ Enlargement of mediastinal and thoracic lymph nodes
  - ○ Septic shock and/or meningitis

Histoplasmosis
- • Manifestations
  - ○ Fever
  - ○ Dyspnea
  - ○ Cough
  - ○ Weight loss
  - ○ Ulcerations of the mouth and oropharynx
  - ○ Muscle wasting
  - ○ Hepatomegaly
  - ○ Splenomegaly

Blastomycosis
- • Manifestations
  - ○ Fever
  - ○ Dyspnea
  - ○ Pleuritic chest pain
  - ○ Cough

Aspergillosis
- • Manifestations
  - ○ Dyspnea

Rupture of this area leaves a cavity filled with air or fluid in a process known as cavitation.

34. Manifestations include productive cough, chills and fever, pleuritic chest pain, malaise, anorexia, and temperature elevation. When the abscess ruptures, the client may expectorate large amounts of foul-smelling, purulent, and blood-streaked sputum.

TUBERCULOSIS

35. Tuberculosis (TB) is a chronic, recurrent infectious disease that usually affects the lungs, although any organ can be affected. The causative agent is *Mycobacterium tuberculosis*.

36. TB is spread through droplet nuclei produced when an infected person coughs, sneezes, speaks, or sings.

37. As inhaled bacteria multiply, a granulomatous lesion called a tubercle is formed. When the infected tissue within the tubercle dies, a cheese-like center is formed. This process is called caseation necrosis.

38. If the immune response is adequate, scar tissue develops around the tubercle and walls off the bacilli. The client is infected, but does not develop tuberculosis disease.

39. If the immune response is inadequate, the disease tuberculosis can develop rapidly.

40. Reactivation tuberculosis can occur when the immune system is suppressed due to age, disease, or use of immunosuppressive drugs.

41. Manifestations of TB include fatigue, weight loss, anorexia, low-grade afternoon fever, dry cough, and night sweats. The cough often becomes productive of purulent and/or blood-tinged sputum.

INHALATION ANTHRAX

42. Inhalation anthrax is caused by the spore-forming rod *Bacillus anthracis* and is thought to be a potential biologic weapon of terrorism. Anthrax spores can be aerosolized so they remain suspended in the air, allowing them to be inhaled into the lungs. Person-to-person transmission of inhalation anthrax does not occur.

43. Manifestations are initially flulike, and include malaise, dry cough, and fever. As the infection progresses, there is an abrupt onset of severe dyspnea, stridor, and cyanosis. Lymph nodes in the mediastinum and thorax enlarge; septic shock and/or meningitis may develop. Death results from hemorrhagic thoracic lymphadenitis and hemorrhagic mediastinitis.

HISTOPLASMOSIS

44. Histoplasmosis is an infectious disease caused by *Histoplasma capsulatum* and is the most common fungal lung infection in the United States. The organism is found in the soil and is linked to exposure to bird dropping and bats.

- ○ Nonproductive cough
- ○ Pleuritic chest pain
- ○ Chills, and fever. Hemoptysis may occur if the organism invades a pulmonary blood vessel

Pleuritis
- • Manifestations
  - ○ Pain aggravated by deep breathing, coughing, and movement
  - ○ Rapid shallow respirations
  - ○ Limitation of chest wall movement on affected side
  - ○ Diminished breath sounds
  - ○ Pleural friction rub

Spontaneous Pneumothorax
- • Manifestations
  - ○ Pain
  - ○ Shortness of breath
  - ○ Increased heart rate
  - ○ Increased respiratory rate
  - ○ Asymmetrical chest wall movement
  - ○ Diminished or absent breath sounds

Traumatic Pneumothorax
- • Manifestations
  - ○ Similar to those of spontaneous pneumothorax
  - ○ May be overlooked if subtle
  - ○ May be masked by the primary injury

Tension Pneumothorax
- • Manifestations
  - ○ Like pneumothorax
  - ○ Presence of hypotension
  - ○ Distention of the neck veins
  - ○ Displacement of trachea to unaffected side
  - ○ Shock

Hemothorax
- • Manifestations
  - ○ Similar to pneumothorax or pleural effusion
  - ○ Risk of shock exists

Rib Fracture
- • Manifestations
  - ○ Pain on inspiration
  - ○ Coughing
  - ○ Diminished breath sounds with rapid and shallow respirations
  - ○ Bruising over the fracture
  - ○ Crepitus

Flail Chest
- • Manifestations
  - ○ Dyspnea
  - ○ Pain
  - ○ Paradoxic chest wall movement
  - ○ Diminished breath sounds
  - ○ Palpable crepitus

45. Histoplasmosis infections develop into latent asymptomatic disease or primary acute histoplasmosis. Chronic progressive disease is usually seen in older adults.
46. Disseminated histoplasmosis occurs in the immunocompromised host when macrophages remove the fungi, but are unable to destroy them. This form is often fatal.
47. Manifestations include fever, dyspnea, cough, weight loss, ulcerations of the mouth and oropharynx, muscle wasting, hepatomegaly, and splenomegaly.

COCCIDIOIDOMYCOSIS

48. Coccidioidomycosis is an infectious disease caused by the fungus *Coccidioides immitis* which grows in the soil of the arid Southwest, Mexico, and Central and South America.
49. The disease is usually acute and self-limited with manifestations that resemble influenza.
50. Disseminated disease can occur in immunocompromised clients. When it occurs, mortality is high.

BLASTOMYCOSIS

51. Blastomycosis is caused by the fungus *Blastomyces dermatitidis*. The disease occurs primarily in the south central and Midwestern regions of the United States and Canada.
52. The lungs are the primary site of infection, but it may spread to the skin, bones, GU system, and, rarely, to the central nervous system.
53. Manifestations include fever, dyspnea, pleuritic chest pain, and cough. If untreated the disseminated disease is slowly progressive and ultimately fatal.

ASPERGILLOSIS

54. Aspergillus spores are common, but rarely cause disease except in immunocompromised individuals. The spores invade the blood vessels and cause venous or arterial thrombosis. In the lungs, the infection can cause an acute, diffuse, self-limited pneumonitis.
55. Manifestations of pulmonary aspergillus are dyspnea, nonproductive cough, pleuritic chest pain, chills, and fever. Hemoptysis may occur if the organism invades a pulmonary blood vessel.

PLEURITIS

56. Pleuritis is inflammation of the pleura and produces a characteristic unilateral, well-localized, sharp, or stabbing pain.
57. Pleural inflammation usually occurs secondarily to another process, such as a viral respiratory illness, pneumonia, or rib injury.
58. Manifestations of pleurisy are pain aggravated by deep breathing, coughing, and movement. Respirations are rapid and shallow and chest wall movement may be limited on the affected side. Breath sounds are diminished and a pleural friction rub may be audible over the site.

Pulmonary Contusion
- Manifestations (may not occur until 12–24 hours after injury)
  ○ Shortness of breath
  ○ Restlessness
  ○ Apprehension
  ○ Chest pain
  ○ Copious sputum
  ○ Tachycardia
  ○ Tachypnea
  ○ Dyspnea
  ○ Cyanosis

Smoke Inhalation
- Manifestations of carbon monoxide poisoning
  ○ Headache
  ○ Dizziness
  ○ Dyspnea
  ○ Nausea
  ○ Characteristic "cherry-red" color to the skin
  ○ Confusion
  ○ Visual disturbances
  ○ Irritability
  ○ Hallucinations
  ○ Hypotension
  ○ Seizures
  ○ Coma

Lung Cancer
- Manifestations
  ○ Chronic cough
  ○ Hemoptysis
  ○ Wheezing, shortness of breath
  ○ Dull, aching chest pain or pleuritic pain
  ○ Hoarseness and/or dysphagia
  ○ Weight loss, anorexia
  ○ Fatigue, weakness
  ○ Bone pain
  ○ Clubbing of the fingers and toes
  ○ Endocrine, neuromuscular, cardiovascular, hematologic symptoms

PLEURAL EFFUSION

59. Pleural effusion is the collection of excess fluid in the pleural space that results from either systemic or local disease.
60. Systemic disorders that may lead to pleural effusion include heart failure, liver or renal disease, and connective tissue disorders.
61. Local diseases that may cause pleural effusion are pneumonia, atelectasis, tuberculosis, lung cancer, and trauma.
62. The pleural fluid may be transudate or exudate.
63. Transudate is formed when capillary pressure is high or plasma proteins are low.
64. Exudate is the result of increased capillary permeability.
65. Empyema is pus in the pleural cavity.
66. Hemothorax is the presence of blood in the cavity; hemorrhagic pleural effusion is a mixture of blood and pleural fluid.
67. Chylothorax is a collection of lymph in the pleural space and may result from thoracic surgery or placement of a central line.
68. Manifestations include dyspnea, pain, diminished breath sounds, and a dull percussion tone over the affected area.

PNEUMOTHORAX

69. Pneumothorax is accumulation of air in the pleural space and can occur spontaneously, as a result of blunt or penetrating trauma, or from an iatrogenic cause.
70. Pressure gradients in the thoracic space are vital to the process of breathing. When the visceral or parietal pleura is breached, air enters the pleural space, and equalizes the normal pressure gradient. Lung expansion is impaired and the lung tissue collapses.

SPONTANEOUS PNEUMOTHORAX

71. Spontaneous pneumothorax develops when an air-filled bleb, or blister, on the lung surface ruptures, allowing air from the airways to enter the pleural space. Spontaneous pneumothorax is classified as primary (simple) or secondary (complicated).
72. Manifestations of spontaneous pneumothorax depend upon the size and extent of the lung collapse. Typical manifestations include pain, shortness of breath, increased heart rate, increased respiratory rate, asymmetrical chest wall movement, and diminished or absent breath sounds on the affected side.

TRAUMATIC PNEUMOTHORAX

73. Blunt or penetrating trauma of the chest wall and pleura can cause pneumothorax.
74. Open pneumothorax (sucking chest wound) results from penetrating chest trauma such as a stab wound, gunshot wound, or impalement injury. Air moves freely between the pleural space and the atmosphere

through the wound, which results in rapid lung collapse and significant hypoventilation.

75. Iatrogenic pneumothorax may result from puncture or laceration of the visceral pleura during central-line placement, thoracentesis, or lung biopsy. Overdistention and rupture of the alveoli can occur secondary to anesthesia, resuscitation procedures, or mechanical ventilation.

76. Manifestations of traumatic pneumothorax are similar to those of spontaneous pneumothorax, but may be overlooked if subtle or may be masked by the primary injury.

TENSION PNEUMOTHORAX

77. Tension pneumothorax develops when injury to the chest wall or lungs allows air to enter the pleural space but prevents it from escaping. Pressures rise rapidly with each breath. The lung on the affected side collapses and pressure on the mediastinum shifts thoracic organs to the unaffected side. Ventilation is severely compromised and venous return to the heart is impaired.

78. Manifestations include those of pneumothorax, presence of hypotension, distention of the neck veins, and displacement of the trachea to the unaffected side. Shock may be present.

HEMOTHORAX

79. Hemothorax is a collection of blood in the pleural space and usually occurs as a result of chest trauma, surgery, or diagnostic procedures.

80. Manifestations are similar to pneumothorax or pleural effusion. With significant hemorrhage, a risk of shock exists.

TRAUMA OF THE CHEST OR LUNG

81. Chest injury is the leading cause of death from trauma.
82. These injuries may be minor with little effect on respiratory status or may be severe and fatal.
83. Rapid and continuous assessment of the airway, breathing, and circulation is vital in chest or lung injuries.
84. Acceleration-deceleration injury and direct mechanisms of injury are the most common causes of thoracic injury.

RIB FRACTURE

85. Rib fractures are generally well-tolerated and heal rapidly in young, previously healthy individuals.
86. Clients with preexisting lung disease may develop pneumonia, atelectasis, or respiratory failure secondary to a rib fracture.
87. Manifestations are pain on inspiration, coughing, diminished breath sounds with rapid and shallow respirations, bruising over the fracture, and crepitus.

FLAIL CHEST

88. Flail chest results from multiple rib fractures (two or more consecutive ribs fractured in multiple places)

that impair chest wall stability and normal chest wall function.

89. Physiologic function of the chest wall is impaired. The flail segment is sucked inward during inhalation and moves outward during exhalation. This is known as paradoxic movement.

90. Flail chest can significantly affect ventilation and gas exchange.

91. Manifestations are dyspnea, pain, paradoxic chest wall movement, diminished breath sounds, and palpable crepitus.

PULMONARY CONTUSION

92. Pulmonary contusion frequently occurs with blunt chest trauma. It may occur unilaterally or bilaterally.

93. In pulmonary contusion, alveoli and pulmonary arterioles rupture, causing intra-alveolar hemorrhage and interstitial and bronchial edema.

94. Inflammation and edema impair the production of surfactant within the alveoli, which decreases compliance and results in airway obstruction, atelectasis, and impaired gas diffusion.

95. Manifestations include shortness of breath, restlessness, apprehension, chest pain, copious sputum, tachycardia, tachypnea, dyspnea, and cyanosis. These manifestations may not be apparent until 12–24 hours after injury.

96. Even with appropriate treatment, pulmonary contusion can lead to acute respiratory distress and death.

SMOKE INHALATION

97. Pulmonary injury due to inhalation of hot air, toxic gases, or particulate matter is the leading cause of death in burn injury.

98. The three mechanisms of injury in smoke inhalation are thermal damage to the airways, which leads to impaired ventilation; carbon monoxide or cyanide poisoning, which results in tissue hypoxia; and chemical damage to the lung from noxious gases, which can impair gas exchange.

99. Manifestations of carbon monoxide poisoning include headache, dizziness, dyspnea, nausea, and a characteristic "cherry-red" color to the skin. As levels increase, confusion, visual disturbances, irritability, hallucinations, hypotension, seizures, and coma develop. Permanent neurologic deficit can occur in survivors.

100. Inhalation of toxic chemicals causes bronchospasm and edema of the airways and alveoli. Acute respiratory distress syndrome may develop in 1–2 days.

101. Pneumonia is common following smoke inhalation.

NEAR-DROWNING

102. Asphyxiation and aspiration are the primary problems associated with drowning and near-drowning.

103. Dry drowning occurs when victims do not aspirate water, but a laryngeal spasm causes asphyxia.

104. Loss of consciousness can occur with 3–5 minutes of total immersion. Circulatory impairment, brain injury, and brain death can occur within 5–10 minutes.

105. Survival may be prolonged if the victim is immersed in very cold water. The associated dive reflex slows the heartbeat, constricts peripheral vessels, and shunts blood to the brain and heart.

106. Water aspiration can cause delayed death from near-drowning.

107. Aspiration of fresh water leads to hypervolemia and hemodilution. The resultant electrolyte imbalances can result in cardiac dysrhythmias and death. Hemolysis can lead to tubular necrosis and acute renal failure. Fresh water also impairs pulmonary surfactant and damages the alveolar-capillary membrane, which leads to respiratory failure.

108. Salt water aspiration results in hypovolemia and hemoconcentration. Hemolysis is insignificant and the small elevations in serum sodium and chloride levels rarely cause life-threatening effects.

109. With either type of near-drowning, inhalation of microorganisms and debris can lead to pneumonia.

LUNG CANCER

110. Lung cancer develops as damaged bronchial epithelial cells mutate over time to become neoplastic.

111. The vast majority of primary lung lesions are bronchogenic carcinoma, which are tumors of the airway epithelium. These tumors are further differentiated by cell type: small-cell carcinoma and non-small cell carcinomas (adenocarcinoma, squamous cell carcinoma, and large-cell carcinoma.)

112. Small-cell carcinomas grow rapidly and spread early. They have paraneoplastic properties and produce manifestations at sites that are not directly affected by the tumor.

113. Adenocarcinoma produces early metastasis to the central nervous system, skeleton, and adrenal glands.

114. Squamous cell carcinoma spreads by local invasion.

115. Large cell carcinoma produces early metastasis.

116. Clients with lung cancer may present with symptoms related to the primary tumor, manifestations of metastatic disease, or with systemic symptoms. Chronic cough, hemoptysis, wheezing and shortness of breath are common respiratory symptoms. There may be a dull, aching chest pain or pleuritic pain. Hoarseness and/or dysphagia indicates pressure on the trachea or esophagus. Other systemic manifestations include weight loss, anorexia, fatigue, weakness, bone pain, clubbing of the fingers and toes and various endocrine, neuromuscular, cardiovascular, and hematologic symptoms.

117. Complications include: superior vena cava syndrome, SIADH, Cushing's syndrome, venous thrombosis, pulmonary embolism, and thrombotic endocarditis.

SUGGESTIONS FOR CLASSROOM ACTIVITIES

- Use anatomical models to review the anatomy of the lower respiratory tract. Using these models explain how the development of pathology in these areas impairs gas exchange.
- Demonstrate airflow through various sizes of common tubules, such as soda straws, coffee stirrers, oxygen tubing, or corrugated oxygen delivery tubes. Consider having students inhale through a soda straw or coffee stirrer to experience the difference in airflow. Relate the pathophysiology of impairment of airway size to that experience.
- Have students group commonly occurring disorders of the lower respiratory system into disorders of air delivery to the aveoli, gas exchange in the alveoli, or both.

SUGGESTIONS FOR CLINICAL ACTIVITIES

- Assign students to the care of clinical clients with lower respiratory disorders. Have students assess for manifestations of those disorders. Have students discuss the experience of air hunger with appropriate clients.

LEARNING OUTCOME 2

Compare and contrast the etiology, risk factors, and vulnerable populations for lower respiratory infections, lung cancer, chest wall disorders, and trauma.

CONCEPTS FOR LECTURE
ACUTE BRONCHITIS

1. Acute bronchitis is relatively common in adults. Impaired immune defenses and cigarette smoking increase the risk for development of bronchitis.
2. Acute bronchitis may follow a viral upper respiratory infection.
3. Chronic bronchitis is a component of chronic obstructive pulmonary disease.

PNEUMONIA

4. Pneumonia remains the seventh leading cause of death in the United States and the leading cause of death from infectious disease.

LEGIONNAIRE'S DISEASE

5. Smokers, older adults, and people with chronic disease or impaired immune systems are most susceptible to Legionnaire's disease.

PRIMARY ATYPICAL PNEUMONIA

6. Young adults—college students and military recruits in particular—are the primary affected population. Primary atypical pneumonia is highly contagious and often has mild manifestations. It is often called "walking pneumonia."

VIRAL PNEUMONIA

7. Viral pneumonia is typically a mild disease that often affects older adults and people with chronic conditions. It usually occurs in community epidemics.

POWERPOINT LECTURE SLIDES

Acute Bronchitis
- Relatively common in adults
- Risk factors
  - Impaired immune defenses
  - Cigarette smoking
- Acute bronchitis
  - Follow a viral URI
- Chronic bronchitis
  - Component of COPD

Lung Abscess
- Most common etiology: aspiration, resultant pneumonia
- At-risk population
  - Decreased level of consciousness
    - Anesthesia
    - Injury
    - Disease of the central nervous system
    - Seizure
    - Excessive sedation
    - Alcohol abuse
    - Swallowing disorders
    - Dental caries
    - Debilitation

Tuberculosis
- United States
  - The incidence fell until the mid-1980s
  - Resurgence late 1980s and early 1990s
  - Incidence is now declining
- Worldwide
  - Continues to be a significant health problem
  - Accounts for an estimated 2 million deaths each year

PNEUMOCYSTIS PNEUMONIA

8. People with acquired immune deficiency syndrome (AIDS) and others with significant immunocompromise are at risk for developing an opportunistic pneumonia caused by *Pneumocystis*, which is a common parasite found worldwide.

ASPIRATION PNEUMONIA

9. Risk factors for aspiration pneumonia include emergency surgery or obstetric procedures, depressed cough and gag reflexes, impaired swallowing, enteral nutrition, and silent regurgitation.

SEVERE ACUTE RESPIRATORY SYNDROME

10. The majority of cases of severe acute respiratory syndrome have been reported in China in previously healthy adults aged 25 to 70 years. The etiology is unknown.

LUNG ABSCESS

11. The most common etiology of lung abscess is aspiration and resulting pneumonia.
12. At-risk clients include those with decreased level of consciousness due to anesthesia, injury, or disease of the central nervous system, seizure, excessive sedation, or alcohol abuse; swallowing disorders; dental caries; and debilitation secondary to cancer or chronic disease.

TUBERCULOSIS

13. The incidence of tuberculosis fell steadily in the United States until the mid-1980s. A resurgence of the disease occurred in the late 1980s and early 1990s. The incidence is now declining.
14. Worldwide, TB continues to be a significant health problem. TB accounts for an estimated 2 million deaths each year.
15. Risk for development of TB includes impaired immune function and prolonged contact with infected persons.

FUNGAL LUNG DISEASES

16. Many fungal lung diseases have a geographic distribution pattern. The spores that cause fungal lung disease are present in the air that everyone breathes. Normal respiratory and immune defenses prevent infection in most people. If infection occurs, it is generally mild and self-limiting. Absence of an adequate immune system places a person at risk for development of these illnesses.

SPONTANEOUS PNEUMOTHORAX

17. Primary pneumothorax is of unknown etiology and affects previously healthy people, usually tall, slender men.

- Risk
  - Impaired immune function
  - Prolonged contact with infected persons

Spontaneous Pneumothorax
- Unknown etiology
- Population
  - Previously healthy people
  - Usually tall, slender men
- Risk factors primary pneumothorax
  - Smoking
  - Familial factors
  - High altitude flying
  - Rapid decompression
- Risk factors secondary pneumothorax
  - Overdistention and rupture of an alveolus
    - COPD
    - Asthma
    - Cystic fibrosis
    - Pulmonary fibrosis
    - TB
    - ARDs

Smoke Inhalation
- Suspect conditions
  - Burn occurs in an enclosed space
  - Burns to the face or upper torso
  - Singed nasal hairs
  - Sputum contains ash-like material
  - Dyspnea, wheezing, rales, or rhonchi
- Carbon monoxide poisoning suspected
  - Burn occurred in a closed space
  - Evidence of inhalation injury
  - Dyspnea develops

Near-drowning
- Leading preventable cause of accidental deaths in US
- Alcohol ingestion major risk factor

Lung Cancer
- Leading cause of cancer deaths in US
- Population
  - Age over 50
  - Exposure to tobacco smoke
  - Exposure to ionizing radiation and inhaled irritants
  - Exposure to radon

18. Risk factors for primary pneumothorax are smoking and familial factors.
19. High altitude flying and rapid decompression during scuba diving may also increase risk of spontaneous pneumothorax.
20. Secondary pneumothorax is generally caused by overdistention and rupture of an alveolus. This disorder develops in clients with underlying lung disease such as COPD, asthma, cystic fibrosis, pulmonary fibrosis, TB, and ARDS. This type of pneumothorax is more serious and is potentially life-threatening.

SMOKE INHALATION

21. Smoke inhalation is suspected whenever a burn occurs in an enclosed space; if there are burns to the face or upper torso or singed nasal hairs; if sputum contains ash-like material; and when manifestations such as dyspnea, wheezing, rales, or rhonchi develop.
22. Carbon monoxide poisoning is suspected if the burn occurred in a closed space, if there is evidence of inhalation injury, or if dyspnea develops.

NEAR-DROWNING

23. Drowning is the leading preventable cause of accidental deaths in the United States.
24. Alcohol ingestion is a factor in about 25% of adult drowning deaths.

LUNG CANCER

25. Lung cancer is the leading cause of cancer deaths in all racial groups in the United States. Most people with lung cancer die within 1 year of the initial diagnosis.
26. The incidence of lung cancer increases with age over 50, exposure to tobacco smoke, exposure to ionizing radiation and inhaled irritants, and exposure to radon.
27. Tobacco use and exposure to cigarette smoke are the leading risk factors for lung cancer.

SUGGESTIONS FOR CLASSROOM ACTIVITIES

• Have students create a chart listing common respiratory disorders covered. Include in the chart an area for etiology of the disorder, risk factors for the development of the disorder, and the vulnerable populations. Help students draw conclusions about similarities in risk behavior and vulnerability.

SUGGESTIONS FOR CLINICAL ACTIVITIES

• Have students identify clinical clients who may be at risk for the development of ventilation disorder. Discuss the care necessary for these clients.

LEARNING OUTCOME 3

Describe interdisciplinary care and the nursing role in health promotion and caring for clients with lower respiratory infections, lung cancer, chest wall disorders, and trauma.

CONCEPTS FOR LECTURE

ACUTE BRONCHITIS

1. Treatment of acute bronchitis is symptomatic and includes rest, increased fluid intake, and use of ASA or acetaminophen to relieve fever and malaise. A broad-spectrum antibiotic may be prescribed, along with expectorant cough medication during the day and a cough suppressant at night.
2. Nursing interventions are primarily educational.

PNEUMONIA

3. Prevention is a key management strategy.
4. Pneumococcal vaccine is recommended for people over age 65 and those with chronic cardiac or respiratory conditions, diabetes mellitus, alcoholism, or other chronic diseases, and immunocompromised people. Influenza vaccine is also recommended for these high-risk populations.
5. Medications used to treat pneumonia may include antibiotics, bronchodilators, and agents to liquefy mucus.
6. Oxygen therapy and chest physiotherapy are used to treat pneumonia.
7. Nursing diagnoses include: Ineffective Airway Clearance; Ineffective Breathing Pattern; and Activity Intolerance.

SEVERE ACUTE RESPIRATORY SYNDROME

8. Prompt identifications of SARS, infection control measures, and reporting of the disease are vital to control this potentially fatal disease.
9. Healthcare workers are at risk for developing SARS after caring for infected clients. Infection control precautions should be immediately instituted when SARS is suspected.
10. Treatment is supportive and may include intubation and mechanical ventilation if respiratory failure or ARDS develops.
11. Nursing diagnoses include: Impaired Gas Exchange and Risk for Infection.

LUNG ABSCESS

12. Lung abscess is treated with antibiotic therapy, postural drainage, bronchoscopy for drainage of abscess, and placement of chest tube.
13. Nursing diagnoses include: Risk for Ineffective Airway Clearance; Impaired Gas Exchange; Hyperthermia; and Anxiety.

POWERPOINT LECTURE SLIDES

Acute Bronchitis
- Treatment
  ○ Symptomatic
  ○ Rest
  ○ Increased fluid intake
- Medications
  ○ ASA or acetaminophen
  ○ Broad-spectrum antibiotic
  ○ Expectorant cough medication
  ○ Cough suppressant
- Nursing interventions
  ○ Teaching

Pneumonia
- Interdisciplinary care
  ○ Prevention
  ○ Pneumococcal vaccine
  ○ Influenza vaccine
- Medications
  ○ Antibiotics
  ○ Bronchodilators
  ○ Agents to liquefy mucus
- Treatments
  ○ Oxygen therapy
  ○ Chest physiotherapy
- Nursing diagnoses
  ○ Ineffective Airway Clearance
  ○ Ineffective Breathing Pattern
  ○ Activity Intolerance

Severe Acute Respiratory Syndrome
- Interdisciplinary care
  ○ Prompt identifications of SARS
  ○ Infection control measures
    – Healthcare workers are at risk
    – IC measures immediately when suspected
  ○ Reporting of the disease
- Treatment
  ○ Supportive
  ○ Intubation and mechanical ventilation
- Nursing diagnoses
  ○ Impaired Gas Exchange
  ○ Risk for Infection

Fungal Lung Diseases
- Diagnosis
  ○ Microscopic examination of sputum specimen
- Treatment
  ○ Oral antifungal agents
  ○ Lobectomy
- Nursing care focus
  ○ Preventative education
  ○ Maintaining good general health

TUBERCULOSIS

14. Interdisciplinary care of TB includes early detection, accurate diagnosis, effective disease treatment, and preventing spread to others.
15. The tuberculin test is used to screen for tuberculosis infection. Methods of tuberculin testing include intradermal PPD (Mantoux) test and multiple-puncture (tine) testing.
16. Goals of pharmacologic treatment are to make the disease noncommunicable to others, reduce symptoms of the disease; and to affect a cure in the shortest possible time.
17. Regular visits to a healthcare provider are necessary during TB treatment, both to monitor the client for adverse side effects and to ensure compliance with the long course of therapy.
18. Major nursing strategies to maintain public health and to prevent TB include education and TB screening.
19. Nursing diagnoses include: Deficient Knowledge; Ineffective Therapeutic Regimen Management; and Risk for Infection.

INHALATION ANTHRAX

20. Because death can quickly result from inhalational anthrax, people who are known or suspected to have been exposed are often treated prophylactically. Ciprofloxacin (Cipro) or doxycycline (Adoxa) is administered. An anthrax vaccine does exist, but it is considered experimental.

FUNGAL LUNG DISEASES

21. Diagnosis is achieved by microscopic examination of a sputum specimen for the fungus.
22. Treatment includes oral antifungal agents. Lobectomy may be required.
23. Nursing care focuses on preventive education, maintaining good general health, and provision of information regarding medication regimens.

PLEURITIS

24. Analgesics and NSAIDs may help to relieve the pain of pleurisy. Codeine may be ordered to relieve pain and to suppress associated cough.
25. Nursing care is directed toward promoting comfort by medication administration, positioning, and splinting the chest while coughing.

PLEURAL EFFUSION

26. Pleural effusion can typically be seen on x-ray. Thoracentesis aspiration of fluid for analysis may be performed if the cause of the effusion is not apparent.
27. If the pleural effusion is large and interferes with respiration, thoracentesis may be performed to remove

- ○ Provision of information regarding medication regimens

Pneumothorax
- • Treatment
  - ○ Depends on the severity of the problem
  - ○ Simple, small pneumothorax
    - – Monitoring for resolution
  - ○ A large pneumothorax
    - – Thoracostomy
    - – Placement of chest tubes
- • Tension pneumothorax
  - ○ Medical emergency
  - ○ Requires immediate intervention
- • Nursing diagnoses
  - ○ Impaired Gas Exchange
  - ○ Risk for Injury

Hemothorax
- • Treatment
  - ○ Thoracentesis or thoracostomy
  - ○ Autotransfusion
- • Priority nursing diagnoses
  - ○ Impaired gas exchange
  - ○ Ineffective breathing pattern
  - ○ Decreased cardiac output
  - ○ Risk for deficient fluid volume

Rib Fracture
- • Treatment
  - ○ Typically heal uneventfully
  - ○ Comfort measures
  - ○ Use of rib belts, binders, taping no longer recommended

Flail Chest
- • Treatment
  - ○ Intubation and mechanical ventilation
  - ○ Pain management
  - ○ Internal or external fixation of the flail segment may be necessary

Lung Cancer
- • Interdisciplinary care
  - ○ Teaching abstinence from tobacco use
  - ○ Staged by TNM
- • Treatments
  - ○ Surgery
    - – Remove all of involved tissue
    - – Preserving as much functional lung as possible
  - ○ Radiation therapy
    - – Cure
    - – Palliation
    - – Debulking
- • Nursing diagnoses
  - ○ Ineffective Breathing Pattern
  - ○ Activity Intolerance
  - ○ Pain
  - ○ Anticipatory Grieving

fluid to allow the lung to expand. Cardiovascular collapse and pneumothorax are possible complications of thoracentesis.

28. Interdisciplinary care focuses on supporting respirations and treating the underlying disease process.

29. Depending upon the etiology of the pleural effusion, repeated drainage, thoracotomy, or surgical excision of tissue may be necessary. In the case of recurrent pleural effusions, an irritant may be instilled into the pleural space to cause adhesion of the parietal and visceral pleura. This procedure is called pleurodesis.

30. Nursing care is directed at supporting respiratory function and assisting with procedures to evacuate collected fluid.

31. Nursing diagnoses may include: Impaired Gas Exchange and Activity Intolerance.

THORACIC INJURY

32. Interdisciplinary care of clients with thoracic injuries is focused on pain control, promoting adequate ventilation, and alveolar gas exchange.

33. Health promotion includes use of safety devices in motor vehicles and appropriate protective equipment and gear for people who engage in potentially hazardous activities.

34. Nursing diagnoses include: Acute Pain, Ineffective Airway Clearance; and Impaired Gas Exchange.

PNEUMOTHORAX

35. Treatment for pneumothorax depends on the severity of the problem. Simple, small pneumothorax may only require monitoring for resolution. A large pneumothorax with significant symptomology requires treatment with a thoracostomy, or placement of chest tubes.

36. Tension pneumothorax is a medical emergency and requires immediate intervention.

37. Health promotion activities to prevent spontaneous and traumatic pneumothorax primarily involve health teaching.

38. Nursing diagnoses include: Impaired Gas Exchange and Risk for Injury.

HEMOTHORAX

39. Thoracentesis or thoracostomy with chest tube drainage is used to remove blood from the pleural space.

40. If hemorrhage is significant, the blood may be collected for subsequent autotransfusion.

41. Priority nursing diagnoses include: Impaired Gas Exchange; Ineffective Breathing Pattern; Decreased Cardiac Output; and Risk for Deficient Fluid Volume.

RIB FRACTURE

42. Simple rib fractures typically heal uneventfully. Measures to promote comfort will also promote breathing, coughing, and moving.

43. Use of rib belts, binders, and taping to stabilize the rib cage is no longer recommended.

FLAIL CHEST

44. The preferred treatment for flail chest is intubation and mechanical ventilation. Pain management may require intercostal nerve blocks or continuous epidural analgesia. In some cases, internal or external fixation of the flail segment may be necessary.

PULMONARY CONTUSION

45. Clients with pulmonary contusion are often critically ill and require intensive care management. Treatment is supportive, directed at maintaining adequate ventilation and alveolar gas exchange.

INHALATION INJURY

46. Inhalation injuries include injury from smoke inhalation and from drowning.
47. Nursing diagnoses include: Ineffective Airway Clearance; Impaired Gas Exchange; and Ineffective Tissue Perfusion: Cerebral.

SMOKE INHALATION

48. Prevention is the most effective treatment of smoke inhalation. Nurses should encourage the use of working smoke detectors in all homes.
49. Intubation may be necessary to establish an airway. Oxygen should be administered as soon as possible. External cardiac defibrillation may be necessary to reestablish an effective cardiac rhythm.
50. Treatment of inhalation injury is generally supportive. Hyperbaric oxygen therapy may be used to treat carbon monoxide poisoning.
51. Other treatment measures for inhalation injury may include bronchodilator therapy; encouraging coughing; and providing suctioning, chest physiotherapy with percussion, and postural drainage.

NEAR-DROWNING

52. Learning to swim safely is important to prevent drowning.
53. Intubation may be necessary to establish an airway. Oxygen should be administered as soon as possible. External cardiac defibrillation may be necessary to reestablish an effective cardiac rhythm.
54. The basic rule in cold water near-drowning is that the client is not declared dead until the body has been rewarmed and life signs remain absent.
55. With near-drowning victims, measures such as inducing hypothermia or barbiturate-induced coma and administering corticosteroids and osmotic diuretics may be employed to help prevent neurologic damage.

LUNG CANCER

56. Prevention by abstinence from tobacco use is the primary goal of healthcare providers.
57. Lung cancer is staged by tumor size, location, degree of invasion of the primary tumor, and the presence of metastatic disease.
58. Surgery offers the only real chance for a cure in non-small-cell lung cancer. The type of surgery performed depends on the location and size of the tumor, as well as the client's pulmonary and general health. The goal of surgery is to remove all of the involved tissue while preserving as much functional lung as possible.
59. The treatment goal of radiation therapy may be either cure or palliation. Radiation may be used to "debulk" tumors prior to surgery. Radiation therapy may be delivered by external beam, by intraluminal radiation, or brachytherapy.
60. Nursing diagnoses include: Ineffective Breathing Pattern; Activity Intolerance, Pain, and Anticipatory Grieving.

SUGGESTIONS FOR CLASSROOM ACTIVITIES

- Divide the class into small groups and assign each group one of the major categories of disorders discussed in this chapter. Have each group work through the nursing process as it would be associated with that disease process. Share the work in a compare and contrast format.

SUGGESTIONS FOR CLINICAL ACTIVITIES

- Assign clinical students to the care of clients who have one of the disorders covered in the chapter. Have the students develop a plan of care for that client.
- In post-conference, have students compare lists of nursing diagnoses chosen for this clinical client. Compare and contrast the interventions appropriate to the nursing diagnoses, because they vary from client to client.

LEARNING OUTCOME 4

Discuss surgery and other invasive procedures used to treat lung cancer, chest wall disorders, and trauma, and nursing responsibilities in caring for clients undergoing these procedures.

CONCEPTS FOR LECTURE
THORACENTESIS

1. Preprocedure care includes verification of signed informed consent; assessing knowledge and understanding of the procedure and its purpose; medication administration as required; positioning the client leaning over an anchored overbed table; and teaching about the level of discomfort to expect.
2. Procedure care includes monitoring pulse, color, oxygen saturation; applying a dressing; positioning the client on the unaffected side; and sending specimens to the laboratory.
3. Postprocedure care includes monitoring vital signs; oxygen saturations; and respiratory status.

CHEST TUBES

4. Preprocedure care includes verification of signed informed consent; providing information about the

POWERPOINT LECTURE SLIDES

Thoracentesis
- Preprocedure care
  - Verification of signed informed consent
  - Assessing knowledge and understanding of the procedure and its purpose
  - Medication administration as required
  - Positioning the client leaning over an anchored overbed table
  - Teaching about the level of discomfort to expect
- Procedure care
  - Monitoring pulse, color, oxygen saturation
  - Applying a dressing
  - Positioning the client on the unaffected side
  - Sending specimens to the laboratory
- Postprocedure care
  - Monitoring vital signs
  - Oxygen saturations
  - Respiratory status

procedure; positioning the client; and assisting with the procedure as necessary.

5. Postprocedure care includes assessment of respiratory status; maintaining the closed chest tube drainage apparatus; and assisting with position changes. After the chest tube is removed, a sterile occlusive petroleum jelly dressing should be applied.

LUNG SURGERY

6. Preprocedure care includes routine preoperative care; taking a history; providing emotional support; instructing about postoperative procedures; and establishing a means of communication if necessary for postop care.

7. Postprocedure care includes provision of routine postoperative care; assessing for pain control; frequent assessment of respiratory status; assisting with effective coughing technique; monitoring and maintaining effective mechanical ventilation; maintaining patent chest tubes and drainage system; assessing for development of infection; assisting with early ambulation; and maintaining nutritional status.

Chest Tubes
- Preprocedure care
  - Verification of signed informed consent
  - Providing information about the procedure
  - Positioning the client
  - Assisting with the procedure as necessary
- Postprocedure care
  - Assessment of respiratory status
  - Maintaining the closed chest tube drainage apparatus
  - Assisting with position changes
  - Sterile occlusive petroleum jelly dressing post chest-tube removal

Lung Surgery
- Preprocedure care
  - Routine preoperative care
  - Taking a history
  - Providing emotional support
  - Instructing about postoperative procedures
  - Establishing a means of communication if necessary for postop care
- Postprocedure care
  - Provision of routine postoperative care
  - Assessing for pain control
  - Frequent assessment of respiratory status
  - Assist with effective coughing technique
  - Monitoring and maintaining effective mechanical ventilation
  - Maintaining patent chest tubes and drainage system
  - Assessing for development of infection
  - Assisting with early ambulation
  - Maintaining nutritional status

SUGGESTIONS FOR CLASSROOM ACTIVITIES

- Divide the students into three groups. Assign one group the preoperative care of a case study client. Assign the second group the interoperative care of the same case study client. Assign the third group the postoperative care of the same case study client. Have the students identify nursing interventions that are appropriate for each phase of the perioperative experience. Share the findings, and emphasize the collaboration necessary among the three levels of care.

SUGGESTIONS FOR CLINICAL ACTIVITIES

- Ask an RN with trauma training to come to post-conference to discuss emergency nursing treatment of the client with chest wall trauma.
- Review the clinical facility policy and procedure manual associated with thoracentesis and chest tube insertion. Have students identify assessment findings that would indicate development of an emergency situation. Discuss nursing interventions necessary in those events.
- Assign clinical students to the care of a client who has experienced thoracic surgery or chest tube placement.

LEARNING OUTCOME 5

Describe the nursing implications for oxygen therapy and medications used to treat respiratory disorders.

CONCEPTS FOR LECTURE

PNEUMONIA

1. Typically a broad-spectrum antibiotic such as a macrolide, a penicillin, or a second- or third-generation cephalosporin, or a fluoroquinolone is ordered until the results of sputum culture and sensitivity tests are available.
2. Bronchodilators may be ordered to improve ventilation and reduce hypoxia. Two major groups of bronchodilators are the sympathomimetic drugs or the methylxanthines.
3. An agent to "break up" mucus or to reduce its viscosity may be prescribed. Acetylcysteine (Airbron), potassium iodide (Pima), and guaifenesin (Amonidrin) are commonly ordered.

SEVERE ACUTE RESPIRATORY SYNDROME

4. No medications have been proven to be effective in controlling SARS. Antibiotic and/or antiviral therapy may be administered if the diagnosis is unclear.

TUBERCULOSIS

5. Single-drug therapy is effective for prophylactic treatment for those who have a recent skin test conversion to positive. For adults, isoniazid (INH) is the drug of choice.
6. Bacillus Calmette-Guerin (BCG) vaccination may be prescribed for some specialized populations if isoniazid (INH) therapy is contraindicated. It is not widely used in the United States.
7. Two or more drugs are used if active disease is suspected. Currently four drugs, isoniazid (INH), rifampin (Rifadin), pyrazinamide (PZA), and ethambutol (Myambutol) are typically prescribed for newly-diagnosed TB. Drug therapy continues for 4–9 months.
8. If a drug-resistant strain of TB is suspected, therapy is tailored to that resistance.

LUNG CANCER

9. Combination chemotherapy is the treatment of choice for small-cell lung cancer. Used in combination, chemotherapeutic drugs allow tumor cells to be attacked at different parts of the cell cycle and in different ways, which increases the effectiveness of therapy.

POWERPOINT LECTURE SLIDES

Pneumonia
- Broad-spectrum antibiotic
  - Macrolide
  - Penicillin
  - Second- or third-generation cephalosporin
  - Fluoroquinolone
- Bronchodilators
  - Sympathomimetic drugs
  - Methylxanthines
- An agent to "break up" mucus
  - Acetylcysteine
  - Potassium iodide
  - Guaifenesin

Severe Acute Respiratory Syndrome
- No medications have been proven to be effective in controlling SARS
- Antibiotic and/or antiviral therapy

Tuberculosis
- Single-drug therapy
  - Isoniazid (INH)
- Bacillus Calmette-Guerin (BCG) vaccination
  - Not widely used in the United States
- Two or more drugs therapy
  - Isoniazid
  - Rifampin
  - Pyrazinamide
  - Ethambutol
- If a drug resistance strain of TB
  - Therapy is tailored to that resistance

Lung Cancer
- Combination chemotherapy treatment of choice for small-cell lung cancer

SUGGESTIONS FOR CLASSROOM ACTIVITIES

- Have students identify medications that are commonly used for treatment of ventilation disorders. Have the students group the medications by class and identify major nursing implications in administration.

SUGGESTIONS FOR CLINICAL ACTIVITIES

- Have students review clinical client medication administration records for medications that are frequently administered for ventilatory problems. Have students write medication information sheets about those medications, including dosages, nursing implications, safety implications, and teaching implications.

CHAPTER 39
NURSING CARE OF CLIENTS WITH GAS EXCHANGE DISORDERS

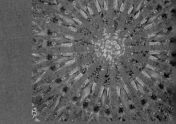

RESOURCE LIBRARY

 PRENTICE HALL NURSING MEDIALINK DVD-ROM

Audio Glossary
NCLEX-RN® Review
Animation/Video
   ARDS
   Asthma
   Metered-Dose Inhalers
   Using a Nebulizer

📖 **IMAGE LIBRARY**

Figure 39.1 The pathogenesis of an acute episode of asthma.

Figure 39.2 The pathogenesis of chronic obstructive pulmonary disease.

Figure 39.3 Typical appearance of a client with emphysema.

Figure 39.4 Ventilation-perfusion relationships.

Figure 39.5 Clubbing of fingers caused by chronic hypoxemia.

Figure 39.6 A thromboembolism lodged in a pulmonary vessel.

 COMPANION WEBSITE

Audio Glossary
NCLEX-RN® Review
Care Plan Activity: Acute Asthma Attack
Case Study: Acute Asthma Attack
Exercise: Compare and Contrast
MediaLink Application: Respiratory Disorders
Links to Resources

Figure 39.7 Causes and manifestations of respiratory failure.

Figure 39.8 Nasal endotracheal (nasotracheal) intubation.

Figure 39.9 *A,* Positive-pressure ventilator and *B,* the control panel used to set the mode, rate, limits, and percentage of oxygen delivered.

Figure 39.10 A T-piece, or "blow-by" unit, for weaning from mechanical ventilation.

Figure 39.11 The pathogenesis of ARDS.

LEARNING OUTCOME 1

Relate the pathophysiology and manifestations of obstructive, pulmonary vascular, and critical respiratory disorders to their effects on ventilation and respiration (gas exchange).

CONCEPTS FOR LECTURE
ASTHMA

1. Asthma is a chronic inflammatory disorder of the airways characterized by recurrent episodes of wheezing, breathlessness, chest tightness, and coughing.
2. Most asthma episodes are relatively brief; however, some clients with asthma may experience longer episodes with some degree of airway impairment daily.
3. Acute asthma may be fatal.
4. In asthma, the airways are in a persistent state of inflammation. Common triggers for an acute asthma attack include exposure to allergens, respiratory tract infection, exercise, inhaled irritants, and emotional upsets.
5. The acute or early response of asthma produces bronchoconstriction, edema, and mucus production.
6. The late phase response may occur 4 to 12 hours after exposure to a trigger and produces mucosal edema, impaired mucociliary clearance, and bronchoconstriction.

POWERPOINT LECTURE SLIDES

Asthma
- Chronic inflammatory disorder of the airways
- Generally brief, but acute asthma may be fatal
- Persistent inflammation of the airways
  - Triggers
    - Allergens
    - Respiratory tract infection
    - Exercise
    - Inhaled irritants
    - Emotional upsets
    - Secondhand smoke
    - Some medications
    - The acute or early response of asthma produces bronchoconstriction, edema, and mucus production.

Pathophysiology
- Inflammatory mediators are released
- Activation of inflammatory cells
- Bronchoconstriction

7. In an acute asthma attack, inflammatory mediators are released, followed by activation of inflammatory cells. These events lead to airway narrowing, which limits airflow and increases the work of breathing; trapped air mixes with inhaled air, which impairs gas exchange.

8. Manifestations include chest tightness, cough, dyspnea, and wheezing. Tachycardia, tachypnea, and prolonged expiration are common.

9. As the attack progresses, fatigue, anxiety, apprehension, and severe dyspnea may occur. As respiratory failure occurs, breath sounds may become inaudible with reduced wheezing and an ineffective cough. Without careful assessment, this apparent relief of symptoms may be misinterpreted as an improvement.

10. Status asthmaticus is severe, prolonged asthma that does not respond to routine treatment.

11. Clients with cough-variant asthma have persistent cough without wheezing or dyspnea. These clients have significant airway inflammation and demonstrate the pathophysiologic features of asthma.

CHRONIC OBSTRUCTIVE PULMONARY DISEASE

12. Clients with chronic airflow obstruction due to chronic bronchitis and/or emphysema are said to have chronic obstructive pulmonary disease (COPD).

13. COPD is characterized by slowly progressive obstruction of the airways.

14. COPD causes airways to narrow, resistance to airflow to increase, and expiration to become slow or difficult. This results in a mismatch between alveolar ventilation and perfusion and impaired gas exchange.

15. Chronic bronchitis is a disorder in which inhaled irritants cause a chronic inflammatory process. This chronic inflammation results in production of thick, tenacious mucus and narrowing of the airways. Recurrent infection is common due to inability to clear this mucus and inhaled pathogens.

16. Emphysema is characterized by destruction of the walls of the alveoli, with resulting enlargement of abnormal air spaces. This enlargement eventually results in airway collapse and the loss of alveolar surface area for gas exchange.

17. COPD is classified according to severity into stages from 0 to 4.

18. Manifestations of COPD include a morning cough, dyspnea with activity, and presence of a barrel-shaped chest.

19. Chronic bronchitis manifests as a cough productive of copious amounts of thick, tenacious sputum; cyanosis; and evidence of right-sided heart failure.

20. Emphysema has an insidious onset, but progresses to manifest severe dyspnea even at rest, barrel chest shape, tachypnea, use of accessory muscles to breathe, and prolongation of the expiratory phase of the respiratory cycle. Breath sounds are diminished and a hyperresonant percussive tone may be heard.

- Airway edema
- Impaired mucociliary clearance
- Work of breathing increases
- Trapping of air impairs gas exchange

Manifestations
- Chest tightness
- Cough, dyspnea, and wheezing
- Tachycardia, tachypnea, prolonged expiration
- Fatigue, anxiety, apprehension
- Respiratory failure
  - Breath sounds may "improve" right before failure

Status Asthmaticus
- Severe, prolonged asthma
- Does not respond to routine treatment

Cough-Variant Asthma
- Persistent cough without wheezing or dyspnea
- Significant airway inflammation

Cystic Fibrosis
- Autosomal recessive disorder
  - Lack of CFTR protein
  - Abnormal electrolyte transfer
- Affects epithelial cells
  - Respiratory
  - Gastrointestinal
  - Reproductive tracts
- Abnormal exocrine gland secretions

Pathophysiology
- Respiratory
  - Excess mucus production
  - Impaired ability to clear secretions
  - Progressive COPD
  - Pulmonary hypertension
  - Right ventricular hypertrophy
  - Cor pulmonale
- Gastrointestinal
  - Pancreatic enzyme deficiency
  - Impaired digestion
  - Elevation of sodium/chloride in sweat
- Reproductive/endocrine
  - Diabetes mellitus
  - Liver failure
  - Males usually sterile
  - Women have difficulty conceiving

Manifestations
- Respiratory
  - History of chronic lung disease
  - Recurrent pneumonia
  - Exercise intolerance
  - Chronic cough
  - Clubbing of fingers and toes
  - Barrel chest
  - Hyperresonant percussion tone
  - Basilar crackles

CYSTIC FIBROSIS

21. Cystic fibrosis (CF) is an autosomal recessive disorder that affects epithelial cells of the respiratory, gastrointestinal, and reproductive tracts and leads to abnormal exocrine gland secretions.
22. The genetic abnormality of CF leads to a lack of the CFTR protein, with resulting abnormal electrolyte transport across epithelial cell membranes.
23. Hallmarks of CF include: excess mucus production in the respiratory tract with impaired ability to clear secretions and progressive COPD; pancreatic enzyme deficiency and impaired digestion; and abnormal elevation of sodium and chloride concentrations in sweat.
24. Severe airway obstruction and chronic hypoxemia lead to pulmonary hypertension, right ventricular hypertrophy, and eventual cor pulmonale.
25. Pancreatic insufficiency and impaired enzyme secretion lead to impaired digestion and absorption of proteins, carbohydrates, and fats.
26. Respiratory manifestations of CF include history of chronic lung disease, recurrent pneumonia, exercise intolerance, chronic cough, clubbing of fingers and toes, barrel chesting, hyperresonant percussion tone, and basilar crackles. Right-sided heart failure may develop.
27. Gastrointestinal manifestations may include abdominal pain and steatorrhea.
28. Growth and development are often retarded, which results in small stature.

ATELECTASIS

29. Atelectasis is a state of partial or total lung collapse and is associated with many respiratory disorders.
30. Manifestations include diminished or absent breath sounds over the affected area, tachypnea, tachycardia, dyspnea, cyanosis, and fever.

BRONCHIECTASIS

31. Bronchiectasis is characterized by permanent abnormal dilation of one or more large bronchi and destruction of bronchial walls. Infection is often present.
32. Chronic cough productive of large amounts of mucopurulent sputum is characteristic. Other manifestations include hemoptysis, recurrent pneumonia, wheezing and shortness of breath, malnutrition, right-sided heart failure, and cor pulmonale.

OCCUPATIONAL LUNG DISEASE

33. Occupational lung diseases are directly related to inhalation of noxious substances in the work environment.
34. Two major classifications of occupational lung disease are pneumoconiosis, which is a chronic fibrotic lung disease caused by inhalation of inorganic dusts and particulate matter; and hypersensitivity pneumonitis, which is an allergic pulmonary disease caused by exposure to inhaled organic dusts.

- Gastrointestinal
  - Abdominal pain
  - Steatorrhea
- Endocrine
  - Small stature

Pulmonary Embolism (Thromboembolism)
- Obstruction of blood flow in part of pulmonary vascular system by embolus
- A medical emergency
  - Fifty percent of deaths occur within first 2 hours following embolization

Effects
- Large pulmonary artery occlusion
  - May cause sudden death
- Significant portion of smaller vessels
  - Lung tissue infarction
- Obstruction of small segment of pulmonary circulation
  - May cause no permanent injury

Manifestations
- Depend upon size and location
- Small emboli may be asymptomatic
- Common manifestations
  - Dyspnea
  - Pleuritic chest pain
  - Anxiety
  - Sense of impending doom
  - Cough
  - Diaphoresis
  - Hemoptysis

Manifestations of Fat Emboli
- Sudden onset dyspnea
- Tachypnea
- Tachycardia
- Confusion
- Delirium
- Decreased level of consciousness
- Petechiae

Acute Respiratory Failure
- Consequence of severe respiratory dysfunction
- Defined by arterial blood gas values
  - An arterial oxygen level of less than 50 to 60 mmHg
  - Arterial carbon dioxide level of greater than 50 mmHg
- In COPD
  - Acute drop in blood oxygen levels
  - Increased carbon dioxide levels
- Failure of oxygenation: hypoxemia without a rise in carbon dioxide levels
- Hypoventilation: hypoxemia with hypercapnia

Manifestations
- Dyspnea
- Restlessness, apprehension

35. Inhaled substances damage alveolar epithelium, which leads to an inflammatory process of the alveoli and interstitial tissue of the lung. This inflammation produces scarring of the lung tissue which causes the lung to become stiff and noncompliant. Lung volumes decrease, the work of breathing increases, and alveolar-capillary diffusion is impaired, which leads to hypoxemia.

36. Asbestosis is a diffuse interstitial fibrotic disease that involves the terminal airways, alveoli, and pleurae. Lung cancer and mesothelioma are associated with asbestos exposure.

37. Manifestations of asbestosis are exertional dyspnea, exercise intolerance, and inspiratory crackles. Respiratory failure and marked hypoxemia may develop.

38. Silicosis is a nodular pulmonary fibrosis that is caused by inhalation of silica dust.

39. Simple silicosis is asymptomatic. Complicated silicosis is characterized dyspnea and productive cough which progresses to severe disability, cor pulmonale, and death.

40. Coal worker's pneumoconiosis or "black lung disease" is caused by inhalation of coal dust which results in "coal macules" in lung tissue.

41. Coal worker's pneumoconiosis generally is asymptomatic, but may progress into massive fibrosis that destroys the pulmonary vascular bed and airways of the upper lungs.

42. Hypersensitivity pneumonitis is an allergic pulmonary disease that affects the airways and alveoli, and develops in workers exposed to organic dusts and gases.

43. In acute hypersensitivity pneumonitis, manifestations develop 4–8 hours after exposure and are heralded by sudden onset of malaise, chills and fever, dyspnea, cough, and nausea. The subacute syndrome is characterized by an insidious onset of chronic cough, progressive dyspnea, anorexia, and weight loss.

SARCOIDOSIS

44. Sarcoidosis is a chronic, multisystem disease characterized by an exaggerated cellular immune response in involved tissues. This response leads to granuloma formation in the lungs, lymph nodes, liver, eyes, skin, and other organs.

45. Manifestations vary according to the organ system affected.

PULMONARY VASCULAR DISORDERS

46. An effective match of alveolar ventilation and capillary perfusion is essential to maintain tissue oxygenation and function of all organ systems.

47. Many lower respiratory system disorders have a secondary effect on lung perfusion, because breakdown or fibrosis of alveolar walls destroys the capillary network as well.

- Impaired judgment
- Motor impairment
- Tachycardia
- Hypertension
- Cyanosis
- Dysrhythmias
- Hypotension
- Decreased cardiac output

Acute Respiratory Distress Syndrome
- Characterized by noncardiac pulmonary edema and refractory hypoxemia
- Mortality due to multiple organ system dysfunction

Pathophysiology
- Acute lung injury
- Unregulated systemic inflammatory response
- Tissue hypoxia
- Metabolic acidosis

Manifestations
- Develop 24–48 hours after the initial insult
- Dyspnea, tachypnea, and anxiety
- Progressive respiratory distress
- Cyanosis does not improve with oxygen administration

PULMONARY EMBOLISM

48. A pulmonary embolism (or thromboembolism) is obstruction of blood flow in part of the pulmonary vascular system by an embolus.

49. Pulmonary embolism is a medical emergency. Fifty percent of deaths from pulmonary embolism occur within the first two hours following embolization.

50. The impact of pulmonary embolism depends upon the extent to which pulmonary blood flow is obstructed, the size of the embolus, its nature, and secondary effects of the obstruction.

51. Occlusion of a large pulmonary artery may cause sudden death. Lung tissue infarction may occur from occlusion of a significant portion of smaller vessels. Obstruction of a small segment of pulmonary circulation may cause no permanent injury. Chronic or recurrent small emboli may be present in multiples.

52. Manifestations of pulmonary embolism depend upon its size and location. Small emboli may be asymptomatic. The most common symptoms are dyspnea and pleuritic chest pain. Anxiety, a sense of impending doom, cough, diaphoresis, and hemoptysis may occur. Large emboli may result in syncope and cyanosis.

53. Characteristic manifestations of fat emboli include sudden onset dyspnea, tachypnea, tachycardia, confusion, delirium, decreased level of consciousness, and petechiae.

PULMONARY HYPERTENSION

54. Pulmonary hypertension is abnormal elevation of the pulmonary arterial pressure. It can develop as a primary disorder, but usually occurs secondarily to another condition. Changes in the pulmonary artery lead to abnormal growth and remodeling of pulmonary vessels.

55. Once initiated, pulmonary hypertension is self-sustaining, because pulmonary vessels undergo changes that further narrow the pulmonary bed.

56. Manifestations are progressive dyspnea, fatigue, angina, and syncope with exertion. Primary pulmonary hypertension is a progressive disorder that generally causes a steady decline to death within 3–4 years.

57. Cor pulmonale is a condition of right ventricular hypertrophy and failure that results from long-standing pulmonary hypertension.

58. Manifestations of cor pulmonale include chronic productive cough, progressive dyspnea, wheezing, peripheral edema, distention of the neck veins, warm and moist skin, and a ruddy and cyanotic color.

ACUTE RESPIRATORY FAILURE

59. Respiratory failure is a consequence of severe respiratory dysfunction and can be defined by arterial blood gas values. An arterial oxygen level of less than 50 to 60 mmHg and an arterial carbon dioxide level of greater than 50 mmHg are generally accepted as indicators of respiratory failure.

60. In clients with COPD, respiratory failure is indicated by an acute drop in blood oxygen levels along with increased carbon dioxide levels.
61. Manifestations are dyspnea, restlessness, apprehension, impaired judgment, motor impairment, tachycardia, hypertension, cyanosis, dysrhythmias, hypotension, and decreased cardiac output.

ACUTE RESPIRATORY DISTRESS SYNDROME

62. Acute respiratory distress syndrome (ARDS) is characterized by noncardiac pulmonary edema and progressive refractory hypoxemia. Mortality associated with ARDS often is due to multiple organ system dysfunction related to ineffective tissue oxygenation.
63. The underlying pathophysiology of ARDS is acute lung injury that results from an unregulated systemic inflammatory response to acute injury or inflammation. Carbon dioxide exchange and oxygen exchange is impaired, which leads to combined respiratory and metabolic acidosis.
64. Manifestations of ARDS typically develop 24–48 hours after the initial insult. Early manifestations include dyspnea, tachypnea, and anxiety. Progressive respiratory distress develops. The cyanosis that develops does not improve with oxygen administration.

SUGGESTIONS FOR CLASSROOM ACTIVITIES

- Divide the students into small groups. Assign one of the major disorders covered in the chapter. Have the group identify the pathophysiology and manifestations of the disorder.
- Share the work, and emphasize commonalities and differences.
- View the animations about ARDS and asthma that are provided on the textbook DVD-ROM.

SUGGESTIONS FOR CLINICAL ACTIVITIES

- Assign clinical students to the care of a client with one of the disorders discussed in this chapter. Have the students identify the assessment findings that are expected with the disorder and contrast those findings to those manifested in the client.

LEARNING OUTCOME 2

Compare and contrast the etiology, risk factors, and vulnerable populations for disorders affecting ventilation and gas exchange within the lungs.

CONCEPTS FOR LECTURE
ASTHMA

1. After several years of increase, the prevalence of asthma currently is relatively stable. Hospitalizations and deaths due to asthma have decreased in recent years.
2. Risk factors for the development of asthma include allergies, family history, air pollution, occupational exposures, respiratory viruses, exercise in cold air, and emotional stress.

CHRONIC OBSTRUCTIVE PULMONARY DISEASE

3. Cigarette smoking is clearly implicated as the primary cause of COPD. Irritants in cigarette smoke impair

POWERPOINT LECTURE SLIDES

Asthma
Incidence
- Prevalence of asthma currently relatively stable
- Hospitalizations and deaths due to asthma decreasing

Risk Factors
- Allergies
- Family history
- Air pollution
- Occupational exposures
- Respiratory viruses

ciliary movement, inhibit the function of alveolar macrophages, and cause mucus-secreting glands to hypertrophy. It also produces emphysema or airway destruction and constricts smooth muscle, which increases airway resistance.

4. Other contributing factors include air pollution, occupational exposure to noxious dusts and gases, airway infection, and familial and genetic factors.

CYSTIC FIBROSIS

5. Cystic fibrosis (CF) is the most common lethal genetic disease in Caucasian Americans. The disease is less common in African Americans and rare in Asians.

ATELECTASIS

6. The most common etiology for the development of atelectasis is obstruction of the bronchus that ventilates a segment of lung tissue.
7. Other causes include compression of the lung by pneumothorax, pleural effusion, or tumor; or loss of pulmonary surfactant and inability to maintain open alveoli.
8. Clients at high risk for atelectasis are those with COPD, smokers undergoing surgery, and people on prolonged bedrest or mechanical ventilation.

BRONCHIECTASIS

9. About half of all cases of bronchiectasis are related to cystic fibrosis. Other causes include infections, lung abscess, exposure to toxic gases, abnormal lung or immunologic defenses, and localized airway obstruction due to foreign body or tumor.

OCCUPATIONAL LUNG DISEASE

10. Exposure to asbestos fibers occurs during mining, milling, manufacturing, and application of asbestos products.
11. Those who are at risk for the development of silicosis are hard-rock miners, foundry workers, sandblasters, pottery makers, and granite cutters.

SARCOIDOSIS

12. Sarcoidosis is of unknown etiology and primarily affects young adults between the ages of 20 and 40. In the United States the incidence is highest in African Americans.

PULMONARY EMBOLISM

13. Thromboemboli that develop in the venous system (deep vein thrombosis or DVT) or right side of the heart are the most frequent cause of pulmonary embolism.
14. Pulmonary embolism is the third leading cause of death in hospitalized clients. Risk factors for pulmonary embolism are stasis of venous flow, vessel

- Exercise in cold air
- Emotional stress

Chronic Obstructive Pulmonary Disease
Risk Factors
- Cigarette smoking
- Air pollution
- Occupational exposures
- Airway infection
- Familial and genetic factors

Atelectasis
- Etiology
- Obstruction of the bronchus
- Pneumothorax
- Pleural effusion
- Tumor
- Loss of pulmonary surfactant

Risk Factors
- COPD
- Smokers undergoing surgery
- Prolonged bedrest
- Mechanical ventilation

Pulmonary Embolism
Etiology
- Thromboemboli
  - Venous system
  - Right side of the heart
- Tumors
- Fat or bone marrow
- Amniotic fluid
- Intravenous injection of air or other foreign substances

Risk Factors
- Status of venous flow
- Vessel wall damage
- Altered blood coagulation
- Prolonged immobility
- Trauma
- Surgery
- Myocardial infarction
- Obesity
- Advanced age
- Oral contraceptive use
- Estrogen therapy

wall damage, and altered blood coagulation. Prolonged immobility, trauma, surgery, myocardial infarction, obesity, and advanced age are risk factors for DVT as are oral contraceptive and estrogen therapy.

PULMONARY HYPERTENSION

15. Primary pulmonary hypertension occurs in familial and sporadic patterns. This disorder primarily affects women in the 30s and 40s.

ACUTE RESPIRATORY FAILURE

16. Respiratory failure can result from inadequate alveolar ventilation, impaired gas exchange, or a significant ventilation-perfusion mismatch. COPD is the most common cause of respiratory failure.

ACUTE RESPIRATORY DISTRESS SYNDROME

17. The exact cause of ARDS is unknown, but it is known that ARDS does not occur as a primary process. It may follow conditions producing direct or indirect lung injury.

SUGGESTIONS FOR CLASSROOM ACTIVITIES

• Have the students identify risk factors that are common to the disorders covered in this chapter. Identify how those risk factors manifest in vulnerable populations. Discuss health promotion implications of the presence of these risk factors.

SUGGESTIONS FOR CLINICAL ACTIVITIES

• Assign clinical students to the care of a client who has one of the disorders covered in this chapter. Have the students review the chart for information that would identify risk factors. Discuss the nursing implication of not knowing that a risk factor exists.

LEARNING OUTCOME 3

Describe interdisciplinary care and the nursing role in health promotion and caring for clients with disorders that affect the ability to ventilate the lungs and exchange gases with the environment.

CONCEPTS FOR LECTURE
ASTHMA

1. Treatment goals are controlling symptoms and preventing acute attacks. When acute attack occurs, therapy is directed toward restoring airway patency and alveolar ventilation.
2. Peak expiratory flow rate (PEFR) is used on a day-to-day basis to evaluate the severity of bronchial hyperresponsiveness. This value is used to evaluate the severity of airway obstruction.
3. Asthma attacks often can be prevented by avoiding allergens and environmental triggers.
4. Nursing diagnoses include: *Ineffective Airway Clearance; Ineffective Breathing Pattern; Anxiety;* and *Ineffective Therapeutic Regimen Management.*

POWERPOINT LECTURE SLIDES

Asthma
Interdisciplinary Care
  • Control of symptoms
  • Prevention of acute attacks
  • Restoring airway patency
  • Restoring alveolar ventilation

Treatments
  • Peak expiratory flow rate (PEFR)
  • Prevention

Nursing Diagnoses
  • *Ineffective Airway Clearance*
  • *Ineffective Breathing Pattern*
  • *Anxiety*
  • *Ineffective Therapeutic Regimen Management*

Chronic Obstructive Pulmonary Disease
Interdisciplinary Care

CHRONIC OBSTRUCTIVE PULMONARY DISEASE

5. Treatment of COPD generally focuses on relieving symptoms, minimizing obstruction, and slowing disability.
6. Diagnosis is made through pulmonary function tests, ventilation-perfusion scanning, serum alpha 1-antitrypsin levels, arterial blood gases, pulse oximetry, capnogram, CBC with WBC differential, and chest x-ray.
7. Smoking cessation can prevent COPD from developing and can also improve lung function once the disease has been diagnosed.
8. Treatments include avoidance of airway irritants and allergens, pulmonary hygiene measures, maintaining adequate hydration, regular aerobic exercise if applicable, and breathing exercises. Instruction about "huffing" coughs should be provided.
9. Long-term oxygen therapy is used for severe and progressive hypoxemia.
10. Acute exacerbation of COPD may necessitate oxygenation and inspiratory positive pressure assistance with a face mask or intubation and mechanical ventilation.
11. When medical therapy is no longer effective, lung transplantation may be an option.
12. Complementary therapies may include herbal teas, minimizing intake of dairy products and salt, licorice root, acupuncture, hypnotherapy, and guided imagery.
13. Nursing diagnoses include: *Ineffective Airway Clearance; Imbalanced Nutrition: Less than Body Requirements; Compromised Family Coping;* and *Decisional Conflict: Smoking.*

CYSTIC FIBROSIS

14. The goals of the multidisciplinary treatment plan is to prevent or treat respiratory complications and maintain adequate nutrition.
15. Diagnosis is confirmed by analysis of chloride concentrations in the sweat. ABGs and oxygen saturation levels may indicate hypoxemia. Pulmonary function testing and alveolar-capillary diffusion are abnormal.
16. Treatments include chest physiotherapy with percussion and postural drainage; oxygen therapy; liberal fluid intake; and a high-protein, high-fat, high-calorie diet.
17. Lung transplantation currently offers the only definitive treatment for CF. Transplants may be single-lung, double-lung, or heart-lung.
18. Nursing diagnoses include: *Ineffective Airway Clearance* and *Anticipatory Grieving.*

ATELECTASIS

19. Chest x-ray shows an area of airless lung.
20. Primary therapy for atelectasis is prevention. After development, treatment focuses on reversing the underlying cause. Bronchoscopy may be necessary to remove mucous plugs. Antibiotic therapy is ordered to treat infections.

- Symptom relief
- Minimization of obstruction
- Slowing development of disability

Diagnosis
- Pulmonary function tests
- Ventilation-perfusion scanning
- Serum alpha 1-antitrypsin levels
- ABGs
- Pulse oximetry
- Capnogram
- CBC with WBC differential
- Chest x-ray

Treatments
- Smoking cessation
- Avoidance of airway irritants and allergens
- Pulmonary hygiene measures
- Adequate hydration
- Regular aerobic exercise if applicable
- Breathing exercises
- Long-term oxygen therapy
- Nursing diagnoses
  - *Ineffective Airway Clearance*
  - *Imbalanced Nutrition: Less than Body Requirements*
  - *Compromised Family Coping*
  - *Decisional Conflict: Smoking*

Cystic Fibrosis
Interdisciplinary Care
- Preventing or treating respiratory complications
- Maintaining adequate nutrition
- Diagnosis
- Analysis of chloride concentrations in the sweat
- ABGs and oxygen saturation levels
- Pulmonary function testing
- Alveolar-capillary diffusion

Treatments
- Chest physiotherapy with percussion and postural drainage
- Oxygen therapy
- Liberal fluid intake
- High protein, high fat, high calorie diet

Surgery
- Organ transplantation
  - Single lung
  - Double lung
  - Heart lung
- Nursing diagnoses
  - *Ineffective Airway Clearance*
  - *Anticipatory Guidance*

Atelectasis
Interdisciplinary Care
- Prevention
- Reversing underlying cause
- Bronchoscopy

21. Nursing care is directed toward airway clearance.

BRONCHIECTASIS

22. Collaborative care focuses on maintaining optimal pulmonary function and preventing progression of the disorder.
23. Diagnosis is typically based on history and physical examination. Chest x-ray and CT scan may help determine the extent of the lung damage.
24. Treatments include chest physiotherapy, percussion, postural drainage, and bronchoscopy.
25. Surgery may be necessary to resect areas of localized lung tissue that is unresponsive to conservative therapy.
26. Nursing diagnoses include: *Ineffective Airway Clearance; Ineffective Breathing Pattern; Impaired Gas Exchange; Imbalanced Nutrition: Less than Body Requirements;* and *Self-Care Deficit.*

OCCUPATIONAL LUNG DISEASE

27. Prevention is the key strategy for all occupational lung disorders.
28. Diagnosis is achieved by chest x-ray, pulmonary function studies, bronchoscopy, pulmonary function tests, ABGs, lung scans, and lung biopsy.
29. There is no specific therapy for occupational lung diseases, but elimination of further exposure is vital.
30. Nursing diagnoses include: *Activity Intolerance; Impaired Gas Exchange; Ineffective Breathing Pattern; Anticipatory Grieving, Low Self-Esteem;* and *Caregiver Role Strain.*

SARCOIDOSIS

31. Leukopenia, eosinophilia, and an elevated erythrocyte sedimentation rate typically are noted in sarcoidosis. Chest x-ray, pulmonary function tests, and biopsy of granulomatous lesions may be used to confirm diagnosis.
32. Nursing care is directed by the involved organ systems and related manifestations.

PULMONARY EMBOLISM

33. Prevention is the primary goal in treating pulmonary embolism. Early ambulation of medical and surgical clients, external pneumatic compression of the legs, elevating the legs, and active and passive exercising may be effective in the prevention of pulmonary embolism.
34. Treatment is supportive and includes oxygen therapy, analgesics, pulmonary artery wedge pressure monitoring, and cardiac output monitoring. Cardiac rhythm is monitored.
35. Diagnostic studies include plasma D-dimer levels, chest CT with contrast, lung scans, pulmonary angiography, chest x-ray, electrocardiogram, ABGs, exhaled carbon dioxide levels, and coagulation studies.

- Antibiotic therapy
- Diagnosis
- Chest x-ray

Nursing Care
- Directed toward airway clearance

Bronchiectasis
Interdisciplinary Care
- Maintaining optimal pulmonary function
- Preventing progression

Diagnosis
- Based on history and physical
- Chest x-ray
- CT scan

Treatments
- Chest physiotherapy
- Percussion
- Postural drainage
- Bronchoscopy

Surgery
- Resection of areas of localized lung tissue

Nursing Diagnoses
- *Ineffective Airway Clearance*
- *Ineffective Breathing Pattern*
- *Impaired Gas Exchange*
- *Imbalanced Nutrition: Less than Body Requirements*
- *Self-care deficit*

Occupational Lung Disease
Interdisciplinary Care
- Prevention
- Diagnosis
- Chest x-ray
- Pulmonary function studies
- Bronchoscopy
- Pulmonary function tests
- ABGs
- Lung scans
- Lung biopsy

Treatments
- No specific therapy
- Elimination of further exposure is vital

Nursing Diagnoses
- *Activity Intolerance*
- *Impaired Gas Exchange*
- *Ineffective Breathing Pattern*
- *Anticipatory Grieving*
- *Low Self-Esteem*
- *Caregiver Role Strain*

Sarcoidosis
Diagnosis
- WBC with diff
- ESR

36. When anticoagulant therapy fails to prevent recurrent emboli or is contraindicated, an umbrella-like filter may be inserted into the inferior vena cava to trap large emboli while allowing continued blood flow.
37. Nursing diagnoses include: *Impaired Gas Exchange; Decreased Cardiac Output; Ineffective Protection;* and *Anxiety.*

PULMONARY HYPERTENSION

38. Interdisciplinary care focuses on slowing the course of the disease, preventing thrombus formation, and reducing pulmonary vasoconstriction.
39. Diagnosis is achieved by analysis of CBC, ABGs, oxygen saturation, chest x-ray, electrocardiogram, Doppler ultrasonography, and heart catheterization.
40. Treatment includes oxygen therapy and phlebotomy for polycythemia if it exists. When cor pulmonale is present, salt and water restriction and diuretic therapy are used.
41. Bilateral lung or heart-lung transplant is the most effective long-term treatment for primary pulmonary hypertension.
42. Nursing diagnoses include: *Anticipatory Grieving; Hopelessness; Decreased Cardiac Output; Excess Fluid Volume,* and *Ineffective Individual Coping.*

- Chest x-ray
- Pulmonary function tests
- Biopsy of granulomatous lesions

Nursing Care
- Directed by the involved organ systems and related manifestations

Pulmonary Embolism
Interdisciplinary Care
- Prevention
  - Early ambulation of medical and surgical clients
  - External pneumatic compression of the legs
  - Elevating the legs
  - Active and passive exercising
- Treatments
- Oxygen therapy
- Analgesics
- Pulmonary artery wedge pressure monitoring
- Cardiac output monitoring
- Cardiac rhythm monitoring

Diagnosis
- Plasma D-dimer levels
- Chest CT with contrast
- Lung scans
- Pulmonary angiography
- Chest x-ray
- Electrocardiogram
- ABGs
- Exhaled carbon dioxide levels
- Coagulation studies

Surgery
- Umbrella-like filter insertion

Nursing Diagnoses
- *Impaired Gas Exchange*
- *Decreased Cardiac Output*
- *Ineffective Protection*
- *Anxiety*

Pulmonary Hypertension
Interdisciplinary Care
- Slowing the course of the disease
- Preventing thrombus formation
- Reducing pulmonary vasoconstriction

Diagnosis
- CBC
- ABGs
- Oxygen saturation
- Chest x-ray
- Electrocardiogram
- Doppler ultrasonography
- Heart catheterization

Treatment
- Oxygen therapy
- Phlebotomy for polycythemia

- Salt and water restriction
- Diuretic therapy

Surgery
- Bilateral lung or heart-lung transplant

Nursing Diagnoses
- *Anticipatory Grieving*
- *Hopelessness*
- *Decreased Cardiac Output*
- *Excess Fluid Volume*
- *Ineffective Individual Coping*

SUGGESTIONS FOR CLASSROOM ACTIVITIES

- Divide the students into small groups. Assign each group a nursing diagnosis problem statement that is frequently appropriate for clients who have ventilatory disorders. Have students investigate how the nursing diagnosis applies to the various disorders covered in this chapter. Share the work.
- Use the information in the case study about acute asthma attack that is provided on the textbook Companion Website as a basis for discussion of the care of clients with these disorders.

SUGGESTIONS FOR CLINICAL ACTIVITIES

- Assign students to the care of clients with identified ventilatory disorders. Have the students develop a plan of care for the client, and identify appropriate alterations in standard assessment and necessary interventions.

LEARNING OUTCOME 4

Discuss interdisciplinary interventions to provide airway and ventilatory support for the client with respiratory failure, and nursing responsibilities in caring for clients requiring airway and ventilatory support.

CONCEPTS FOR LECTURE
ACUTE RESPIRATORY FAILURE

1. Treatment of respiratory failure focuses on correcting the underlying cause or disease; supporting ventilation; and correcting hypoxemia and hypercapnia.
2. Diagnostic testing includes exhaled carbon dioxide and ABGs.
3. Drugs used in treating respiratory failure depend upon the underlying cause of the failure and the need for intubation and mechanical failure. Common medications include bronchodilators, corticosteroids, antibiotics, sedatives, analgesics, and neuromuscular blocking agents.
4. Oxygen is administered to reverse hypoxemia. The goal of treatment is to achieve an oxygen saturation of 90% or greater without oxygen toxicity.
5. Continued high oxygen concentrations impair the synthesis of surfactant, which reduces lung compliance. Acute respiratory distress syndrome or atelectasis may occur.

AIRWAY MANAGEMENT

6. If the upper airway is obstructed or positive pressure mechanical ventilation is necessary, an endotracheal tube may be inserted. To maintain positive pressure

POWERPOINT LECTURE SLIDES

Acute Respiratory Distress Syndrome
Interdisciplinary Care
- Identifying and treating its underlying cause
- Providing aggressive respiratory support

Diagnosis
- ABGs
- Chest x-ray
- Pulmonary function tests
- Pulmonary artery pressure monitoring

Medication
- No definitive drug therapy
- Inhaled nitric oxide
- Surfactant
- NSAIDs
- Corticosteroids

Treatments
- Endotracheal intubation
- Mechanical ventilation
- Prone positioning
- Careful fluid replacement
- Nutrition
- Treatment of infection
- Correction of underlying condition

ventilation, the tube is cuffed with an air-filled or foam sac just above the end of the tube. This cuff obstructs the upper airway and prevents air leakage back into the nose or mouth.

7. Long-term mechanical ventilation requires placement of a tracheostomy tube.

8. Close observation for respiratory distress is necessary after extubation. While sore throat and voice hoarseness are common postextubation, respiratory stridor may indicate need for reintubation. The client's gag reflex must be carefully assessed before oral intake is reestablished.

MECHANICAL VENTILATION

9. Specific indications for mechanical ventilation are: apnea or acute ventilatory failure, hypoxemia unresponsive to oxygen therapy alone, and increased work of breathing with progressive client fatigue.

10. Mechanical ventilators are classified into two broad categories. Negative-pressure ventilators create negative (subatmospheric) pressure externally to draw the chest outward and air into the lungs. The iron lung, curiass ventilator, and PulmoWrap are examples of negative-pressure ventilators. Positive-pressure ventilators are more commonly used and work by pushing air into the lungs.

11. Positive-pressure ventilators have several variables to trigger, cycle, and limit airflow. The trigger prompts the ventilator to deliver a breath. Ventilator-assisted breaths are triggered by the client's inspiratory effort. Ventilator-controlled breaths are triggered by a preset time.

12. Common modes of ventilation are continuous positive airway pressure, bilevel airway pressure support, assist-control mode ventilation, synchronized intermittent mandatory ventilation, positive end-expiratory ventilation, pressure support ventilation, and pressure-control ventilation.

13. Noninvasive ventilation provides ventilator support using a tight-fitting facemask and does not require intubation. Its primary use is to support clients with obstructive sleep apnea, neuromuscular disease, or impending respiratory failure.

14. Continuous positive airway pressure (CPAP) applies positive pressure to the airways of a spontaneously breathing client. All breathing is client-initiated and pressure-controlled.

15. Bilevel ventilators (BiPAP) provide inspiratory positive airway pressure as well as airway support during expiration. BiPAP modes are spontaneous breathing (S), timed breathing (T), and spontaneous/timed (S/T).

16. Assist-control mode ventilation (ACMV or AC) provides assisted breaths triggered by inspiratory effort; however, if the respiratory rate falls below a preset level, ventilator-controlled breaths are delivered.

17. Synchronized intermittent mandatory ventilation (SIMV) allows the client to breathe spontaneously, without ventilator assistance, between delivered ventilator breaths.

Nursing Diagnoses
- Decreased Cardiac Output
- Dysfunctional Ventilatory Weaning Response

18. Positive end-expiratory pressure (PEEP) requires intubation. Positive pressure is maintained in the airways during exhalation and between breaths.

19. Pressure support ventilation (PSV) delivers ventilator-assisted breaths when the client initiates an inspiratory effort.

20. Pressure-control ventilation (PCV) controls pressure within the airways to reduce the risk of airway trauma.

21. Other ventilator parameters set to meet individual client needs are rate, tidal volume, and percentage of oxygen delivered.

22. Complications of mechanical ventilation are nosocomial pneumonia, barotrauma, decreased cardiac output, and development of gastric stress ulcers.

23. The process of removing ventilator support and reestablishing spontaneous, independent respirations is called weaning. This process can begin only when the underlying condition that causes respiratory failure has been corrected or stabilized.

24. Processes for weaning include T-piece or CPAP, SIMV, and PSV.

25. When an illness is terminal or irreversible with a poor prognosis, terminal weaning may occur. Terminal weaning is the gradual withdrawal of mechanical ventilation when survival without assisted ventilation is not expected.

26. Fluid and electrolyte balance are closely monitored in the ventilator client. Nutrition is often provided by enteral or parenteral means.

27. Nursing diagnoses include: Impaired Spontaneous Ventilation; Ineffective Airway Clearance; Risk for Injury; and Anxiety

ACUTE RESPIRATORY DISTRESS SYNDROME

28. ARDS management is directed toward identifying and treating its underlying cause and providing aggressive respiratory support.

29. Diagnostic testing includes ABGs, chest x-ray, pulmonary function tests, and pulmonary artery pressure monitoring.

30. There is no definitive drug therapy for ARDS. Some medications used symptomatically include inhaled nitric oxide, surfactant, NSAIDs, and corticosteroids.

31. The mainstay of ARDS management is endotracheal intubation and mechanical ventilation. Prone positioning in conjunction with mechanical ventilation reduces the pressure of surrounding tissues on dependent regions and improves oxygenation.

32. Additional management strategies include careful fluid replacement, attention to nutrition, treatment of infection, and correction of underlying condition.

33. Nursing diagnoses include: Decreased Cardiac Output and Dysfunctional Ventilatory Weaning Response.

<table>
<tr><td>

SUGGESTIONS FOR CLASSROOM ACTIVITIES

- Have students identify settings common to most mechanical ventilators. Have students identify the nursing implications associated with those settings. Include emergency care in the discussion.

</td><td>

SUGGESTIONS FOR CLINICAL ACTIVITIES

- Arrange for clinical students to visit the hospital department responsible for mechanical ventilators. Look at various types of ventilators and discuss their application in the clinical area. Discuss nursing implications of caring for these clients.
- Arrange for students to work or observe in a facility where clients are maintained on long-term mechanical ventilation. Compare and contrast the nursing care required for these clients and clients who are on short-term ventilators.

</td></tr>
</table>

LEARNING OUTCOME 5

Describe the nursing implications for medications used to promote ventilation and gas exchange.

CONCEPTS FOR LECTURE

ASTHMA

1. Drugs used for long-term control of asthma are anti-inflammatory agents, long-acting bronchodilators; and leukotriene modifiers.
2. Quick-relief medications provide prompt relief of bronchoconstriction and airflow obstruction with associated wheezing, cough, and chest tightness. Short-acting adrenergic stimulants, anticholinergic drugs, and methylxanthines fall into this category.
3. Many drugs used for asthma management can be administered by metered-dose inhaler (MDI), dry powder inhaler (DPI), or nebulizer.

CHRONIC OBSTRUCTIVE PULMONARY DISEASE

4. Medications include immunizations against pneumococcal pneumonia and influenza, broad-spectrum antibiotics, bronchodilators, corticosteroids, and alpha 1-antitrypsin replacement therapy.

CYSTIC FIBROSIS

5. Medications include immunization against respiratory infections, bronchodilators, antibiotics, and dornase alfa.

BRONCHIECTASIS

6. Medications include antibiotics, inhaled bronchodilators, and oxygen.

OCCUPATIONAL LUNG DISEASE

7. Medications include anti-inflammatories and immunizations.

SARCOIDOSIS

8. Medications include corticosteroids, anti-inflammatories, or immune-modifiers.

POWERPOINT LECTURE SLIDES

Asthma
Long-Term Control
- Anti-inflammatory agents
- Long-acting bronchodilators
- Leukotriene modifiers

Quick Relief
- Short-acting adrenergic stimulants
- Anticholinergic drugs
- Methylxanthines

Administration Methods
- Metered-dose inhaler (MDI)
- Dry powder inhaler (DPI)
- Nebulizer

Chronic Obstructive Pulmonary Disease
- Immunizations against pneumococcal pneumonia and influenza
- Broad-spectrum antibiotics
- Bronchodilators
- Corticosteroids
- Alpha 1-antitrypsin replacement therapy

Cystic Fibrosis
- Immunization against respiratory infections
- Bronchodilators
- Antibiotics
- Dornase alfa

Bronchiectasis
- Antibiotics
- Inhaled bronchodilators
- Oxygen

Occupational Lung Disease
- Anti-inflammatories
- Immunizations

Sarcoidosis
- Corticosteroids
- Anti-inflammatory
- Immune-modifiers

PULMONARY EMBOLISM

9. Medication therapy includes anticoagulation with intravenous heparin and warfarin sodium. Bleeding is an associated risk. Massive pulmonary embolus and hypotension are treated with thrombolytic therapy. Streptokinase, urokinase, or tissue plasminogen activator are used to lyse the embolus, restore pulmonary blood flow, and reduce pulmonary artery and right heart pressures.

PULMONARY HYPERTENSION

10. Medications include calcium channel blockers, short-acting direct vasodilators, and oral anticoagulants.

NURSING IMPLICATIONS

11. The nurse should provide client and family education regarding use of all medications.
12. Many medications used for respiratory disorders also effect other body systems so the nurse must be aware of possible side effects.
13. The nurse must be aware of the need to monitor medication peak and trough levels and the desired therapeutic blood levels of many common respiratory medications.
14. Some medications are incompatible with other medications and fluids given intravenously.

Pulmonary Embolism
- Heparin
- Warfarin sodium
- Thrombolytic therapy
  ○ Streptokinase
  ○ Urokinase
  ○ Tissue plasminogen activator

Pulmonary Hypertension
- Calcium channel blockers
- Short-acting direct vasodilators
- Oral anticoagulants

Nursing Implications
- Client and family education
- Effects on other bodily systems
- Peak and trough levels
- Therapeutic blood levels
- IV compatibility

SUGGESTIONS FOR CLASSROOM ACTIVITIES

- Have students identify medications that are commonly used for treatment of ventilation disorders. Have the students group the medications by class and identify major nursing implications in administration.

SUGGESTIONS FOR CLINICAL ACTIVITIES

- Have students review clinical client medication administration records for medications that are frequently administered for ventilatory problems. Have students write medication information sheets about those medications, including dosages, nursing implications, safety implications, and teaching implications.

CHAPTER 40

ASSESSING CLIENTS WITH MUSCULOSKELETAL DISORDERS

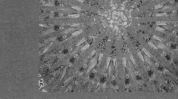

RESOURCE LIBRARY

PRENTICE HALL NURSING MEDIALINK DVD-ROM

Audio Glossary
NCLEX-RN® Review
Animation
  Joint Movement

COMPANION WEBSITE

Audio Glossary
NCLEX-RN® Review
Care Plan Activity: Musculoskeletal Disorders
Case Study: Knee Pain
MediaLink Application: Musculoskeletal Injuries of
  Health Care Providers
Links to Resources

IMAGE LIBRARY

Figure 40.1 Bones of the human skeleton.
Figure 40.2 The microscopic structure (Haversian system) of compact bone.
Figure 40.3 Classification of bones according to shape.
Figure 40.4 Parts of a long bone.
Figure 40.5 *A,* Muscles of the anterior body. *B,* Muscles of the posterior body.
Figure 40.6 Structure of a synovial joint (knee).

Figure 40.7 Using a goniometer to measure joint ROM.
Figure 40.8 Palpating the temporomandibular joints.
Figure 40.9 *A,* Forward flexion of spine. *B,* Lateral flexion of spine. *C,* Rotation of spine.
Figure 40.10 Phalen's test.
Figure 40.11 Checking for the bulge sign.
Figure 40.12 Checking for ballottement.
Figure 40.13 McMurray's test.
Figure 40.14 Thomas test for hip contracture.

LEARNING OUTCOME 1

Describe the anatomy, physiology, and functions of the musculoskeletal system.

CONCEPTS FOR LECTURE
THE SKELETON

1. The musculoskeletal system is composed of bones of the skeletal system; ligaments, tendons, and muscles of the muscular system; and joints.
2. Bones support soft tissues, protect vital organs from injury, serve to move body parts by providing points of attachment for muscles, store minerals, and serve as a site for hematopoiesis.
3. The 206 bones of the body are divided into the axial and appendicular skeleton. The axial skeleton includes the bones of the skull, ribs, sternum, and vertebral column. The appendicular skeleton consists of all the bones of the limbs, the shoulder girdles, and the pelvic girdle.
4. Bone cells include osteoblasts, osteocytes, and osteoclasts.
5. Bone matrix consists of collagen fibers, minerals, proteins, carbohydrates, and ground substance. Ground substance is a gelatinous material that facilitates

POWERPOINT LECTURE SLIDES

The Skeleton
- Composed of bones of the skeletal system
- Ligaments
- Tendons
- Muscles of the muscular system
- Joints

Bone Functions
- Support soft tissues
- Protect vital organs from injury
- Move body parts
- Store minerals
- Hematopoiesis

Anatomy
- 206 Bones
  - Axial skeleton
  - Appendicular skeleton

Physiology
- Bone cells
- Bone matrix

diffusion of nutrients, wastes, and gases between blood vessels and bone tissue.

6. Periosteum is the double-layered connective tissue that covers the bone.

7. Compact bone is smooth and dense and the basic structural unit is the Haversian system.

8. Spongy bone contains spaces between meshworks of bone and has no Haversian systems. The spongy sections of long bones and flat bones contain tissue (red marrow) for hematopoiesis.

9. Bones are classified by shape. Long bones are longer than they are wide and consist of a shaft called a diaphysis and two broad ends called epiphyses. Short or cuboid bones are spongy bone covered by compact bone and are found in the wrist and ankle. Flat bones are thin and flat and most are curved. Irregular bones are of various shapes and sizes.

10. Although the bones of adults do not normally increase in length and size, constant remodeling of bones, as well as repair of damaged bone tissue, occurs throughout life.

11. Bones that are in use and are subjected to stress increase their osteoblastic activity to increase ossification or bone development.

12. Bones that are inactive undergo increased osteoclast activity and bone resorption.

13. The hormonal stimulus for bone remodeling involves the interaction of parathyroid hormone and calcitonin.

14. Bone remodeling is also regulated by the response of bones to gravitational pull and to mechanical stress from the pull of muscles. Wolff's law states that bone develops and remodels itself to resist the stresses placed on it.

THE MUSCLES

15. Three types of muscle tissue are skeletal, smooth, and cardiac. Skeletal muscles promote body movement, help maintain posture, and produce body heat.

16. Typically functional properties of skeletal muscle are: excitability, contractility, extensibility, and elasticity.

17. Skeletal muscle movement is triggered when motor neurons release acetylcholine, which produces an action potential that causes muscle contraction. Prolonged strenuous activity causes continuous nerve impulses and eventually results in buildup of lactic acid and reduced energy in the muscle, or muscle fatigue.

18. Continuous nerve impulses are responsible for maintaining muscle tone. Lack of use results in muscle atrophy. Regular exercise increases the size and strength of muscles.

JOINTS, LIGAMENTS, AND TENDONS

19. Joints are the regions where two or more bones meet. Joints hold the bones together, but allow for movement.

- Periosteum
- Compact bone
- Spongy bone

Shape Classification
- Long bones
- Short or cuboid bones
- Flat bones
- Irregular bones

Bone Remodeling
- Occurs throughout life
- Use and stress increase osteoblastic activity
- Inactivity increases osteoclast activity
- Hormonal stimulus
- Also regulated by response to gravitational pull/mechanical stress

The Muscles
Types
- Skeletal
- Smooth
- Cardiac

Physiology
- Functional properties of skeletal muscle
- Muscle movement trigger

Joints, Ligaments, and Tendons
- Regions where two or more bones meet
- Hold the bones together
- Allow for movement

20. Ligaments are dense bands of connective tissue that connect bones to bones. Ligaments limit or enhance movement, provide joint stability, and enhance joint strength.
21. Tendons are fibrous connective tissue bands that connect muscles to the periosteum of bones. The increased pressure of muscle movement causes tendons to pull, push, or rotate the bone to which it is connected.

SUGGESTIONS FOR CLASSROOM ACTIVITIES

• Using anatomical models, review the anatomy and function of the musculoskeletal system.

LEARNING OUTCOME 2

Explain the normal movements allowed by synovial joints.

CONCEPTS FOR LECTURE

1. Fibrous joints permit little or no movement. Examples are the sutures of the skull.
2. Cartilaginous joints may be fixed (sternocostal joints of the rib cage) or movable (intervertebral discs).
3. Synovial joints are enclosed by a cavity that contains synovial fluid. They are freely movable. Bursae are small sacs of synovial fluid that cushion and protect bony areas that are at high risk for friction.
4. The fibrous capsules that surround synovial joints are supported by ligaments, which are dense bands of connective tissue. Tendons connect muscle to the periosteum of bones and enable movement.

POWERPOINT LECTURE SLIDES

Types of Joints
- Fibrous joints
  - Permit little or no movement
  - Sutures of the skull
- Cartilaginous joints
  - May be fixed (sternocostal joints of the rib cage)
  - Movable (intervertebral discs)
- Synovial joints
  - Enclosed by a cavity that contains synovial fluid
  - Freely moveable
  - Bursae
- Ligaments
  - Dense bands of connective tissue
  - Support fibrous capsules
- Tendons
  - Connect muscle to the perioteum of bones
  - Enable movement

SUGGESTIONS FOR CLASSROOM ACTIVITIES

• Using anatomical models review the movement of joints.
• View the joint movement animation provided on the textbook DVD-ROM.

SUGGESTIONS FOR CLINICAL ACTIVITIES

• Have students provide range of motion exercises as appropriate to clinical clients.

LEARNING OUTCOME 3

Identify specific topics for consideration during a health history interview of the client with health problems involving the musculoskeletal system.

CONCEPTS FOR LECTURE

1. Health problems that affect the neurologic system may manifest as problems with musculoskeletal function and an assessment of both systems may be necessary.
2. Genetic influences on the musculoskeletal system may include presence of arthritis, abnormally long bones, muscular dystrophy, and amyotrophic lateral sclerosis.
3. The primary manifestations of altered function of the musculoskeletal system are pain and limited mobility. Changes in weight, rash, and/or swelling may also be manifestations of altered function.
4. The nurse should also collect information about lifestyle, employment, exercise patterns, use of alcohol or drugs, nutrition, past trauma history, and measures to self-treat pain.
5. Physical examination of the musculoskeletal system includes assessment of gait and posture; inspection and palpation of bones; measurement of extremities for length and circumference; assessment of muscle mass; and assessment of joints for swelling, pain, redness, warmth, crepitus, and ROM.

POWERPOINT LECTURE SLIDES

Health Assessment Interview
- Assess both musculoskeletal and neurologic systems
- Genetic influences
  - Arthritis
  - Abnormally long bones
  - Muscular dystrophy
  - Amyotrophic lateral sclerosis
- The primary manifestations of altered function
  - Pain and limited mobility
  - Changes in weight
  - Rash and/or swelling
- Lifestyle
- Employment
- Exercise patterns
- Use of alcohol or drugs
- Nutrition
- Past trauma history
- Measures to self-treat pain

Physical Examination
- Assessment of gait and posture
- Inspection and palpation of bones
- Measurement of extremities for length and circumference
- Assessment of muscle mass
- Assessment of joints
  - Swelling
  - Pain
  - Redness
  - Warmth
  - Crepitus
  - ROM

SUGGESTIONS FOR CLASSROOM ACTIVITIES

- Using the case study about knee pain that is provided in the MediaLink application section of the Companion Website for the textbook, identify appropriate health history questions for a client.

SUGGESTIONS FOR CLINICAL ACTIVITIES

- Have students complete a health history interview for a client with a musculoskeletal disorder.

LEARNING OUTCOME 4

Describe normal variations in assessment findings for the older adult.

CONCEPTS FOR LECTURE

1. Aging may cause decrease in bone mass and mineralization. Calcium may be reabsorbed. Vertebrae may shorten and intervertebral disks may thin. Bone spurs may develop as cartilage on the bone surfaces deteriorates.

POWERPOINT LECTURE SLIDES

Bones and Joints
- Decrease in bone mass and mineralization
- Calcium reabsorption
- Vertebral shortening

2. As a result of these bone and joint changes, the older adult may become shorter and have thinner, weaker bones. Movement may become more painful, limiting mobility.
3. Aging may cause atrophy of muscle fibers and slow replacement of muscle tissue with fibrous tissue. Muscle mass and strength may reduce, range of motion decreases, and muscle cramping may occur.

- Intervertebral disk thinning
- Joint cartilage deterioration

Muscles
- Atrophy of muscle fibers
- Fibrotic replacement of muscle tissue

SUGGESTIONS FOR CLASSROOM ACTIVITIES

- Have students review the assessment of an older adult and identify age-related changes.

LEARNING OUTCOME 5

Identify manifestations of impairment of the musculoskeletal system.

CONCEPTS FOR LECTURE

1. Blood tests include alkaline phosphatase, calcium, uric acid, and creatine kinase.
2. Radiologic examinations include x-rays, CT scans, MRIs, and bone scans.
3. Bone mineral density measurements include dual energy x-ray absorptiometry (DEXA), quantitative ultrasound (QUS), and bone mineral density (BMD).
4. Arthroscopy uses a fiberoptic endoscope to examine the joint interior, to diagnose disease, and to perform surgery. Arthrocentesis is done to withdraw fluid from a joint by needle aspiration.
5. Electrical activity is tested by electromyogram (EMG) and somatosensory evoked potential (SSEP).
6. Gait and body posture assessment may reveal joint stiffness, pain, deformities, or muscle weakness.
7. Curvature of the spine may exist. Lordosis is an increased lumbar curve. Scoliosis is a lateral, S-shaped curvature. Kyphosis is an exaggerated thoracic curvature that is common in older adults.
8. Assessment of the joints may reveal deformity, swelling, and redness; tissue loss, tissue overgrowth, contractures, or irreversible shortenings of muscle or tendons; edema; pain; or crepitation.
9. Range of motion assessment may reveal decreased ROM, pain, swelling, or presence of structural changes in the joint. Examples of these changes include Heberden's nodes and Bouchard's nodes.
10. Tendonitis (inflammation of a tendon), bursitis (inflammation of a bursa), or synovitis (inflammation of the synovial membrane) may be present and noted on ROM assessment.
11. Special tests include: Phalen's test for carpal tunnel syndrome, the bulge test for small amounts of fluid on the knee, the ballottement test for large amounts of fluid on the knee, McMurray's test for injury to the meniscus, and the Thomas test for hip flexion contracture.

POWERPOINT LECTURE SLIDES

Blood Tests
- Alkaline phosphatase
- Calcium
- Uric acid
- Creatine kinase

Radiologic Examinations
- X-rays
- CT scans
- MRIs
- Bone scans

Bone Mineral Density Measurements
- Dual energy X-ray absorptiometry (DEXA)
- Quantitative ultrasound (QUS)
- Bone mineral density (BMD)

Arthroscopy
- Use of fiber optic endoscope
  - To examine the joint interior
  - To diagnose disease
  - To perform surgery

Arthrocentesis
- Withdrawal of fluid from a joint by needle aspiration

Electrical Activity Tested by
- Electromyogram (EMG)
- Somatosensory evoked potential (SSEP)

Gait and Body Posture Assessment
- Joint stiffness
- Pain
- Deformities
- Muscle weakness

Curvature of the Spine
- Lordosis is an increased lumbar curve
- Scoliosis is a lateral, S-shaped curvature
- Kyphosis is an exaggerated thoracic curvature

Assessment of the Joints
- Deformity
- Swelling and redness
- Tissue loss
- Tissue overgrowth
- Contractures
- Edema
- Pain
- Crepitation

Range of Motion
- Decreased ROM
- Pain
- Swelling
- Presence of structural changes in the joint
  - Heberden's nodes
  - Bouchard's nodes
- Tendinitis
- Bursitis
- Synovitis

Special Tests Include
- Phalen's test for carpal tunnel syndrome
- Bulge Test for small amounts of fluid on the knee
- Ballottement for large amounts of fluid on the knee
- McMurray's test for injury to the meniscus
- Thomas test for hip flexion contracture

SUGGESTIONS FOR CLASSROOM ACTIVITIES

- Review the manifestations of impairment that are listed in the textbook. Have students identify nursing implications of caring for clients with these manifestations.

SUGGESTIONS FOR CLINICAL ACTIVITIES

- Have students review the medical records of clinical clients with musculoskeletal disorders. Help them identify the assessment findings that are associated with the documented disorder.

CHAPTER 41
NURSING CARE OF CLIENTS WITH MUSCULOSKELETAL TRAUMA

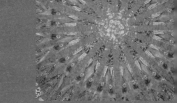

RESOURCE LIBRARY

 PRENTICE HALL NURSING MEDIALINK DVD-ROM

Audio Glossary
NCLEX-RN® Review
Animation/Video
   Bone Healing
   Crutch Instruction

 COMPANION WEBSITE

Audio Glossary
NCLEX-RN® Review
Care Plan Activity: Below-the-Knee Amputation
Case Study: A Client with Fractures
MediaLink Applications
   Compartment Syndrome
   Preventing Musculoskeletal Injuries
Links to Resources

IMAGE LIBRARY

Figure 41.1 *A,* An open fracture. *B,* A closed fracture.
Figure 41.2 Types of fractures.
Figure 41.4 Traction is the application of a pulling force to maintain bone alignment during fracture healing.
Figure 41.5 Examples of types of casts used to immobilize fractures.
Figure 41.6 In external fixation, pins are placed through the bone above and below the fracture site to immobilize the bone.
Figure 41.7 Internal fixation hardware is entirely within the body.

Figure 41.9 Regions where hip fractures may occur.
Figure 41.10 Surgical fixation of hip fractures.
Figure 41.11 Bivalving is the process of splitting the cast down both sides to alleviate pressure on or allow visualization of the extremity.
Figure 41.12 Common sites of amputation.
Figure 41.13 Stump dressings increase venous return, decrease edema, and help shape the stump for a prosthesis.

LEARNING OUTCOME 1

Compare and contrast the causes, risk factors, pathophysiology, manifestations, interdisciplinary care, and nursing care of contusions, strains, sprains, joint dislocations, and fractures.

CONCEPTS FOR LECTURE
CONTUSION, STRAINS, AND SPRAINS

1. Contusion, strains, and sprains are among the most commonly reported injuries. Lower back injury is the most commonly reported occupational injury.
2. A contusion is the least serious form of musculoskeletal injury. Blunt force causes bleeding into the soft tissue but the skin remains intact. A contusion with a large amount of bleeding is referred to as a hematoma.
3. Manifestations of contusion are swelling and discoloration of the skin.
4. A strain is a stretching injury to a muscle or a muscle-tendon unit that is caused by mechanical overloading. The most common sites for muscle strain are the lower back and cervical regions of the spine.

POWERPOINT LECTURE SLIDES

Contusion
- Least serious form of musculoskeletal injury
- Blunt force
- Bleeding into the soft tissue
- Skin remains intact
- Hematoma

Manifestations
- Swelling
- Discoloration of the skin

Strain
- Stretching injury to a muscle or a muscle-tendon unit
- Mechanical overloading

5. Manifestations of a strain include pain, limited motion, muscle spasms, swelling, and possible muscle weakness.
6. A sprain is a stretch and/or tear of one or more ligaments that surround a joint. The ankle and knee are the most common areas of sprain.
7. Manifestations of sprain include loss of the ability to move or use the joint, a feeling of a "pop" or tear, discoloration, pain, and rapid swelling.
8. The goal of the initial stage of treating soft-tissue trauma is to reduce swelling and pain. For the first 24 to 48 hours, the client is advised to follow a regimen of rest, ice, compression, and elevation (RICE).
9. Immobilization of the joint and limitations on weight bearing may be necessary. Severe sprains may require surgery.
10. The second stage of treatment is provision of physical therapy for rehabilitation.
11. Nursing diagnoses include: *Acute Pain* and *Impaired Physical Mobility*.

JOINT DISLOCATION

12. A dislocation is an injury of a joint in which the ends of bones are forced from their normal position. These injuries most commonly occur in the shoulder and acromioclavicular joints.
13. A subluxation is a partial dislocation in which the bone ends are still partially in contact with each other.
14. Dislocations may be congenital, traumatic, or pathologic.
15. Manifestations include pain, deformity, and limited motion.
16. Care of the client with a dislocation focuses on relieving pain, correcting the dislocation, and preventing complications.
17. The joint is most often reduced (bone ends realigned) by manual traction. Only the most severely dislocated shoulder joints are surgically reduced. Dislocations of the hip require immediate reduction to prevent necrosis of the femoral head and injury to the sciatic and femoral nerve. Surgery may be necessary if the hip dislocation is accompanied by a fracture.
18. Nursing diagnoses include: *Acute Pain* and *Risk for Injury*.

TRAUMATIC INJURIES OF THE BONES

19. A fracture is any break in the continuity of a bone and varies in severity according to the location and type of fracture.
20. A fracture occurs when the bone is subjected to more kinetic energy than it can absorb. This force may be from a direct blow (compression), a sudden twisting motion (torsion), a severe muscle contraction, or disease that has weakened the bone (stress or pathologic fracture).

- Common sites
  - Lower back
  - Cervical spine
    - Manifestations
- Pain
- Limited motion
- Muscle spasms
- Swelling
- Muscle weakness

Sprain
- Stretch and/or tear of ligaments surrounding joint
- Common sites
  - Ankle
  - Knee

Manifestations
- Loss of the ability to move or use the joint
- Feeling a "pop" or tear
- Discoloration
- Pain
- Rapid swelling

Joint Dislocation
- Injury of a joint
  - Ends of bones are forced from normal position
- Most common
  - Shoulder
  - Acromioclavicular joints
- Subluxation
  - Partial dislocation
- May be congenital, traumatic, or pathologic

Manifestations
- Pain
- Deformity
- Limited motion

Types of Fracture
- Closed or simple fractures
- Open or compound fractures
- Oblique
- Spiral
- Avulsed
- Comminuted
- Compressed
- Impacted
- Depressed
- Complete
- Incomplete
- Stable
- Unstable

Interdisciplinary Care
- Stabilize the fractured bone(s)
- Maintain bone immobilization
- Prevent complications
- Restore function

21. Closed or simple fractures are ones in which the overlying skin is intact. Open or compound fractures are ones in which the skin integrity is interrupted.
22. Fractures are often accompanied by soft tissue injuries that involve muscles, arteries, veins, nerves, and skin.
23. A fracture requires treatment to stabilize the fractured bone(s), maintain bone immobilization, prevent complications, and restore function.
24. Emergency care of the client with a fracture includes immobilizing the fracture, maintaining tissue perfusion, and preventing infection.
25. Medications prescribed for clients with fractures include pain medications, stool softeners, antacids, NSAIDs, antibiotics, and anticoagulants.
26. Surgery is indicated for the client who has a fracture that requires direct visualization and repair, a fracture with common long-term complication(s), or a fracture that is severely comminuted and threatens vascular supply.
27. The simplest form of surgery is done by external fixation with an external fixation device. Pin site care is similar to that of skeletal traction pins.
28. Internal fixation can be accomplished through a surgical procedure called an open reduction and internal fixation (ORIF). In this procedure, the fracture is reduced and held in place with nails, screws, plates, or pins that are surgically placed.
29. Electrical bone stimulation is the application of an electrical current at the fracture site and can be either externally or internally delivered. The electrical stress provided by this painless procedure increases the migration of osteoblasts and osteoclasts to the fracture site.

SPECIFIC FRACTURES

30. The skull may be fractured as a result of a fall or a direct blow. The client must be assessed for neurologic damage and any loss of consciousness must be documented.
31. Facial fractures may result from a direct blow. Manifestations are hematomas, pain, edema, and bony deformity. The client must be observed for neurologic deficits. Nursing care focuses on maintaining the airway, treating pain, and addressing body image disturbances.
32. Spinal fractures can be cervical, thoracic, lumbar, or sacral. Injury to the spinal cord is the most severe complication of spinal fracture. Pressure on the spinal cord may result in permanent paralysis.
33. Fracture of the clavicle commonly results from a direct blow or a fall. The most common area is midclavicular. Injuries to the clavicle may be associated with skull or cervical fractures. Treatment focuses on immobilizing the fractured bone in normal anatomic position by applying a clavicular strap. Surgical repair may be necessary.

Emergency Care
- Immobilizing the fracture
- Maintaining tissue perfusion
- Preventing infection

Medications
- Pain medications
- Stool softeners
- Antacids
- NSAIDs
- Antibiotics
- Anticoagulants

34. Fractures of the humerus are treated by immobilizing the fractured bone in normal anatomic position. Common complications are nerve and ligament damage, frozen or stiff joints, and malunion. Fractures of the proximal humerus are common in older adults and require surgery if complicated.

35. The most common location of an elbow fracture is the distal humerus. These fractures usually result from a fall or direct blow to the elbow. Complications of an elbow fracture include nerve or artery damage and hemarthrosis.

36. Fractures of the radius and ulna may occur as a result of either indirect injury, such as twisting or pulling of the arm, of direct injury, such as from a fall. When both bones are broken, the fracture is usually displaced. Complications after a radius and/or ulnar fracture include compartment syndrome, delayed healing, and decreased wrist and finger movement. Nursing interventions focus on alleviating pain, maintaining immobilization, educating clients in neurovascular assessment, and the importance of elevation.

37 A common type of wrist fracture is a Colles's fracture, in which the distal radius fractures after a fall onto an outstretched hand. The client presents with a bony deformity, pain, numbness, weakness, and decreased ROM of the fingers. The most common bones involved in hand fractures are the metacarpals and phalanges. Complications of wrist and hand fractures are compartment syndrome, nerve damage, ligament damage, and delayed union.

38. Rib fractures commonly result from blunt chest trauma. Fractures of the first through third ribs may result in injury to the subclavian artery or vein. Fractures of the lower rib may result in spleen and liver injuries. A complication of rib fracture is flail chest which is the result of fracture of two or more adjacent ribs in two or more places. Simple rib fracture is treated with pain medication and instructions for coughing, deep breathing, and splinting.

39. Pelvic fractures are often caused by trauma. A single fracture in the pelvis is treated conservatively with bed rest on a firm mattress. A pelvic fracture with two sites is considered unstable and treated with surgery. Common complications include hypovolemia, spinal injury, bladder injury, urethral injury, kidney damage, and gastrointestinal trauma. Nursing management includes alleviating discomfort, maintaining immobilization, and preparing the client for surgery if indicated.

40. Clients with fractures to the femoral shaft should be assessed for other trauma because a large amount of force is required to cause that injury. Manifestations are edema, deformity, and pain in the thigh with inability to move the hip or knee. Assessment should also include pedal pulses and capillary refill. Complications of femoral shaft fracture include hypovolemia due to blood loss, fat embolism, dislocation of the hip or knee, muscle atrophy, and ligament damage. Skeletal traction

is used initially to separate the bony fragments and re-duce and immobilize the fracture. Internal or external fixation may be used to stabilize the fracture for heal-ing. Nursing management includes providing pain medication, providing reassurance and decreasing anxiety, and assisting with exercises as indicated.

41. Hip fractures are intracapsular (involving the head or neck of the femur) or extracapsular (involving the trochanteric region). Hip fractures are common in the elderly and may be spontaneous, which results in a fall or may occur as a result of a fall.

42. Manifestations of hip fracture may be subtle with no change in ability to ambulate, or the client may pre-sent with pain, inability to walk, and shortening and external rotation of the affected limb. Treatment may include traction followed by surgery, or there may be immediate surgery. Surgical treatment may be open reduction with internal fixation or replacement of the femoral head or acetabulum (hemiarthroplasty) or the entire joint (total hip arthroplasty). Nursing care focuses on maintaining skin integrity, preventing in-fection, alleviating pain, maintaining circulation to the injury extremity, and increasing mobility.

43. Clients with fracture of the tibia and/or fibula gener-ally present with edema, pain, bony deformity, and a hematoma at the level of the injury. Complications in-clude peroneal nerve damage, tibial artery damage, compartment syndrome, hemarthrosis, and ligament damage. Treatments of closed injury include closed reduction and casting. An open fracture may require open reduction and internal fixation. Nursing care is designed to increase comfort, monitor neurovascular status, and prevent complications.

44. Clients with ankle fractures present with pain, limited ROM, hematoma, edema, and difficulty ambulating. Clients with foot fractures present with similar find-ings; however, ROM of the ankle is usually not af-fected. Simple fractures of both areas are treated with closed reduction and casting. More complicated frac-tures of either area may require surgery. Nursing care focuses on increasing comfort, increasing mobility, and client education.

NURSING CARE

45. The best treatment of traumatic injuries is preven-tion. Regular screening for osteoporosis, regular exer-cise, and education about trip hazards may help prevent hip fracture in the older adult. All adults should be educated in a regular exercise program, avoiding obesity, and adequate calcium intake to pre-vent fracture.

46. Nursing diagnoses may include: *Acute Pain, Risk for Infection, Risk for Peripheral Neurovascular Dys-function; Impaired Physical Mobility,* and *Risk for Disturbed Sensory Perception: Tactile.*

SUGGESTIONS FOR CLASSROOM ACTIVITIES

SUGGESTIONS FOR CLINICAL ACTIVITIES

- Divide the students into small groups. Assign each group a set of disorders that are covered in this chapter. Have the students prepare a chart that lists the common causes and risk factors for the development of the disorders assigned. Share the findings and look for commonalities.
- On the board, list manifestations that are common to the disorders covered in this chapter. Help students identify the commonalities among these disorders. Relate the disorders to the pathophysiologic basis.
- Review the case study about a client with fractures that is provided on the textbook Companion Website. Use this case study to help students prepare a plan of care for this client.

- Have students review the medical records of clients who have suffered a disorder that is covered in this chapter. Look for the manifestations and the client's risk factors for developing the disorder.

LEARNING OUTCOME 2

Describe the stages of bone healing.

CONCEPTS FOR LECTURE

1. Fracture healing progresses over three phases: the inflammatory phase, the reparative phase, and the remodeling phase.
2. The fracture causes inflammation, bleeding, and hematoma formation. The presence of the hematoma clot causes the osteocytes at the bone ends to die. Necrosis of the cells heightens the inflammatory response. Fibroblasts, lymphocytes, macrophages, and osteoblasts from the bone migrate to the fracture site and promote growth of granulation tissue and capillary buds. Calcium begins to be deposited.
3. Once calcium is deposited, a callus begins to form, which signals the beginning of the reparative stage. Collagen formation and calcium deposition continues.
4. In the remodeling stage, excess callus is removed and new bone is laid down along the fracture line. Eventually the fracture site is calcified, and the bone is reunited.

POWERPOINT LECTURE SLIDES

Three Phases of Fracture Healing
- Inflammatory phase
- Reparative phase
- Remodeling phase

Inflammatory Phase
- Inflammation, bleeding, and hematoma formation
- Osteocytes at the bone ends die
- Necrosis of cells heightens inflammatory response
- Fibroblasts, lymphocytes, macrophages, and osteoblasts migrate to fracture site
- Promote growth of granulation tissue and capillary buds
- Calcium deposited

Reparative Stage
- Begins when callus begins to form
- Collagen formation
- Calcium deposition

Remodeling
- Excess callus is removed
- New bone is laid down
- Fracture site calcifies
- Bone is reunited

SUGGESTIONS FOR CLASSROOM ACTIVITIES

- Review the animation/video about bone healing that is provided on the textbook DVD-ROM.
- Using anatomical models, demonstrate the phases of bone healing. Compare these structures to those of an uninjured bone.

SUGGESTIONS FOR CLINICAL ACTIVITIES

- Discuss the nursing implications of caring for a client with a fracture as the client moves through the phases of bone healing. Identify nursing interventions appropriate for each phase and emphasize assessment and safety.

LEARNING OUTCOME 3

Explain the pathophysiology, manifestations, and related treatments for complications of bone fractures: compartment syndrome, fat embolism syndrome, deep venous thrombosis, infection, delayed union and nonunion, and reflex sympathetic dystrophy.

CONCEPTS FOR LECTURE

1. Complications of musculoskeletal trauma are associated with pressure from edema and hemorrhage, development of fat emboli, deep venous thrombosis, infection, loss of skeletal integrity, or involvement of nerve fibers.

COMPARTMENT SYNDROME

2. Compartment syndrome occurs when excess pressure constricts the structures within a compartment, which reduces circulation to muscles and nerves. A compartment is a space enclosed by fibrous membrane or fascia and is nonexpendable.
3. Early manifestations of compartment syndrome are pain and either normal or decreased peripheral pulse. Later manifestations include cyanosis, paresthesias, paresis, severe pain, and eventually renal failure.
4. Interventions to alleviate pressure must be implemented. External pressure from a tight cast can be relieved by removal of the cast. Internal pressure may require a fasciotomy, after which the incision is left open.
5. Volkmann's contracture is a common complication of elbow fracture and can result from unresolved compartment syndrome. Arm mobility is impaired and the client is unable to fully extend the arm.

FAT EMBOLISM SYNDROME

6. Fat emboli occur when fat globules lodge in the pulmonary vascular bed or peripheral circulation. Fat embolism syndrome is characterized by neurologic dysfunction; pulmonary insufficiency; and petechiae rash on the chest, axilla, and upper arms.
7. Long bone fractures and other major trauma are the principle risk factors for fat emboli; hip replacement is also a risk.
8. Bone fracture results in a rise of pressure in the bone marrow and fat globules enter the bloodstream. They combine with platelets and travel throughout the body, which occludes small blood vessels and causes tissue ischemia.
9. Manifestations of fat embolism include confusion, changes in level of consciousness, pulmonary edema, impaired surfactant production, atelectasis, petechiae, and ARDS. Manifestations may occur within a few hours to a week after injury.
10. Prevention of fat embolism requires early stabilization of long bone fracture. Treatment may include intubation and mechanical ventilation to prevent hypoxemia. Fluid balance must be closely monitored. Corticosteroids may be administered to decrease the inflammatory response of lung tissues, stabilize lipid metabolism, and reduce bronchospasm.

POWERPOINT LECTURE SLIDES

Complications of Musculoskeletal Trauma
- Pressure from edema and hemorrhage
- Development of fat emboli
- Deep vein thrombosis
- Infection
- Loss of skeletal integrity
- Involvement of nerve fibers

Compartment Syndrome
- Physiology
- Entrapment of the blood vessels limits tissue perfusion
- Results in edema within the compartment
- Edema causes further pressure

Early Manifestations
- Pain
- Normal or decreased peripheral pulse

Later Manifestations
- Cyanosis
- Paresthesias, paresis
- Severe pain
- Renal failure

Treatment
- Interventions to alleviate pressure
- Removal of the cast
- Fasciotomy

Complication
- Volkmann's contracture

Fat Embolism Syndrome
Pathophysiology
- Bone fracture results in a rise of pressure in the bone marrow
- Fat globules enter the bloodstream
- Combine with platelets
- Travel throughout the body
- Occluding small blood vessels
- Causes tissue ischemia

Manifestations
- Confusion
- Changes in level of consciousness
- Pulmonary edema
- Impaired surfactant production
- Atelectasis
- Petechiae
- ARDS
- Prevention
- Early stabilization of long bone fracture

DEEP VENOUS THROMBOSIS

11. A deep venous thrombosis is a blood clot that forms along the intimal lining of a large vein.

12. Precursors linked to DVT are venous stasis, injury to the blood vessel walls, and altered blood coagulation.

13. Manifestations of DVT include swelling, leg pain, tenderness, or cramping. Some DVTs are asymptomatic.

14. Diagnosis is often made by Doppler ultrasound of the extremity.

15. Treatment includes bed rest and thrombolytic agents. Heparin may be administered to prevent subsequent clots. A vena cava filter may be inserted. Thrombectomy may be necessary.

16. Prevention is the best treatment for DVT. Early immobilization of fractures and early mobilization of the client are imperative.

INFECTION

17. Infection may result from contamination at the time of injury or during surgery. *Clostridium* infection is particularly serious because it may lead to gas gangrene and cellulitis. Any infection may delay healing and result in osteomyelitis.

DELAYED UNION AND NONUNION

18. Delayed union is the prolonged healing of bones beyond the usual time period.

19. Risks for delayed union include poor nutrition, inadequate immobilization, prolonged reduction time, infection, necrosis, age, immunosuppression, and severe bone trauma with multiple fragments.

20. Delayed union may lead to nonunion, which can cause persistent pain and movement at the fracture site. Nonunion may require surgical intervention.

REFLEX SYMPATHETIC DYSTROPHY

21. Reflex sympathetic dystrophy may occur after musculoskeletal or nerve trauma. Manifestations include persistent pain, hyperesthesias, swelling, changes in skin color and texture, changes in temperature, and decreased motion.

22. Treatment modalities include administration of a sympathetic nervous system blocking agent.

Treatment
- Intubation and mechanical ventilation
- Fluid balance
- Corticosteroids

Deep Vein Thrombosis
- Manifestations
  ○ Swelling
  ○ Leg pain
  ○ Tenderness
  ○ Cramping
  ○ Some are asymptomatic
- Diagnosis
  ○ Doppler ultrasound
- Treatment
  ○ Bed rest
  ○ Thrombolytic agents
  ○ Heparin
  ○ Vena cava filter
  ○ Thrombectomy
- Prevention is the best treatment
  ○ Early immobilization of fractures
  ○ Early mobilization of the client

Reflex Sympathetic Dystrophy
- May occur after musculoskeletal or nerve trauma
- Manifestations
  ○ Persistent pain
  ○ Hyperesthesias
  ○ Swelling
  ○ Changes in skin color and texture
  ○ Changes in temperature
  ○ Decreased motion
- Treatment
  ○ Administration of sympathetic nervous system blocking agent

---

SUGGESTIONS FOR CLASSROOM ACTIVITIES

- Use the information in the case study about a client with fractures that is provided on the textbook Companion Website to develop a plan of care for a client who has sustained a fracture.

SUGGESTIONS FOR CLINICAL ACTIVITIES

- Assign students to the care of a client who has sustained a fracture. Have the students list the specific assessment details they will look for when monitoring for development of complications. Have students identify nursing interventions appropriate if complications occur.

LEARNING OUTCOME 4

Discuss the purposes and related nursing interventions for casts, traction, and stump care.

CONCEPTS FOR LECTURE

TRACTION

1. Traction is the application of a straightening or pulling force to return or maintain the fractured bones in normal anatomic position.
2. In manual traction, the hand directly applies the pulling force.
3. In skin traction, the traction apparatus is applied to the client's skin. Buck's traction is an example of skin traction. The advantages of skin traction are the relative ease of use and ability to maintain comfort. The disadvantage is that the weight required to maintain normal body alignment or fracture alignment cannot exceed the tolerance of the skin.
4. Balanced suspension traction involves more than one force of pull. The advantage of this type of traction is that it increases mobility without threatening joint continuity. The disadvantage is that the increased use of multiple weights makes the client more likely to slide in bed.
5. Skeletal traction is the application of a pulling force through placement of pins into the bone. The advantage of this type of traction is that more weight can be used to maintain the proper anatomic alignment if necessary. The disadvantage includes increased anxiety, increased risk of infection, and increased discomfort.
6. Nursing interventions include careful management of traction weights and ropes, assessment of the skin or pin sites, frequent neurovascular assessment, and monitoring for the hazards associated with immobility.

CASTS

7. A cast is a rigid device applied to immobilize the injured bones and promote healing. The cast is applied to immobilize the joint above and joint below the fractured area.
8. Casts may be plaster or fiberglass and are applied over a thin cushion of padding. The cast is molded to the shape of the body.
9. Nursing responsibilities include performing frequent neurovascular assessment, monitoring for the development of "hot spots" that indicate infection, and monitoring for drainage on the cast. The nurse also teaches the client and family regarding cast care.
10. No pressure should be applied to the cast until it is dry and nothing should be inserted into the cast. The cast should be kept dry.

POWERPOINT LECTURE SLIDES

Traction
- In manual traction, hand directly applies the pulling force
- In skin traction, the traction apparatus is applied to the client's skin
- Balanced suspension traction involves more than one force of pull
- Skeletal traction—application of a pulling force through placement of pins into the bone
- Nursing interventions—careful management of traction weights and ropes, assessment of the skin or pin sites, frequent neurovascular assessment, and monitoring for the hazards associated with immobility

Casts
- Rigid device applied to immobilize the injured bones
- Immobilize the joint above and joint below
- Application
  - Plaster or fiberglass
  - Applied over padding
  - Molded to shape of body
- Nursing responsibilities
  - Frequent neurovascular assessment
  - Monitoring for the development of "hot spots"
  - Monitoring for drainage
  - Cast care teaching
- Cast care
  - No pressure to cast
  - Nothing should be inserted into cast
  - Cast should be kept dry

LEARNING OUTCOME 5

Explain the causes, levels, types, and potential complications (infection, delayed healing, chronic stump pain, phantom pain, and contractures) of an amputation.

CONCEPTS FOR LECTURE

1. An amputation is the partial or total removal of a body part and may be the result of an acute event or a chronic condition.
2. Peripheral vascular disease is the major cause of amputation of the lower extremities. Risk factors include hypertension, diabetes, smoking, peripheral neuropathy, and hyperlipidemia.
3. Upper extremity amputation often results from a traumatic event such as motor vehicle crashes, workplace machinery accidents, frostbite, burns, and electrocutions.
4. Amputations result from the interruption of blood flow. Following acute amputations, replantation of fingers, small body parts, and entire limbs has been successful. Chronic disease progression begins with circulation impairment and edema development. Status ulcers develop and become infected, which further compromises circulation. Development of gangrene requires amputation.
5. Amputation above or below the elbow are both termed as arm amputation. Amputation of the leg is designated as below the knee (BKA) or above the knee (AKA). An open amputation (Guillotine) is performed perpendicularly to the extremity and leaves an open wound. Open amputation is often used in the face of infection. Closed (flap) amputation leaves a flap of skin to cover the end of the wound.
6. Following amputation a rigid or compression dressing is applied to prevent infection and minimize edema. Proper healing of the amputation site is essential for the prosthesis to fit well.
7. Complications of amputation include infection, delayed healing, chronic stump pain and phantom pain, and contracture.
8. Traumatic amputation generally results in a higher risk of infection than a planned amputation, but risk is related to the client's general health status. Infection may

POWERPOINT LECTURE SLIDES

Amputation
- Partial or total removal of a body part
- May be the result of an acute event or a chronic condition

Risk Factors
- Peripheral vascular disease
- Hypertension
- Diabetes
- Smoking
- Peripheral neuropathy
- Hyperlipidemia
- Trauma

Pathophysiology
- Interruption of blood flow
- Circulation impairment
- Edema development
- Status ulcers develop/become infected
- Development of gangrene

Types of Amputation
- Above or below the elbow: arm amputation
- Leg amputation
  - Below the knee (BKA)
  - Above the knee (AKA)
- Open amputation (Guillotine)
- Closed (flap) amputation

Post Amputation Care
- Rigid or compression dressing is applied
  - Prevents infection
  - Minimize edema

Complications
- Infection
- Delayed healing
- Chronic stump pain
- Phantom pain
- Contracture

be localized or systemic and manifests as drainage, odor, redness, or increased discomfort at the wound site, fever, increased heart rate, decreased blood pressure, chills, and positive blood or wound cultures.

9. Delayed healing will result from infection or compromise of circulation.

10. Chronic stump pain is the result of neuroma formation, which causes severe burning pain. Medications, nerve blocks, transcutaneous electrical nerve stimulation, and surgical stump reconstruction are used as treatment.

11. Phantom limb sensation is the common experience of sensations such as tingling, numbness, cramping, or itching in an amputated body part. When this sensation is painful, it is called phantom limb pain. Treatments include pain management, TENS, and surgical procedures.

12. A contracture is an abnormal flexion and fixation of a joint that is caused by muscle atrophy and shortening. Contracture of the joint above the amputation is common and can be lessened by educating the client to extend the joint.

13. Nursing diagnoses commonly applicable to a client with an amputation include: *Acute Pain; Risk for Infection; Risk for Impaired Skin Integrity; Impaired Physical Mobility;* and *Disturbed Body Image.*

SUGGESTIONS FOR CLASSROOM ACTIVITIES

- Review the care plan activity about below the knee amputation that is provided on the textbook Companion Website. Use this activity to help students design a plan of care for a client who has experienced amputation.
- Discuss the psychologic support of a client who is undergoing amputation.
- Have students explore the internet for types of prostheses.

SUGGESTIONS FOR CLINICAL ACTIVITIES

- Have an RN who has cared for clients with amputation talk to students regarding stump care.
- Have students practice dressing an amputation stump on anatomic models.
- Have students identify risk factors that are present in clinical clients that might someday lead to amputation. Have students identify health promotion activities to help clients avoid that eventuality.

LEARNING OUTCOME 6

Describe the pathophysiology, interdisciplinary care, and nursing care for repetitive use injuries: carpal tunnel syndrome, bursitis, and epicondylitis.

CONCEPTS FOR LECTURE

1. Repeatedly twisting and turning the wrist, pronating and supinating the forearm, kneeling, or raising the arms over the head can result in repetitive use injuries.

2. Carpal tunnel syndrome is caused by narrowing of the carpal tunnel through the wrist and irritation of the flexor tendon and median nerve that pass through that tunnel. Manifestations are numbness and tingling of the thumb, index finger, and lateral ventral surface of the middle finger. History of computer use, jackhammer operation, mechanical work, or gymnastics, radial bone fracture, or rheumatoid arthritis is common.

POWERPOINT LECTURE SLIDES

Carpal Tunnel Syndrome
- Narrowing of the carpal tunnel through the wrist
  ○ Irritation of the flexor tendon and median nerve
- Manifestations
  ○ Numbness and tingling
    - Thumb
    - Index finger
    - Lateral ventral surface of the middle finger

3. Bursitis is an inflammation of a bursa. The bursae that most commonly become inflamed are in the shoulder, hip, leg, and elbow. Manifestations include a warm, edematous, reddened area around the involved joint. Movement of the joint is painful.
4. Epicondylitis is the inflammation of the tendon at its point of origin into the bone. It is also known as tennis elbow and golfer's elbow. Exact pathophysiology is unknown, but may be related to microvascular trauma or inflammation of the tendon. Manifestations are point tenderness, pain radiating down the dorsal surface of the forearm, and a history of repetitive use.
5. Treatment of repetitive use injuries is first by conservative management such as immobilization and rest. Ice may be applied for the first 24 to 48 hours of treatment, followed by heat application every 4 hours.
6. Surgical treatment for carpal tunnel syndrome includes resection of the carpal ligament to enlarge the tunnel. In epicondylitis and bursitis, calcified deposits may be removed from the area around the tendon or bursa.
7. Nursing diagnoses include: *Acute Pain* and *Impaired Physical Mobility*.

- Risk factors
  - Computer use
  - Jackhammer operation
  - Mechanical work
  - Gymnastics
  - Radial bone fracture history
  - Rheumatoid arthritis

Bursitis
- Inflammation of a bursa
  - Shoulder, hip, leg, and elbow
- Manifestations
  - Warm, edematous, reddened area around joint
  - Movement of joint is painful

Epicondylitis
- Inflammation of tendon at point of origin into bone
  - Tennis elbow
  - Golfer's elbow
- Pathophysiology
  - Unknown
  - Microvascular trauma
  - Inflammation of the tendon
- Manifestations
  - Point tenderness
  - Pain radiating down dorsal surface of forearm
  - History of repetitive use

Treatment
- Conservative management
  - Immobilization and rest
  - Ice for the first 24 to 48 hours
  - Followed by heat application every 4 hours

Surgical Treatment
- Carpal tunnel syndrome
  - Resection of the carpal ligament
  - Enlarges the tunnel
- Epicondylitis and bursitis
  - Removal of calcified deposits

Nursing Diagnoses
- Acute pain
- Impaired physical mobility

SUGGESTIONS FOR CLASSROOM ACTIVITIES

- Have students identify risk factors for the development of repetitive use injuries. Discuss how nursing teaching interventions can help clients avoid those risk factors.
- Have students research the treatment options for repetitive use injuries.
- Use anatomic models to demonstrate the pathophysiology of repetitive use injuries. Using the same models, demonstrate treatment options.

SUGGESTIONS FOR CLINICAL ACTIVITIES

- Have students assess clinical clients for risk factors for development of repetitive use injuries.
- Discuss nursing interventions specific to repetitive use injuries. Help students implement interventions as appropriate.

Chapter 42
Nursing Care of Clients with Musculoskeletal Disorders

Resource Library

PRENTICE HALL NURSING MEDIALINK DVD-ROM

Audio Glossary
NCLEX-RN® Review
Animations
  Arthritis
  Carpal Tunnel
  Muscular Dystrophy
  Osteoporosis

COMPANION WEBSITE

Audio Glossary
NCLEX-RN® Review
Care Plan Activity: Lower Back Pain
Case Studies:
  Diet and Gout
  Hip Replacement
  Rheumatoid Arthritis
MediaLink Applications
  Compartment Syndrome
  Osteoporosis Prevention
Links to Resources

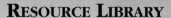 IMAGE LIBRARY

Figure 42.1 Spinal changes caused by osteoporosis.
Figure 42.2 Typical interphalangeal joint changes associated with osteoarthritis.
Figure 42.3 Total hip prosthesis.
Figure 42.4 Total knee replacement.
Figure 42.5 Joint inflammation and destruction in rheumatoid arthritis.
Figure 42.6 Typical hand deformities associated with rheumatoid arthritis.
Figure 42.7 The butterfly rash of systemic lupus erythematosus.

Figure 42.8 Osteomyelitis.
Figure 42.9 Characteristic skin changes of scleroderma.
Figure 42.10 Location of "tender points" in fibromyalgia.
Figure 42.11 Common deformities of the spinal column.
Figure 42.12 Hallux valgus (bunion).
Figure 42.13 Morton's neuroma.

Learning Outcome 1

Explain the pathophysiology, manifestations, complications, interdisciplinary care, and nursing care of metabolic, degenerative, autoimmune, inflammatory, infectious, neoplastic, connective tissue, and structural musculoskeletal disorders.

Concepts for Lecture
Gout

1. Gout is a metabolic disease that occurs from an inflammatory response to the production or excretion of uric acid that results in high levels of uric acid in the blood and in other body fluids, including synovial fluid.
2. Gout has an acute onset, usually at night, and often involves the first metatarsophalangeal joint (great toe). Deposits in the synovial fluids cause acute inflammation of the joint (gouty arthritis). Urate deposits in subcutaneous tissues cause the formation of small white nodules or tophi.

PowerPoint Lecture Slides

Osteomalacia
  • Adult rickets
  • Characterized by inadequate/delayed mineralization of bone
    ○ Results in softening of bones

Etiology
  • Insufficient calcium absorption
    ○ Due to a lack of calcium
  • Resistance to the action of vitamin D
  • Increased losses of phosphorus through the urine

3. Manifestations of gout are hyperuricemia, recurrent attacks of inflammation of a single joint, tophi in and around the joint, renal disease, and renal stones. Manifestations occur in three stages.

4. Asymptomatic hyperuricemia manifests serum levels that average 9–10 mg/dL. Most clients will not progress past this stage of the disease.

5. Acute gouty arthritis is the second stage. An acute attack or "flare" occurs unexpectedly, usually at night and affecting only one joint. It may be triggered by trauma, alcohol ingestion, dietary excess, or a stressor such as surgery. The attack may be accompanied by fever and elevation of WBC and sedimentation rate. Acute attacks last from several hours to several weeks and typically subside spontaneously.

6. After the initial gouty arthritis attack, an "intercritical period" occurs that may last up to 10 years before disease progression.

7. Tophaceous or chronic gout occurs when hyperuricemia is not treated. Tophi develop in cartilage, synovial membranes, tendons, and soft tissues. The skin over the tophi may ulcerate and exude chalky material that contains inflammatory cells and urate crystals.

8. Complications of gout include kidney disease.

9. Diagnostic testing includes measurement of serum uric acid, WBC count, eosinophil sedimentation levels, 24-hour urine collection for uric acid production and excretion, and analysis of fluid aspirated from acutely inflamed joint or material aspirated from a tophus.

10. Dietary management of gout may include a low-purine diet. High purine foods include all meats and seafood, yeast, beans, peas, lentils, oatmeal, spinach, asparagus, cauliflower, and mushrooms. The obese client is encouraged to lose weight. Fluid intake should be liberal.

11. Bed rest is prescribed during an acute attack of gouty arthritis and should be continued for 24 hours after the attack has subsided.

12. Nursing diagnoses include: Acute Pain and Impaired Physical Mobility.

OSTEOMALACIA

13. Osteomalacia, or adult rickets, is a metabolic bone disorder characterized by inadequate or delayed mineralization of bone matrix in mature compact and spongy bone, which results in softening of bones.

14. The two main causes of osteomalacia are insufficient calcium absorption in the intestine due to a lack of calcium or resistance to the action of vitamin D and increased losses of phosphorus through the urine.

15. Vitamin D is inactive when it is absorbed from the intestine or synthesized from exposure to ultraviolet light. The two step process necessary for vitamin D to become active includes 1) the transport of vitamin D in the blood to the liver where it is converted to calcidiol, and 2) transport of the calcidiol to the kidney where it is transformed to an active form, calcitriol.

Incidence
- Almost nonexistent in United States
  - Vitamin D fortified foods
- Incidence increasing
  - Older adults
  - Very-low-birth-weight infants
  - Strict vegetarian diets

Pathophysiology
- Vitamin D is inactive when absorbed
- Activation process
  - Transport of vitamin D to liver
    - Conversion to calcidiol
  - Transport of the calcidiol to kidney
    - Transformation to calcitriol

Manifestations
- Bone pain
- Tenderness
- Pathologic fractures, commonly
  - Distal radius
  - Proximal femur

Diagnostic Testing
- Serum calcium
- Parathyroid hormone
- Alkaline phosphatase

Nursing Management
- Assessing current diet
- Exposure to ultraviolet light
- Pain level
- Fracture status
- Muscle weakness
- Client education

Muscular Dystrophy
- Group of inherited muscle diseases
- Cause progressive muscle degeneration and wasting

Duchenne's Muscular Dystrophy
- Most common form
- Inherited as recessive single gene defect on X chromosome
- Transmitted from mother to male children

Manifestations
- Early childhood onset
- Average lifespan 15 years

Pathophysiology
- Vascular and neurogenic theories
- Membrane theory

Progression of Illness
- Progressive muscle weakness
- Difficulty with ambulation
  - Wheelchair and bed-bound
- Cardiac, endocrine, and mental function abnormalities

16. Inadequate mineralization of bone results in gross deformities of the long bones, spine, pelvis, and skull.
17. Manifestations include bone pain and tenderness and pathologic fractures of commonly weakened areas such as the distal radius and proximal femur.
18. Laboratory testing includes serum calcium, parathyroid hormone, and alkaline phosphatase levels.
19. Nursing management includes assessing the client's current dietary intake of vitamin D, calcium and phosphorus, exposure to ultraviolet light, pain level, fracture status, and muscle weakness. Client education should include sources of vitamin D, calcium, and phosphorus, safety measures to prevent falls, and use of assistive devices such as walkers, canes, or crutches.

MUSCULAR DYSTROPHY

20. Muscular dystrophy (MD) is a group of inherited muscle diseases that cause progressive muscle degeneration and wasting. The differences in types of MD relate to age at onset, gender affected, muscles involved, and rate at which the disease progresses.
21. Duchenne's muscular dystrophy is the most common form of MD. It is inherited as a recessive single gene defect on the X chromosome and is transmitted from the mother to male children. Manifestations begin early in childhood with the average lifespan being about 15 years after onset.
22. Three theories of pathophysiology have been proposed. The vascular and neurogenic theories suggest that the cause is a lack of blood supply to the muscle or a disturbance in the interaction between the nerve and muscle. The membrane theory suggests that an alteration in the cell membranes of the muscle causes them to degenerate.
23. All forms of MD exhibit manifestations of muscle weakness. As the disease progresses, the person develops difficulty with ambulation and eventually becomes wheelchair and bed-bound. Cardiac, endocrine, and mental function abnormalities may also be involved.
24. Since there is no cure or specific treatment for MD, care focuses on preserving and promoting mobility.
25. The primary nursing diagnosis is *Self-Care Deficit.*

ANKYLOSING SPONDYLITIS

26. Ankylosing spondylitis (AS) is a chronic inflammatory arthritis that primarily affects the axial skeleton, which leads to pain and progressive stiffening and fusion of the spine.
27. The cause of AS is unknown. Early inflammatory changes often are first noted in the sacroiliac joints. The joints of the spine are also affected with gradual calcification and ossifications that leads to ankylosis, or joint consolidation and immobility. The eyes, lungs, heart, and kidneys may also be affected.
28. AS is generally of slow and insidious onset. Initial manifestations may include persistent or intermittent

- Interdisciplinary care
- No cure or specific treatment
- Care focuses on preserving and promoting mobility

Nursing Diagnoses
- *Self-Care Deficit*

bouts of back pain that are worse at night, followed by morning stiffness that is relieved by activity. As the disease progresses, back motion becomes limited, the lumbar curve is lost, and the thoracic curvature is accentuated. The entire spine may become fused, which prevents any motion.

29. Systemic manifestations include anorexia, weight loss, fever, and fatigue. Many clients develop uveitis, which is inflammation of the iris and middle vascular layer of the eye.

30. Diagnostic testing reveals elevation of the ESR during periods of active disease and a positive HLA-B27 antigen. The diagnosis is generally confirmed by x-ray.

31. Disease management focuses on maintaining mobility and pain relief. Severe cases may require total hip replacement.

32. Nursing care is focused on supportive care and education.

REACTIVE ARTHRITIS

33. Reactive arthritis (ReA; also known as Reiter's syndrome) is an acute, nonpurulent inflammatory arthritis that is believed to be a response to an exposure or infection with certain types of bacteria.

34. The initial manifestation of ReA is often nonbacterial urethritis. Conjunctivitis and inflammatory arthritis follow. Large weight-bearing joints such as the knees and ankles are often affected. Manifestations generally occur 2–4 weeks after infection and subside in 3–12 months.

35. Systemic manifestations of ReA include inflammation of the glans penis, mouth ulcers, and skin lesions. The heart and aorta may also be involved.

36. Diagnosis of ReA is generally based on client history and presenting symptoms. The disease tends to recur.

37. When chlamydia is suspected as the causative agent, the client and sexual partners are treated with tetracycline (Achromycin) or erythromycin (Akne-Mycin). NSAIDs are also used to treat arthritic manifestations.

38. The nursing role is primarily educative.

SYSTEMIC LUPUS ERYTHEMATOSUS

39. Systemic lupus erythematosus (SLE) is a chronic inflammatory connective tissue disease. It affects all body systems.

40. SLE can range from a mild episodic disorder to a rapidly fatal disease process.

41. The exact etiology of SLE is unknown. Genetic, environmental, and hormonal factors may play a role in its development.

42. The pathophysiology of SLE involves the production of a large variety of autoantibodies against normal body components such as nucleic acids, erythrocytes, coagulation proteins, lymphocytes, and platelets.

43. These autoantibodies react with their corresponding antigen to form immune complexes which are then

deposited in the connective tissues of blood vessels, lymphatic vessels, and other tissues. The kidneys are a frequent site of this deposition and damage.

44. A number of drugs may produce a syndrome that mimics SLE. Procainamide (Procan), hydralazine (Alazine), and isoniazid (INH) are the most common drugs implicated.

45. Early manifestations include fever, anorexia, malaise, weight loss, arthralgias, and polyarthritis. Skin manifestations are common, with a characteristic red butterfly rash across the cheeks and the bridge of the nose. Alopecia is common.

46. Diagnosis can be difficult because of the variety of body systems involved. Typically diagnostic testing includes anti-DNA antibody testing, ESR rates, serum complement levels, CBC, UA, and kidney biopsy.

47. Because of the photosensitivity associated with SLE, the client should be cautioned to avoid sun exposure.

48. There may be a link between estrogen in oral contraceptives and acute episodes of SLE.

49. Nursing diagnoses include: *Impaired Skin Integrity; Ineffective Protection;* and *Impaired Health Maintenance.*

POLYMYOSITIS

50. Polymyositis is a systemic connective-tissue disorder characterized by inflammation of connective tissue and muscle fibers that leads to muscle weakness and atrophy. When muscle fiber inflammation is accompanied by skin lesions, the disease is known as dermatomyositis.

51. The immune mechanism that causes this inflammatory response is not clear, but autoantibodies can be identified in most clients. The activation of complement is also thought to contribute to the inflammatory process.

52. Initial manifestations include muscle pain, tenderness, and weakness; rash; arthralgias; fatigue; fever; and weight loss. Skeletal muscle weakness is the predominant manifestation.

53. A characteristic dusky red rash may be present on the face and upper trunk.

54. Other manifestations include Raynaud's phenomenon, dysphagia, dyspnea, and cough. Risk for malignancy is increased.

55. A combination of rest and corticosteroid therapy is prescribed for the client with polymyositis.

56. Nursing care is predominantly supportive and educative.

LYME DISEASE

57. Lyme disease is an inflammatory disorder caused by the spirochete *Borrelia burgdorferi*, which is transmitted primarily by ticks. It is the most commonly reported tick-borne illness in the United States.

58. After an incubation period of up to 30 days, a characteristic lesion called erythema migrans forms. This lesion is flat or slightly raised and red. It expands over several days with a central clear area as it expands. The infection may also spread via lymph or blood to other skin sites, nodes, or organs.

59. The inflammatory joint changes of Lyme disease closely resemble those of rheumatoid arthritis.

60. The typical progression of Lyme disease is an initial flu-like illness and a skin rash, followed weeks or months later by Bell's palsy or meningitis, and months to years later by arthritis.

61. Complications of Lyme disease include chronic recurrent arthritis, meningitis, encephalitis, neuropathies, myocarditis, and heart block.

62. Antibodies to *B. burgdorferi* can be detected by either ELISA or Western blot methods within 2–4 weeks of the initial skin lesion.

63. Early diagnosis and proper antibiotic treatment of Lyme disease are important to preventing the complications of infections.

64. Nursing care focuses on prevention of the disease through protection from tick bites and management of tick bite should it occur.

Osteomyelitis

65. Osteomyelitis is an infection of the bone and may occur as an acute, subacute, or chronic process.

66. The cause of osteomyelitis is usually bacterial.

67. Direct contamination of the bone from an open wound is the most common cause.

68. Bacterial invasion of the bone results in a destruction of bone tissue and development of pus, edema, and vascular congestion. Ischemia and eventual necrosis occurs. Blood and antibiotics cannot reach the bone tissue once pressure compromises the vascular and arteriolar systems.

69. Hematogenous osteomyelitis is caused by pathogens that are carried in the blood from sites of infection elsewhere in the body. The spine is the usual site of infection in adults.

70. Osteomyelitis from a contiguous infection is a classification of osteomyelitis in which the infection is caused by an extension of infection from adjacent soft tissues. This is the most common cause of osteomyelitis in adults. This condition may be difficult to diagnosis because of the local tissue inflammation already present. Failure to heal a surgical wound or fracture or development of a sinus tract infection may be initial indicators of infection.

71. Osteomyelitis associated with vascular insufficiency is often associated with people who have diabetes and peripheral vascular disease.

72. Manifestations of osteomyelitis vary according to age of the client; cause and site of involvement; and whether the infection is acute, subacute, or chronic.

73. The care of the client with osteomyelitis focuses on relieving pain, eliminating the infection, and preventing or minimizing complications.

74. Diagnosis is based on bone scans, magnetic resonance imaging, blood tests, and biopsy.

75. Surgical debridement is the primary treatment for the client with chronic osteomyelitis.

76. Nursing diagnoses include: *Risk for Infection; Hyperthermia; Impaired Physical Mobility;* and *Acute Pain.*

SEPTIC ARTHRITIS

77. Septic arthritis can develop if a joint space is invaded by a pathogen. The primary risk factors are persistent bacteremia and previous joint damage.

78. The most common bacteria implicated in septic arthritis are *gonococci, Staphylococcus aureus,* and *streptococci. E. coli* and *Pseudomonas* are evolving as causative agents, especially in those who inject recreational drugs or are immunocompromised.

79. Joint infection may result in abscesses in synovial tissues or the bone underlying joint cartilage.

80. Manifestations include abrupt onset of pain and stiffness in the affected joint. The joint appears red and swollen and is hot and tender to touch. Effusion is generally present.

81. Septic arthritis is a medical emergency that requires prompt treatment to preserve joint function.

82. Cultures of joint aspirate and from likely sources of infection are obtained.

83. Treatment is rest, immobilization, and elevation of the infected joint, along with systemic antibiotic therapy.

84. Frequent joint aspirations or surgical drainage of the joint may be necessary.

85. Nursing care is supportive and educative.

BONE TUMORS

86. Bone tumors may be either benign or malignant. Benign bone tumors tend to grow slowly and do not often destroy surrounding tissues. Malignant tumors grow rapidly and metastasize.

87. Primary malignancies of the bone are rare. The most common metastatic bone tumors originate from primary tumors in the prostate, breast, kidney, thyroid, and lung.

88. Primary malignancies are most common during peak growth as in adolescence or Paget's disease. Osteolysis occurs which weakens the bone and results in fracture.

89. Malignant tumors invade and destroy adjacent bone structures.

90. Benign tumors often result in pathologic fracture.

91. The three manifestations of bone tumor are pain, presence of a mass, and impaired function.

92. Treatment and care of clients with bone tumors focuses on prompt diagnosis, removal of the tumor, prevention of complications, and client education.

93. Diagnosis may be achieved by x-ray, CT scan, MRI, and needle biopsy. Laboratory tests include alkaline phosphatase and calcium levels.

94. Chemotherapeutic agents are administered to shrink the tumor before surgery, to control recurrence of tumor growth after surgery, or to treat metastasis of the tumor.

95. Radiation therapy may be used in combination with chemotherapy and is often used as a method of pain control.

96. The goal of surgery in the treatment of primary bone tumors is to eliminate the tumor completely.

97. Nursing diagnoses include: *Risk for Injury; Acute Pain; Chronic Pain; Impaired Physical Mobility;* and *Decisional Conflict.*

SCLERODERMA

98. Systemic sclerosis or scleroderma is a hardening of the skin. This is a chronic disease characterized by the formation of excess fibrous connective tissue and diffuse fibrosis of the skin and internal organs.

99. The etiology of scleroderma is unknown. Genetic, immune, and environmental factors are thought to play a role.

100. Scleroderma may be either localized and affect the skin only, or generalized (systemic scleroderma) with both skin and visceral organ involvement.

101. Those clients with limited systemic disease may manifest CREST syndrome. CREST syndrome is a combination of <u>c</u>alcinosis, <u>R</u>aynaud's phenomenon, <u>e</u>sophageal dysfunction, <u>s</u>clerodactyly, and <u>t</u>elangiectasia.

102. Initial manifestations are usually noted in the skin which thickens markedly. Diffuse, nonpitting edema is also noted. As the disease progresses, the skin atrophies and becomes taut, shiny, and hyperpigmented. This skin tightness may limit mobility and ability to take oral nutrition.

103. Visceral symptoms include dysphagia, exertional dyspnea, pericarditis, dysrhythmias, bowel changes with cramping, proteinuria, hematuria, hypertension, and renal failure.

104. There is no specific test for systemic sclerosis. An ANA titer of 1:40 or higher is the most sensitive test for diagnosis. Other tests are CBC and ESR. A skin biopsy may be done to confirm diagnosis.

105. Physical therapy is an important part of the management of systemic sclerosis to maintain mobility of affected tissues, the hands and face in particular.

106. Nursing care focuses on maintaining skin integrity, support of nutritional intake, support of mental health, and support of respiratory function.

SJOGREN'S SYNDROME

107. Sjogren's syndrome is an autoimmune disorder that causes inflammation and dysfunction of exocrine glands throughout the body.

108. Exocrine glands in many areas of the body are destroyed by the infiltration of lymphocytes and deposition of immune complexes. The salivary and lacrimal glands are particularly affected.
109. Manifestations include xerophthalmia, xerostomia, parotid gland enlargement arthritis, dysphagia, pancreatitis, pleuritis, migraine, and vasculitis.
110. Clients with Sjogren's syndrome have a greatly increased risk of developing malignant lymphoma.
111. Diagnosis is often based upon the client's history and clinical presentation. Schirmer's test, which measures the quantity of tears produced in 5 minutes in response to irritation, ocular staining, and slit-lamp examination of the eye may be performed. Definitive diagnosis may result from biopsy of either the lacrimal or salivary gland.
112. Medications that increase mouth dryness, such as atropine and decongestants, should be avoided.
113. Nursing care focuses on symptom relief and education regarding protection of the eyes and oral mucosa.

FIBROMYALGIA

114. Fibromyalgia is a common rheumatic syndrome characterized by musculoskeletal pain, stiffness, and tenderness.
115. The etiology of fibromyalgia is unknown, but possible causes are sleep disorders, depression, infections, and an altered perception of normal stimuli.
116. No inflammatory, structural, or physiologic muscle changes have been demonstrated in fibromyalgia.
117. A gradual onset of chronic, achy muscle pain is typical, although the onset may be sudden, occasionally following a viral illness. Pain may be localized or systemic and can be produced by palpating localized "tender points." Systemic manifestations include fatigue, sleep disruptions, headaches, morning stiffness, painful menstrual periods, and problems with thinking and memory.
118. Criteria for diagnosis are a history of widespread pain that has been present for at least 3 months and pain at 11 of the 18 tender points on palpation.
119. This disorder may resolve spontaneously or become chronic and recurrent. Treatment measures include local heat applications, massage, stretching exercises, and sleep improvement.
120. Amitriptyline (Amitril) has been shown to promote better sleep and relieve manifestations of fibromyalgia.
121. Nursing care is supportive and educational. Validation of the client's concerns is important.

SPINAL DEFORMITIES

122. Scoliosis and kyphosis are the two most common deformities of the spinal column.
123. Scoliosis is a lateral curvature of the spine.
124. Scoliosis is classified as postural when the small curve corrects with bending and structural when the curve does not correct with bending. The lateral curve is

usually evident in the thoracic, lumbar, or thoracolumbar regions of the spine.

125. Manifestations of scoliosis are one shoulder that is higher than the other, a prominent hip, or a projecting scapula. Pain, shortness of breath, and GI disturbances may be present.

126. Kyphosis is excessive angulation of the normal posterior curve of the thoracic spine and is also classified as postural or structural.

127. Postural kyphosis is caused by a slumping posture. Structural kyphosis may result from congenital malformations, rickets, poliomyelitis, vertebral tuberculosis, Paget's disease, osteoporosis, or osteomalacia. Kyphosis may also occur from surgical removal or radiation of intervertebral discs.

128. Manifestations include moderate back pain and increased curvature of the spine or a "hunchback" appearance. Impaired mobility and respiratory problems may occur.

129. Interdisciplinary care focuses on screening for development and accurate diagnosis. A scoliometer is used to quantify the amount of curvature.

130. Conservative therapy includes braces, electrical stimulation, and traction in children and weight reduction, active and passive exercises and the use of braces in adults.

131. Surgery may include attaching metal reinforcing rods to the spine.

132. Nursing diagnoses include: *Risk for Injury* and *Risk for Peripheral Neurovascular Dysfunction.*

LOW BACK PAIN

133. Acute and chronic low back pain involves the lumbar, lumbosacral, or sacroiliac areas of the back and is generally due to abnormal stress or overuse.

134. There are five general causes of low back pain. Local pain is caused by compression or irritation of sensory nerves. Referred pain may originate from abdominal or pelvic viscera. Pain of spinal origin may be referred to the buttocks, groin, or legs. Radicular back pain is sharp, and radiates from the back to the leg along a nerve route. Muscle spasm pain is dull and may be accompanied by abnormal posture and taut spinal muscles.

135. Manifestations are pain that ranges from mild discomfort to chronic debilitating pain.

136. Care of the client with low back pain focuses on relieving pain, correcting the condition if possible, preventing complications, and educating the client.

137. Conservative treatment is often focused on rest, combined with appropriate exercise and education. Pain may be relieved by an ice bag or hot water bottle applied to the back.

138. Physical therapy procedures include diathermy, ultrasonography, hydrotherapy, and TENS units.

139. Nursing care include health promotion activities. Nursing diagnoses include: *Acute Pain; Deficient Knowledge;* and *Risk for Impaired Adjustment.*

FOOT DISORDERS

140. Hallux valgus, hammertoe, and Morton's neuroma are common foot disorders that cause pain or difficulty walking. All are caused by wearing ill-fitting footwear.

141. Hallux valgus (bunion) is the enlargement and lateral displacement of the first metatarsal. Bunions may be a congenital disorder, but most are caused by wearing pointed, narrow-toed shoes or high heels.

142. Bunion develops when chronic pressure against the great toes causes the connective tissue in the sole of the foot to lengthen so that the stabilizing action of the great toe is gradually lost.

143. In severe cases, the lateral displacement of the great toe may approach 70–90 degrees and the second toe may be forced upward, which causes hammertoe.

144. Manifestations of bunion are the obvious physical deformity and pain.

145. Hammertoe, or "claw toe," is the dorsiflexion of the first phalanx with accompanying plantar flexion of the second and third phalanges. This condition most commonly affects the second toe.

146. As the deformity progresses, the dorsiflexed joint rubs against the overlying shoe, and causes painful corns to develop.

147. Morton's neuroma is a tumor-like mass formed within the neurovascular bundle of the intermetatarsal spaces. These tumors occur most often in the third web space.

148. Morton's neuroma develops when repeated compression of the toes causes irritation and scarring of tissues that surround the plantar digital nerve. This nerve becomes inflamed and swells, becomes fibrotic, and forms a neuroma.

149. Manifestations of Morton's neuroma are a burring pain at the web space of the affected foot that radiates into the tips of the involved toes. A palpable mass may be present.

150. Care of the client with common foot disorders focuses on relieving the pain, correcting the structural deformity, and preventing reoccurrence.

151. Conservative treatment for common foot disorders usually involves the use of corrective shoes. Analgesics may be prescribed to relieve pain and inflammation. Corticosteroid drugs may be injected into the affected joints or surrounding tissues.

152. Surgery is reserved for clients with intractable toe deformities or pain.

153. Nursing diagnoses include: *Chronic Pain* and *Risk for Infection.*

SUGGESTIONS FOR CLASSROOM ACTIVITIES

- Divide the students into small groups. Assign each group one division of the disorders covered in the Learning Outcome. Have the students identify the manifestations, complications, and nursing care of the disorders in the division assigned. Emphasize the commonalities in nursing care. Share the findings among all groups.
- Using small groups as described previously, have students search the internet for current statistics and treatment options for clients with these disorders.
- View the animation/video about muscular dystrophy that is provided on the textbook DVD-ROM. Use the information from this activity to devise nursing interventions for clients with this disorder.

SUGGESTIONS FOR CLINICAL ACTIVITIES

- Have students assess clinical clients for manifestations of the disorders covered in this chapter. Emphasize that the client may manifest these disorders even if that is not the primary reason for hospitalization.
- Discuss modifications in assessment and intervention that would be made necessary for clients with musculoskeletal disorders. Help students implement these modified techniques.

LEARNING OUTCOME 2

Compare and contrast the pathophysiology, manifestations, diagnosis, and treatments for osteoporosis, osteoarthritis, Paget's disease, and rheumatoid arthritis.

CONCEPTS FOR LECTURE
OSTEOPOROSIS

1. Osteoporosis is a metabolic bone disorder characterized by loss of bone mass, increased bone fragility, and an increased risk for fractures. Osteoporosis is most often associated with aging, but may result from an endocrine disorder or a malignancy. Risk factors are unmodifiable or modifiable.

2. Unmodifiable risk factors include aging (bone mass peaks at age 35), race, and presence of endocrine disorders such as hyperthyroidism, hyperparathyroidism, Cushing's syndrome, or diabetes mellitus.

3. Modifiable risk factors include insufficient intake of calcium, cigarette smoking, excess alcohol intake, a sedentary lifestyle, and prolonged use of medications that increase calcium excretion.

4. The exact pathophysiology of osteoporosis is unknown, but does involve an imbalance between the activity of osteoblasts that form bone and osteoclasts that resorb bone. The bone diameter increases, which thins the outer supporting cortex to the point that minimal stress will cause fracture.

5. The most common manifestations are loss of height; progressive curvature of the spine; low back pain; and fractures of the forearm, spine, or hip. The most common complication is fracture.

6. Acute episodes of vertebral body collapse are painful, with radiation of the pain around the flank into the abdomen. Slowly-occurring vertebral collapse is accompanied by little discomfort. Characteristic dorsal

POWERPOINT LECTURE SLIDES

Osteoporosis
Pathophysiology
- Exact pathophysiology unknown
  ○ Imbalance between osteoblasts and osteoclasts
  ○ Bone diameter increases
  ○ Thins outer supporting cortex
  ○ Minimal stress causes fracture

Manifestations
- Loss of height
- Progressive curvature of spine
- Low back pain
- Fractures of forearm, spine, hip
- Development of "dowager's hump"
  ○ Dorsal kyphosis
  ○ Cervical lordosis

Vertebral Body Collapse
- Acute episodes painful
- Radiation of pain around flank into abdomen
- Slowly occurring accompanied by little discomfort

Diagnosis
- Dual-energy x-ray absorptiometry (DEXA)
- Alkaline phosphatase measurement
- Serum bone GLa-protein

Nursing Care
- Prevention
  ○ Calcium intake
  ○ Exercise

kyphosis and cervical lordosis develop causing a characteristic "dowager's hump."

7. Diagnosis of osteoporosis is achieved by dual-energy x-ray absorptiometry (DEXA) measurement, alkaline phosphatase measurement, and serum bone Glaprotein testing.

8. Nursing care focuses primarily on prevention. Health promotion activities include focus on calcium intake, exercise, and health-related behaviors.

9. Nursing diagnoses include: *Health-Seeking Behaviors; Risk for Injury; Imbalanced Nutrition: Less than Body Requirements;* and *Acute Pain.*

OSTEOARTHRITIS

10. Osteoarthritis (OA) is the most common of all forms of arthritis. The disease is characterized by loss of articular cartilage in articulating joints and hypertrophy of the bones of the articular margins. OA may be idiopathic or secondary to other factors.

11. Idiopathic OA most commonly affects the terminal interphalangeal joints (Heberden's nodes) and, less often, the proximal interphalangeal joints (Bouchard's nodes), the joints of the thumb, the hip, the knee, the metatarsophalangeal joint of the big toe, and the cervical or lumbar spine.

12. Secondary OA may occur in any joint from an articular injury.

13. Idiopathic OA is associated with increasing age. The disease may be inherited as an autosomal recessive trait, with genetic defects causing premature destruction of the joint cartilage.

14. Secondary OA is associated with trauma, mechanical stress, inflammation of joint structures, joint instability, neurologic disorders, endocrine disorders, and selected medications.

15. Risk factors for the development of OA are excess weight, inactivity, strenuous or repetitive exercise, decreased estrogen, excessive growth hormone, and increased parathyroid hormone.

16. The pathophysiology of OA centers on the degradation of the cartilage that lines the joints. This degradation results in the loss of a large area of the articular cartilage and exposure of the underlying bone. Cysts can develop in the bone and cartilage-coated osteophytes change the anatomy of the joint.

17. The onset of OA is generally slow and insidious. Pain and stiffness in one or more joints are the first manifestations. The pain is generally aggravated by use or motion of the joint and relieved by rest. Joints may stiffen with immobility. Bony overgrowths may cause joint enlargement and flexion contractures may occur because of joint instability.

18. Complications of OA include degenerative disk disease with herniation, increased risk of falling, and increased risk of debilitation.

19. No treatment is available to arrest the process of joint degeneration. Appropriate management includes pain

Nursing Diagnoses
- *Health-Seeking Behaviors*
- *Risk for Injury*
- *Imbalanced Nutrition: Less than Body Requirements*
- *Acute Pain*

Osteoarthritis
Pathophysiology
- Degradation of cartilage lining joints
- Results in loss of articular cartilage, exposure of bone
- Cysts can develop in bone
- Osteophytes change joint anatomy

Manifestations
- Onset of OA generally slow and insidious
- Joint pain, stiffness
  - Aggravated by use or motion
  - Relieved by rest
  - Stiffen with immobility
- Joint enlargement
- Flexion contractures

Complications
- Degenerative disk disease with herniation
- Increased risk of falling
- Increased risk of debilitation

Interdisciplinary Treatment
- No treatment available to arrest process
- Pain control
- Maintenance of function and mobility

Conservative Treatment
- ROM exercises
- Muscle strengthening exercises
- Heat and ice
- Balance between exercise and rest
- Use of cane, crutches, or a walker
- Weight loss if indicated
- Analgesics and anti-inflammatory medications

Invasive Procedures
- Viscosupplementation

Complementary Therapies
- Biomagnetic therapy
- Acupuncture
- Elimination of nightshade foods
- Nutritional supplementation
- Herbal therapy
- Massage therapy
- Osteopathic manipulation
- Vitamin therapy
- Yoga

Nursing Diagnoses
- *Chronic Pain*
- *Impaired Physical Mobility*
- *Self-Care Deficit*

control and maintenance of the client's function and mobility.

20. OA is initially treated conservatively with ROM exercises; muscle strengthening exercises; heat and ice; a balance between exercise and rest; using a cane, crutches, or a walker; weight loss if indicated; and analgesics and anti-inflammatory medications.

21. Viscosupplementation is a new treatment for OA of the knee. Hyaluronan, a natural component of synovial fluid, is injected directly into the knee joint.

22. Complementary therapies include biomagnetic therapy; acupuncture; elimination of nightshade foods (potatoes, tomatoes, peppers, eggplant, tobacco); nutritional supplementation with glucosamine, chrondroitin, boron, zinc, copper, selenium, manganese, flavonoids, and/or SAM-e; herbal therapy; massage therapy; osteopathic manipulation; vitamin therapy; and yoga.

23. Nursing diagnoses include: *Chronic Pain; Impaired Physical Mobility;* and *Self-Care Deficit.*

PAGET'S DISEASE

24. Paget's disease is also called osteitis deformans and is a progressive metabolic skeletal disorder of the osteoclast that results from excessive metabolic activity in bone, with excessive bone resorption followed by excessive bone formation. The disorder affects bones of the axial skeleton, especially the femur, pelvis, vertebrae, and skull.

25. As the disease progresses, bones become larger and softer. Fracture is common.

26. Manifestations are bone pain, arthritis, obvious skeletal deformities, and fractures. The pain is aggravated by pressure and weight bearing, but is more noticeable at night or at rest.

27. Complications are nerve palsy syndrome, pathologic fractures, mental deterioration, tetraplegia, cardiovascular disease, and osteogenic sarcoma.

28. Diagnosis can be achieved by x-ray and bone scans.

29. Nursing diagnoses include *Chronic Pain* and *Impaired Mobility.*

RHEUMATOID ARTHRITIS

30. Rheumatoid arthritis is a chronic systemic autoimmune disease that causes inflammation of connective tissue, primarily in the joints.

31. The cause of RA is unknown, but a combination of genetic, environmental, hormonal, and reproductive factors are thought to play a role in its development.

32. It is speculated that infectious agents, such as bacteria, mycoplasmas, and viruses (especially Epstein-Barr virus) may play a role in initiating the autoimmune processes in RA. The characteristic transformed antibodies usually present in people with RA are called rheumatoid factors (RFs).

33. In RA, the synovial membrane is damaged by the inflammatory and immune processes. As the

Paget's Disease
Pathophysiology
- Results from excessive metabolic activity in bone
- Excessive bone resorption
- Followed by excessive bone formation
- Bones become larger and softer
- Fracture is common

Manifestations
- Bone pain
- Arthritis
- Obvious skeletal deformities
- Fractures

Complications
- Nerve palsy syndrome
- Pathologic fractures
- Mental deterioration
- Tetraplegia
- Cardiovascular disease
- Osteogenic sarcoma

Diagnosis
- X-ray
- Bone scans
- Nursing diagnoses
- Chronic pain
- Impaired mobility

Rheumatoid Arthritis
Pathophysiology
- Synovial membrane damaged by inflammatory, immune processes
- Synovial blood vessels are involved
- Blood supply to synovial tissue
- Hemorrhage, coagulation, deposits of fibrin
  - Synovial membrane
  - Intracellular matrix
  - Synovial fluid

Systemic Manifestations
- Fatigue
- Anorexia
- Weight loss
- Nonspecific aching and stiffness
- Fever
- Rheumatoid nodules

Joint Manifestations
- Swelling
- Stiffness
- Warmth
- Tenderness
- Pain
- "Boggy" feel
- Limitation of range of motion
- Bony deformities

Deformities
- Ulnar deviation of the fingers
- Subluxation at the MCP joints

inflammation spreads, the synovial blood vessels are involved and blood supply to the synovial tissue decreases.

34. Joint manifestations of RA are often preceded by systemic manifestations of inflammation, including fatigue, anorexia, weight loss, and nonspecific aching and stiffness. Clients report joint swelling with associated stiffness, warmth, tenderness, and pain.

35. The proximal interphalangeal (PIP) and metacarpophalangeal (MCP) joints of the fingers, the wrists, the knees, the ankles, and the toes are most frequently involved.

36. Swollen, inflamed joints feel "boggy" or sponge-like on palpation because of synovial edema. Range of motion is limited in affected joints, and weakness may be evident.

37. Persistent inflammation causes deformities of the joint and supporting structures. Characteristic changes in the hands and fingers include ulnar deviation of the fingers and subluxation at the MCP joints.

38. Swan-neck deformity is characterized by hyperextension of the PIP joint with compensatory flexion of the distal interphalangeal (DIP) joints.

39. Boutonniere deformity is characterized by flexion of the PIP joints with extension of the DIP joint.

40. Wrist involvement limits movement, and causes deformity and carpal tunnel syndrome.

41. Knee involvement manifests as swelling and instability of the knee joint along with quadriceps atrophy, contractures, and valgus deformities.

42. Typical deformities of the feet and toes include subluxation, hallux valgus, lateral deviation of the toes, and cock-up toes.

43. Extra-articular manifestations include fatigue, weakness, anorexia, weight loss, and low-grade fever. Rheumatoid nodules may develop in subcutaneous tissues or in the viscera.

44. People with autoimmune disease have an increased risk of developing coronary heart disease (CAD), which increases the risk of MI and death.

45. Once the diagnosis of RA has been made, the goals of therapy are to relieve pain, reduce inflammation, slow or stop joint damage, and improve well-being and ability to function.

46. Because a cure is not available and traditional therapies are not always effective, the client with RA is vulnerable to quackery.

47. Laboratory tests used to diagnose RA are rheumatoid factors (RFs) and the erythrocyte sedimentation rate (ESR). In a newer blood test, clients are tested for antibodies to cyclic citrullinated peptide (CCP) with accurate detection of early RA.

48. The primary objectives in treating RA are to reduce pain and inflammation, preserve function, and prevent deformity.

49. A balanced program of rest and exercise are important.

50. Physical and occupational therapists can design and monitor individualized activity and rest programs.

- Swan-neck deformity
- Boutonniere deformity
- Wrist deformity with carpal tunnel syndrome
- Instability of the knee
- Toe subluxation, hallux valgus, lateral deviation of toes, cock-up toes

Complications
- Increased risk of developing coronary heart disease
- Quackery

Interdisciplinary Care
- Goals of care
  ○ Reduce pain and inflammation
  ○ Preserve function
  ○ Prevent deformity
- Laboratory tests
  ○ Rheumatoid factors (RFs)
  ○ ESR
  ○ Antibodies to cyclic citrullinated peptide (CCP)

Treatment
- Balanced program of rest and exercise
- Physical and occupational therapy referral
- Heat and cold application
- Use of assistive devices
- Plasmapheresis
- Total lymphoid irradiation

Nursing Diagnoses
- *Chronic Pain*
- *Fatigue*
- *Disturbed Body Image*
- *Ineffective Role Performance*

51. Heat and cold are used for their analgesic and muscle-relaxing effects. Moist heat is most effective.
52. Assistive devices, such as a cane, walker, or raised toilet seat, are most useful for clients with significant hip or knee arthritis. Splints provide joint rest and prevent contractures.
53. Plasmapheresis has been used to remove circulating antibodies, which moderates the autoimmune response. Total lymphoid irradiation has had limited success.
54. Nursing diagnoses include: *Chronic Pain; Fatigue; Disturbed Body Image;* and *Ineffective Role Performance.*

SUGGESTIONS FOR CLASSROOM ACTIVITIES

- View the animation/video about arthritis that is provided on the textbook DVD-ROM. Use the information provided as a basis for discussion of the disorder.
- Use anatomic models to demonstrate the pathologic changes associated with the disorders listed.
- Ask a person who is living with severe rheumatoid arthritis to come to speak to the class about that experience.
- View the animation/video about osteoporosis that is provided on the textbook DVD-ROM. Use the information provided as a basis for discussion of the disorder.
- Review the care plan about lower back pain that is provided on the textbook DVD-ROM. Using the information provided, have students develop a plan of care for a client with this disorder.
- Review the care study about rheumatoid arthritis that is provided on the textbook DVD-ROM. Using the information provided, have students develop a plan of care for a client with this disorder.

SUGGESTIONS FOR CLINICAL ACTIVITIES

- Have students review clinical client medical records for risk factors for development of the disorders listed in this outcome. Also, have students assess the client for manifestations of these disorders. Compare the manifestations found with the risk factors noted. Share these findings in post-conference.
- Have an RN who works in dialysis speak to the group. Ask students why nurses from this specialty would be involved in caring for clients with musculoskeletal disorders.

LEARNING OUTCOME 3

Discuss the purposes, nursing implications, and health education for the client and family for medications used to treat osteoporosis, Paget's disease, gout, osteomalacia, osteoarthritis, rheumatoid arthritis, systemic lupus erythematosus, osteomyelitis, bone tumors, scleroderma, and low back pain.

CONCEPTS FOR LECTURE
OSTEOPOROSIS

1. Estrogen replacement therapy reduces bone loss, increases bone density in the spine and hip, and reduces the risk of fractures in postmenopausal women.
2. Raloxifene (Evista) is a selective estrogen receptor modulator (SERM) that appears to prevent bone loss by mimicking estrogen's beneficial effects on bone density in postmenopausal women.
3. Alendronate (Fosamax) and risedronate (Actonel) are from a class of drugs that are potent inhibitors of bone resorption.
4. Teriparatide (Forteo) is a synthetic parathyroid hormone that is administered subcutaneously to stimulate new bone formation and mass.

POWERPOINT LECTURE SLIDES

Osteoporosis
- Estrogen replacement therapy
  - Reduces bone loss
  - Increases bone density in spine/hip
  - Reduces risk of fracture in postmenopausal women
- Raloxifene
  - Selective estrogen receptor modulator (SERM)
  - Mimics estrogen's effects on bone density
- Alendronate and risedronate
  - Potent inhibitors of bone resorption
- Teriparatide
  - Synthetic parathyroid hormone
  - Administered subcutaneously
  - Stimulates new bone formation and mass

5. Ibandronate sodium (Boniva) is the first monthly osteoporosis medication and is used for both treatment and prevention of postmenopausal osteoporosis.
6. Calcitonin (Cibacalcin) is a hormone that increases bone formation and decreases bone resorption.
7. Sodium fluoride stimulates osteoblast activity and increases bone formation.

PAGET'S DISEASE

8. NSAIDs and aspirin (ASA) may relieve mild symptoms.
9. Calcitonin or a bisphosphonate are often also prescribed to retard bone resorption.

GOUT

10. Medications are used to terminate an acute attack, prevent further attacks, and to reduce serum uric acid levels.
11. It is important to treat the acute attack of gouty arthritis before initiating treatment to reduce serum uric acid levels, because an abrupt decrease in serum uric acid may lead to further acute manifestations.
12. Acute attacks are treated with NSAIDs; indomethacin (Indameth) being the NSAID of choice. Colchicine (Novocolchine) can dramatically diminish joint pain. Corticosteroids may also be prescribed for the client with acute gouty arthritis. Analgesics are also prescribed.
13. Prophylactic therapy may include daily colchicine. Uricosuric agents are used for clients who do not eliminate uric acid adequately; allopurinol (Alloprim) is prescribed for clients who produce excessive amounts of uric acid.
14. Complementary and alternative therapies include vitamin E and selenium, amino acids, ingestion of dark reddish-blue berries, and acupuncture.

OSTEOMALACIA

15. Most clients are placed on vitamin D therapy. Calcium and phosphate supplements may also be indicated.

OSTEOARTHRITIS

16. Pain management of OA is often achieved by the use of analgesics such as aspirin, acetaminophen, NSAIDs, or COX-2 inhibitors.
17. Topical medications include counterirritants, salicylates, and capsaicin.
18. Research is ongoing on a new class of medications called disease-modifying osteoarthritis drugs (DMOADs) and gene therapy.

RHEUMATOID ARTHRITIS

19. ASA and NSAIDs and mild analgesics are used to reduce the inflammatory process and manage the manifestations of RA.

- Ibandronate sodium
  - First monthly osteoporosis medication
  - Used for both treatment and prevention
- Calcitonin
  - Hormone that increases bone formation
  - Decreases bone resorption
- Sodium fluoride
  - Stimulates osteoblast activity

Paget's Disease
- NSAIDs, and ASA
- Calcitonin or a bisphosphonate

Gout
- Treat acute attacks before treatment to reduce serum uric acid levels
  - Abrupt decrease in serum uric acid may lead to further acute manifestations
- NSAIDs
  - Indomethacin
- Colchicine
- Corticosteroids
- Analgesics
- Uricosuric
- Allopurinol

Complementary and Alternative Therapies
- Vitamin E
- Selenium
- Amino acids
- Dark reddish-blue berries
- Acupuncture

Osteomalacia
- Vitamin D therapy
- Calcium and phosphate supplements

Osteoarthritis
- Analgesics
- Topical counterirritants, salicylates, and capsaicin
- Disease-modifying osteoarthritis drugs (DMOADs)
- Gene therapy

Rheumatoid Arthritis
- ASA and NSAIDs and mild analgesics
- Low-dose corticosteroids
- Gold compounds, D-penicillamine, antimalarial agents, infliximab, and sulfasalazine
- Immunosuppressive and cytotoxic drugs
- Intra-articular corticosteroids

Systemic Lupus Erythematosus
- ASA and NSAIDs
- Antimalarial drugs
- High dose corticosteroid therapy
- Immunosuppressive agents

Osteomyelitis
- Antibiotic therapy

20. Low-dose corticosteroids may be used to reduce pain and inflammation.
21. Gold compounds, D-penicillamine, antimalarial agents, infliximab (Remicade), and sulfasalazine (Azulfidine) appear to alter the course of the disease and reduce its destruction of joints. This class of drugs also includes immunosuppressive and cytotoxic drugs.
22. Intra-articular corticosteroids may be used to provide temporary relief in clients for whom other therapies have failed to control inflammation.

SYSTEMIC LUPUS ERYTHEMATOSUS

23. ASA and NSAIDs may be used to manage arthralgias, arthritis, fever, and fatigue.
24. Antimalarial drugs such as hydroxychloroquine (Plaquenil Sulfate) may be prescribed to manage skin and arthritic manifestations.
25. Clients with severe and life-threatening manifestations such as nephritis, hemolytic anemia, myocarditis, pericarditis, or CNS lupus may require corticosteroid therapy in high doses.
26. Immunosuppressive agents such as cyclophosphamide (Cytoxan) or azathioprine (Azasan) may be used, alone or in combination with corticosteroids, to treat clients with active SLE or lupus nephritis.

OSTEOMYELITIS

27. Antibiotic therapy is mandatory to prevent acute osteomyelitis from progressing to the chronic phase. Therapy is parenteral, and may be changed to oral dosages as the course of therapy progresses. Since many cases of osteomyelitis are caused by *Staphylococcus aureus,* a penicillinase-resistant semisynthetic penicillin is often given until culture and sensitivity results are known.

SCLERODERMA

28. Medication therapy is focused on control of symptoms. Medications may include immunosuppressives, corticosteroids, penicillamine, calcium channel blockers, H2 receptor blockers, tetracycline, and ACE inhibitors.

LOW BACK PAIN

29. Medications include NSAIDs and analgesics. Muscle relaxants such as cyclobenzaprine (Flexeril), methocarbamol (Robaxin), or carisoprodol (Soma) may be used, but there is little evidence to support their efficacy.
30. Epidural steroid injections may be used to help reduce intense, intractable pain.

Scleroderma
- Immunosuppressives
- Corticosteroids
- Penicillamine
- Calcium channel blockers
- H2 receptor blockers
- Tetracycline
- ACE inhibitors

Low Back Pain
- NSAIDs and analgesics
- Muscle relaxants
- Epidural steroid injections

LEARNING OUTCOME 4

Describe the surgical procedures used to treat clients with arthritis.

CONCEPTS FOR LECTURE
OSTEOARTHRITIS

1. Arthroscopy is a surgical procedure in which an arthroscope is inserted into a joint to diagnose or perform debridement and lavage. Arthroscopy can also be useful to repair torn cartilage.

2. Osteotomy is an incision into or transaction of the bone. It is used to realign an affected joint or to shift the joint load toward areas of less severely damaged cartilage.

3. Joint arthroplasty is the reconstruction or replacement of a joint. Arthroplasty may involve partial joint replacement or reshaping of the bones of a joint. In total joint replacement, both surfaces of the affected joint are replaced with prosthetic parts. Joints that may be replaced are the hip, knee, shoulder, elbow, ankle, wrist, and the joints of the fingers and toes.

4. In total hip replacement, the articular surfaces of the acetabulum and femoral head are replaced. Potential complications are blood clots in the leg veins, dislocations within the prosthesis, loosening of joint components from surrounding bone, and infection. If recurrent or ineffectively treated, these complications may necessitate removal of the prosthesis.

5. In total knee replacement, the femoral side of the joint is replaced with a metallic surface, and the tibial side with polyethylene. Joint failure is more common with knee replacement than with a total hip replacement. Loosened joint components, often on the tibial side, are the most common cause of failure.

6. Total shoulder replacement is indicated for unremitting pain and marked limitation of range of motion. Post replacement, the joint is immobilized in a sling or abduction splint for 2–3 weeks. Dislocation, loosening of the prosthesis, and infections are potential problems.

7. Total elbow replacement involves replacement of the humeral and ulnar surfaces of the elbow joint with a metal and polyethylene prosthesis. Complications include dislocation, fracture, triceps weakness, loosening, and infection.

POWERPOINT LECTURE SLIDES

Osteoarthritis
Surgical Procedures
- Arthroscopy
- Osteotomy
- Joint arthroplasty
- Total hip replacement
- Total knee replacement
- Total shoulder replacement
- Total elbow replacement
- Post-operative physical therapy

Rheumatoid Arthritis
- Synovectomy
- Arthrodesis
- Arthroplasty

8. Recovery from all types of joint replacement requires postoperative physical therapy that focuses on building back strength and regaining joint flexibility.

RHEUMATOID ARTHRITIS

9. Early in the course of the disease, synovectomy (excision of the synovial membrane) can provide temporary relief.
10. Arthrodesis (joint fusion) can be used to stabilize joints.
11. Arthroplasty may be necessary in cases of gross deformities and joint destruction.

SUGGESTIONS FOR CLASSROOM ACTIVITIES

- Review the case study about hip replacement that is provided on the textbook Companion Website. Have students use the information provided to develop a plan of care for the preoperative and postoperative care of the client undergoing hip replacement.
- Have a person who has had a joint replacement come to the classroom to speak about their experience of the surgery and recovery.

SUGGESTIONS FOR CLINICAL ACTIVITIES

- Have students identify ancillary health services that are crucial in the recovery of a post-joint replacement client. Discuss the interdisciplinary planning that would best benefit the client.
- Visit the physical therapy or occupational therapy departments of the clinical site. Discuss postoperative rehabilitation with the professionals who work there.

Chapter 43

Assessing Clients with Neurologic Disorders

RESOURCE LIBRARY

PRENTICE HALL NURSING MEDIALINK DVD-ROM

Audio Glossary
NCLEX-RN® Review
Video
  Testing Reflexes

COMPANION WEBSITE

Audio Glossary
NCLEX-RN® Review
Case Study: Assessing an Unconscious Client
MediaLink Application: NIH Stroke Scale
Links to Resources

📖 IMAGE LIBRARY

LEARNING OUTCOME 1

Describe the anatomy, physiology, and functions of the nervous system.

CONCEPTS FOR LECTURE
BASIC CONCEPTS

1. The nervous system consists of the central nervous system (CNS) and the peripheral nervous system (PNS).
2. There are only two types of cells in the nervous system. Neurons are cells that receive impulses and send them on to other cells. Neuroglia are cells that protect and nourish the neurons.
3. Neurons consist of a dendrite, a cell body, and an axon. Dendrites conduct impulses toward (afferent) the cell body and the axon conducts impulses away from (efferent) the cell body.
4. The dendrites and cell bodies make up the gray matter of the CNS. The axons, which are covered with a white lipid substance called the myelin sheath, make up the white matter. The myelin sheath serves to increase the speed of nerve impulse conduction.
5. Action potentials are impulses that allow neurons to communicate with other neurons and body cells.
6. Afferent, or sensory, neurons have receptors in the skin, muscles, and other organs and relay impulses to

POWERPOINT LECTURE SLIDES

Basic Concepts
- The nervous system
  - Central nervous system (CNS)
  - Peripheral nervous system (PNS)
- Cells in the nervous system
  - Neurons receive impulses
  - Neuroglia protect and nourish the neurons
- Neurons consist of a dendrite, a cell body, and an axon
- Action potentials: impulses that allow neurons to communicate with other neurons and body cells
- Neurotransmitters: chemicals that move impulses across the synaptic cleft; may be inhibitory or excitatory

The Central Nervous System
- Brain and spinal cord
- Brain
  - Control center
  - Thoughts

the CNS. Efferent, or motor, neurons transmit impulses from the CNS to cause some type of action.

7. Nerve impulses occur when a stimulus reaches a point great enough to generate a change in electrical charge across the cell membrane of a neuron. The chief regulators of membrane potential are sodium and potassium.

8. Neurotransmitters are chemicals that move impulses across the synaptic cleft. These neurotransmitters may be inhibitory or excitatory.

9. Acetylcholine (ACh) is an excitatory neurotransmitter. Nerves that transmit impulses through the release of ACh are called cholinergic.

10. Norepinephrine (NE) is another major neurotransmitter and can be excitatory or inhibitory. Nerves that transmit impulses through the release of NE are called adrenergic. Adrenergic receptors are further divided into alpha and beta types. Beta-adrenergic fibers may be either beta1 or beta2 receptors.

11. Other neurotransmitters include gamma aminobutyric acid (GABA), dopamine, and serotonin.

THE CENTRAL NERVOUS SYSTEM

12. The CNS consists of the brain and spinal cord.
13. The brain is the control center of the nervous system and also generates thoughts, emotions, and speech. The brain has four major regions: the cerebrum, the diencephalon, the brainstem, and the cerebellum.
14. The cerebrum interprets sensory input, controls skeletal muscle activity, processes intellect and emotions, and contains skills memory.
15. The diencephalon consists of the thalamus, hypothalamus, and epithalamus. The thalamus serves as a sorting, processing, and relay station for input into the cortical region. The hypothalamus regulates temperature, water metabolism, appetite, emotional expressions, part of the sleep-wake cycle, and thirst. The epithalamus includes the pineal body which is part of the endocrine system that affects growth and development.
16. The brainstem consists of the midbrain, the pons, and the medulla oblongata. The midbrain is a center for auditory and visual reflexes and also serves as a nerve pathway between the cerebral hemispheres and lower brain. The pons contains nuclei that control respiration. The medulla oblongata plays an important role in controlling cardiac rate, blood pressure, respiration, and swallowing.
17. The cerebellum coordinates skeletal muscle activity, maintains balance, and controls fine movements.
18. The brain contains four ventricles, which are chambers filled with cerebrospinal fluid (CSF). CSF is formed by the choroid plexus and serves as a cushion for the brain tissue, protects the brain and spinal cord from trauma, helps provide nourishment for the brain, and removes waste products of cerebrospinal cellular metabolism.

- ○ Emotions
- ○ Speech
- Four regions of the brain
  - ○ Cerebrum
  - ○ Diencephalon
  - ○ Brainstem
  - ○ Cerebellum

Anatomy/Physiology
- Meninges
- Blood flow to brain
- Blood vessels
- Blood-brain barrier
- Limbic system
- Reticular formation
- Spinal cord
- Messages conduction
- Upper motor neurons
- Lower motor neurons

The Peripheral Nervous System
- Links CNS to rest of body
- Nerves, ganglia, and sensory receptors
- 31 pairs of spinal nerves
- 12 pairs of cranial nerves

Reflexes
- Rapid, involuntary, predictable motor responses to stimulus
- Somatic reflexes
- Autonomic reflexes

The Autonomic Nervous System
- Division of the PNS that regulates the normal environment
- Sympathetic division
- Parasympathetic division

19. The brain and spinal cord are covered and protected by three connective tissue membranes called meninges. The outermost membrane is the dura mater and is attached to the inner surface of the skull. The middle layer is the arachnoid mater which encloses the entire CNS. The innermost layer is the pia mater which clings to the brain, spinal cord, and segmental nerves and is filled with small blood vessels.

20. The brain uses about 20% of the body's total oxygen uptake. Blood flow to the brain is mostly controlled by autoregulatory or local mechanisms that respond to the brain's metabolic needs. Carbon dioxide in the major stimulus for vasodilation with resultant increased cerebral blood flow.

21. The anterior part of the brain is supplied with blood by the two internal carotid arteries. The posterior part is supplied by the vertebral arteries.

22. The capillaries of the brain have low permeability and are therefore protected from many harmful substances in the blood. This protection is called the blood-brain barrier.

23. The limbic system consists of structures that form a ring of tissue in the medial side of each hemisphere. This system integrates and modulates input to make up the affective part of the brain, and provides emotional and behavioral responses to stimuli.

24. The reticular formation has widespread connections throughout the brain and relays sensory input from all body systems to all levels of the brain. The reticular activation system (RAS) is part of the reticular formation.

25. The spinal cord serves as a center for conducting messages to and from the brain and as a reflex center. The gray matter of the cord in on the inside and the white matter is on the outside (reverse of the brain).

26. Messages to and from the brain are conducted through ascending (sensory) pathways and descending (motor) pathways.

27. Upper motor neurons carry impulses from the cerebral cortex to the anterior gray column of the spinal cord. Lower motor neurons begin in the anterior gray column and end in the muscle.

THE PERIPHERAL NERVOUS SYSTEM

28. The peripheral nervous system (PNS) links the CNS to the rest of the body. The PNS consists of nerves, ganglia, and sensory receptors. It is divided into a sensory (afferent) division and a motor (efferent) division.

29. There are 31 pairs of spinal nerves, 8 pairs are cervical, 12 pairs are thoracic, 5 pairs are lumbar, 5 pairs are sacral, and 1 pair is coccygeal. Each spinal nerve contains both sensory and motor fibers.

30. There are 12 pairs of cranial nerves that originate in the forebrain and brainstem.

31. Reflexes are rapid, involuntary, predictable motor responses to a stimulus and are organized as either somatic or autonomic.

32. Somatic reflexes result in skeletal muscle contraction. Somatic reflexes that are mediated by the spinal cord are called spinal reflexes.
33. Autonomic reflexes activate cardiac muscle, smooth muscle, and glands.

THE AUTONOMIC NERVOUS SYSTEM

34. The autonomic nervous system (ANS) is a division of the PNS that regulates the normal environment of the body. The ANS is primarily controlled by the reticular formation in the brainstem.
35. The ANS has sympathetic and parasympathetic divisions. The action of these two divisions is opposite in effect and they serve to counterbalance each other.
36. The sympathetic division of the ANS prepares the body to handle situations that are perceived as harmful or stressful and to participate in strenuous activity. The primary neurotransmitter of the sympathetic nervous system is norepinephrine.
37. The parasympathetic division of the ANS operates during nonstressful situations. Acetylcholine is the primary neurotransmitter of the parasympathetic division.

SUGGESTIONS FOR CLASSROOM ACTIVITIES

• Using anatomic models, review the anatomy of the nervous system.

LEARNING OUTCOME 2

Identify specific topics for consideration during a health history assessment interview of the client with neurologic disorders.

CONCEPTS FOR LECTURE

1. Health problems that affect the neurologic system may manifest as problems with musculoskeletal function.
2. If the client has problems with neurologic structure or function, the nurse should analyze its onset, characteristics, course, severity, precipitating and relieving factors, and any associated symptoms.
3. Information about numbness, tingling sensations, tremors, problems with coordination or balance, or loss of movement in any part of the body are important considerations in the client with health problems that affect the neurologic system.
4. Information about perception difficulties such as visual and/or auditory disturbances is important in the assessment of this client. Information about cognitive difficulties such as memory disturbances, anxiety, depression, and sleep disturbances are important.
5. A medication review of all prescribed and over-the-counter medications should be completed. Herbal and complementary therapies should be included in this review.

POWERPOINT LECTURE SLIDES

Health History Assessment Topics
- Information about neurologic changes
  - Numbness, tingling, tremors, coordination, loss of movement
- Information about perception difficulties
  - Visual and/or auditory disturbances, cognitive difficulties
- A medication review
- Personal past history
  - Seizures, fainting, dizziness, headaches, trauma, tumors
  - Surgery of the nervous system, cardiac disease, diabetes
  - Hypertension, stroke, anemia, sinus infections
  - Liver disease, and/or renal failure
  - Family history
- Occupational hazards
- Use of tobacco, drugs, alcohol
- Safety measures
  - Seatbelt use
  - Bike helmet use

6. Past history of seizures, fainting, dizziness, headaches, trauma, tumors, surgery of the nervous system, cardiac disease, diabetes, hypertension, stroke, anemia, sinus infections, liver disease, and/or renal failure should be investigated. Family history of any of these conditions should also be investigated.
7. Other concerns are occupational hazards, use of tobacco, drugs, alcohol, and safety measures such as seatbelts and bike helmets.

SUGGESTIONS FOR CLASSROOM ACTIVITIES

- Have students search the internet for ideas for safety measures to prevent neurologic injury.
- Have students identify occupational hazards for development of neurologic disorders.

SUGGESTIONS FOR CLINICAL ACTIVITIES

- Have students review clinical client medical records for risk factors for the development of neurologic disorders.

LEARNING OUTCOME 3

Explain techniques for assessment of neurologic function, including examinations of mental status, cranial nerves, sensory nerves, motor nerves, cerebellar function, and reflexes.

CONCEPTS FOR LECTURE

1. The neurologic assessment begins with an overall evaluation of mental and physical status.
2. Complete neurologic assessment is lengthy. A brief version of neurologic assessment can be performed in a shorter period of time when the client requires frequent ongoing assessment. This "neuro check" includes assessment of LOC, vital signs, pupillary response to light, strength of hand grips, movement of extremities, and ability to sense pain.
3. The Glasgow Coma Scale can be used to quantify level of consciousness.
4. Cranial nerve I is the olfactory nerve. Note the client's ability to smell scents with each nostril.
5. Cranial nerve II is the optic nerve. Vision in each eye should be assessed using a Snellen chart.
6. CN III, IV, and VI are the oculomotor, trochlear, and abducens nerves. Assess extraocular movements by asking the client to follow your finger as you write H in the air. Assess PERRL. Assess for ptosis.
7. CN V is the trigeminal nerve. Assess ability to feel light, dull, and sharp sensations on the face. Assess corneal reflex.
8. CN VII is the facial nerve. Assess ability to taste sweet, sour, and salt. Assess ability to frown, show teeth, blow out checks, raise eyebrows, smile, and close eyes tightly.
9. CN VIII is the acoustic nerve. Assess ability to hear the ticking of a watch and whispered or spoken words.
10. CN IX and X are the glossopharyngeal and vagus nerves. Assess gag reflex, symmetry in rise of soft palate, and uvula as client says "ah."
11. CN XI is the accessory nerve. Assess client's ability to shrug shoulders and turn head against resistance.

POWERPOINT LECTURE SLIDES

Neurologic Assessment
- Overall evaluation of mental and physical status
- "Neuro check"
- Glasgow Coma Scale
- Cranial nerve assessment
- Sensory function assessments
- Motor function assessment
- Cerebellar functions assessment
- Reflex assessment
- Additional assessments

12. CN XII is the hypoglossal nerve. Assess the client's ability to stick out the tongue and move the tongue from side to side.
13. Sensory function assessments include ability to perceive sensations, sense of position, and ability to discriminate fine touch.
14. Motor function assessment includes assessment for bilateral symmetry and size of muscles, presence of tremors, and muscle tone.
15. Cerebellar functions assessment includes assessment of the gait, performance of Romberg's test, and assessment of coordination.
16. Reflex assessment includes assessment of the patellar, biceps, brachioradialis, triceps, and Achilles deep-tendon reflexes; assessment for presence of clonus; assessment for presence of superficial abdominal and cremasteric reflexes, and assessment for Babinski reflex.
17. Other assessments include presence of Brudzinski's sign, Kernig's sign, and posturing.

SUGGESTIONS FOR CLASSROOM ACTIVITIES

- View the video about testing reflexes that is provided on the textbook DVD-ROM. Have students practice the techniques on classmates.
- View the case study about assessing the unconscious client that is provided on the textbook Companion Website. Use information from that case study to help students identify nursing strategies to use when assessing a client who is unconscious.

SUGGESTIONS FOR CLINICAL ACTIVITIES

- Have students assess the reflexes of clinical clients. In post-conference, have students compare findings from clients of different ages who have different disorders.
- Have students assess the cranial nerve function of clinical clients. Help students identify reasons for any variations from normal that might arise.

LEARNING OUTCOME 4

Identify manifestations of impairment of neurologic function.

CONCEPTS FOR LECTURE

1. Assessment of appearance may reveal unilateral neglect or abnormal gait or posture.
2. Changes in speech pattern may manifest as aphasia (defective or absent language function), dysphonia (change in the tone of the voice), or dysarthria (difficulty speaking).
3. A score of 15 on the Glasgow Coma Score indicates that the client is alert and oriented.
4. Anosmia is the inability to smell.
5. Ptosis is drooping of the eyelids.
6. Dysphagia is difficulty swallowing.
7. Fasciculations are twitches of the tongue.
8. Kinesthesia is the sense of position.
9. Tremors are rhythmic movements of muscles or muscle groups.
10. Flaccidity is a condition in which muscle tone is decreased.
11. Spasticity is a condition in which muscle tone is increased.

POWERPOINT LECTURE SLIDES

Abnormal Neurologic Findings
- Unilateral neglect
- Abnormal gait or posture
- Aphasia
- Dysphonia
- Dysarthria
- Anosmia
- Ptosis
- Dysphagia
- Fasciculations
- Tremors
- Flaccidity
- Spasticity
- Ataxia
- Decorticate posturing
- Decerebrate posturing

12. Ataxia is a lack of coordination and a clumsiness of movement.
13. Decorticate posturing is a response in which the upper arms are close to the sides; the elbows, wrists, and fingers are flexed; the legs are extended with internal rotation; and the feet are plantar flexed.
14. Decerebrate posturing is a response in which the neck is extended; the jaw is clenched; the arms are pronated, extended, and close to the sides; the legs are extended straight out; and the feet are plantar flexed.

SUGGESTIONS FOR CLASSROOM ACTIVITIES

- Have students assume the decorticate and decerebrate postures as you describe them.
- Have students describe findings that would indicate that the client is experiencing unilateral neglect.

SUGGESTIONS FOR CLINICAL ACTIVITIES

- Have students identify manifestations of neurologic disorders in clinical clients. Help students relate the pathophysiology of these manifestations to the underlying disorder.

LEARNING OUTCOME 5

Describe normal variations in assessment findings for the older adult.

CONCEPTS FOR LECTURE

1. Aging may result in a decrease in the number of brain cells, cerebral blood flow, and metabolism. Nerve conduction may slow and retrieval of information from long-term memory may take longer. This may result in delayed response to multiple stimuli and slower reflexes. There may be some age-related forgetfulness.
2. Aging may result in a slower response to changes in balance with resultant increased risk for falls.
3. Aging may result in less readiness to learn and greater distractability.

POWERPOINT LECTURE SLIDES

Age-Associated Assessment Findings
- Slowed nerve conduction
- Slowed retrieval of information from long-term memory
- Slowed response to multiple stimuli
- Slower reflexes
- Slowed response to balance changes
- Decreased readiness to learn
- Greater distractability

SUGGESTIONS FOR CLINICAL ACTIVITIES

- Have students review the assessment of an older adult and identify age-related changes of the neurologic system.

CHAPTER 44
NURSING CARE OF CLIENTS WITH INTRACRANIAL DISORDERS

RESOURCE LIBRARY

 PRENTICE HALL NURSING MEDIALINK DVD-ROM

Audio Glossary
NCLEX-RN® Review
Animations/Videos
   Complex Seizure
   Coup-Contrecoup Injury
   Epilepsy
   Grand Mal Seizure

📖 IMAGE LIBRARY

Figure 44.1 Doll's eye movements characteristic of altered LOC.
Figure 44.2 Forms of brain herniation due to intracranial hypertension.
Figure 44.3 Types of intracranial pressure monitoring.
Figure 44.4 Tonic-clonic seizures in grand mal seizures.
Figure 44.5 Coup-contrecoup head injury.

COMPANION WEBSITE

Audio Glossary
NCLEX-RN® Review
Care Plan Activity: Subdural Hematoma
Case Study: Bacterial Meningitis
MediaLink Applications
   Meningitis Prevention
   Paralysis
Links to Resources

Figure 44.6 Three types of hematomas: epidural hematoma, subdural hematoma, and intracerebral hematoma.
Figure 44.7 Possible locations of burr holes.
Figure 44.8 Ommaya reservoir for medication administration.
Figure 44.9 In a craniotomy, a portion of the skull and overlying scalp is removed to allow access to the brain.

LEARNING OUTCOME 1

Compare and contrast the pathophysiology, manifestations, interdisciplinary care, and nursing care of clients with alterations in level of consciousness and increased intracranial pressure.

CONCEPTS FOR LECTURE
ALTERATIONS OF LEVEL OF CONSCIOUSNESS

1. Consciousness is a condition in which the person is aware of self and environment and is able to respond appropriately to stimuli. It is a dynamic state.
2. Full consciousness requires both normal arousal and full cognition.
3. Arousal or alertness depends on the reticular activating system (RAS).
4. Cognition is a complex process that involves all mental activities controlled by the cerebral hemispheres, including thought processes, memory, perception, problem solving, and emotion.
5. Major causes of changes in level of consciousness are (1) lesions or injuries that affect the cerebral hemispheres directly and widely or that compress or destroy the neurons of the RAS and (2) metabolic disorders.

POWERPOINT LECTURE SLIDES

Alterations of Level of Consciousness
- Consciousness
- Full consciousness
- Etiology of changes in LOC
  - Lesions or injuries
  - Metabolic disorders
- Initial impairment
  - Difficult to arouse
  - Agitated and confused
  - Orientation impaired
  - Eventually nonresponsive
  - Yawning and sighing
- Progressive respiratory changes
  - Cheynes-Stokes respirations
  - Neurogenic hyperventilation
  - Apneustic respirations
  - Ataxic/apneic respirations

6. The function of the brain depends upon continuous blood flow that supplies oxygen and glucose.

7. With deterioration of neurologic function, the client becomes more difficult to arouse and may become agitated and confused. Orientation is impaired. Increasing amounts of stimulation are required to arouse the client. Eventually, the client does not respond, even with deep, painful stimuli.

8. Progressive impairment of neural function causes predictable changes in respiratory function. Initial manifestations of deteriorating brain function are yawning and sighing. Progressive respiratory changes include: Cheyne-Stokes respirations (damage to diencephalon); neurogenic hyperventilation (damage to the midbrain); apneustic respirations (damage to the pons); and ataxic/apneic respirations (damage to the medulla).

9. A predictable progression of pupillary and oculomotor responses occurs as LOC deteriorates toward coma. With localized disorders, effects may be seen in the ipsilateral pupil. With generalized or systemic processes, pupil effects are bilateral.

10. Spontaneous eye movement and ocular reflexes may be altered. Changes may include the presence of Doll's eyes movements or fixation.

11. In altered LOC, motor responses to stimuli range from an appropriate response to a command to flaccidity. Reflexive responses include decorticate and decerebrate posturing.

12. Possible outcome of altered LOC and coma include full recovery with no long-term residual effects, recovery with residual damage, or more severe consequences such as persistent vegetative state or brain death.

INCREASED INTRACRANIAL PRESSURE

13. Increased intracranial pressure is the sustained elevation (10 mm Hg or higher) within the cranial cavity.

14. Interruption of the cerebral blood flow leads to ischemia and disruption of cellular metabolism.

15. Increased ICP may result from an increase in intracranial contents from a space-occupying lesion, hydrocephalus, cerebral edema, excess cerebrospinal fluid, or intracranial hemorrhage.

16. Manifestations of increased ICP are: mental status changes and decreased LOC; hemiparesis, hemiplegia, and posturing; alterations in vision; changes in vital signs; headache; papilledema; and vomiting without nausea.

17. Cushing's triad is a trio of manifestations (increased mean arterial pressure, increased pulse pressure, and bradycardia) and represents the brainstem's final effort to maintain cerebral perfusion.

- Pupillary/oculomotor responses
  - Ipsilateral pupil changes with localized problem
  - Bilateral pupil changes with generalized problems
  - Doll's eyes movements
  - Pupil fixation
- Motor responses
  - Range from appropriate to flaccid
  - Decorticate posturing
  - Decerebrate posturing
- Outcomes
  - Full recovery with no long-term residual effects
  - Recovery with residual damage
  - Persistent vegetative state
  - Brain death

Increased Intracranial Pressure
- Sustained elevation (10 mm Hg or higher)
- The Monro-Kellie hypothesis
- Pathophysiology
  - Interruption of the cerebral blood flow
  - Leads to ischemia
  - Disruption of cellular metabolism
- Etiology
  - Space-occupying lesion
  - Hydrocephalus
  - Cerebral edema
  - Excess CSF
  - Intracranial hemorrhage
- Manifestations
  - Mental status changes
  - Decreased LOC
  - Hemiparesis
  - Hemiplegia
  - Posturing
  - Alterations in vision
  - Vital sign changes
  - Headache
  - Papilledema
  - Vomiting without nausea
  - Cushing's triad

Cerebral Edema
- Abnormal accumulation of fluid

Hydrocephalus
- Progressive dilatation of ventricular system

Brain Herniation
- Displacement of brain tissue

Management of IICP
- Identifying and treating underlying cause
- Controlling ICP to prevent herniation

18. Cerebral edema is an increase in the volume of brain tissue due to abnormal accumulation of fluid. Cerebral edema is identified as vasogenic or cytotoxic in origin.

19. Hydrocephalus is a progressive dilation of the ventricular system, which becomes dilated as the production of CSF exceeds its absorption. It is generally classified as either noncommunicating or communicating hydrocephalus.

20. Brain herniation is the displacement of brain tissue from an area of increased pressure to a more compliant area. This syndrome is generally categorized as supratentorial or infratentorial.

21. Management of the client with increased intracranial pressure is directed toward identifying and treating the underlying cause of the disorder, and controlling ICP to prevent herniation syndrome.

22. Diagnosis of increased ICP is made on the basis of observation and neurologic assessment; even subtle changes may be clinically significant. Testing may include CT scan or MRI, serum osmolality, and ABGs. Lumbar puncture is not performed.

23. Treatments include careful assessment of ICP with monitors that measure cerebral blood flow, cerebral perfusion pressure, and oxygen levels of brain tissue. Basic monitoring systems include an intraventricular catheter, subarachnoid bolt or screw, and epidural probe.

24. Clients with IICP often require intubation and mechanical ventilation.

25. Nursing diagnoses include: *Ineffective Tissue Perfusion: Cerebral* and *Risk for Infection*.

Diagnosis
- Observation and neurologic assessment
- CT scan or MRI
- Serum osmolality
- ABGs
- Lumbar puncture is not performed

Treatments
- Careful assessment of ICP
- Intubation, mechanical ventilation

Nursing Diagnoses
- *Ineffective Tissue Perfusion: Cerebral*
- *Risk for Infection*

SUGGESTIONS FOR CLASSROOM ACTIVITIES

- Introduce the nursing diagnosis, *Ineffective Tissue Perfusion: Cerebral* to the student group. Use this nursing diagnosis as a basis for discussion of levels of consciousness and increased intracranial pressure. Discuss the pathophysiologic findings and the manifestations as they apply to changes in cerebral tissue perfusion.

SUGGESTIONS FOR CLINICAL ACTIVITIES

- Have students identify clinical clients who have some alteration in level of consciousness. Have students investigate the etiology of this alteration, its manifestations, and what nursing interventions are being used to care for the client.
- Share this information in post-conference discussion.

LEARNING OUTCOME 2

Explain the pathophysiology, manifestations, complications, interdisciplinary care, and nursing care of intracranial disorders, including headaches, epilepsy, traumatic brain injury, central nervous system infections, and brain tumors.

CONCEPTS FOR LECTURE
ALTERATIONS IN LEVEL OF CONSCIOUSNESS

1. Age, general medical condition, underlying cause, and pathologic process are all factors in the prognosis of clients with altered level of consciousness (LOC).

POWERPOINT LECTURE SLIDES

Alterations in LOC
Prognosis
- Depends upon
  - Age
  - General medical condition

2. Recovery of consciousness within 2 weeks is associated with a favorable outcome.
3. The focus of management of the client with altered LOC is to identify the underlying cause, preserve function, and prevent deterioration. Immediate treatment focuses on the ABCs and treatment is often by protocol.
4. Diagnostic testing includes CT, MRI, cerebral angiography, brain scan, transcranial Doppler, lumbar puncture, blood glucose, serum electrolytes, serum osmolality, ABGs, liver function tests, and toxicology.
5. Treatments may include airway placement, mechanical ventilation, and enteral or parenteral nutrition.
6. Nursing diagnoses include: *Ineffective Airway Clearance; Risk for Aspiration; Risk for Impaired Skin Integrity; Impaired Physical Mobility;* and *Risk for Imbalanced Nutrition: Less than Body Requirements.*

HEADACHES

7. Headache is pain within the cranial vault and may occur as a result of benign or pathologic conditions; intracranial or extracranial conditions; disease of other body systems; stress; musculoskeletal tension; or a combination of these factors.
8. Headache is experienced when there is traction, pressure, displacement, inflammation, or dilation of nociceptors in areas sensitive to pain.
9. The most common types of headache are tension, migraine, and cluster headaches.
10. Tension headache is characterized by bilateral pain, with a sensation of a band of tightness or pressure around the head. This type of headache is caused by sustained contraction of the muscles of the head and neck.
11. Migraine headache is a recurring vascular headache that lasts from 4 to 72 hours, often initiated by a triggering event and usually accompanied by a neurologic dysfunction. The two types of migraine headaches are common (no aura) migraine and classic (aura) migraine.
12. Cluster headaches are extremely severe, unilateral, and burning in quality. The headaches occur in groups or "clusters" of 1 to 8 each day for several weeks or months, followed by remission that lasts months to years.
13. The initial focus of the interdisciplinary care of headaches is identification of the underlying cause. Accurate diagnosis of the type of headache is key to treatment. Therapeutic management for migraine headaches includes a combination of client teaching, medications, and measures to control contributing factors. Treatment protocols for cluster headaches include eliminating aggravating factors, medications, and oxygen inhalation. Tension headache management is directed toward reducing the client's level of stress and relieving pain with ice and medications.

- ○ Underlying cause
- ○ Pathologic process
- Recovery of consciousness within 2 weeks favorable

Interdisciplinary Care
- Identification of underlying cause
- Preservation of function
- Prevention of deterioration

Immediate Treatment
- ABCs
- Treatment by protocol

Diagnostic Testing
- CT, MRI
- Cerebral angiography, brain scan
- Transcranial doppler
- Lumbar puncture
- Serum glucose, electrolytes, molality
- ABGs, liver function tests, toxicology

Treatments
- Airway placement
- Mechanical ventilation
- Enteral or parenteral nutrition

Nursing Diagnoses
- *Ineffective Airway Clearance*
- *Risk for Aspiration*
- *Risk for Impaired Skin Integrity*
- *Impaired Physical Mobility*
- *Risk for Imbalanced Nutrition: Less Than Body Requirements*

Headaches
- Pain within the cranial vault

Etiology
- Benign or pathologic conditions
- Intracranial or extracranial conditions
- Disease of other body systems
- Stress
- Musculoskeletal tension

Types
- Tension
- Migraine headache
- Cluster headaches

Interdisciplinary Care
- Identification of cause
- Accurate diagnosis
- Client teaching
- Medications
- Control of contributing factors

Primary Nursing Diagnosis
- *Acute Pain*

14. Diagnosis and treatment are based on history, the identification of triggering or precipitating events, and the type of headache.
15. The primary nursing diagnosis is *Acute Pain.*

Epilepsy

16. Epilepsy is a chronic disorder of abnormal recurring, excessive, and self-terminating electrical discharge from the neuron(s) that causes the seizure.
17. Isolated seizure episodes may occur in otherwise healthy people secondary to an acute febrile state, infection, metabolic or endocrine disorder, or exposure to toxins. Epilepsy may be idiopathic, or may be due to birth injury, infection, vascular abnormalities, trauma, or tumors. There is a strong genetic component.
18. Most seizures arise from a few unstable, hypersensitive, and hyperreactive neurons in the brain. Abnormal neuronal activity may remain localized and cause a partial or focal seizure, or it may spread to involve the entire brain and cause generalized seizure activity. More than one type of seizure in an individual client is called mixed seizure.
19. Metabolic needs of the brain increase dramatically during seizure activity. As long as oxygenation, blood glucose levels, and cardiac function remain normal, cerebral blood flow can respond to this increase. If cerebral blood flow cannot meet these needs, cellular exhaustion and cellular destruction may occur.
20. The manifestations of simple partial seizures may include involvement of the motor portion of the cortex, abnormal sensations or hallucinations, tachycardia, flushing, hypotension, hypertension, or psychic manifestations.
21. During a complex partial seizure, consciousness is impaired and the client may engage in repetitive, non-purposeful activity.
22. Generalized seizures involve both hemispheres of the brain as well as deeper brain structures, such as the thalamus, basal ganglia, and upper brainstem. Absence and tonic-clonic seizures are common forms of generalized seizure activity.
23. Absence (petit mal) seizures are characterized by sudden, brief cessation of all motor activity accompanied by a blank stare and unresponsiveness. These seizures are more common in children than in adults.
24. Tonic-clonic seizures are the most common type of seizure in adults. The seizure is preceded by a warning aura and then begins with sudden loss of consciousness and sharp muscle contractions (the tonic phase) which are followed by alternating contraction and relaxation of the muscles of all the extremities along with hyperventilation (the clonic phase). The postictal phase follows the seizure and is characterized by a period of unconsciousness and unresponsiveness.

Epilepsy
- Chronic seizure disorder

Etiology
- Isolated seizure episodes

Pathophysiology
- Arise from unstable, hypersensitive, hyperreactive neurons in brain
- May remain localized, causing a partial or focal seizure
- May spread to involve entire brain, causing generalized seizure activity
- May cause exhaustion and destruction of brain cells

Manifestations
- Simple partial seizures
- Complex partial seizure
- Absence (petit mal) seizures
- Tonic-clonic seizures
- Status epilepticus

Diagnostic Testing
- MRI, CT scans, skull x-rays
- EEG
- Lumbar puncture
- CBC, electrolytes, blood urea, blood glucose

Nursing Diagnoses
- *Risk for Ineffective Airway Clearance*
- *Anxiety*

Traumatic Brain Injury
- Any injury of the scalp, skull, or brain
- Leading cause of death and disability in the United States
- Penetrating (open) or closed (blunt trauma)

Acceleration
- Head is struck by a moving object

Deceleration
- Head hits a stationary object

Acceleration-Deceleration Injury
- Coup-contrecoup phenomenon
- Head hits an object, brain "rebounds" within skull

Deformation Injuries
- Skull fracture
- Linear fractures
- Comminuted and depressed skull fractures
- Basal skull fractures

Nursing Care
- Focuses on risk for infection and teaching for nonhospitalized clients

Closed Head Injuries
- Primary injury results from impact
- Secondary injury is progression of the initial injury

25. Status epilepticus is a situation in which seizure activity becomes continuous with only very short periods of calm between intense and persistent seizures. This is considered a life-threatening medical emergency that requires immediate treatment.

26. Diagnostic testing is performed to confirm the seizure diagnosis and to determine any treatable causes and precipitating factors. Common diagnostic tests include MRI, CT scans, skull x-rays, EEG, lumbar puncture, blood count, electrolytes, blood urea, and blood glucose.

27. Nursing diagnoses include: *Risk for Ineffective Airway Clearance* and *Anxiety*.

TRAUMATIC BRAIN INJURY

28. Traumatic brain injury refers to any injury of the scalp, skull, or brain. It is the leading cause of death and disability in the United States.

29. TBIs are classified as penetrating (open) or closed (blunt trauma).

30. Acceleration injury is sustained when the head is struck by a moving object. Deceleration injury occurs when the head hits a stationary object. Acceleration-deceleration injury (coup-contrecoup phenomenon) occurs when the head hits an object and the brain "rebounds" within the skull. Deformation injuries are those in which the force deforms and disrupts the integrity of the body.

31. A skull fracture is a break in the continuity of the skull and may occur with or without damage to the brain.

32. Linear fractures are the most common and typically extend from the point of impact toward the base of the skull. Subdural or epidural hematomas frequently underlie the fracture. Treatment is bed rest and observation.

33. Comminuted and depressed skull fractures increase the risk of direct damage to brain tissue from contusion and bone fragments. These fractures require surgical intervention, usually within 24 hours of the injury, to debride the wound completely and remove bone fragments.

34. Basal skull fractures involve the base of the skull and usually are extensions of adjacent fractures. Complicated basal skull fractures are those that involve the sinuses of the frontal bone or the petrous portion of the temporal bone and often result in leakage of CSF. This leakage may manifest as rhinorrhea or otorrhea. Basal skull fractures do not require surgery unless CSF leakage persists.

35. Nursing care focuses on the client's risk for infection and teaching for nonhospitalized clients.

36. Closed head injuries may result in either diffuse or focal damage to the brain. Primary injury results from the impact. Secondary injury is the progression of the initial injury from events that affect perfusion

Focal Brain Injuries
- Confined to one area of the brain
- Intracranial hemorrhage
- Contusion
- Epidural hematoma
- Subdural hematoma

Intracerebral Hematoma
- Single or multiple
- Associated with contusions
- Headache
- Decreased LOC
- Hemiplegia
- Dilation of the ipsilateral pupil

Diffuse Brain Injury (DBI)
- Affects the entire brain
- Caused by a shaking motion
- Rotational acceleration is primary mechanism of injury
- Mild concussion
- Classic cerebral concussion

Postconcussion Syndrome
- May last several weeks up to a year
- Manifestations
  - Persistent headache
  - Dizziness
  - Irritability
  - Insomnia
  - Impaired memory and concentration
  - Learning problems

Diffuse Axonal Injury (DAI)
- Widespread disruption of white matter axons
- Prognosis is poor
- Most die or remain in a persistent vegetative state

Interdisciplinary Care
- Rapid recognition of injury
- Transport to an ED
- Support of ABCs
- Detection and management of IICP

Nursing Diagnoses
- *Decreased Intracranial Adaptive Capacity*
- *Ineffective Airway Clearance*
- *Ineffective Breathing Pattern*

Central Nervous System Infections
- Meningitis, encephalitis, and brain abscesses
- Etiology
  - Bacteria, viruses, fungi
  - Protozoans, rickettsiae
  - Bacterial toxins
- Pathophysiology
- Inflammation and ICCP

Meningitis
- Inflammation of pia mater, arachnoid, and subarachnoid space

and oxygenation of brain cells. These events include intracranial edema, hematoma, infection, hypoxia, or ischemia.

37. Focal brain injuries are specific, grossly observable brain lesions confined to one area of the brain. They include contusions, lacerations, and intracranial hemorrhage.

38. Intracranial hemorrhage can result directly from trauma or from shearing forces on cerebral arteries and veins that occur with acceleration-deceleration. Manifestations may appear immediately or may not become evident for hours or weeks.

39. A contusion is a bruise of the surface of the brain, and is typically accompanied by small, diffuse, venous hemorrhages. Manifestations depend on the size and location of the brain injury, but usually include an initial loss of consciousness. Focal effects may cause loss of reflexes, hemiparesis, or abnormal posturing.

40. An epidural hematoma develops in the potential space between the dura and the skull. The etiology is often a skull fracture that tears an artery and results in rapid development of the hematoma. Manifestations include an initial loss of consciousness with a brief return to the lucid state. Consciousness then rapidly declines.

41. Subdural hematoma is a condition in which a localized mass of blood collects between the dura mater and the arachnoid mater.

42. Acute subdural hematomas develop rapidly after head injury. Manifestations are drowsiness, confusion, and enlargement of the ipsilateral pupil. Hemiparesis and respiratory pattern changes may occur.

43. Chronic subdural hematomas may develop over weeks to months. Manifestations are slowed thinking, confusion, drowsiness, lethargy, headache, dilation and sluggishness of the ipsilateral pupil, and possible seizures. They develop slowly and may be mistaken for the onset of dementia in the older adult.

44. Intracerebral hematoma may be single or multiple and are associated with contusions. Manifestations vary according to location, but may include headache, decreased LOC, hemiplegia, and dilation of the ipsilateral pupil.

45. Diffuse brain injury (DBI) affects the entire brain and is caused by a shaking motion with rotational acceleration being the primary mechanism of injury. Categories of DBI include mild concussion, classic cerebral concussion, and diffuse axonal injury.

46. Mild concussion is a momentary interruption of brain function with or without loss of consciousness. Manifestations include possible brief loss of consciousness, retrograde and antegrade amnesia, headache, drowsiness, confusion, dizziness, and visual disturbances. Treatment includes 1–2 hours of observation

- Bacterial meningitis
- Acute viral meningitis
- Encephalitis
- Arbovirus encephalitis
- A brain abscess
- Brain tumors
  - Growths within the cranium
  - Etiology
    - Unknown
    - Heredity
    - Cranial irradiation
    - Chemical exposure
  - Manifestations
    - Change in cognition or consciousness
    - Headache, seizures, vomiting
  - Treatment
    - Chemotherapy
    - Radiation therapy
    - Surgery
  - Diagnostic tests
    - CT scan, MRI
    - Arteriography, EEC
    - Endocrine studies
  - Radiation therapy
    - May be primary treatment
    - May be adjunctive therapy
  - Nursing diagnoses
    - *Anxiety*
    - *Risk for Infection*
    - *Ineffective Protection*
    - *Disturbed Self-Esteem*

and discharge home with instructions for further observation.

47. A classic cerebral concussion involves diffuse cerebral disconnection from the brainstem RAS. Immediate loss of consciousness occurs and lasts less than 6 hours.

48. Postconcussion syndrome may develop and last for several weeks, or up to one year. Manifestations are persistent headache, dizziness, irritability, insomnia, impaired memory and concentration, and learning problems.

49. Diffuse axonal injury (DAI) is a brain injury in which a high-speed acceleration-deceleration injury causes a widespread disruption of axons in the white matter. Prognosis is poor; most clients with severe DAI either die or remain in a persistent vegetative state.

50. The interdisciplinary care of the client with TBI includes rapid recognition of injury and transport to an ED. Support of the ABCs is essential, as is detection and management of IICP.

51. Nursing diagnoses include: *Decreased Intracranial Adaptive Capacity; Ineffective Airway Clearance;* and *Ineffective Breathing Pattern.*

CENTRAL NERVOUS SYSTEM INFECTIONS

52. The major CNS infections include meningitis, encephalitis, and brain abscesses. These infections may be caused by bacteria, viruses, fungi, protozoans, rickettsiae, and by toxins from bacterial infections.

53. The pathology of CNS infections includes the invading pathogens, the subsequent inflammation, and the increase in intracranial pressure that may result from the inflammatory process.

54. Meningitis is the inflammation of the pia mater, the arachnoid, and the subarachnoid space. Meningitis may be acute or chronic, and it may be bacterial, viral, fungal, or parasitic in origin. Infection causes an inflammatory response that involves both the brain and the spinal cord and results in IICP.

55. Bacterial meningitis can develop secondary to head trauma with a basal skull fracture, otitis media, mastoiditis, sinusitis, neurosurgery, systemic sepsis, or immunocompromise. Mortality rate reaches 25%, even with appropriate antibiotic use.

56. Manifestations of bacterial meningitis are fever and chills, headache, back and abdominal pain, nausea and vomiting, and nuchal rigidity. Brudzinski's sign and Kernig's sign are positive. The client is often photophobic. With meningococcal meningitis, a rapidly-spreading petechial rash that involves the skin and mucous membranes may be evident.

57. Complications of bacterial meningitis are arthritis, cranial nerve damage, and hydrocephalus. Bacterial meningitis is a medical emergency that can be fatal within days.

58. Acute viral meningitis is also called aseptic meningitis and is less severe than bacterial meningitis. It most commonly appears after a case of mumps.

59. Manifestations of viral meningitis are similar to those of bacterial meningitis, although usually milder. Recovery is usually uneventful. Treatment focuses on managing symptoms and is supportive.

60. Encephalitis is an acute inflammation of the parenchyma of the brain or spinal cord. It may be viral, bacterial, fungal, or caused by other organisms.

61. The pathology of encephalitis includes local necrotizing hemorrhage, which ultimately becomes generalized, with prominent edema. There is progressive degeneration of nerve cell bodies. Manifestations are similar to those of meningitis.

62. Arbovirus encephalitis is a result of arbovirus infection from a mosquito or tick. West Nile virus is an arbovirus encephalitis. Manifestations include fever, malaise, sore throat, nausea and vomiting, stiff neck, tremors, paralysis of extremities, exaggerated deep tendon reflexes, seizures, and altered LOC.

63. A brain abscess is an infection with a collection of purulent material within the brain tissue. Causes are open trauma and neurosurgery; infections of the mastoid, middle ear cavity, nasal cavity, or nasal sinuses; metastatic spread from distant foci; and arising from other associated areas of infection. Immunosuppression raises risk for brain abscess.

64. Manifestations of brain abscess are general symptoms of infection that worsen and produce seizure, alterations in LOC, and manifestations of IICP. Treatment focuses on prompt initiation of antibiotic therapy.

65. Diagnosis is achieved by analysis of CSF obtained by lumbar puncture.

66. Nursing diagnoses include: *Ineffective Protection* and *Risk for Deficient Fluid Volume*.

BRAIN TUMORS

67. Brain tumors are growths within the cranium, including tumors in brain tissue, meninges, the pituitary gland, or blood vessels. The cause of many brain tumors is unknown; however, heredity, cranial irradiation, and exposure to some chemicals may be a factor.

68. Brain tumors may be benign or malignant. A tumor that is histologically benign but surgically inaccessible can still cause death.

69. Brain tumors may be primary or metastatic. Primary brain tumors rarely metastasize outside the CNS. Common primary sites are the breast, kidney, lung, and GI tract.

70. Manifestations include a change in cognition or consciousness, a headache, seizures, or vomiting. Compression of brain tissue secondary to growth and invasion may lead to changes typically seen with cerebral edema or IICP.

71. Treatment for brain tumor may involve chemotherapy, radiation therapy, surgery, or any combination of these.
72. Diagnostic tests include: CT scan, MRI, arteriography, EEC, and endocrine studies.
73. Radiation therapy may be administered alone or as adjunctive therapy with surgery.
74. Nursing diagnoses include: *Anxiety; Risk for Infection; Ineffective Protection;* and *Disturbed Self-Esteem.*

SUGGESTIONS FOR CLASSROOM ACTIVITIES

- Divide the students into small groups. Assign each group one of the disorders covered in the chapter. Have the group investigate the pathophysiology, manifestations, complications, interdisciplinary care, and nursing care of that disorder. Share the group findings.
- Have students create a chart of the major disorders covered in the chapter. In the chart, allow room for pathophysiology, manifestations, complications, interdisciplinary care focus, and nursing diagnoses. Use these charts to draw conclusions about the similarities and differences in the care of clients with these disorders.
- Review the care plan activities about subdural hematoma and tension headache that are provided on the textbook Companion Website. Use this information to assist the group in developing a nursing plan of care for the clients presented.

SUGGESTIONS FOR CLINICAL ACTIVITIES

- Assign students to the care of clinical clients who have one of the intercranial disorders covered in the chapter. In post-conference, have students share what was learned about caring for clients with the various disorders.

LEARNING OUTCOME 3

Describe criteria for diagnosing persistent vegetative state and brain death.

CONCEPTS FOR LECTURE
PERSISTENT VEGETATIVE STATE

1. Persistent vegetative state (also called irreversible coma) is a permanent condition of complete unawareness of self and the environment and loss of all cognitive functions.
2. The condition results from death of the cerebral hemispheres with continued function of the brainstem and cerebellum.
3. The diagnosis of persistent vegetative state requires that the condition has continued for at least one month.
4. Assessment reveals sleep-wake cycles, the ability to chew, swallow, and cough; and the inability to interact with the environment. When awake, the eyes may wander back and forth, but no tracking is evident.

LOCKED-IN SYNDROME

5. Locked-in syndrome is a condition in which the client is alert and fully aware of the environment and has intact cognitive abilities, but is unable to communicate through speech or movement because of blocked efferent pathways from the brain.

POWERPOINT LECTURE SLIDES

Persistent Vegetative State
- Irreversible coma
- Permanent condition of complete unawareness
- Loss of all cognitive functions
- Etiology
  - Death of the cerebral hemispheres
  - Continued function of brainstem/cerebellum
- Diagnosis
  - Requires one month continuation
- Assessment
  - Sleep-wake cycles
  - Ability to chew, swallow, and cough
  - No ability to interact with environment
  - Eyes may wander back and forth
    - No tracking is evident

Locked-In Syndrome
- Alert and fully aware of the environment
- Intact cognitive abilities
- Unable to communicate through speech
- Unable to move

BRAIN DEATH

6. Brain death is the cessation of all brain functions, including the brainstem.
7. General diagnostic criteria are: unresponsive coma with absent motor and reflex movements; no spontaneous respirations; pupils fixed and dilated; absent ocular responses to head turning and caloric stimulation; flat EEG; and no cerebral blood flow on angiography. These manifestations must be persistent for 30 minutes to 1 hour and for 6 hours after onset of coma and apnea.
8. Apnea in the comatose client is determined by the apnea test.

Brain Death
- Cessation of all brain functions
  - Including the brainstem
- General criteria
  - Unresponsive coma
  - Absent motor and reflex movements
  - No spontaneous respirations
  - Pupils fixed and dilated
  - Absent ocular responses
  - Flat EEG
  - No cerebral blood flow
  - Must be persistent 30 minutes–1 hour
  - Must be persistent for 6 hours after coma/apnea onset

SUGGESTIONS FOR CLASSROOM ACTIVITIES

- Have students research the internet for information about diagnosis of persistent vegetative state and brain death. Look for differences between and among states. Look for differences in definition between children and adults.

SUGGESTIONS FOR CLINICAL ACTIVITIES

- Discuss the differences in clinical assessment of the client in a persistent vegetative state and the client who is brain dead.
- Discuss the issue of organ harvest.

LEARNING OUTCOME 4

Discuss the purposes, nursing implications, and health education for the client and family for medications used to treat altered cerebral function, headaches, epilepsy, traumatic brain injury, central nervous system infections, and brain tumors.

CONCEPTS FOR LECTURE
ALTERED LOC

1. Fluid balance is supported via infusion of an isotonic or slightly hypertonic solution.
2. If hypoglycemia is present, 50% glucose is administered intravenously.
3. Insulin is administered to the client with hyperglycemia.
4. Naloxone (Narcan) is administered to the client with narcotic overdose.
5. Thiamine may be administered with glucose to prevent exacerbation of Wernicke's encephalopathy.
6. Underlying fluid and electrolyte imbalances are managed by administering appropriate electrolytes and diuretics.
7. Antibiotics are given for clients who have suspected or confirmed meningitis.

INCREASED INTRACRANIAL PRESSURE

8. Osmotic diuretics are commonly administered to decrease ICP. Loop diuretics may also be prescribed.
9. Sedation and paralysis (with a neuromuscular blocking agent) are used as chemical restraints to control restlessness and agitation.
10. Antipyretics, anticonvulsants, and intravenous histamine H_2 antagonists or proton pump inhibitors are also frequently prescribed.

POWERPOINT LECTURE SLIDES

Altered LOC
- Infusion of an isotonic or slightly hypertonic solution
- Intravenous 50% glucose
- Insulin
- Naloxone
- Thiamine
- Electrolytes and diuretics as appropriate
- Antibiotics

Increased Intracranial Pressure
- Osmotic diuretics
- Loop diuretics
- Neuromuscular blocking agent for sedation and paralysis
- Antipyretics, anticonvulsants
- Histamine H2 antagonists or proton pump inhibitors
- IV fluids

Headaches
- Migraine
  - Prophylactic medications
    - Methysergide maleate
    - Propranolol hydrochloride
    - Topiramate
    - Valproic acid

11. IV fluids are administered to maintain fluid and electrolyte balances and vascular volume.

HEADACHES

12. Management of migraine headaches includes administering medications prophylactically and well as when the headache occurs. Prophylactic medications include methysergide maleate (Sansert), propranolol hydrochloride (Inderal), topiramate (Topamax), and valproic acid (Depakote). Medications to abort migraine are ergotamine tartrate (Cafergot), sumatriptan (Imitrex), and zolmitriptan (Zolmig). Narcotic analgesics and antiemetics may be prescribed to control pain and nausea once migraine has occurred.

13. Many of the same medications can also treat or prevent cluster headaches. Inhaling 100% oxygen may also relieve cluster headache.

14. Tension headaches are treated with nonnarcotic analgesics. Tranquilizers to reduce muscle tension may be required.

15. Alternative and complementary therapies include vitamin, acupuncture, relaxation, herbal therapy, magnetic field therapy, and osteopathic manipulation.

EPILEPSY

16. Antiepileptic drugs do not cure the disorder, but can help in management of its manifestations. These drugs help by raising the seizure threshold or by limiting the spread of abnormal activity within the brain.

17. Newly recommended drugs for monotherapy include gabapentin (Neurontin), lamotrigine (Lamictal), oxcarbazepine (Trileptal), and topiramate (Topamax).

18. Status epilepticus requires immediate intervention with airway protection and establishment of intravenous access. Diazepam (Valium) or lorazepam (Ativan) are given IV to stop seizure activity. Phenytoin (Dilantin) and phenobarbital may also be used.

TRAUMATIC BRAIN INJURY

19. Antibiotics may be administered prophylactically in the event of basal skull fractures.

CENTRAL NERVOUS SYSTEM INFECTIONS

20. Immediate intravenous administration of a broad-spectrum antibiotic that crosses the blood-brain barrier into the subarachnoid space is instituted in cases of bacterial meningitis. Cephalosporin antibiotics are preferred.

21. Steroids may be prescribed to suppress inflammation.

22. Anticonvulsant medications are often prescribed.

23. Analgesics that have a depressant effect on the CNS are avoided to prevent masking early manifestations of deteriorating LOC.

- ○ To abort migraine
  - – Ergotamine tartrate
  - – Sumitryptan
  - – Zolmitriptan
  - – Narcotic analgesics
  - – Antiemetics

Cluster Headaches
- • Many are same as for migraines
- • Inhaling 100% oxygen

Tension Headaches
- • Nonnarcotic analgesics
- • Tranquilizers

Alternative and Complementary Therapies
- • Vitamins
- • Acupuncture
- • Relaxation
- • Herbal therapy
- • Magnetic field therapy
- • Osteopathic manipulation

Epilepsy
- • Antiepileptic drugs
- • Monotherapy
  - ○ Gabapentin
  - ○ Lamotrigine
  - ○ Oxcarbazepine
  - ○ Topiramate

Status Epilepticus
- • Immediate intervention
  - ○ Airway protection
  - ○ Establishment of IV
  - ○ Diazepam or lorazepam
  - ○ Phenytoin and phenobarbital

Traumatic Brain Injury
- • Antibiotics for basal skull fracture

Central Nervous System Infections
- • Immediate IV administration of broad-spectrum antibiotic
- • Steroids
- • Anticonvulsants
- • Avoid depressant analgesics

Brain Tumors
- • Based on the type, location, response to therapy
- • Corticosteroids and anticonvulsants

BRAIN TUMORS

24. The choice of drug treatment is based on the type of tumor, its location, and the client's response to therapy.
25. Other drugs commonly prescribed include cortico-steroids and anticonvulsants.

SUGGESTIONS FOR CLASSROOM ACTIVITIES

- Have students group the medications commonly prescribed for clients with neurologic disorders according to class. Compare the classes of medications for indications and side effects. Look for commonalities and differences.

SUGGESTIONS FOR CLINICAL ACTIVITIES

- Have students review medication administration records for medications that are given for neurologic disorders. Have students develop medication information sheets that include dosages, indications for use, contraindications to use, nursing implications, side effects, and teaching necessary when administering these medications.

LEARNING OUTCOME 5

Discuss surgical options for the treatment of increased intracranial pressure, epilepsy, traumatic brain injury, and brain tumors.

CONCEPTS FOR LECTURE
INCREASED INTRACRANIAL PRESSURE

1. Clients with IICP may undergo various intracranial surgical techniques to treat the underlying cause.
2. Infarcted or necrotic tissue may be removed.
3. A drainage catheter or shunt may be inserted via a burr hole to drain excess CSF.

EPILEPSY

4. When all attempts to control the client's seizures fail, excision of the tissue involved may be an effective and safe treatment alternative.
5. Vagal nerve stimulation is approved as a treatment for clients with partial-onset seizures who do not respond to medication therapy.

TRAUMATIC BRAIN INJURY

6. Surgery for depressed skull fractures include debridement and removal of bone fragments.
7. For deeply depressed fractures, cranioplasty with insertion of acrylic bone may be performed.
8. Small, subdural hematomas can frequently be reabsorbed and may be treated conservatively. The treatment of choice for epidural hematomas and large acute subdural hematomas is surgical evacuation of the clot.

CENTRAL NERVOUS SYSTEM INFECTIONS

9. Surgical drainage of encapsulated brain abscesses may be necessary.

POWERPOINT LECTURE SLIDES

Increased Intracranial Pressure
- Variety of procedures
- Infarcted or necrotic tissue may be removed
- Drainage catheter or shunt insertion

Epilepsy
- Excision of involved tissue
- Vagal nerve stimulation

Traumatic Brain Injury
- Debridement and removal of bone fragments.
- Cranioplasty with insertion of acrylic bone
- Surgical evacuation of clot

Central Nervous System Infections
- Surgical drainage of encapsulated brain abscesses

Brain Tumors
- Remove tumors
- Debulk tumor
- Symptom relief
- Burr holes
- Craniotomy
- Craniectomy
- Cranioplasty

BRAIN TUMORS

10. Surgery can be used to remove tumors, reduce the size of the tumor, or for symptom relief. Some common surgical approaches include Burr holes, craniotomy, craniectomy, and cranioplasty.

SUGGESTIONS FOR CLASSROOM ACTIVITIES

- Using anatomic models, explain the surgical procedures often used in treatment of clients with intracranial disorders. Explain the pathophysiologic reason the procedure is used and the effects expected in the client.

SUGGESTIONS FOR CLINICAL ACTIVITIES

- Arrange for students to tour a neurointensive care area where clients are recovering from neurologic surgery.
- Have a client who has had neurologic surgery speak to the post-conference student group.

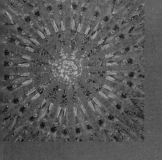

CHAPTER 45
NURSING CARE OF CLIENTS WITH CEREBROVASCULAR AND SPINAL CORD DISORDERS

RESOURCE LIBRARY

 PRENTICE HALL NURSING MEDIALINK DVD-ROM

Audio Glossary
NCLEX-RN® Review

 COMPANION WEBSITE

Audio Glossary
NCLEX-RN® Review
Care Plan Activity: Hemorrhagic Stroke
Case Study: Spinal Cord Injury
MediaLink Applications
  Intracranial Pressure
  Spinal Cord Injury
  Stroke
  Stroke Lifestyle Changes
Links to Resources

IMAGE LIBRARY

Figure 45.1 Abnormal visual fields.
Figure 45.2 Types of paralysis.
Figure 45.3 Carotid endarterectomy.
Figure 45.4 Positioning the client with hemiplegia is important in preventing deformity of the affected extremities.
Figure 45.5 Spinal cord injury mechanisms.

Figure 45.6 Examples of traction or external fixation devices.
Figure 45.7 Cervical traction may be applied by several methods, including Gardner-Wells tongs.
Figure 45.8 The halo external fixation device.
Figure 45.9 A herniated intervertebral disk.

LEARNING OUTCOME 1

Identify prevalence, incidence, and risk factors responsible for disorders of cerebral blood flow and spinal cord structure and function.

CONCEPTS FOR LECTURE
STROKE

1. Stroke is the third leading cause of death and disability in North America. The highest incidence occurs in people over 65 years of age.
2. Risk factors for the development of stroke include: hypertension, heart disease, diabetes mellitus, sleep apnea, increased blood cholesterol levels, smoking, sickle cell disease, substance abuse, and living in the stroke belt.
3. Other risk factors include a family history of stroke, obesity, a sedentary lifestyle, recent viral and bacterial infections, and previous transient ischemic attacks.
4. Risk factors specific to women include oral contraceptive use, pregnancy, childbirth, menopause, migraine headaches with aura, autoimmune disorders, and clotting disorders.

POWERPOINT LECTURE SLIDES

Stroke
- Third leading cause of death/disability in North America
- Highest incidence over 65
- Risk factors
  ○ Hypertension, heart disease
  ○ Diabetes mellitus
  ○ Sleep apnea
  ○ Hyperlipedemia
  ○ Smoking
  ○ Sickle cell disease
  ○ Substance abuse
  ○ Living in the "stroke belt"
  ○ Family history of stroke
  ○ Obesity, sedentary lifestyle
  ○ Recent viral and bacterial infections
  ○ Previous TIA

5. About 5–14% of people who have a stroke and recover have another stroke within 1 year.

INTRACRANIAL ANEURYSM

6. Approximately 5 million North Americans have intracranial aneurysms; most are asymptomatic. Rupture of an intracranial aneurysm will occur in about 30,000 people each year, and two-thirds of the survivors will have serious disabilities.

SPINAL CORD INJURY

7. The major causes of spinal cord injury (SCI) are contusion, laceration, transaction, hemorrhage, and damage to blood vessels that supply the spinal cord.
8. The three major risk factors for SCIs are age, gender, and alcohol or drug abuse.

HERNIATED INTERVERTEBRAL DISK

9. A herniated intervertebral disk can occur at any adult age, but is more prevalent as people enter middle-age and age-related changes occur.
10. The majority of herniated disks occur in the lumbar region (L4, L5 to S1). Cervical herniations most commonly occur at C6 to C7.

- Risk factors specific to women
  - Oral contraceptive use
  - Pregnancy
  - Childbirth
  - Menopause
  - Migraine headaches with aura
  - Autoimmune disorders
  - Clotting disorders

Intracranial Aneurysm
- 5 million North Americans have intracranial aneurysms
  - Most are asymptomatic
- 30,000 ruptured each year
  - Two-thirds of survivors will have serious disabilities

Spinal Cord Injury
- Major causes
  - Contusion
  - Laceration
  - Transaction
  - Hemorrhage
  - Damage to blood supply
- Major risk factors
  - Age
  - Gender
  - Alcohol or drug abuse

Herniated Intervertebral Disk
- Most common as people enter middle-age
- Most are L4, L5 to S1
- Cervical herniation most common at C6/C7

SUGGESTIONS FOR CLASSROOM ACTIVITIES

- Have student access the internet for information regarding the prevalence of stroke in the U.S.
- Discuss the risk factors for development of stroke. Have students identify three teaching topics pertinent for inclusion in an education session about risk factor avoidance.
- Discuss risk taking behaviors as a cause of spinal cord injury. Have students identify teaching techniques that might be useful in teaching the high-risk populations.

SUGGESTIONS FOR CLINICAL ACTIVITIES

- Have students review their clinical client's medical record and identify risk factors for development of stroke. In post-conference, share the risk factors and discuss prevention strategies.

LEARNING OUTCOME 2

Explain the pathophysiology, manifestations, complications, interdisciplinary care, and nursing care of clients with stroke, ruptured intracranial aneurysm, arteriovenous malformation, spinal cord injury, herniated intervertebral disk, and spinal cord tumor.

CONCEPTS FOR LECTURE
STROKE

1. A stroke (cerebral vascular accident or brain attack) is a condition in which neurologic deficits result from a

POWERPOINT LECTURE SLIDES

Stroke
- Pathophysiology
  - Ischemia
  - Necrosis of cells

sudden decrease in blood flow to a localized area of the brain.
2. Strokes may be ischemic or hemorrhagic.
3. When blood flow to and oxygenation of cerebral neurons are decreased or interrupted, pathophysiologic changes at the cellular level take place in 4 to 5 minutes. Severe or prolonged ischemia leads to cellular death.
4. Strokes lead to loss or impairment of sensory-motor functions on the side of the body opposite the side of the brain that is damaged. This is known as a contralateral deficit.
5. Ischemic strokes result from blockage of a cerebral artery, which decreases or stops blood flow and ultimately causes a brain infarction. This blockage may result from a blood clot or from stenosis of a vessel that results from a buildup of plaque. Ischemic strokes are classified as transient, thrombotic, or embolic.
6. A transient ischemic attack (TIA) is a brief period of localized cerebral ischemia that causes neurologic deficits lasting for less than 24 hours. TIAs are often warning signals of an ischemic thrombotic stroke.
7. A thrombotic stroke is caused by occlusion of a large cerebral vessel by a thrombus. These strokes most often occur in older people who are resting or sleeping. A thrombotic stroke occurs rapidly but progresses slowly. They continue to worsen over 1–2 days as a stroke in evolution.
8. An embolic stroke occurs when a blood clot or clump of matter that is traveling through the cerebral blood vessels becomes lodged in a vessel too narrow to permit further movement. Embolic strokes are of sudden onset and cause immediate deficits.
9. Hemorrhagic stroke, or intracranial hemorrhage, occurs when a cerebral blood vessel ruptures. These strokes occur most often in people with sustained increase in blood pressure. They occur suddenly, often when the affected person is engaged in activity.
10. In a stroke, the blood entering the brain compresses adjacent tissues and causes vessel spasm and cerebral edema. Blood irritates the meninges and brain tissue, which causes an inflammatory response. Onset of manifestations is rapid.
11. The most common manifestation of stroke is weakness that involves the face and arm, and sometimes the leg. Other common manifestations include numbness on one side, loss of vision, speech difficulties, sudden severe headache, and difficulties with balance.
12. Sensory-perceptual deficits associated with stroke are: hemianopia, agnosia, apraxia, and neglect syndrome.
13. A change in consciousness that ranges from mild confusion to coma is a common manifestation of a stroke. Behavior changes include emotional lability, loss of self-control, and decreased tolerance for stress. Intellectual changes may include memory loss, decreased attention span, poor judgment, and an inability to think abstractly.

- ○ Contralateral deficit
- Ischemic strokes
- Transient Ischemic Attack (TIA)
- Thrombotic stroke
- Embolic stroke
- Hemorrhagic stroke
- Manifestations of stroke
- Sensory-perceptual deficits
- Behavior changes
- Intellectual changes
- Disorders of communication
- Motor deficits
- Elimination changes
- Treatment
  - ○ Stroke prevention
  - ○ Acute care
  - ○ Rehabilitation
- Diagnosis
  - ○ Diagnostic imaging
  - ○ Lumbar puncture
  - ○ PLAC blood testing
  - ○ NIH stroke scale
- Nursing diagnoses include
  - ○ *Ineffective Tissue Perfusion: Cerebral*
  - ○ *Impaired Physical Mobility*
  - ○ *Self-care Deficit*
  - ○ *Impaired Verbal Communication*
  - ○ *Impaired Urinary Elimination*
  - ○ *Risk for Constipation*
  - ○ *Impaired Swallowing*

Ruptured Intracranial Aneurysm
- Etiology
  - ○ Developmental defect in vessel wall
  - ○ Hypertension
  - ○ Atherosclerosis
  - ○ Connective tissue disease
  - ○ Abnormal blood flow
- Types
  - ○ Berry
  - ○ Saccular
  - ○ Fusiform
  - ○ Dissecting
  - ○ Mycotic
- Manifestations
  - ○ Asymptomatic until rupture
  - ○ Small leakages
    - – Headache
    - – Nausea, vomiting
    - – Pain
    - – Visual deficits
    - – Dilation of a pupil
  - ○ At rupture
    - – Sudden, explosive headache
    - – Loss of consciousness
    - – Nausea and vomiting
    - – Stiff neck
    - – Photophobia

14. Depending on the area of the brain involved, strokes may cause weakness, paralysis, and/or spasticity. Deficits include hemiplegia, hemiparesis, flaccidity, and spasticity.

15. The three treatment stages of stroke are stroke prevention, acute care immediately after a stroke, and rehabilitation after a stroke.

16. Diagnosis is achieved by diagnostic imaging, lumbar puncture if there is no increase in intracranial pressure, and PLAC blood testing. The NIH stroke scale is used to assess neurological outcomes and recovery.

17. The treatments used in management of stroke include surgery and rehabilitation. Rehabilitation includes physical therapy, occupational therapy, and speech therapy.

18. Nursing care of clients experiencing stroke is often complex and multidimensional, and requires consideration of continuity of care for clients in acute care settings, long-term care settings, rehabilitation centers, and the home.

19. Nursing diagnoses include: *Ineffective Tissue Perfusion (Cerebral); Impaired Physical Mobility; Self-Care Deficit; Impaired Verbal Communication; Impaired Urinary Elimination; Risk for Constipation;* and *Impaired Swallowing.*

RUPTURED INTRACRANIAL ANEURYSM

20. An intracranial aneurysm is a saccular outpouching of a cerebral artery that occurs at the site of a weakness in the vessel wall. A ruptured cerebral aneurysm is the most common cause of a hemorrhagic stroke.

21. Causes of intracranial aneurysm may include a developmental defect in the vessel wall and degeneration of fragility of the vessel wall due to conditions such as hypertension, atherosclerosis, connective tissue disease, or abnormal blood flow. Hypertension and cigarette smoking may be contributing factors.

22. Types of aneurysm include berry (probably congenital); saccular (probably traumatic); fusiform (probably from changes of arteriosclerosis); dissecting (probably from atherosclerosis, inflammation, or trauma) and mycotic (emboli from infections).

23. Intracranial aneurysms are usually asymptomatic until rupture. Small leakages may cause headache, nausea, vomiting, and pain in the head and neck. Prodromal manifestation such as headache, eye pain, visual deficits, and dilation of a pupil may occur. At rupture, the client experiences a sudden, explosive headache, loss of consciousness, nausea and vomiting, stiff neck, photophobia, cranial nerve deficits, stroke syndrome manifestations, and pituitary manifestations.

24. Major complications of a ruptured intracranial aneurysm are rebleeding, vasospasm, and hydrocephalus.

25. Manifestations of rebleeding are sudden severe headache, nausea and vomiting, decreasing LOC, and new neurologic deficits.

  - Cranial nerve deficits
  - Stroke syndrome manifestations
  - Pituitary manifestations
- Hunt-Hess Classification of Subarachnoid Manifestations
- Rebleeding
- Cerebral vasospasm
- Hydrocephalus
- Interdisciplinary care
- Diagnostic testing
  - Cerebral angiogram
  - CT scan and lumbar puncture
- Major nursing diagnosis
  - *Ineffective Tissue Perfusion: Cerebral*

Arteriovenous Malformations
- Pathophysiology
  - Spontaneous bleeding into subarachnoid space
  - Vascular "steal" phenomenon
- Manifestations
  - Small malformations: neurologic deficits
  - Large malformations: seizure
- Treatment
  - Accessible malformations
    - Surgery
  - Inaccessible malformations
    - Radiation therapy
    - Laser therapy
  - Nursing Care
    - Preventative education
    - After hemorrhage, same as stroke

Spinal Cord Injury
- Pathophysiology
  - Primary injury: microscopic hemorrhages/edema
  - Secondary injury: increase size of primary injury
  - Necrosis of both the white and gray matter
- Etiology
  - Excessive force
  - Abnormal movements
  - Penetrating injury
- Diagnostic testing
  - X-ray
  - CT or MRI
  - Somatosensory evoked potential studies
- Nursing diagnoses
  - *Impaired Physical Mobility*
  - *Impaired Gas Exchange*
  - *Ineffective Breathing Patterns*
  - *Dysreflexia*
  - *Altered Urinary Elimination*
  - *Constipation*
  - *Sexual Dysfunction*
  - *Low Self-Esteem*

Herniated Intervertebral Disk
- Lumbar disk manifestations
  - Pain

26. Cerebral vasospasm is a common complication that occurs 3–10 days after a subarachnoid hemorrhage and is associated with a large number of deaths and disability. Regional manifestations may include focal deficits (hemiplegia), whereas global alterations cause loss of consciousness.
27. Hydrocephalus is an abnormal accumulation of CSF within the cranial vault that results in dilation of the ventricles. Manifestations are those of increased intracranial pressure.
28. The care of the client with a ruptured intracranial aneurysm includes determining the location of the aneurysm, treating the manifestations of the hemorrhage, and preventing rebleeding and vasospasm.
29. A cerebral angiogram is the gold standard for evaluating cerebral aneurysm. CT scan and lumbar puncture may also be performed.
30. The major nursing diagnosis is *Ineffective Tissue Perfusion (Cerebral)*.

ARTERIOVENOUS MALFORMATIONS

31. An arteriovenous (AV) malformation is a congenital intracranial lesion, formed by a tangled collection of dilated arteries and veins that allows blood to flow directly from the arterial system into the venous system.
32. Clients with this condition develop manifestations before age 40. Manifestations are a result of spontaneous bleeding from the lesion into the subarachnoid space or brain tissue. Altered cerebral perfusion results from vascular "steal" phenomenon.
33. Manifestations of small malformations are due to hemorrhage that causes neurologic deficits. Large malformations usually manifest with seizure activity.
34. Accessible malformations are treated surgically. Inaccessible malformations are treated with radiation therapy or laser therapy.
35. Nursing care of the client whose has not experienced hemorrhage focuses on preventive education. If hemorrhage has occurred, nursing care is the same as for any client who has had a hemorrhagic stroke.

SPINAL CORD INJURY

36. Nursing care of clients with a spinal cord injury takes place from the acute management phase through ongoing rehabilitation in a variety of settings.
37. When the spinal cord is injured, the primary injury causes microscopic hemorrhages in the gray matter of the cord and edema of the white matter of the cord. Secondary injury increases the area of injury. When ischemia is prolonged, necrosis of both the white and gray matter begins.
38. SCIs are the result of application of excessive force to the spinal column. Abnormal movements that produce deformation of the spinal cord include acceleration, deceleration, hyperflexion, hyperextension, axial loading, and excessive rotation.

- ○ Sciatica
- ○ Postural deformity
- ○ Motor deficits
- ○ Sensory deficits
- ○ Changes in reflexes
- Cervical disk manifestations
  - ○ Pain the shoulder, neck, arm
  - ○ Paresthesia
  - ○ Muscle spasms, stiff neck
  - ○ Decreased or absent arm reflexes
- Central cervical herniation manifestations
  - ○ Mild, intermittent pain
  - ○ Lower extremity weakness
  - ○ Unsteady gait
  - ○ Muscle spasms
  - ○ Urinary elimination problems
  - ○ Altered sexual function
  - ○ Hyperactive lower extremity reflexes
- Interdisciplinary care
  - ○ Identifying location of herniation
  - ○ Conservative treatment
    - – Pain relief
    - – Healing by fibrosis
  - ○ Surgery
- Diagnosis
  - ○ X-ray
  - ○ CT scan
  - ○ Electromyoraphy
  - ○ Myelogram
- Nursing diagnoses
  - ○ *Acute Pain*
  - ○ *Chronic Pain*
  - ○ *Constipation*

Spinal Cord Tumor
- Pathophysiology
  - ○ Compression
  - ○ Invasion
  - ○ Ischemia
- Manifestations
  - ○ Pain
  - ○ Motor and sensory deficits
  - ○ Changes in bowel/bladder function
  - ○ Changes in sexual function
- Diagnostic testing
  - ○ X-ray
  - ○ CT
  - ○ MRI
  - ○ Myelogram
  - ○ Examination of CSF
- Radiation therapy
  - ○ Treatment for metastatic spinal cord tumors
- Nursing care
  - ○ Monitoring for neurologic changes
  - ○ Provision of pain management
  - ○ Preservation of quality of life

39. The spinal cord may also be injured by penetration by bullets, other foreign objects, or by bone fragments from vertebral fractures.
40. Diagnostic testing includes x-ray of the spine, CT or MRI, and somatosensory evoked potential studies.
41. Nursing care of the client with SCI is focused on prevention of secondary complications of immobility and altered body functions, promotion of self-care, and education. Common nursing diagnoses are: *Impaired Physical Mobility; Impaired Gas Exchange; Ineffective Breathing Patterns; Dysreflexia; Altered Urinary Elimination; Constipation; Sexual Dysfunction;* and *Low Self-Esteem*.

HERNIATED INTERVERTEBRAL DISK

42. A herniated intervertebral disk is also called a ruptured disk, a herniated nucleus pulposus, or a slipped disk. It is a rupture of the cartilage that surrounds the intervertebral disk with protrusion of the nucleus pulposus.
43. This herniation may occur spontaneously or as a result of trauma. They may be abrupt or gradual.
44. The classic manifestation of a ruptured lumbar disk is a recurrent episode of pain in the lower back.
45. Cervical disks that herniate laterally cause pain in the shoulder, neck, and arm. Paresthesia, muscle spasms, and stiff neck; and decreased or absent arm reflexes may also occur.
46. Central cervical herniation results in mild, intermittent pain, but the client may also experience lower extremity weakness, unsteady gait, muscle spasms, urinary elimination problems, altered sexual function, and hyperactive lower extremity reflexes.
47. Interdisciplinary care includes identifying the location of herniation and determining whether conservative treatment or surgery is necessary.
48. Diagnosis is determined by x-ray, CT scan, electromyography, and myelogram.
49. The goals of conservative treatment are pain relief and healing of the involved disk by fibrosis.
50. Nursing diagnoses include: *Acute Pain; Chronic Pain;* and *Constipation*.

SPINAL CORD TUMOR

51. Spinal cord tumors may be benign or malignant, primary or metastatic.
52. Intramedullary tumors arise from within the neural tissues of the spinal cord and include astrocytomas, ependymomas, glioblastomas, and medulloblastomas.
53. Extra medullary tumors arise from the tissues outside the spinal cord and include neurofibromas, meningiomas, sarcomas, chordomas, and vascular tumors.
54. Depending upon their anatomic location, spinal cord tumors result in pathologic changes as a result of compression, invasion, or ischemia secondary to arterial or venous obstruction.

55. General manifestations include pain, motor and sensory deficits, changes in bowel and/or bladder function, and changes in sexual function. Pain is often the initial manifestation.

56. Diagnostic testing includes x-ray, CT, MRI, and myelogram. Examination of CSF obtained by lumbar puncture may be necessary.

57. Radiation therapy is used to treat metastatic spinal cord tumors. Radiation may be used to treat rapidly progressive neurologic deficits or to reduce pain.

58. Nursing care focuses on monitoring for neurologic changes, providing pain management, and management of motor and sensory deficits in order to preserve quality of life.

SUGGESTIONS FOR CLASSROOM ACTIVITIES

- In class, discuss the statement, "A stroke is like a heart attack in the brain." Discuss the teaching implications of this statement.
- Review the care plan activity about hemorrhagic stroke that is provided on the textbook Companion Website. Use this information to assist students in the development of a nursing plan of care for the client.
- Have students access the internet for information regarding spinal cord injuries. Have students share information about new treatments, prevention, and rehabilitation efforts.
- Review the case study about spinal cord injury that is provided on the textbook Companion Website. Use this information to assist students in the development of a nursing plan of care for the client.

SUGGESTIONS FOR CLINICAL ACTIVITIES

- Have students investigate the NIH Stroke Scale as an instrument for assessing the client who has had a stroke. Help students learn techniques from the scale.
- Arrange for students to tour a physical therapy area where clients who have suffered a stroke or spinal cord injury are being assisted with rehabilitation.

LEARNING OUTCOME 3

Compare and contrast the acute treatment and care of the client with a stroke or ruptured intracranial aneurysm and a spinal cord injury.

CONCEPTS FOR LECTURE
STROKE

1. The goals of stroke care are rapid recognition and reaction to stroke warning signs, rapid emergency medical services dispatch, rapid EMS system transport and hospital prenotification, and rapid diagnosis and treatment in the hospital.

RUPTURED INTRACRANIAL ANEURYSM

2. All people who have sustained trauma to the head or to the spine, or who are unconscious, should be treated as though they have a spinal cord injury.

3. Prehospital management includes rapid assessment of the ABCs, immobilizing and stabilizing the head and neck, removing the person from the site of the injury, and rapid transport to the appropriate facility.

4. Emergency department treatment includes respiratory support, inserting a nasogastric tube to treat developing

POWERPOINT LECTURE SLIDES

Stroke
- Goals of stoke care
  - Rapid recognition
  - Rapid reaction
  - Rapid EMS dispatch
  - Rapid EMS system transport
  - Hospital prenotification
  - Rapid diagnosis and treatment

Ruptured Intracranial Aneurysm
- Treat all victims of trauma as if a spinal cord injury exists
- Prehospital management
  - Rapid assessment of ABCs
  - Immobilizing and stabilizing head/neck
  - Rapid transport
- Emergency department treatment
  - Respiratory support

paralytic ileus, inserting an indwelling urinary catheter to prevent overdistention of an atonic bladder, and continuous assessment of cardiovascular status.

SPINAL CORD INJURY

5. The client with an acute SCI requires emergency assessment and care. The client is first assessed and stabilized at the scene of the accident, initially treated in the emergency room, and then admitted to the hospital intensive care unit.
6. It is critically important not to complicate the initial injury by allowing the fractured vertebrae to damage the cord further during transport to the hospital.
7. Prehospital management includes rapid assessment of ABGs, immobilizing and stabilizing the head and neck, removing the person from the site of the injury, stabilizing other life-threatening injuries, and rapidly transporting the person to the appropriate facility.
8. Guidelines for emergency care are: avoid flexing, extending, or rotating the neck; immobilizing the neck; secure the head; maintain the client in the supine position; and transfer from the stretcher with backboard in place to the hospital bed.
9. In the emergency department the client is treated for respiratory problems, paralytic ileus, atonic bladder, and cardiovascular alterations.

- ○ Insertion of a nasogastric tube
- ○ Insertion of an indwelling urinary catheter
- ○ Continuous cardiac assessment

Spinal Cord Injury
- Prehospital management
  - ○ Rapid assessment of ABCs
  - ○ Immobilizing and stabilizing head/neck
  - ○ Rapid transport
- Guidelines for emergency care
  - ○ Avoid flexing, extending, or rotating neck
  - ○ Immobilize neck
  - ○ Secure head
  - ○ Maintain supine position
  - ○ Transfer with backboard in place
- Emergency department management
  - ○ Respiratory problems
  - ○ Paralytic ileus
  - ○ Atonic bladder
  - ○ Cardiovascular alterations

SUGGESTIONS FOR CLASSROOM ACTIVITIES

- Arrange for a paramedic and an emergency department RN to come to the class to discuss the management of the client who has suffered a spinal cord injury.
- Discuss the important assessment warning signs of impending stroke and the actions that are appropriate secondary to those signs.

SUGGESTIONS FOR CLINICAL ACTIVITIES

- Assign students to work in an emergency department or to tour an emergency department. Talk with staff in the department about safety measures taken with clients who may have sustained a spinal cord injury.
- Discuss rapid assessment of the client who may be experiencing a stroke.

LEARNING OUTCOME 4

Discuss the pathophysiologic effects of injuries and tumors of the spinal cord by level of injury.

CONCEPTS FOR LECTURE

1. SCIs are classified as complete or incomplete cord injury, cause of injury, and level of injury.
2. Complete SCI results in complete interruption of the motor and sensory neural pathways accompanied by total loss of motor and sensory functions below the level of the injury. Incomplete SCI results in partial interruption of the motor and sensory neural pathways. Alterations in function are dependent upon the level of injury.
3. Spinal shock is the temporary loss of reflex function below the level of the injury. Manifestations include flaccid paralysis of skeletal muscles, loss of all spinal reflexes, loss of sensations of pain, touch, temperature,

POWERPOINT LECTURE SLIDES

Spinal Cord Injury
- Complete SCI
  - ○ Complete interruption of motor/sensory neural pathways
  - ○ Total loss of motor/sensory function below level of injury
- Incomplete SCI
  - ○ Partial interruption of motor/sensory neural pathways
  - ○ Alterations in function dependent upon level of injury
- Spinal shock
  - ○ Temporary loss of reflex function below level of injury

and pressure, absence of visceral and somatic sensations, bowel and bladder dysfunction, and loss of the ability to perspire below the level of the injury.

4. Cervical or upper thoracic spinal cord injury may also result in neurogenic shock.

5. Clients with injury to C1 to C4 may experience respiratory insufficiency, hypothermia, paralytic ileus, urinary retention, and oliguria.

6. Complications of an SCI often result in permanent disability and loss of functional health status.

7. When upper motor neurons are interrupted, the client experiences spastic paralysis and hyperreflexia and may be unable to carry out skilled movement.

8. Interruption of lower motor neurons results in muscle flaccidity and extensive muscle atrophy, with loss of both voluntary and involuntary movement. Amount of paresis and hyporeflexia is dependent upon amount of loss of motor neurons.

9. Paraplegia is a paralysis of the lower portion of the body, which sometimes involves the lower trunk. Paraplegia occurs when the thoracic, lumbar, and sacral portions of the spinal cord are injured.

10. Quadriplegia, also called tetraplegia, occurs when cervical segments of the cord are injured, which impairs function of the arms, trunk, legs, and pelvic organs.

11. Autonomic dysreflexia (also call autonomic hyperreflexia) is an exaggerated sympathetic response that occurs in clients with SCIs at or above the T6 level. Manifestations include pounding headache; bradycardia; hypertension; flushed, warm skin with profuse sweating above the lesion and pale, cold, dry skin below it; and anxiety. This condition is a neurologic emergency and requires immediate treatment.

- Neurogenic shock
  - May result from cervical or upper thoracic spinal cord injury
  - Injury to C1 to C4 may result in
    - Respiratory insufficiency
    - Hypothermia
    - Paralytic ileus
    - Urinary retention
    - Oliguria
- Upper motor neuron interruption
  - Spastic paralysis
  - Hyperreflexia
  - Inability to carry out skilled movement
- Lower motor neuron interruption
  - Muscle flaccidity
  - Extensive muscle atrophy
  - Loss of voluntary/involuntary movement
- Paraplegia
  - Paralyis of the lower portion of the body
  - Occurs with thoracic, lumbar, sacral injury
- Quadraplegia
  - Also called tetraplegia
  - Impairs function of arms, trunk, legs, pelvic organs
  - Occurs with cervical injury
- Autonomic dysreflexia
  - Autonomic hyperreflexia
  - Exaggerated sympathetic response
  - Occurs with CIs at or above the T6
  - Manifestations
    - Pounding headache
    - Bradycardia
    - Hypertension
    - Flushed, warm skin with profuse sweating above lesion
    - Pale, cold, dry skin below lesion
    - Anxiety
  - Neurologic emergency
  - Requires immediate treatment

SUGGESTIONS FOR CLASSROOM ACTIVITIES

- Using anatomic models, identify the primary areas of spinal cord injury. Have students identify the deficits that occur at each level. Discuss the care of clients with these deficits.
- Arrange for a person who has sustained a spinal cord injury to speak to the students about living with the deficits sustained.

SUGGESTIONS FOR CLINICAL ACTIVITIES

- Arrange for a student tour of a neurointensive care unit. Discuss the nursing challenges encountered with the unit staff.

LEARNING OUTCOME 5

Discuss the purposes, nursing implications, and health education of the client and family for medications used to treat stroke, ruptured intracranial aneurysm, and spinal cord injury.

CONCEPTS FOR LECTURE

STROKE

1. Antiplatelet agents such as ASA, clopidogrel (Plavix), dipyridamole (Persantine), and ticlopidine (Ticlid), are often used to treat clients with TIAs or who have had a previous stroke.
2. Anticoagulant therapy with warfarin (Coumadin), heparin, and enoxaparin (Lovenox) is often ordered for an ischemic stroke.
3. Thrombolytic therapy such as ft-PA, or tPA is often given concurrently with an anticoagulant to treat a thrombotic stroke.
4. Other classes of medications administered to the stroke client are antihypertensives, corticosteroids, hyperosmolar solutions, diuretics, and anticonvulsants.

RUPTURED INTRACRANIAL ANEURYSM

5. Calcium channel blockers are used to improve neurologic deficits due to vasospasm. Other medications that may be prescribed include anticonvulsants, analgesics, and stool softeners.

SPINAL CORD INJURY

6. High-dose steroid therapy protocol using methylprednisolone (Medrol) is implemented within 8 hours of the injury to improve neurologic recovery.
7. Vasopressors, antispasmodics, analgesics, proton pump inhibitors, anticoagulants, and stool softeners are often prescribed.

HERNIATED INTERVERTEBRAL DISK

8. Medications are administered to relieve pain and reduce swelling and muscle spasms.

SPINAL TUMORS

9. Medications are administered to relieve pain and control edema. An epidural catheter may be inserted for narcotic analgesic administration.

POWERPOINT LECTURE SLIDES

Stroke
- Antiplatelet agents
  - ASA, clopidogrel, dipyridamole, and ticlopidine
- Anticoagulant therapy
  - Warfarin, heparin, and enoxaparin
- Thrombolytic therapy
  - ft-PA, or tPA
- Antihypertensives
- Corticosteroids
- Hyperosmolar solutions
- Diuretics
- Anticonvulsants

Ruptured Intracranial Aneurysm
- Calcium channel blockers
- Anticonvulsants
- Analgesics
- Stool softeners

Spinal Cord Injury
- High-dose steroid therapy protocol within 8 hours of the injury
- GMI ganglioside for 3–4 weeks is experimental
- Vasopressors
- Antispasmodics
- Analgesics
- Proton pump inhibitors
- Anticoagulants
- Stool softeners

Herniated Intervertebral Disk
- Pain relief
- Reduction of swelling and muscle spasms

Spinal Tumors
- Pain relief
  - Epidural catheter may be inserted
- Reduction of edema

SUGGESTIONS FOR CLASSROOM ACTIVITIES

- Have students group the common medications used for cerebrovascular and spinal cord disorders according to pharmacodynamics. Have students identify the commonalities and differences among these medications.

SUGGESTIONS FOR CLINICAL ACTIVITIES

- Have students develop a teaching plan of care for a client who is receiving a medication covered in this chapter.

LEARNING OUTCOME 6

Describe the methods used to stabilize and immobilize spinal cord injuries.

CONCEPTS FOR LECTURE

1. The client with an SCI may be immobilized in some type of traction or external fixation device to stabilize the vertebral column and to prevent any further damage.
2. Gardner-Wells tongs may be used for traction.
3. The halo external fixation device is secured with four pins inserted into the skull. The halo ring is then attached to a rigid plastic vest lined with sheepskin.

POWERPOINT LECTURE SLIDES

Immobilization of SCI
- Traction
  ○ Gardner-Wells tongs
- External fixation
  ○ Halo external fixation device
  ○ Halo ring attached to rigid plastic vest

SUGGESTIONS FOR CLASSROOM ACTIVITIES

- Using anatomic models, describe the techniques used to immobilize a spinal cord injury.
- Discuss the care of an external fixation device.

SUGGESTIONS FOR CLINICAL ACTIVITIES

- Arrange for students to speak with a client who has sustained a spinal cord injury and who has been treated with traction and external fixation. Focus the discussion on techniques that would make the experience more comfortable for the client.

LEARNING OUTCOME 7

Describe the surgical procedures used to treat cerebrovascular and spinal cord disorders.

CONCEPTS FOR LECTURE
STROKE

1. Surgery may be performed to prevent the occurrence of a stroke, to restore blood flow when a stroke has already occurred, or to repair vascular damage or malformations. Examples of such surgical procedures are carotid endarterectomy and extracranial-intracranial bypass.

INTRACRANIAL ANEURYSM

2. Surgical procedures to repair ruptured intracranial aneurysm or to prevent the rupture of an existing large aneurysm include craniotomy with clip placement, placement of Guglielmi detachable coils, stent placement, balloon remodeling, and parent vessel occlusion.

AV MALFORMATION

3. If the malformation is accessible, the ideal treatment is excision of the malformation and removal of any hematoma.
4. Large malformations may be treated by embolization with substances such as Gelfoam or metallic pellets.

SPINAL CORD INJURY

5. Early surgical treatment may be necessary if there is evidence of compression of the spinal cord by bone fragments or a hematoma. Surgery may also be done to stabilize and support the spine.
6. Surgical procedures may include decompression laminectomy, spinal fusion, and insertion of metal rods.

POWERPOINT LECTURE SLIDES

Stroke
- Carotid endarterectomy
- Extracranial-intracranial bypass

Intracranial Aneurysm
- Craniotomy with clip placement
- Placement of Gudlielmi detachable coils
- Stent placement
- Balloon remodeling
- Parent vessel occlusion

AV Malformation
- Excision and removal of hematoma
- Embolization
  ○ Gelfoam
  ○ Metallic pellets

Spinal Cord Injury
- Removal of bone fragments or hematoma
- Stabilization and support of spine
- Decompression laminectomy
- Spinal fusion
- Insertion of metal rods

Herniated Intervertebral Disk
- Indications
  ○ Nonresponsive to conservative treatment
  ○ Serious neurologic defects
- Laminectomy
- Nuclectomy
- Diskectomy
- Spinal fusion

HERNIATED INTERVERTEBRAL DISK

7. Surgery is indicated for clients who do not respond to conservative treatment or who have serious neurologic defects.
8. Surgical interventions include laminectomy, nuclectomy, diskectomy, spinal fusion, foraminotomy, IntraDiskal Electrothermal therapy, and microdiskectomy.

SPINAL TUMORS

9. Intramedullary and extramedullary tumors are excised when possible. Surgical excision is made through a laminectomy. Spinal fusion and rod insertion may be necessary.

- Foraminotomy
- IntraDiskal electrothermal therapy
- Microdiskectomy

Spinal Tumors
- Surgical excision through laminectomy
- Spinal fusion
- Rod insertion

SUGGESTIONS FOR CLASSROOM ACTIVITIES

- Using anatomic models, describe the physiology of the procedures listed.
- Have students search the internet for information about the procedures listed. Share findings in class.

SUGGESTIONS FOR CLINICAL ACTIVITIES

- Arrange for students to observe one of the procedures identified.

CHAPTER 46

NURSING CARE OF CLIENTS WITH NEUROLOGIC DISORDERS

RESOURCE LIBRARY

PRENTICE HALL NURSING MEDIALINK DVD-ROM

Audio Glossary
NCLEX Review
Animations/Videos
  Akinesia
  Alzheimer's Disease
  Bradykinesia
  Dopamine
  Forward Tremor
  Lateral Tremor
  Levodopa
  Multiple Sclerosis
  Parkinson's Disease

IMAGE LIBRARY

Figure 46.1 Neuron with neurofibrillary tangles seen in Alzheimer's disease.
Figure 46.2 Changes in neuroanatomy associated with Alzheimer's disease.
Figure 46.3 In Parkinson's disease, the client's face lacks expression or animation.
Figure 46.4 *A,* A normal neuromuscular junction and *B,* one showing the changes seen in myasthenia gravis.

COMPANION WEBSITE

Audio Glossary
NCLEX–RN® Review
Care Plan Activity: Guillain-Barré Syndrome
Case Studies
  Huntington's Disease
  Parkinson's Disease
MediaLink Application: Alzheimer's Disease
Links to Resources

Figure 46.5 In myasthenia gravis, the client experiences unilateral weakness of the facial muscles.
Figure 46.7 Sensory and motor distribution of the trigeminal nerve.
Figure 46.8 The client with Bell's palsy shows the typical drooping of one side of the face.

LEARNING OUTCOME 1

Identify prevalence, incidence, and risk factors for degenerative neurologic, peripheral nervous system, cranial nerve, and infection- and neurotoxin-caused neurologic disorders.

CONCEPTS FOR LECTURE
DEGENERATIVE NEUROLOGIC DISORDERS

1. Dementia affects multiple cortical functions, calculations, learning capacity, language, and judgment.
2. Impairments of cognitive function are usually accompanied by deterioration in emotional control, social behavior, and motivation.
3. As many as 6.8 million people in the United States have dementia. At least 1.8 million of those are severely affected. Almost half of those 85 and older have some form of dementia. Dementia is not a normal part of aging.
4. Dementia is diagnosed when two or more brain functions such as memory, language skills, perception, reasoning, and judgment are significantly impaired without loss of consciousness.

POWERPOINT LECTURE SLIDES

Degenerative Neurologic Disorders
Dementia
- Affects multiple cortical functions
  - Calculations
  - Learning capacity
  - Language
  - Judgment
  - Emotional control
  - Social behavior
  - Motivation
- Prevalence
  - 6.8 million people in United States have dementia
  - 1.8 million are severely affected

5. Risk factors for development of dementia include advancing age, family history, smoking, alcohol use, atherosclerosis, high cholesterol and plasma homocysteine levels, diabetes, mild cognitive impairment, and Down syndrome.

ALZHEIMER'S DISEASE

6. Alzheimer's disease (AD) is the most common degenerative neurologic disorder and the most common cause of cognitive impairment in older adults.
7. Familial AD follows an inheritance pattern, while sporadic AD has no obvious inheritance pattern. AD is also described as early onset (occurring in people less than 65) and late onset (occurring in people age 65 and over).
8. Risk factors for AD are older age, family history, and female gender.

MULTIPLE SCLEROSIS

9. The onset of multiple sclerosis (MS) is generally between the ages of 20 and 50 and has a peak incidence at age 30.
10. MS is the leading cause of neurologic disability in young adults. Females are affected 2 times more often than males. The disorder occurs more commonly in temperate climates, including the northern United States.

PARKINSON'S DISEASE

11. Parkinson's disease (PD) usually develops after age 65, but 15% of those diagnosed are under 40 years of age.
12. Recent discovery of inherited forms of PD suggest a genetic role in the development of this disease.
13. Parkinson's-like manifestations, called secondary parkinsonism, may result from other disorders such as trauma, encephalitis, tumors, toxins, and drugs.

HUNTINGTON'S DISEASE

14. Huntington's disease (HD) causes destruction of cells in the caudate nucleus and putamen areas of the basal ganglia. Other areas of the brain may also atrophy.
15. HD is a familial disease; each child of an HD parent has a 50% chance of inheriting the HD gene. There is no cure.

AMYOTROPHIC LATERAL SCLEROSIS

16. Amyotrophic lateral sclerosis (ALS) is the most common motor neuron disease in the United States. About 5% to 10% of all cases are inherited in what is termed familial ALS.
17. Most people are between 40 and 60 years of age at diagnosis.
18. Death results in 2–5 years after onset of manifestations, and is generally due to respiratory failure.

MYASTHENIA GRAVIS

19. Women are 3 times more frequently affected than men.
20. Age of onset is generally between 20 and 30.

- ○ Almost half of 85+ affected
- ○ Not a normal part of aging
- • Diagnosis
  - ○ Two or more brain functions significantly impaired
  - ○ No loss of consciousness
- • Risk factors
  - ○ Advancing age
  - ○ Family history
  - ○ Smoking, alcohol use
  - ○ Atherosclerosis
  - ○ High cholesterol and plasma homocysteine levels
  - ○ Diabetes
  - ○ Mild cognitive impairment, Down syndrome
- • Conditions that mimic dementia
  - ○ Age-related cognitive decline
  - ○ Mild cognitive impairment
  - ○ Depression
  - ○ Delirium
    - – Usually caused by treatable physical/mental illness
    - – Treatment can result in full recovery

Alzheimer's Disease
- • Most common degenerative neurologic disorder
- • Most common cause of cognitive impairment in older adults

Etiology
- • Familial
- • Sporadic
- • Early onset
- • Late onset
- • Risk factors
  - ○ Older age
  - ○ Family history
  - ○ Female gender

GUILLAIN-BARRÉ SYNDROME

21. Guillain-Barré syndrome (GBS) is one of the most common peripheral nervous system disorders.
22. Precipitating events include a respiratory or gastrointestinal viral or bacterial infection 1–3 weeks prior to the onset of manifestations, surgery, viral immunizations, and other viral illnesses.
23. *Campylobacter jejuni* is identified as the cause of the preceding infection in 60% of cases.

TRIGEMINAL NEURALGIA

24. Trigeminal neuralgia occurs more commonly in middle and older adults and affects women more often than men.

BELL'S PALSY

25. This disorder is seen most often in adults between 20 and 60.

CREUTZFELDT-JAKOB DISEASE

26. Creutzfeldt-Jakob disease (CJD) is in two forms, classic CJD and new variant CJD. The disease occurs worldwide, but clusters occur in several areas, more often in England, Chile, and Italy.
27. Classic CJD affects adults over the age of 50. New variant CJD affects younger people.
28. The median age of death in classic CJD is 68 years. The median age of death in new variant CJD is 28 years.

POSTPOLIOMYELITIS SYNDROME

29. Nearly 50% of the estimated 1.63 million people in the United States who had poliomyelitis in the 1940s and 1950s are experiencing manifestations of the same acute illness.

RABIES

30. If untreated, rabies is fatal and accounts for 30,000 to 70,000 deaths worldwide each year.
31. Approximately 25,000 to 40,000 people in the United States are treated each year for contact with potentially rabid animals.

SUGGESTIONS FOR CLASSROOM ACTIVITIES

- Assign each student one of the disorders covered in this chapter. Have the student identify the prevalence, incidence, and risk factors for developing that disorder. In class, group students and their disorders according to risk factors.
- Assign someone from the class to call a local veterinarian. Ask this animal health specialist to describe activities taken when someone is bitten by a potential rabid animal. Share the findings in class.

SUGGESTIONS FOR CLINICAL ACTIVITIES

- Assign students to the care of clients with Alzheimer's or Parkinson's disease. After the students have cared for the clients, discuss the similarities and differences in the disease presentation and care.

LEARNING OUTCOME 2

Explain the pathophysiology, manifestations, complications, interdisciplinary care, and nursing care of clients with neurologic disorders.

CONCEPTS FOR LECTURE
ALZHEIMER'S DISEASE

1. Alzheimer's disease (AD) is a form of dementia characterized by progressive, irreversible deterioration of general intellectual functioning.
2. Clients with AD live about 8–10 years following diagnosis. The cause of death is frequently aspiration pneumonia.
3. The first sign of AD is memory loss. This loss may be subtle and initially overlooked.
4. Warning signs for development of AD are: memory loss that affects job skills; difficulty performing familiar tasks; problems with language; disorientation to time and place; poor or decreased judgment; problems with abstract thinking; misplacing things; changes in mood or behavior; changes in personality; and loss of initiative.
5. Characteristic findings in the brains of AD clients are loss of nerve cells and the presence of neurofibrillary tangles and amyloid plaques.
6. AD is characterized by atrophy of the cortical area of the brain and loss of neurons, especially in the parietal and temporal lobes.
7. The exact cause of AD is unknown. Theories include a decrease in choline acetyltransferase activity in the cortex and hippocampus, a mutation for encoding amyloid precursor protein, and alteration in apolipoprotein E. There may be gene defects on chromosomes 14, 19, or 21. The role of protein kinase C, the link between AD and aluminum, viral causes, autoimmune causes, and mitochondrial defects are also being studied.
8. Interdisciplinary care is focused on providing an environment that matches the client's functional abilities. There is no cure.
9. Alzheimer's disease is diagnosed by ruling out causes for the client's manifestations. The only definitive diagnosis is postmortem examination of brain tissue. Mental status is assessed with tests such as the Folstein Mini Mental Status Examination.
10. The diagnosis of Alzheimer's disease requires the documented presence of dementia, onset between

POWERPOINT LECTURE SLIDES

Alzheimer's Disease
- Progressive, irreversible deterioration of general intellectual functioning
- Prognosis
  - 8–10 years following diagnosis
  - Cause of death often aspiration pneumonia
- Manifestations
  - First sign: memory loss
  - This loss may be subtle and initially overlooked
- Warning signs for development
  - Memory loss that affects job skills
  - Difficulty performing familiar tasks
  - Problems with language
  - Disorientation to time and place
  - Poor or decreased judgment
  - Problems with abstract thinking
  - Misplacing things
  - Changes in mood or behavior
  - Changes in personality
  - Loss of initiative
- Pathophysiology
  - Neurofibrillary tangles
  - Amyloid plaques
- Etiology
  - Exact cause unknown
  - Decrease in choline acetyltransferase activity
  - Mutation for encoding amyloid precursor protein
  - Alteration in apolipoprotein E
  - Possible gene defects on chromosomes 14, 19, or 21
  - Protein kinase C
  - Link with aluminum
  - Viral causes
  - Mitochondrial defects
- Interdisciplinary care
  - Provision of environment that matches abilities
  - No cure

40 and 90 years, no loss of consciousness, and absence of systemic or brain disorders that could cause mental changes.

11. Health promotion for the client with AD focuses on maintaining functional abilities and safety.

12. Nursing diagnoses include: *Impaired Memory; Chronic Confusion; Anxiety; Hopelessness;* and *Caregiver Role Strain.*

MULTIPLE SCLEROSIS

13. Multiple sclerosis (MS) is a chronic demyelinating neurologic disorder of the central nervous system associated with an abnormal immune response to an environmental factor.

14. MS is believed to occur as a result of an autoimmune response to a prior viral infection in a genetically susceptible person. Inflammation destroys myelin and oligodendrocytes, which leads to axon dysfunction.

15. Demyelination occurs in patches or plaques and slows, distorts, and sometimes totally eliminates the ability of the nerve to carry impulses.

16. There are four classifications of MS: relapsing-remitting, primary progressive, secondary progressive, and progressive-relapsing. Most individuals with MS present with the relapsing-remitting type.

17. Triggers for development of MS may include febrile states, pregnancy, extreme physical exertion, and fatigue. These triggers may also cause relapse of manifestations during the course of the illness.

18. The manifestations of MS vary according to the areas destroyed by demyelination and the affected body system. Fatigue is one of the most disabling of the manifestations and affects almost all clients with MS. Manifestations are classified as mixed or generalized type, spinal type, cerebellar type, or amaurotic form.

19. Short-lived attacks of neurologic deficits indicate the appearance or worsening of manifestations. These short-lived attacks can be triggered by minor increases in body temperature or serum calcium concentrations and function demands that exceed conduction capacity.

20. Management of the client with MS varies according to the severity of the manifestations. The focus is on retaining the optimal level of functioning possible, given the degree of disability.

21. The diagnosis of MS requires that the client has one of the following: (1) two or more exacerbations separated by 1 month or more and lasting more than 24 hours, followed by recovery; (2) a history of repeated exacerbation and remission with or without complete recovery, followed by progressively more severe manifestations lasting for 6 months or more; or (3) slowly increasing manifestations for at least 6 months.

22. Diagnostic testing includes MRI, CSF analysis, CT scan of the brain, PET scan, and evoked response testing.

23. Surgery may be indicated for clients who experience severe spasticity and deformity.

- Diagnosis
  - Diagnosis of exclusion
  - Definitive diagnosis only on autopsy
  - Mental status testing
    - Folstein Mini Mental Status Examination
- Requirement for diagnosis
  - Documented presence of dementia
  - Onset between 40 and 90 years
  - No loss of consciousness
  - Absence of systemic or brain disorders
- Nursing diagnoses
  - *Impaired Memory*
  - *Chronic Confusion*
  - *Anxiety*
  - *Hopelessness*
  - *Caregiver Role Strain*

Huntington's Disease
- Progressive, degenerative, inherited neurologic disease
  - Characterized by increasing dementia and chorea
- Etiology
  - Unknown
  - Post-mortem examination
    - Decrease in gamma-aminobutyric acid
    - Inhibitory neurotransmitter in basal ganglia
  - Decrease in acetylcholine levels
- Manifestations
  - Abnormal movement and progressive dementia
- Psychologic manifestations
  - Severe depression
  - Memory loss
  - Decreased ability to concentrate
  - Emotional liability
  - Impulsiveness
- Movement
  - "Fidgeting" or restlessness
  - Facial grimaces
  - Tongue protrusion
  - Jerky movements of distal arms/legs
  - Rhythmic, lurching gait
    - Almost resembles a dance
    - Contributes to frequent falls
  - Affects muscles of swallowing, chewing, speaking
- Testing
  - Genetic testing
    - Blood and amniotic fluid
- Nursing diagnoses
  - *Risk for Aspiration*
  - *Imbalanced Nutrition: Less than Body Requirements*
  - *Impaired Skin Integrity*
  - *Impaired Verbal Communication*

Guillain-Barré Syndrome
- Acute onset of motor paralysis
- Usually ascending in nature

24. Physical and rehabilitative therapies are tailored to the client's level of functioning. The long-term goal is to enable the client to retain as much independence as possible.

25. Common nursing diagnoses include: *Self-Care Deficit; Impaired Home Maintenance; Powerlessness; Impaired Physical Mobility; Ineffective Breathing Pattern; Constipation; Functional Urinary Incontinence* and *Fatigue.*

PARKINSON'S DISEASE

26. Parkinson's disease (PD) is a progressive, degenerative neurologic disease characterized by tremor, muscle rigidity, and bradykinesia.

27. A disturbed balance between excitatory and inhibitory neurotransmitters causes disorders of voluntary motor functions, such as PD. The failure to inhibit acetylcholine is the underlying basis for the manifestations of the disorder.

28. Parkinson's disease has five stages. Manifestations are initially subtle but progressively increase in severity.

29. Tremor at rest is usually the first manifestation. Resting tremors of the hand show a "pill rolling" motion of the thumb and fingers.

30. Manifestations related to motor and postural effects include rigidity, bradykinesia, and uncoordinated movements. Cogwheel rigidity is common. Slowed or delayed movements that affect the eyes, mouth, and voice cause a mask-like face and softened or muffled voice.

31. Many manifestations result from the loss of functions controlled by the autonomic nervous system. Such manifestations are constipation, urinary hesitation, urinary frequency, orthostatic hypotension, eczematous skin changes, and seborrhea.

32. Both depression and dementia are pathologies associated with PD. Bradyphrenia may also occur, which results in slow thinking and a decreased ability to form thoughts, plan, and decide.

33. Clients with PD commonly have sleep disturbances. The ability to fall and stay asleep is affected by acetylcholine.

34. Diagnosis of PD is based primarily on a thorough history and physical examination and is made based on having two of the following manifestations: tremor at rest, bradykinesia, rigidity, and postural instability. No test clearly differentiates PD from other neurologic disorders. PET scan will show decreased uptake of 6-[18F]-fluro-dopa.

35. Activa TM tremor control therapy uses an implanted pacemaker-like device to deliver mild electrical stimulation to block the brain impulses that cause tremor, rigidity, stiffness, slowed movement, and problems with walking.

36. Pallidotomy is a surgical technique for PD in which the affected areas of the globus pallidus are destroyed. Results have been helpful for many clients. Long-term effects are still being evaluated.

- 20% of clients require mechanical ventilation
- Pathophysiology
  ○ Destruction of myelin sheaths
  ○ Humoral and cell mediated immunologic response
- Manifestations
  ○ Weakness of muscles, sensory and cranial nerves
  ○ Symmetric muscle weakness in lower extremities
  ○ Ascends to the upper extremities, torso, and cranial nerves
  ○ Cognition and LOC not affected
- Interdisciplinary interventions
  ○ Focus primarily on ventilation
  ○ Preventing complications from immobility
- Diagnosis
  ○ Essential
  ○ Based on manifestations
    – History of a recent viral infection
  ○ Elevations of CSF protein levels
  ○ EMG studies
- Nutritional support
  ○ May include parenteral therapies
- Nursing diagnoses
  ○ *Pain*
  ○ *Risk for Impaired Skin Integrity*
  ○ *Anxiety*
  ○ *Powerlessness*
  ○ *Imbalanced Nutrition: Less than Body Requirements*
  ○ *Impaired Swallowing*
  ○ *Impaired Verbal Communication*
  ○ *Ineffective Airway Clearance*

37. Stereotaxic thalamotomy is another method of destroying brain tissue that causes tremors and rigidity.
38. Fetal tissue transplantation is also being used to treat PD.
39. Depending on individual needs, clients frequently benefit from rehabilitation therapy with a physical therapist, social worker, psychologist, and/or speech therapist.
40. Nursing diagnoses include: *Impaired Physical Mobility; Impaired Verbal Communication; Imbalanced Nutrition;* and *Disturbed Sleep Patterns.*

HUNTINGTON'S DISEASE

41. Huntington's disease is a progressive, degenerative, inherited neurologic disease characterized by increasing dementia and chorea.
42. The exact cause is unknown, but postmortem studies have demonstrated a decrease in gamma-aminobutyric acid, which is an inhibitory neurotransmitter in the basal ganglia. There is also a decrease in acetylcholine levels.
43. Manifestations primarily involve abnormal movement and progressive dementia. Initially the psychologic manifestations are more debilitating than the choreiform movements.
44. Muscles of swallowing, chewing, and speaking are affected.
45. Clients with Huntington's disease face inevitable total multisystem debilitation and require skilled interdisciplinary care.
46. Genetic testing is the only test available to diagnose clients suspected of having Huntington's disease. Both blood and amniotic fluid may be tested.
47. Nurses are faced with a multitude of challenges when caring for families who have Huntington's disease, including physiologic, psychosocial, and ethical problems.
48. Nursing diagnoses include: *Risk for Aspiration; Imbalanced Nutrition: Less than Body Requirements; Impaired Skin Integrity;* and *Impaired Verbal Communication.*

AMYOTROPHIC LATERAL SCLEROSIS

49. Amyotrophic lateral sclerosis (ALS), or Lou Gehrig's disease, is a rapidly progressive and fatal degenerative neurologic disease characterized by weakness and wasting of muscles under voluntary control, without any accompanying sensory or cognitive changes.
50. ALS results from the degeneration and demyelination of both upper and lower motor neurons in the anterior horn of the spinal cord, brainstem, and cerebral cortex.
51. The pathogenesis of ALS is not clear. Abnormal glutamate metabolism and hydrogen peroxide production are being studied as possible causative factors. Viral, environmental, excessive intracellular calcium, and antibodies to calcium channels are being researched as possible factors.
52. Weakness and paresis are common early manifestations. Fasciculations of involved muscles are common

in the early stage. Typically, the disease first affects the hands, then shoulders, upper arms, and finally the legs.

53. Increasing brainstem involvement causes progressive atrophy of the tongue and facial muscles. Vision, hearing, sensation, and cognitive ability usually remain intact.

54. Once ALS is diagnosed, the primary goal is to support the client and family in meeting physical and psychosocial needs.

55. Diagnosis is made based on manifestations and tests to rule out other disorders.

56. Nursing diagnoses include: *Risk for Disuse Syndrome and Ineffective Breathing Pattern*. Special attention should also be made in planning for the client's eventual inability to communicate.

MYASTHENIA GRAVIS

57. Myasthenia gravis (MG) is a chronic autoimmune neuromuscular disorder characterized by fatigue and severe weakness of skeletal muscles. Clients with MG experience periods of remission and exacerbation.

58. In MG, antibodies destroy or block neuromuscular junction receptor sites, which results in a decreased number of acetylcholine receptors. This results in a decrease in the muscle's ability to contract despite a sufficient amount of acetylcholine.

59. Initial manifestations include diplopia or ptosis. Facial, speech, and mastication muscles become weak and dysarthria and dysphagia occur. Muscle weakness spreads to other muscle groups as the disease progresses.

60. Complications are directly related to the degree of muscle weakness and the muscle groups involved. Clients with MG can develop life-threatening emergencies, including myasthenic crisis and cholinergic crisis.

61. Myasthenic crisis is a sudden exacerbation of motor weakness that puts the client at risk of respiratory failure and aspiration. Manifestations include tachycardia, tachypnea, severe respiratory distress, dysphagia, restlessness, impaired speech, and anxiety. The causative factor is almost always undermedication.

62. Cholinergic crisis is the result of overdosage with anticholinesterase medications. GI manifestations, severe muscle weakness, vertigo, and respiratory distress are signs of cholinergic crisis.

63. Diagnostic testing includes anticholinesterase test, nerve stimulation studies, and an analysis of antiacetylcholine receptor antibodies.

64. Common nursing diagnoses are: *Ineffective Airway Clearance, Impaired Swallowing,* and *Fatigue.*

GUILLAIN-BARRÉ SYNDROME

65. Guillain-Barré syndrome (GBS) is an acute inflammatory demyelinating disorder of the peripheral nervous system characterized by an acute onset of motor paralysis which is usually ascending in nature. About 20% of clients have respiratory involvement to the point of requiring mechanical ventilation.

66. The primary pathophysiologic process in GBS is the destruction of myelin sheaths that cover the axons of peripheral nerves. This demyelination is thought to be the result of both a humoral and cell-mediated immunologic response.

67. Manifestations are weakness of muscles, sensory nerves, and cranial nerves. Cognition and level of consciousness are not affected.

68. Interdisciplinary interventions during the acute phase focus primarily on ventilation and preventing complications from immobility.

69. An accurate and rapid diagnosis is needed to ensure prompt, supportive treatment. Diagnosis is made based on manifestations, history of a recent viral infection, elevations of CSF protein levels, and EMG studies that reflect decreased nerve conduction.

70. Nutritional support of the client with GBS is crucial and may include parenteral therapies.

71. Clients with GBS usually require prolonged rehabilitation care, which begins during the acute phase and focuses on preventing complications and limiting the effects of immobility.

72. Common nursing diagnoses include: *Pain; Risk for Impaired Skin Integrity; Anxiety; Powerlessness; Imbalanced Nutrition: Less than Body Requirements; Impaired Swallowing; Impaired Verbal Communication;* and *Ineffective Airway Clearance.*

TRIGEMINAL NEURALGIA

73. Trigeminal neuralgia is also called *tic douloureux.* It is a chronic disease of the trigeminal cranial nerve that causes severe facial pain.

74. The actual cause of trigeminal neuralgia is unknown. Contributing factors include irritation from flu-like illnesses, trauma or infection of the teeth or jaw, pressure on the nerve by an aneurysm or tumor, or arteriosclerotic changes of an artery close to the nerve.

75. Stimulating specific areas of the face, called trigger zones, may initiate the onset of pain.

76. Characteristic manifestations are brief, repetitive episodes of severe unilateral pain.

77. There is no specific diagnostic testing for trigeminal neuralgia.

78. If medications do not control the pain, surgical procedures may be performed, including various types of rhizotomy.

79. Nursing diagnoses include: *Acute Pain and Risk for Altered Nutrition: Less than Body Requirements.*

BELL'S PALSY

80. Bell's palsy is also call facial palsy. It is a disorder of the seventh cranial nerve, characterized by unilateral paralysis of the facial muscles.

81. The exact cause of the disorder is unknown, although inflammation of the nerve and a relationship to the herpes simplex virus have been suggested.

82. Onset of Bell's palsy is usually sudden and is almost always unilateral. Pain behind the ear or along the jaw may precede the paralysis. As the disease progresses, the face becomes obviously asymmetric.

83. Some clients have only mild manifestations, whereas others have complete facial paralysis. Clients often believe they have had a stroke.

84. There are no definitive laboratory or diagnostic tests for Bell's palsy, nor are there any specific treatments. Moist heat applied to the affected side of the face may decrease pain.

85. Nursing care should include education about eye care, pain control, and dietary modifications.

CREUTZFELDT-JAKOB DISEASE

86. Creutzfeldt-Jakob disease (CJD), or spongiform encephalopathy, is a rapidly-progressive, degenerative, neurologic disease that causes brain degeneration without inflammation.

87. CJD is transmissible and is progressively fatal.

88. The causative agent is though to be a prion protein. Transmission is by direct contamination with infected neural tissue, such as during eye or brain surgery. Injection of contaminated human growth hormone from cadaveric pituitaries has also been implicated.

89. New variant CJD (vCJD or mad-cow disease) is also a rare, degenerative, fatal brain disorder, but it is not the same as classic CJD.

90. New variant CJD is thought to be due to consumption of cattle products contaminated with bovine spongiform encephalopathy (BSE).

91. CJD is characterized by degeneration of the gray matter of the brain.

92. Onset of CJD is characterized by memory changes, an exaggerated startle reflex, sleep disturbances, and nervousness. Rapid deterioration in motor, sensor, and language follows. Clients in the terminal state are comatose and exhibit decorticate and decerebrate posturing.

93. There is no specific treatment to stop or slow the progression of CJD.

94. Definitive diagnosis can be made only by postmortem examination.

95. Nursing care focuses on maximizing comfort, preventing injury, preventing transmission, and providing support.

POSTPOLIOMYELITIS SYNDROME

96. Postpoliomyelitis syndrome is a complication of a previous infection by the poliomyelitis virus. The virus destroys motor cells of the anterior horn cells of the spinal cord, which causes neuromuscular effects that range from mild to severe flaccid paralysis and atrophy.

97. Manifestations of motor neuron degeneration and weakness may emerge 10 to 40 years after the initial infection and include fatigue, muscle and joint weakness, loss of muscle mass, respiratory difficulties, and pain.

98. Postpoliomyelitis syndrome is diagnosed by a previous history of polio and the current manifestations.

99. Interdisciplinary management addresses the manifestations and often involves physical therapy and pulmonary rehabilitation programs.

100. Nursing care addresses respiratory dysfunction, impairment of mobility, inability to perform activities of daily living and independent self-care, and psychological issues.

RABIES

101. Rabies is a rhabdovirus infection of the central nervous system transmitted by infected saliva that enters the body through a bite or an open wound. If untreated, rabies is fatal.

102. The virus spreads from the wound to local muscle cells and then invades the peripheral nerves. It eventually travels to the central nervous system.

103. During the initial, or prodromal, stage the site of the wound is painful and the client exhibits various paresthesias. The client is anxious, irritable, depressed, has manifestations of infection, an increased sensitivity to light and sounds, and skin sensitivity to temperature changes.

104. The excitement stage follows and is characterized by alternate periods of excitement and quiet. The client experiences laryngospasms with attempts to swallow. Large amounts of thick, tenacious mucus are present and the client experiences convulsions, muscle spasms, and periods of apnea. Death occurs approximately 7 days after onset of manifestations and is usually due to respiratory failure.

105. Interdisciplinary care includes keeping animals that bite under observation for 7 to 10 days. Sick animals should be euthanized; their brains are examined for presence of the rabies virus.

106. Nursing care focuses on maintaining the airway, maintaining oxygenation, and controlling seizures. Standard precautions are essential.

TETANUS

107. Tetanus is more commonly called lockjaw and is a disorder of the nervous system caused by a neurotoxin elaborated by *Clostridium tetani*. Spores of the bacillus enter the body through open wounds contaminated with dirt, street dust, or feces.

108. When spores enter the open wounds, they germinate and produce a toxin called tetanospasmin. The toxins are absorbed by the peripheral nerves and carried to the spinal cord. The action of inhibitory enzymes at spinal synapses is blocked.

109. Manifestations often begin with pain at the site of the infection, stiffness of the jaw and neck, dysphagia, profuse perspiration, and drooling. Disease progression includes hyperreflexia, spasms of the jaw muscles or facial muscles, and rigidity and spasms of

the abdominal, neck, and back muscles. Generalized tonic seizures occur.

110. Complications include urinary retention, airway obstruction, and cardiac and respiratory failure.

111. There is no specific diagnostic test for tetanus.

112. Nursing care for the client with tetanus is intensive and focuses on assessments and interventions to promote safety, prevent injury, maintain nutrition, and maintain pulmonary and cardiovascular function.

BOTULISM

113. Botulism is food poisoning caused by ingestion of food contaminated with a toxin produced by the bacillus *Clostridium botulinum*, which is found in the soil.

114. Toxin liberated by this bacillus are absorbed by the GI tract and bound to nerve tissue. They block the release of acetylcholine from nerve endings and thus cause respiratory paralysis due to paralysis of skeletal muscles.

115. Manifestations usually appear 12–36 hours after ingestion of contaminated food. Initial manifestations are diplopia, loss of accommodation, and fixed, dilated pupils. Ptosis is often present. GI manifestations include nausea and vomiting, diarrhea, dysphagia, and dry mouth. Paralysis progresses throughout the body.

116. Infection with the Clostridium toxin is verified by laboratory analysis of the serum and stool and of suspected food.

117. Botulism is a reportable disease and all people who may have eaten the contaminated food must be located and observed.

118. Toxins in the GI system are removed by cathartics, enemas, and gastric lavage. Mechanical ventilation and tracheostomy may be necessary. Total parenteral nutrition is used for nutritional support. IV fluids are administered.

119. Nursing care is focused on maintaining oxygenation, nutrition, hydration, and support.

SUGGESTIONS FOR CLASSROOM ACTIVITIES

- Have a family member of a client with Alzheimer's disease address the class regarding the experience of caring for a client with Alzheimer's in the home.
- Review the animation about multiple sclerosis that is provided on the textbook DVD-ROM. Use the information provided as a beginning discussion of the disorder.
- Review the case study about Parkinson's disease that is provided on the textbook Companion Website. View the video about akinesia and bradykinesia that is provided on the textbook DVD-ROM. Use this information to discuss the care of the client who has Parkinson's disease.
- Have students access the internet and look for information about the association of immunizations with development of Guillain-Barré syndrome.

SUGGESTIONS FOR CLINICAL ACTIVITIES

- Assign students to the care of clinical clients who have neuromuscular disorders. After the care experience has ended, have students share their ideas about interventions for these clients. Discuss the frustrations encountered in the care of these clients. Identify the coping mechanisms the client and family use to deal with their frustrations.

LEARNING OUTCOME 3

Compare and contrast the manifestations of the progressive stages of Alzheimer's disease.

CONCEPTS FOR LECTURE

1. Alzheimer's disease is classified into three stages based on the client's manifestations and abilities. Progression of AD is individual and may not follow the model.

2. In stage 1 AD, the client typically appears physically healthy and alert. Cognitive defects can go undetected. Clients may seem restless, forgetful, uncoordinated, may lack spontaneity, and may be disoriented to time and date.

3. In stage 2, memory deficits become more apparent, and the client is less able to behave spontaneously. Although progression of manifestations continues and orientation to place and time deteriorates, AD clients may still have periods of mental lucidity.

4. Stage 2 clients are generally more confused, may demonstrate repetitive behavior, are less able to make simple decisions and to adapt to environmental changes, and are often unable to carry out activities of daily living.

5. Sundowning is a behavior change of stage 2 AD, characterized by increased agitation, time disorientation, and wandering behaviors during afternoon and evening hours. It is accelerated on overcast days.

6. Common language deficits of stage 2 include: paraphasia, echolalia, scanning speech, and eventually total aphasia. Frustration and depression are common.

7. Sensorimotor deficits include apraxia, astereognosis, and agraphia.

8. Problems with malnutrition, fluid balance, and sleep pattern arise.

9. Stage 3 AD brings increasing dependence, inability to communicate, loss of urinary and fecal continence, and progressive loss of cognitive abilities.

10. Common complications of stage 3 include pneumonia, dehydration, malnutrition, falls, depression, delusions, seizures, and paranoid reactions. Average life expectancy is 1–3 years from onset of stage 3.

POWERPOINT LECTURE SLIDES

Three Stages of AD
Stage 1
- Appears physically healthy and alert
- Cognitive defects undetected
- Restlessness
- Forgetfulness
- Lack of coordination
- Lack of spontaneity
- Disorientation to time and date
- Clients/families compensation

Stage 2
- Memory deficits more apparent
- Less able to behave spontaneously
- Orientation to place and time deteriorates
- More confusion
- Demonstrate repetitive behavior
- Less able to make simple decisions
- Less able to adapt to environmental changes
- Often unable to carry out ADLs
- Sundowning
- Language deficits
- Sensorimotor deficits

Stage 3
- Increasing dependence
- Inability to communicate
- Loss of urinary and fecal continence
- Progressive loss of cognitive abilities
- Common complications
  - Pneumonia
  - Dehydration, malnutrition
  - Falls
  - Depression, delusions
  - Seizures
  - Paranoid reactions
- Average life expectancy is 1–3 years

SUGGESTIONS FOR CLASSROOM ACTIVITIES

- Have students access the MediaLink applications about Alzheimer's disease that are provided on the textbook Companion Website. In class, have students share what they have learned about stages of Alzheimer's disease and nursing care strategies pertinent to each stage.

SUGGESTIONS FOR CLINICAL ACTIVITIES

- Assign students to care for clients in an Alzheimer's unit or to tour a unit specifically designed for the care of the clients with Alzheimer's. Discuss the physical structure of the facility and how the architecture might impact nursing care.
- Have students identify safety hazards associated with each stage of Alzheimer's disease and nursing strategies for protection of the client in that stage.

LEARNING OUTCOME 4

Discuss the purposes, nursing implications, and health education for the client and family for medications used to treat Alzheimer's disease, multiple sclerosis, Parkinson's disease, and myasthenia gravis.

CONCEPTS FOR LECTURE
ALZHEIMER'S DISEASE

1. Tacrine hydrocholoride (Cognex) was the first medication specifically approved for the treatment of AD.
2. Donepezil hydrochloride (Aricept), rivastigmine tartrate (Exelon), and galantamine hydrobromide (Reminyl) are used to treat mild to moderate AD.
3. Memantine (Namenda) is used to improve cognitive function in moderate-to-severe AD.
4. Depression is common in AD and is treated with medication. Antihistamines and tricyclic antidepressants are avoided.
5. AD clients may also require tranquilizers.
6. Study medications include vitamin E, antiinflammatory agents, and antihypertensive medications.
7. Alternative and complementary therapies include massage, herbs such as gingko biloba, coenzyme Q10, vitamin supplements, and therapies that involve art, music, sound, and dance.

MULTIPLE SCLEROSIS

8. Medications are used to treat manifestations, to modify the course of the disease, and/or to interrupt the progression of the disease.
9. A combination of adrenocorticotrophic hormone and glucocorticoids may be administered to decrease inflammation and suppress the immune system. Immunosuppressive agents, including azathioprine (Imuran) and cyclophosphamide (Cytoxan), are also used.
10. Interferon and glatiramer acetate (Copaxone) are used to reduce exacerbations in clients with relapsing-remitting MS.
11. Anticholinergics are administered for bladder spasticity; cholinergics are given if the client has a problem with urinary retention related to flaccid bladder.
12. Depression is treated with antidepressant drugs.

PARKINSON'S DISEASE

13. The goal of drug therapy is to control manifestations to the extent possible.
14. Types of drugs used include monoamine oxidase inhibitors, dopaminergics, dopamine agonists, and anticholinergics.
15. Medications used to treat PD include selegiline (Eldepryl), amantadine (Symmetrel), levodopa (Larodopa), carbidopa-levodopa (Sinemet), bromocriptine (Parlodel), pergolide (Permax), COMT inhibitors, and entacapone (Comtan).
16. Response to drugs fluctuates; this phenomenon is called the "on-off" response.
17. Other medications used to treat PD include antidepressants, propranolol (Inderal), and botulism toxin.

POWERPOINT LECTURE SLIDES

Alzheimer's Disease
- Tacrine hydrocholoride
- Donepezil hydrochloride, rivastigmine tartrate, and galantamine hydrobromide
- Memantine
- Antidepressants
  ○ Antihistamines and tricyclic antidepressants are avoided
- Tranquilizers
- Vitamin E, anti-inflammatory agents, and antihypertensive medications
- Complementary therapies
  ○ Massage
  ○ Herbs such as ginko biloba
  ○ Coenzyme Q10
  ○ Vitamin supplements
  ○ Therapies
    – Art
    – Music
    – Sound
    – Dance

Multiple Sclerosis
- A combination of adrenocorticotrophic hormone and glucocorticoids
- Immunosuppressive agents, including azathioprine and cyclophosphamide
- Interferon and glatiramer acetate
- Anticholinergics
- Cholinergics
- Antidepressants

Parkinson's Disease
- Monoamine oxidase inhibitors, dopaminergics, dopamine agonists, and anticholinergics
- Selegiline, amantadine, levodopa, carbidopa, bromocriptine, pergolide, COMT inhibitors, and entacapone
- "On-off" response
- Antidepressants, propranolol, and botulism toxin

Myasthenia Gravis
- Anticholinesterases
- Pyridostigmine
- Glucocorticoids

MYASTHENIA GRAVIS

18. The primary group of medications used to treat MG is the anticholinesterases.
19. Pyridostigmine (Mestinon) is the most commonly used acetylcholinesterase inhibitor used for MG.
20. Glucocorticoids are another therapy aimed at improving muscle strength.

SUGGESTIONS FOR CLASSROOM ACTIVITIES

- Review the Animations, "Dopamine" and "Levodopa" provided on the textbook DVD-ROM. Discuss the nursing implications of administering these medications. Include teaching and observation for side effects.

SUGGESTIONS FOR CLINICAL ACTIVITIES

- Have students review the medical records of clinical clients for medications that are commonly administered to people with chronic neurologic disorders. Require students to develop medication administration information sheets on the medications. Include information regarding dose, side effects, administration implications, and teaching required.

LEARNING OUTCOME 5

Describe the procedures (thymectomy, percutaneous rhizotomy, plasmapheresis) used to treat selected neurologic disorders.

CONCEPTS FOR LECTURE

THYMECTOMY

1. Thymectomy is often recommended for clients with MG who are younger than 60.
2. Two surgical approaches are used for thymectomy.
3. The transcervical approach is considered less invasive.
4. The transternal approach allows a more extensive removal of the gland. It also poses more potential complications because it involves splitting the sternum.

RHIZOTOMY

5. Rhizotomy involves surgically severing a nerve root.
6. Percutaneous rhizotomy involves inserting a needle through the cheek into the foramen ovale at the base of the brain and partially destroying the trigeminal nerve with glycerol, by radio-frequency-induced heat, or by balloon compression of the trigeminal nerve.

PLASMAPHERESIS

7. Plasmapheresis is a procedure used to separate the blood's cellular components from plasma. About 50 mL per minute is withdrawn to the centrifuge in the plasmapheresis.

POWERPOINT LECTURE SLIDES

Thymectomy
- Recommended for clients under 60
- Two surgical approaches
  - Transcervical approach
    - Less invasive
  - The transternal approach
    - Allows more extensive removal
    - More potential complications

Rhizotomy
- Surgical severing of a nerve root
- Percutaneous rhizotomy
  - Inserting a needle through the cheek into the foramen ovale
    - Partially destroying the trigeminal nerve
      · Glycerol
      · Radio-frequency-induced heat
      · Balloon compression

Plasmapheresis
- Procedure used to separate blood cells from plasma
  - 50 mL per minute is withdrawn and treated

SUGGESTIONS FOR CLASSROOM ACTIVITIES

- Using anatomic models, discuss how these procedures are performed. Discuss the nursing implications of care of the clients post-procedure.

SUGGESTIONS FOR CLINICAL ACTIVITIES

- If possible, assign students to observe one of the procedures covered.
- Have an RN who cares for clients who have undergone plasmapheresis come to speak to the students regarding the care of those clients.

CHAPTER 47
ASSESSING CLIENTS WITH EYE AND EAR DISORDERS

LEARNING OUTCOME 1

Describe the anatomy, physiology, and functions of the eye and the ear.

CONCEPTS FOR LECTURE
EYES

1. The eyes are complex structures and contain 70% of the sensory receptors of the body.
2. The primary function of the eye is to encode the patterns of light from the environment through photoreceptors and to carry the coded information to the brain.
3. Extraocular structures of the eye include eyebrows, eyelids, eyelashes, conjunctiva, lacrimal apparatus, and extrinsic eye muscles.
4. The palpebral conjunctiva lines the upper and lower eyelids, whereas the bulbar conjunctiva loosely covers the anterior sclera.
5. The lacrimal apparatus is composed of the lacrimal gland, the puncta, the lacrimal sac, and the nasolacrimal duct.
6. Intraocular structures of the anterior portion of the eye include the sclera, cornea, iris, pupil, and anterior cavity.

POWERPOINT LECTURE SLIDES

Eyes
- Contain 70% of body's sensory receptors
- Primary functions
  - Encode patterns of light
  - Carry coded information to brain
- Extraocular structures
  - Eyebrows, eyelids, eyelashes
  - Conjunctiva
  - Lacrimal apparatus
  - Extrinsic eye muscles
- Anterior intraocular structures
  - Sclera
  - Cornea
  - Iris
  - Pupil
  - Anterior cavity
- Aqueous humor
  - Constantly formed and drained
  - Pressure of 15 to 20 mmHg in eye
  - Canal of Schlemm

7. The sclera is the white portion of the eye. The cornea is transparent, avascular, and sensitive to touch. When the cornea is touched, the eyelids blink (corneal reflex) and tears are secreted.
8. The iris is a disc of muscle tissue that surrounds the pupil and lies between the cornea and the lens. The iris gives the eye its color and regulates light entry by controlling the size of the pupil.
9. The anterior cavity is made of the anterior chamber (the space between the cornea and the iris) and the posterior chamber (the space between the iris and the lens).
10. The aqueous humor, a clear fluid, is constantly formed and drained to maintain a relatively constant pressure of from 15 to 20 mmHg in the eye. The canal of Schlemm is the drainage system for fluid moving between the anterior and posterior chambers.
11. Intraocular structures of the internal chamber of the eye include the lens, posterior cavity, vitreous humor, ciliary body, uvea, and retina.
12. The posterior cavity lies behind the lens and is filled with a clear gelatinous substance, the vitreous humor, which supports the posterior surface of the lens, maintains the position of the retina, and transmits light.
13. The uvea, also called the vascular tunic, is the middle layer of the eyeball. This pigmented layer has three components: the iris, ciliary body, and the choroid.
14. The retina is the innermost lining of the eyeball. The transparent inner layer is made up of millions of light receptors in structures called rods and cones.
15. The optic disc is a cream-colored round or oval area within the retina and is the point at which the optic nerve enters the eye.
16. The slight depression in the center of the optic disc is called the physiologic cup.
17. The fovea centralis is a slight depression in the center of the macula that contains only cones and is the main receptor of detailed color vision.

EARS

18. As sensory organs, the ears have two primary functions: hearing and maintaining equilibrium.
19. Anatomically the ear is divided into the external ear, the middle ear, and the inner ear.
20. The external ear consists of the auricle (or pinna), the external auditory canal, and the tympanic membrane.
21. The external auditory canal serves as a resonator for the range of sound waves typical of human speech.
22. The canal's ceruminous glands secrete a yellow to brown waxy substance called cerumen.
23. The tympanic membrane lies between the external ear and the middle ear. The membrane vibrates as sound waves strike it; these vibrations are transferred as sound waves to the middle ear.
24. The middle ear is an air-filled cavity in the temporal bone and contains three auditory ossicles: the malleus, the incus, and the stapes.

- Intraocular structures of internal chamber
  ○ Lens
  ○ Posterior cavity
  ○ Vitreous humor
  ○ Ciliary body
  ○ Uvea
  ○ Retina
  ○ Optic disc

Ears
- Primary sensory functions
  ○ Hearing
  ○ Maintaining equilibrium
- External ear
  ○ Auricle (or pinna)
  ○ External auditory canal
  ○ Tympanic membrane
- Middle ear
  ○ Auditory ossicles
  ○ Medial side
  ○ Posterior wall
- Ossicles
  ○ Malleus attaches to tympanic membrane
  ○ Articulates with incus
  ○ Articulates with stapes
  ○ Stapes fits into oval window
- Inner ear
  ○ Labyrinth
  ○ Deep within temporal
  ○ Bony labyrinth
  ○ Membranous labyrinth

25. The medial side of the middle ear is a bony wall that contains two membrane-covered openings, the oval window and the round window.
26. The posterior wall of the middle ear contains the mastoid antrum, which communicates with the mastoid sinuses and opens into the eustachian tube.
27. The malleus attaches to the tympanic membrane and articulates with the incus, which in turn articulates with the stapes. The stapes fits into the oval window.
28. The inner ear, also called the labyrinth, is a maze of bony chambers located deep within the temporal bone. The labyrinth is further divided into the bony labyrinth and the membranous labyrinth.
29. The body labyrinth is filled with a fluid similar to cerebrospinal fluid called perilymph that bathes the membranous labyrinth.
30. Within the chambers of the membranous labyrinth is a fluid called endolymph.

SUGGESTIONS FOR CLASSROOM ACTIVITIES

- Using anatomic models, review the anatomy of the eye and the ear.

LEARNING OUTCOME 2

Explain the physiologic processes involved in vision, hearing, and equilibrium.

CONCEPTS FOR LECTURE
VISION

1. The two optic nerves meet at the optic chiasma. Axons from the medial half of each retina cross to the opposite sides to form pairs of axons from each eye and continue on as the right and left optic tracts.
2. The ganglion cells in the optic tracts travel to the thalamus and synapse with neurons, forming pathways called optic radiations.
3. The optic radiations terminate in the visual cortex of the occipital lobe where nerve impulses are interpreted.
4. Depth perception depends upon visual input from two eyes that both focus well.
5. Refraction is the bending of light rays as they pass from one medium to another medium of different optical density. As light passes through the eye, it is bent at several points.
6. Accommodation is the focusing of the image on the retina and is accomplished by contraction of the ciliary muscles.
7. The far point of vision is the distance from the viewed object at which the eyes require no accommodation (normally 20 ft.)
8. The near point of vision is the closest point on which a person can focus and is normally 8–10 inches.
9. Convergence is the medial rotation of the eyeballs so that each is directed toward the viewed object. This convergence allows for focusing of the image on the retinal fovea of each eye.

POWERPOINT LECTURE SLIDES

Vision
- Physiology
  - Optic chiasma
  - Ganglion cells
  - Optic radiations
- Depth perception
- Refraction
- Accomodation
  - Focusing of image on retina
  - Accomplished by contraction of ciliary muscles
- Far point of vision
  - Distance at which eyes require no accommodation
  - Normally 20 ft
- Near point of vision
  - Closest point on which person can focus
  - Normally 8–10 inches
- Convergence
  - Medial rotation of the eyeballs
  - Directs eye toward viewed object
  - Allows for focus

Hearing
- Perception and interpretation of sound
  - Best at between 1000 and 4000 cycles per second
  - Can interpret at between 200 and 20,000 cycles

HEARING

10. Hearing is the perception and interpretation of sound. The human ear is most sensitive to sound waves with frequencies between 1000 and 4000 cycles per second, but can detect sound waves with frequencies between 200 and 20,000 cycles per second.
11. Sound waves enter the external auditory canal and cause the tympanic membrane to vibrate at the same frequency.
12. The ossicles transmit the motion of the tympanic membrane and amplify the energy of the sound wave.
13. As the stapes moves against the oval window, the perilymph in the vestibule is set in motion.
14. The increased pressure of the perilymph is transmitted to fibers of the basilar membrane and then to the organ of Corti. The movements of the fibers of the basilar membrane pull the hair cells of the organ of Corti, which in turn generates action potentials that are transmitted to cranial nerve VIII and then to the brain for interpretation.

EQUILIBRIUM

15. The inner ear also provides information about the position of the head. This information is used to coordinate body movements so that equilibrium and balance are maintained.
16. Types of equilibrium are static balance (affected by changes in position of the head) and dynamic balance (affected by the movement of the head).
17. Receptors called maculae in the utricle and the saccule of the vestibule detect changes in the position of the head.
18. As different patterns of nerve impulses are transmitted to the brain, stimulation of the motor centers initiates actions that coordinate various body movements according to the position of the head.
19. The receptor for dynamic equilibrium is in the crista which is stimulated by rotary head movement.

- Physiology
  - Sound waves enter the external auditory canal
  - Tympanic membrane vibrates
  - Ossicles transmit the motion
  - Movement of stapes against oval window
  - Increases pressure of the perilymph
  - Pressure is transmitted
    - To fibers of the basilar membrane
    - Then to the organ of Corti
    - Interpreted in brain

Equilibrium
- Inner ear provides information about head position
  - Used to coordinate body movements
  - Maintains equilibrium and balance
- Static balance
  - Affected by changes in position of the head
  - Receptors detect changes in the position of the head
  - Body movements are coordinated according to head position
- Dynamic balance
  - Affected by the movement of the head
  - Receptors in the crista are stimulated
    - Rotary head movement

SUGGESTIONS FOR CLASSROOM ACTIVITIES

- Using anatomic models, review the physiology processes of vision, hearing, and equilibrium.

LEARNING OUTCOME 3

Identify specific topics for consideration during a health history interview of the client with health problems of the eye or ear.

CONCEPTS FOR LECTURE
EYES

1. Several diseases of the eye have a genetic component. During the health assessment interview, the nurse should ask about a family history of glaucoma or blindness.

POWERPOINT LECTURE SLIDES

Eyes
- Health history
- Family history
- Specific questions about current problem

2. If the client has a health problem that involves the eyes, specific questions about that problem should be included in the health assessment interview.
3. The nurse should be alert to indications of eye disorders such as squinting, abnormal eye movements, watering or irritation of the eyes, or changes in vision.
4. If the client uses eye medications, questions about type, purpose, frequency, and duration of use should be included in the interview.
5. History of chronic disease and history of previous eye disorders are important in the health assessment.

EARS

6. Several diseases of the ear have a genetic component. During the health assessment interview, the nurse should ask about a family history of congenital deafness, deafness associated with a thyroid goiter, or tumors of the auditory nerve.
7. If the client has a health problem that involves the ears, specific questions about that problem should be included in the health assessment interview.
8. Inappropriate answers to requests to repeat statement may suggest problems with ear function. Explore changes in hearing, ringing in the ears (tinnitus), ear pain, drainage from the ears, or the use of hearing aids.
9. Ask about trauma, surgery, or infections of the ear and the use of medications.

- Observe for
  - Squinting
  - Abnormal eye movements
  - Watering or irritation
  - Changes in vision
- Ask about medication use
- History of chronic disease
- History of previous eye disorders

Ears
- Health history
- Family history
- Specific questions about current problem
- Observe for
  - Inappropriate answers
  - Requests to repeat statements
  - Changes in hearing
- Investigate
  - Reports of tinnitus
  - Ear pain
  - Drainage
  - Use of hearing aids
  - Trauma
  - Surgery
  - Ear infection history
  - Use of medications

SUGGESTIONS FOR CLASSROOM ACTIVITIES

- Assign each student a disorder of the eye or ear to investigate. Divide the students into pairs and have them complete a health history interview pertinent to the assessment of the eyes or ears. Have the "client" of each group provide answers according to the assigned disorder.

SUGGESTIONS FOR CLINICAL ACTIVITIES

- Have students complete a health assessment interview regarding eye and ear health on assigned clinical clients.

LEARNING OUTCOME 4

Describe normal variations in assessment findings for the older adult.

CONCEPTS FOR LECTURE
EYE

1. Aging may result in a decreased elasticity of the lens, along with increased lens density and size. These changes may lead to difficulties with accommodation and to cataract development. The lens may yellow and retinal changes may affect color perception.
2. As fat is deposited around and throughout the cornea, arcus senilis develops. Vision may become blurred. Decrease in corneal sensitivity may increase risk of injury to the eye.
3. Aging results in a decrease in size of the pupil, which also become less responsive to light. The older adult may experience difficulty in seeing in dim light or at night.

POWERPOINT LECTURE SLIDES

Eyes
- Inability to accommodate
- Cataract development
- Changes in color perception
- Arcus senilis
- Blurring of vision
- Increased risk of injury to the eye
- Difficulty seeing in low light
- Glaucoma
- Dry eyes
- Macular degeneration
- Floaters

4. Aging may result in narrowing of the visual field, loss of photoreceptor cells, and distorted depth perception. The rods of the eye work less effectively, adaptation to dark and light take longer, and the risk for macular degeneration increases. The older adult may exhibit a decrease in peripheral or central vision and a progressive vision decline.

5. There is a decrease in the production of tears and decreased reabsorption of intraocular fluid. This results in an increase in the risk for developing glaucoma and reports of dry eyes.

6. Debris and condensation may become visible in the posterior chamber and the vitreous body may pull away from the retina. The client may report blurred or distorted vision with "floaters."

EAR

7. Aging may result in a loss of hair cells, decreased blood supply, a less flexible basilar membrane, degeneration of the spiral ganglion cells, and decrease in the production of endolymph. These changes result in progressive hearing loss and the need for hearing aids.

8. High-frequency sounds are lost and middle and low-frequency sounds may be lost or decreased. Speech may be distorted.

9. There is degeneration of the vestibular structures and the organ of Corti and the cochlea atrophy. This degeneration may cause problems with balance and equilibrium and the risk for falls increases.

10. As the muscles and ligaments of the middle ear weaken and stiffen the acoustic reflex is decreased. The client may have a decreased appreciation for the sounds made from own speech and may begin to speak more loudly.

11. The keratin content of the cerumen increases, resulting in accumulation in the ear canal and associated hearing loss.

Ear
- Progressive hearing loss
- Loss of high frequency sounds
- Speech distortion
- Balance and equilibrium problems
- Speaking more loudly
- Accumulation of cerumen in ear canal

SUGGESTIONS FOR CLINICAL ACTIVITIES

- Assign students to clinical clients of different ages. Have the students assess the client's eyes and ears. In post-conference, share the variations in findings and discuss which findings are a normal part of aging and what may indicate a disorder.

LEARNING OUTCOME 5

Identify abnormal findings that may indicate impairment in the function of the eye and the ear.

CONCEPTS FOR LECTURE
EYE

1. The eyes and vision are primarily assessed through inspection of external structures and assessment of visual fields and visual acuity, extraocular muscle function, and internal structures.

POWERPOINT LECTURE SLIDES

Eye
- Assessment techniques
  - Inspection of external structures
  - Visual field testing
  - Visual acuity testing
  - Extraocular muscle function
  - Assessment of internal structures

2. Visual fields are tested to assess the function of the macula and peripheral vision. The visual fields of the examiner are used as the standard.
3. Central visual field may be assessed with an Amsler grid. This grid is useful for identifying early changes in vision from macular degeneration and diabetes mellitus.
4. Visual acuity is assessed with an eye chart such as a Snellen chart or the E chart for testing far vision and the Rosenbaum chart for testing near vision.
5. When standing 20 feet from the chart, the client should be able to read the smallest line of letters with or without correction. This is recorded as 20/20 vision.
6. Changes in distant vision are most commonly the result of myopia (nearsightedness).
7. Normal near visual acuity is 14/14 with or without correction and is assessed with the Rosenbaum chart held 12 to 14 inches from the client's nose.
8. Changes in near vision can indicate presbyopia or hyperopia.
9. Assessment of the cardinal fields of vision should reveal smooth movement through each field without involuntary movements.
10. The cover-uncover test is a test for strabismus.
11. Convergence testing should reveal the client's ability to follow an object as you move it toward the client's eyes. Failure of the eye to converge equally may indicate a neuromuscular disorder or improper eye alignment.
12. Extraocular eye movements should be symmetrical and even. Failure of this test may indicate extraocular muscle weakness or cranial nerve dysfunction. Involuntary rhythmic movement of the eyes is nystagmus and is associated with neurologic disorders and the use of some medications.
13. Assessment of the corneal light reflex should reveal equal reflection of the light from each eye. If this reflection is not equal, the eyes may be improperly aligned.
14. Observation of pupil size and equality should reveal pupils of equal size about 3–5 mm. Pupils that are unequal may indicate a severe neurologic problem, such as increased intracranial pressure.
15. The normal direct and consensual pupillary response is constriction. Failure of the pupils to respond to light may indicate degeneration of the retina or destruction of the optic nerve. One dilated pupil and one nonresponsive pupil may indicate paralysis of the oculomotor nerve. Some eye medications may cause unequal dilation, constriction, or inequality of pupil size.
16. Testing for accommodation should reveal that pupils constrict and converge as they change focus to follow the object. Failure of accommodation along with lack of pupil response to light may indicate a neurologic problem. Lack of response to light with appropriate accommodation is often seen in diabetes.
17. Abnormality of the eyelids may indicate inflammation, ptosis, exophthalmos, xanthelasma, hordeolum, or chalzion.

- Visual field testing
  - Function of the macula
  - Peripheral vision
  - Examiner is used as standard
- Central visual field
- Visual acuity
- Cardinal fields of vision
- Extraocular eye movements
- Corneal light reflex
- Pupil size and equality
- Response to light
- Accomodation
- Eyelids
- Puncta
- Conjunctiva
- Sclera
- Cornea
- Iris
- Internal structures by ophthalmoscope

Ears
- Assessment techniques
  - Inspection
    - External structures
    - External auditory canal
    - Tympanic membrane
- Weber testing
- Rinne test
- Whisper test
- Tympanogram
- Inspection of auricle
- External auditory canal
- Tympanic membrane
- Mastoid process

18. Unusual redness or discharge from the puncta may indicate an inflammation due to trauma, infection, or allergies.

19. The conjunctiva should be clear, moist, and smooth. Increased erythema or presence of exudate may indicate acute conjunctivitis. A cobblestone appearance may indicate allergies. A fold in the conjunctiva, called a pterygium, may be seen as a clouded area that extends over the cornea.

20. Unusual redness of the sclera may indicate an inflammatory response. Yellow discoloration may indicate liver disorder. Bright red subconjunctival hemorrhages may indicate trauma or a bleeding disorder or may occur spontaneously.

21. Dullness, opacities, or irregularities of the cornea may be abnormal.

22. Corneal arcus is a thin, grayish-white arc seen toward the edge of the cornea. It is normal in older clients.

23. Failure of the corneal reflex may indicate a neurologic disorder.

24. Lack of clarity of the iris may indicate cloudiness of the cornea. Constriction of the pupil accompanied by pain and circumcorneal redness indicates acute iritis.

25. Assessment of the internal structures of the eye is accomplished by use of the ophthalmoscope.

26. Absence of a red reflex may indicate total opacity of the pupil by cataract or a hemorrhage into the vitreous humor.

27. A cataract is an opacity of the lens that may be due to aging, trauma, diabetes, or a congenital defect.

28. Areas of hemorrhage, exudate, and white patches of the retina may be a result of diabetes or long-standing hypertension.

29. Loss of definition of the optic disc is seen in papilledema from increased intracranial pressure.

30. Glaucoma often results in displacement of blood vessels from the center of the optic disc due to increased intraocular pressure. Hypertension may cause an apparent narrowing of the vein where an arteriole crosses over. Engorged veins may occur in diabetes, arthrosclerosis, and blood disorders.

31. Variations in the color or a pale color of the retinal background may indicate disease.

32. Absence of the fovea centralis is common in older clients, but may indicate macular degeneration.

33. Tenderness over the lacrimal glands, puncta, and nasolacrimal duct or drainage from the puncta may indicate an infectious process. Excessive tearing may indicate a blockage of the nasolacrimal duct.

EARS

34. The ears and hearing are assessed primarily through inspection of external structures, the external auditory canal, and the tympanic membrane.

35. Weber testing should reveal sound normally heard equally in both ears. Sound heard in, or lateralized to,

one ear indicates either a conductive loss in that ear or a sensorineural loss in the other ear.

36. Rinne testing should reveal no loss of conductive hearing. The client should hear the sound twice as long by air conduction as by bone conduction.

37. A rough estimate of hearing loss can be established by the whisper test.

38. Abnormal findings on tympanogram testing may indicate fluid in the middle ear, a perforated ear drum, impacted ear wax, or a tumor of the middle ear.

39. Unusual redness or drainage in the auricle may indicate an inflammatory response to infection or trauma.

40. Scales or skin lesions around the rim of the auricle may indicate skin cancer.

41. Small, raised lesions on the rim of the ear are known as tophi and indicate gout.

42. Unusual redness, lesion, or purulent drainage from the external auditory canal may indicate an infection.

43. Cerumen varies in color and texture, but hardened, dry, or foul-smelling cerumen may indicate infection or impaction of cerumen that requires removal.

44. White, opaque areas on the tympanic membrane are often due to previous perforations.

45. Inconsistent texture and color may be due to scarring from previous perforation caused by infection, allergies, or trauma.

46. Bulging tympanic membranes are indicated by loss of bony landmarks and a distorted light reflex. Such bulges may be a result of otitis media or malfunctioning auditory tubes.

47. Retracted tympanic membranes are indicated by accentuated bony landmarks and a distorted light reflex. Such a retraction is often due to an obstructed auditory tube.

48. Tenderness, swelling, or nodules of the auricles or mastoid process may indicate inflammation of the external auditory canal or mastoiditis.

SUGGESTIONS FOR CLASSROOM ACTIVITIES

- Review the case study about otitis media that is provided on the textbook Companion Website. Use the information in the case study as a starting point for the discussion of physical assessment findings associated with the ear and the eye.

SUGGESTIONS FOR CLINICAL ACTIVITIES

- Focus students on the assessment of the eye and the ear. Help them identify changes that are abnormal. Relate functional health pattern changes to physical changes in the eye and ear.

CHAPTER 48
NURSING CARE OF CLIENTS WITH EYE AND EAR DISORDERS

RESOURCE LIBRARY

 PRENTICE HALL NURSING MEDIALINK DVD-ROM

Audio Glossary
NCLEX Review
Animations/Video
  Middle Ear Dynamics
  Pilocarpine

 COMPANION WEBSITE

Audio Glossary
NCLEX-RN® Review
Care Plan Activity: The Client with a Hearing Aid
Case Study: Retinal Detachment
MediaLink Application: Cataracts
Links to Resources

📖 IMAGE LIBRARY

Figure 48.1 The appearance of an eye with conjunctivitis.
Figure 48.2 Entropion.
Figure 48.3 Corneal transplant.
Figure 48.4 Hordeolum.
Figure 48.5 Chalazion.
Figure 48.6 Ectropion.
Figure 48.8 Extracapsular cataract extraction with removal of the lens and anterior capsule, leaving the posterior capsule intact.

Figure 48.10 Forms of primary adult glaucoma.
Figure 48.12 Visual field testing.
Figure 48.15 A red, bulging tympanic membrane of otitis media.
Figure 48.16 An in-ear hearing aid.
Figure 48.17 A behind-ear hearing aid.
Figure 48.18 A cochlear implant for sensorineural hearing loss.

LEARNING OUTCOME 1

Relate knowledge of normal anatomy, physiology, and sensory functions of the eye and ear to the effects of disorders of these organs on the cognitive/perceptual functional health pattern.

CONCEPTS FOR LECTURE
EYE DISORDERS

1. Many disorders of the eye are minor and have little or no effect on vision. Other disorders can result in permanent vision impairment.
2. Disorders and diseases of the outer, visible portion of the eye often cause discomfort and may have cosmetic effects.
3. Disorders of the cornea present the greatest risk to vision of the external disorders.
4. Eye surgery or minor trauma may have either temporary or permanent visual impairment.
5. Disorders that affect the internal structures or the function of the eye are more likely to have adverse effects on vision.

POWERPOINT LECTURE SLIDES

Eye Disorders
- Minor
  - Have little or no effect on vision
- More serious
  - Permanent vision impairment
- Outer, visible portion of the eye
  - Cause discomfort
  - May have cosmetic effects
- Corneal disorder
  - Greatest risk to vision of external disorders
- Eye surgery/minor trauma
  - May result in temporary or permanent impairment
- Internal structure disorder
  - More likely to have adverse effects on vision

EAR DISORDERS

6. Hearing requires that sound waves enter the external auditory meatus and travel through the ear canal to vibrate the tympanic membrane and body structures of the middle ear, which in turn activate the receptors of the cochlea.
7. Tinnitus is the perception of sound such as ringing, buzzing, or roaring in the ears.
8. Disorders of the external ear, including the auricle, auditory meatus, and ear canal, can affect the conduction of sound waves and hearing.
9. Obstruction of the external auditory canal or damage to the tympanic membrane can lead to conductive hearing loss.
10. Infection, inflammation, trauma, or obstruction of the ear canal are the most common conditions that affect the external ear.
11. Disorders of the middle ear may be acute or chronic and can result in permanent hearing loss.

Ear Disorders
- Hearing requires transfer of sound waves to cochlea and brain
- Tinnitus
  - Ringing, buzzing, or roaring in ears
- Disorders of conduction
  - Disorders of the external ear
  - Obstruction of external auditory canal
  - Damage to the tympanic membrane
- External ear
  - Infection, inflammation, trauma, and obstruction
- Middle ear
  - Disorders may be acute or chronic
  - Can result in permanent hearing loss

SUGGESTIONS FOR CLASSROOM ACTIVITIES

- Review the normal anatomy and physiology of the eye. Discuss how changes in the anatomy or physiology affects the sensory function of the eye.

LEARNING OUTCOME 2

Describe the pathophysiology of commonly occurring disorders of the eyes and ears, relating their manifestations to the pathophysiologic process.

CONCEPTS FOR LECTURE
CONJUNCTIVITIS

1. Conjunctivitis is the inflammation of the conjunctiva and is the most common eye disease. Its usual cause is a bacterial or viral infection.
2. Infection conjunctivitis may be bacterial, viral, or fungal in origin. Bacterial conjunctivitis is also known as "pink eye" and is highly contagious.
3. Adenovirus infection is the leading cause of conjunctivitis in adults.
4. Gonococcal conjunctivitis is a medical emergency that can lead to corneal perforation.
5. Manifestations of conjunctivitis include redness, itching of the eye, photophobia, tearing, and discharge. Pain is uncommon. Associated systemic manifestations may include pharyngitis, fever, malaise, and swollen preauricular lymph nodes.
6. Trachoma is chronic conjunctivitis and is caused by *Chlamydia trachomatis* and is a significant preventable cause of blindness worldwide. It is contagious.
7. Early manifestations of trachoma include redness, eyelid edema, tearing, and photophobia. Small conjunctival follicles develop on the upper lids, and ultimately

POWERPOINT LECTURE SLIDES

Common Disorders of the Eye
- Conjunctivitis
- Corneal disorders
- Keratitis
- Corneal ulcer
- Corneal dystrophy
- Keratoconus
- Uveitis
- Cataracts
- Glaucoma
- Age-related macular degeneration
- Diabetic retinopathy
- Retinal detachment
- Retinitis pigmentosa
- HIV infection

Common Disorders of the Ear
- Otitis externa
- Impacted cerumen or foreign body
- Otitis media
- Acute mastoiditis
- Chronic otitis media
- Otosclerosis

cause scarring of the lid and entropion. Corneal ulceration and scarring then occurs, which leads to corneal opacity and blindness.

CORNEAL DISORDERS

8. The cornea can be affected by a variety of disorders, including infection and trauma. The cornea heals quickly after minor injuries or abrasions, but injury to deeper layers may delay healing or result in scarring.

9. Refractive errors are the most common problem that affects visual acuity and result from abnormal curvature of the cornea or alteration in the shape of the eyeball.

10. Myopia (nearsightedness) occurs when the curvature of the cornea is excessive or the eyeball is elongated. The image focuses in front of the retina, instead of on it.

11. Hyperopia (farsightedness) occurs when the eyeball is too short. The image focuses behind the retina.

12. Astigmatism develops due to an irregular or abnormal curvature of the cornea. As a result, light rays focus on more than one area of the retina, which distorts both near and distance vision.

13. Keratitis is inflammation of the cornea. Keratoconjunctivitis is inflammation of both the conjunctiva and the cornea. Keratitis is caused by infection, hypersensitivity, ischemia, tearing defects, trauma, and impaired innervation of the cornea. Scarring secondary to keratitis is a leading cause of blindness worldwide.

14. In nonulcerative keratitis all layers of corneal epithelium are affected, but remain intact. This condition may be a result of viral infections, TB, and autoimmune disorders.

15. Ulcerative keratitis affects the epithelium and stroma of the cornea, and leads to tissue destruction and ulceration.

16. Manifestations include tearing, pain, decreased visual acuity, and blepharospasm. Discharge may be present and corneal ulceration may be visible.

17. A corneal ulcer, which is local necrosis of the cornea, may be caused by infection, exposure trauma, or misuse of contact lenses.

18. Complications include fibrous tissue development and perforation. Partial or total vision loss may occur.

19. A corneal dystrophy is an accumulation of cloudy material in part or parts of the normally clear cornea, and potentially affects visual acuity. Corneal dystrophies are typically inherited disorders that progress gradually and affect both eyes. Keratoconus is a progressive thinning of the cornea.

20. Corrective lenses either in the form of eyeglasses or contact lenses, generally are prescribed to restore visual acuity for clients with refractory errors. Specially-fitted contact lenses to reduce visual distortion are ordered for clients with keratoconus.

- ○ Inner ear disorders
- ○ Vertigo
- ○ Labyrinthitis
- ○ Ménière's disease
- ○ Acoustic neuroma
- ○ Hearing loss

Disorders that Affect the Eyelids

21. The most common disorder that affects the eyelids is marginal blepharitis, which is an inflammation of the glands and lash follicles on the margin of the eyelids.
22. This inflammatory disorder can be caused by a staphylococcal infection or it may be seborrheic in origin.
23. Manifestations are irritation, burning, itching of eyelid with crusting or scaling of lid margins.
24. A hordeolum (sty) is a staphylococcal abscess that may occur on either the external or internal margin of the lid.
25. Initial manifestations of external hordeolum are acute pain at the lid margin and redness. A small, tender, raised area appears, and is accompanied by photophobia, tearing, and the sensation of a foreign body in the affected eye.
26. An internal hordeolum is seen on the conjunctival side of the lid and may have more severe manifestations.
27. Chronic inflammation of a meibomian gland may lead to formation of a chalazion, a granulomatous cyst, or nodule of the lid.
28. Manifestations of chalazion are the presence of a hard, painless swelling on the lid. The chalazion may eventually require removal, but may also spontaneously resolve.
29. Entropion is inversion of the lid margin and may be associated with the normal aging process (senile entropion) or result from an infectious process such as trachoma.
30. Ectropion is eversion of the lid margin and occurs primarily as an effect of aging.

Eye Trauma

31. All eye injuries should be considered medical emergencies that require immediate evaluation and intervention.
32. Foreign bodies, abrasions, and lacerations are the most common types of eye injury. Traumatic injury may be due to a burn, penetrating objects, or blunt force.
33. Corneal abrasion is a disruption of the superficial epithelium of the cornea. Superficial abrasions are extremely painful, but generally heal rapidly without complications or scarring. Deeper abrasions increase the risk of infection, slowed healing, and scar formation.
34. The outer surface of the eye may be subjected to burns caused by heat, radiation, or explosion, but chemical burns are the most common.
35. Manifestations include eye pain and decreased vision. Eyelids are often swollen, and the conjunctiva is reddened and edematous with sloughing possible. Corneas are often cloudy or hazy and ulcerations may be evident.
36. In penetrating injuries, the layers of the eye spontaneously reapproximate after entry of a sharp-pointed object into the globe. Injuries may not be readily apparent.

37. In a perforating injury, the layers do not spontaneously reapproximate, which results in rupture of the globe and potential loss of ocular contents.

38. Blunt trauma may lead to a minor eye injury such as lid ecchymoses or subconjunctival hemorrhage. A well-defined bright area of erythema appears under the conjunctiva. No pain or discomfort is associated with the hemorrhage and no treatment is necessary. The blood typically resolves within 2–3 weeks.

39. Hyphema is bleeding into the anterior chamber of the eye and is a potential result of blunt eye trauma.

40. Orbital blowout fracture is another potential result of blunt eye trauma. The most commonly involved area is the ethmoid bone. Orbital contents, including fat, muscles, and the eye itself may herniate.

UVEITIS

41. Uveitis is inflammation of all or part of the middle vascular layer of the eye, including the choroid, the ciliary body, and the iris. Iritis is inflammation of the iris only and occurs more commonly than uveitis.

42. Causes of uveitis include autoimmune processes, infection, parasitic disease, and trauma. Uveitis may also be idiopathic.

43. Manifestations include pupillary constriction and erythema around the limbus. Photophobia, blurred vision, and severe eye pain may be present.

CATARACTS

44. A cataract is an opacification of the lens of the eye which can significantly interfere with light transmission to the retina.

45. The majority of cataracts are senile cataracts, formed as a result of the aging process.

46. Clouding generally begins at the periphery and moves toward the center of the lens. If only a portion of the lens is clouded, the cataract is described as immature. A mature cataract is opacity of the entire lens.

47. Manifestations include cloudy appearance to the lens and loss of visual acuity.

GLAUCOMA

48. Glaucoma is a condition characterized by optic neuropathy with gradual loss of peripheral vision and, usually, increased intraocular pressure.

49. The only manifestation may be narrowing of the visual field that occurs so gradually that it often goes unnoticed.

50. The normal intraocular pressure of 12–15 mmHg is maintained by a balance between the production of aqueous humor in the ciliary body, its flow through the pupil from the posterior to the anterior chamber of the eye, and its outflow or absorption through the trabecular meshwork and canal of Schlemm.

51. As intraocular pressure increases, the optic nerve is damaged and optic cupping occurs. These changes are visible before visual field changes can be detected.

52. Open-angle glaucoma is the most common form in adults, and accounts for approximately 90% of all glaucomas. It is thought to have a hereditary component.

53. In open-angle glaucoma, the anterior chamber angle between the iris and cornea is normal, but the outflow of aqueous humor is relatively obstructed.

54. Manifestations of open-angle glaucoma are subtle with painless and gradual loss of visual fields. Intraocular pressure is usually, but not always, elevated.

55. Acute angle-closure glaucoma is a less common form of primary glaucoma in adults. Narrowing of the anterior chamber angle occurs because of corneal flattening or bulging of the iris into the anterior chamber. This narrowing may progress to closure of the angle which blocks the outflow of aqueous humor. If this abrupt increase in intraocular pressure is not treated promptly, rapid and permanent loss of vision can occur.

56. Manifestations include severe eye and face pain, general malaise, nausea and vomiting, seeing colored halos around lights, and an abrupt decrease in visual acuity. The conjunctiva may be reddened and the cornea clouded with corneal edema. The pupil may be fixed at midpoint.

AGE-RELATED MACULAR DEGENERATION

57. Age-related macular degeneration (AMD) is the leading cause of legal blindness and impaired vision in people over the age of 65.

58. The two types of AMD identified are nonexudative or dry form and exudative or wet form.

59. Nonexudative macular degeneration is the more common form. It is a gradual process that begins with accumulation of drusen beneath the pigment epithelium of the retina. The pigment epithelium detaches in small areas, which interferes with sensory function of the macula. Vision loss is generally not significant.

60. Exudative macular degeneration is characterized by the formation of new, weak blood vessels in the potential space between the choroid and the retina. As these vessels leak, the retina is elevated from the choroid, which causes vision disturbances. As scar tissue forms, central vision is lost.

61. Manifestations include blurring of the central vision with intact peripheral vision.

DIABETIC RETINOPATHY

62. Diabetic retinopathy is a vascular disorder that affects the capillaries of the retina. These capillaries become sclerotic and lose the ability to transport sufficient oxygen and nutrients to the retina.

63. The four stages of diabetic retinopathy are: (1) mild nonproliferative or background retinopathy; (2) moderate nonproliferative retinopathy; (3) severe nonproliferative retinopathy; and (4) proliferative retinopathy.

64. Nonproliferative retinopathy is typically the initial form. Retinal edema or small hemorrhages into the retina occur. Few symptoms may occur unless edema or large hemorrhage develops.

65. Diabetic retinopathy may progress to the proliferative form which includes large areas of retinal ischemia and neovascularization with fine, fragile vessels that are prone to rupture. Retinal edema and hemorrhage into the vitreous body may occur. The vessels attach to the vitreous body, which increases risk for retinal detachment.

RETINAL DETACHMENT

66. Separation of the retina or sensory portion of the eye from the choroid, the pigmented vascular layer, is known as retinal detachment.

67. Interruption of this neural layer of the eye interferes with light perception and image transmission, and potentially results in blindness.

68. Detachment may be preceded by trauma, but it usually occurs spontaneously.

69. A break or tear in the retina allows fluid from the vitreous cavity to enter the defect, which contributes to the separation of the retina from the choroid. The detached area may rapidly increase in size. Unless contact between the retina and choroid is reestablished, permanent vision loss can occur. Retinal detachment is a true medical emergency.

70. Manifestations include floaters, lines or flashes of light, or a sensation of having a curtain drawn across the vision. The client feels no pain and the eye appears normal to visual inspection.

RETINITIS PIGMENTOSA

71. Retinitis pigmentosa is a hereditary degenerative disease characterized by retinal atrophy and loss of retinal function that progresses from the periphery to the central region of the retina.

72. The genetic effect causes production of an unstable form of rhodopsin in the rod cells. Rod cells degenerate, beginning at the periphery of the retina. The areas of degeneration expand, which causes central vision to fail.

73. The initial manifestation is difficulty with night vision. Progression of the disease brings a slow loss of visual fields, photophobia, and disrupted color vision. Progression to tunnel vision and blindness are gradual.

HIV INFECTION

74. HIV retinopathy, seen as cotton-wool spots around the optic nerve, is the most common noninfectious ophthalmic lesion in AIDS.

75. Neoplasms, such as Kaposi's lesions, which are common in the client with AIDS can also affect the eye.

76. The most serious and frequent opportunistic eye infection associated with HIV infection is cytomegalovirus (CMV) retinitis.
77. Corneal ulcers from opportunistic bacterial, fungal, protozoal, or viral infections are also associated with HIV infection. Toxoplasmic and fungal retinal infections may occur.
78. Manifestations of disorders depend upon the amount of retinal damage.

OTITIS EXTERNA

79. Otitis externa is inflammation of the ear canal.
80. This disorder may be due to a bacterial or fungal infection, mechanical trauma, or a local hypersensitivity reaction.
81. Disruption of the normal environment within the external auditory canal typically precedes the inflammatory process.
82. Manifestations include a feeling of fullness in the ear, pain, odorless watery or purulent drainage, and an inflamed or edematous ear canal.
83. Cellulitis is a possible complication.

IMPACTED CERUMEN OR FOREIGN BODY

84. The curved shape and narrow lumen of the ear canal make it particularly vulnerable to obstruction.
85. Cerumen impaction can occur as cerumen dries and moves down and out of the ear.
86. When the ear canal becomes occluded, the client experiences a conductive hearing loss. Manifestations include a sensation of fullness, tinnitus, pain, and coughing due to stimulation of the vagal nerve.

OTITIS MEDIA

87. Otitis media, which is inflammation or infection of the middle ear, primarily affects infants and young children but may also occur in adults.
88. There are two primary forms of otitis media: serous and acute or suppurative. Both forms are associated with upper respiratory infection and eustachian tube dysfunction.
89. Serous otitis media (otitis media with effusion) occurs when the eustachian tube is obstructed for a prolonged time, which impairs equalization of air pressure in the middle ear. Negative pressure in the middle ear causes sterile serous fluid to move from the capillaries into the space, which forms a sterile effusion of the middle ear.
90. In barotraumas or barotitis media, the client's abnormally narrowed or edematous eustachian tube cannot adapt to rapid changes in barometric pressure.
91. Manifestations of serous otitis media include decreased hearing and complaints of "snapping" or "popping" in the ear. The tympanic membrane demonstrates decreased mobility and may appear retracted or bulging.

92. Barotrauma may cause acute pain, hemorrhage into the middle ear, rupture of the tympanic membrane, rupture of the round window with sensory hearing loss, and vertigo.

93. Hemotympanum is bleeding into or behind the tympanic membrane.

94. Acute otitis media occurs when pathogens enter the normally sterile middle ear. The infection and resultant migration of white blood cells cause pus formation. Accumulated pus causes increased middle ear pressure and the tympanic membrane may rupture.

95. Complications are mastoiditis, brain abscess, bacterial meningitis or, more commonly, persistent conductive hearing loss.

96. Manifestations include mild to severe pain, fever, diminished hearing, dizziness, vertigo, and tinnitus.

ACUTE MASTOIDITIS

97. Acute mastoiditis is bacterial infection of the mastoid process. The bony septa between mastoid air cells are destroyed and cells coalesce to form large spaces.

98. An abscess may form, or bony sclerosis of the mastoid may result.

99. Manifestations usually develop 2–3 weeks after an episode of acute otitis media and include recurrent earache and hearing loss. Tenderness is present over the mastoid process.

CHRONIC OTITIS MEDIA

100. Chronic otitis media involves permanent perforation of the tympanic membrane, with or without recurrent pus information. It usually is the result of recurrent acute otitis media and eustachian tube dysfunction, but may also result from trauma or other disease.

101. Cholesteatoma is a cyst or mass filled with epithelial cell debris that forms when squamous epithelium migrate from the ear canal or into the middle ear. Progressive disease destroys adjacent bone and impairs blood supply to the stapes, which causes its destruction and conductive hearing loss.

OTOSCLEROSIS

102. Otosclerosis is abnormal bone formation in the osseous labyrinth of the temporal bone. This bony growth causes the stapes to become fixed or immobile in the oval window, which results in conductive hearing loss.

103. Manifestations include asymmetric hearing loss. Bone conduction of sound is retained. The client may experience tinnitus.

104. The tympanic membrane may appear a reddish or pinkish-orange color.

INNER EAR DISORDERS

105. Inner ear disorders affect equilibrium and may also affect sensorineural hearing, the perception of sound.

106. Vertigo is a sensation of movement when there is none and is a disorder of equilibrium. This sensation can be a result of disorders of the labyrinth, vestibular nerve or nuclei, eyes, cerebellum, brainstem, or cerebral cortex. Vertigo may be disabling, and result in falls and difficulty walking. Episodes are often accompanied by nausea and vomiting, nystagmus, pallor, sweating, hypotension, and salivation.

107. Labyrinthitis, also called otitis interna, is a rare inflammation of the inner ear. Bacteria, viruses, and other organisms may enter and infect the inner ear through the oval window during acute otitis media.

108. Manifestations include vertigo, sensorineural hearing deficit, and nystagmus.

109. Ménière's disease, also known as endolymphatic hydrops, is a chronic disorder characterized by recurrent attacks of vertigo with tinnitus and a progressive unilateral hearing loss. It results from an excess of endolymph.

110. The cause is unclear, although the most common form of the disease is thought to result from viral injury to the fluid transport system of the inner ear. There may be a genetic link in some clients.

111. Manifestations include vertigo, gradual loss of hearing, and tinnitus. The attacks are recurrent and may be preceded by a feeling of fullness in the ears and a roaring or ringing sensation. Attacks are often accompanied by hypotension, sweating, and nystagmus.

ACOUSTIC NEUROMA

112. An acoustic neuroma or schwannoma is a benign tumor of cranial nerve VIII. It typically occurs in adults between the ages of 40 and 50.

113. These tumors generally occur in the internal auditory meatus, and compress the auditory nerve. If allowed to grow, the tumor eventually destroys the labyrinth and may grow large enough to impinge on the inferior cerebellar artery.

114. Early manifestations include tinnitus, unilateral hearing loss, and nystagmus.

115. As the tumor grows, the client experiences neurologic signs related to the area of the brain involved.

HEARING LOSS

116. A hearing deficit may be partial or total, congenital or acquired, unilateral or bilateral, and may affect all or only partial frequencies.

117. Manifestations of hearing loss may include increase in voice volume, positioning the head with the good ear toward the speaker, asking speakers to repeat what they have said, or responding inappropriately to questions or statements.

118. Lesions in the outer ear, middle ear, inner ear, or central auditory pathways can result in hearing loss. Aging is also a significant factor in hearing loss. Profound deafness can be congenital.

119. Hearing loss can be classified as conductive, sensorineural, or mixed.

120. Conductive hearing loss occurs as a result of anything that disrupts the transmission of sound from the external auditory meatus to the inner ear. The most common cause is obstruction of the external ear canal.

121. Conductive hearing loss causes an equal loss of hearing at all sound frequencies. These clients benefit from amplification by a hearing aid.

122. Sensorineural hearing loss occurs as a result of loss or damage of receptor cells, changes in the cochlear apparatus, or auditory nerve abnormalities that decrease or distort the ability to receive and interpret stimuli.

123. A significant cause of sensorineural hearing deficit is damage to the hair cells of the organ of Corti. Noise exposure is a major contributing factor. Ototoxic drugs also damage the hair cells.

124. Neural hearing loss may be caused by tumors, vascular disorders, demyelinating or degenerative diseases, infections, or trauma.

125. Sensorineural hearing losses typically affect the ability to hear high-frequency tones more than low-frequency tones. Hearing aids are often not useful because they amplify both speech and background noise.

126. Presbycusis is a gradual hearing loss associated with aging. Higher-pitched tones and conversational speech are lost initially. Hearing aids and other amplification devices are useful for most clients with presbycusis.

127. Tinnitus is the perception of sound or noise in the ears without stimulus from the environment. Tinnitus is usually associated with hearing loss. It is often an early symptom of noise-induced hearing damage and drug-related toxicity.

128. Types of hearing aids include: canal hearing aids, in-ear style hearing aids, behind-the-ear hearing aids, and body hearing aids.

129. An assistive listening device, or "pocket talker," with a microphone and earpieces may also help the client to hear.

130. Clients with tinnitus may find a white-noise masking device helpful to promote concentration and rest.

SUGGESTIONS FOR CLASSROOM ACTIVITIES

- View the animations about middle ear dynamics that are provided on the textbook DVD-ROM. Use this information to explain the pathophysiology of middle ear disorder.
- View the care plan activity about hearing aid care that is provided on the textbook Companion Website. Discuss the care of these devices.
- Divide the class into small groups. Assign each group a type of eye or ear disorder covered in this chapter. Have the group create a visual presentation of the disorder's pathophysiology. Share the work in class.

LEARNING OUTCOME 3

Explain the risk factors for selected disorders of the eyes and ears, identifying the nursing implications for these risk factors.

CONCEPTS FOR LECTURE

CORNEAL DISORDERS

1. Contact lens use is a risk factor for corneal infections and ulcers.

EYE TRAUMA

2. Teaching individuals and groups how to prevent eye injuries is an important nursing role, especially for people involved in hazardous occupations and activities.

CATARACTS

3. Age is the greatest single risk factor for cataract development. Genetic factors may also contribute to the risk. Long-term exposure to sunlight, cigarette smoking, heavy alcohol use, eye trauma, and diabetes mellitus are associated with cataract development. Drugs such as systemic or inhaled corticosteroids, chlorpromazine, and busulfan also prompt the formation of cataracts.

GLAUCOMA

4. Glaucoma is usually a primary condition without an identified cause. Primary glaucoma is most common in adults over 60, but may be a congenital defect in infants and children.
5. Secondary glaucoma can develop as a result of infection, inflammation, cataract, tumor, hemorrhage, or eye trauma.

AGE-RELATED MACULAR DEGENERATION

6. Evidence suggests that the risk for developing AMD may be reduced by consumption of certain antioxidant nutrients, including vitamin C, vitamin E, beta-carotene, and zinc.

DIABETIC RETINOPATHY

7. The risk of developing diabetic retinopathy is related to the duration of the diabetes and the degree of glycemic control.
8. Hypertension is also a risk factor.

RETINAL DETACHMENT

9. Common risk factors for development of retinal detachment are aging, myopia, and aphakia.

RETINITIS PIGMENTOSA

10. Retinitis pigmentosa is inherited as an autosomal dominant, autosomal recessive, or X-linked trait and may be associated with other genetic defects.

POWERPOINT LECTURE SLIDES

Corneal Disorders
- Improper contact lens use
  - Corneal infections
  - Corneal ulcerations

Eye Trauma
- Hazardous occupations
- Hazardous activities

Cataracts
- Sunlight exposure
- Cigarette smoking
- Heavy alcohol use
- Eye trauma
- Diabetes mellitus
- Some medications

Glaucoma
- Primary
  - Unknown cause
- Secondary glaucoma
  - Infection
  - Inflammation
  - Cataract
  - Tumor
  - Hemorrhage
  - Eye trauma

Age-Related Macular Degeneration
- Risk reduction
  - Antioxidant nutrients
  - Vitamin C
  - Vitamin E
  - Beta-carotene
  - Zinc

Diabetic Retinopathy
- Glycemic control
- Hypertension

Retinal Detachment
- Aging
- Myopia
- Aphakia

Retinitis Pigmentosa
- Genetic defects

Otitis Externa
- Significant time in water
- Wearing ear plugs
- Wearing hearing aid

Impacted Cerumen or Foreign Body
- Aging

OTITIS EXTERNA

11. Since otitis externa, or swimmer's ear, is prevalent in people who spend significant time in the water, swimmers, divers, and surfers are particularly prone to the disorder.
12. Wearing ear plugs or a hearing aid is an additional risk factor.

IMPACTED CERUMEN OR FOREIGN BODY

13. Aging is a risk factor for development of impacted cerumen.

OTITIS MEDIA

14. Upper respiratory infections or allergies predispose the client to serous otitis media.
15. Barotrauma tends to occur during descent in an airplane and underwater diving.

OTOSCLEROSIS

16. Otosclerosis is a hereditary disorder with an autosomal dominant pattern of inheritance. It is most common in Caucasians and in females.

HEARING LOSS

17. Awareness of the effects of noise exposure, especially when combined with the ototoxic effects of aspirin or other drugs, is important to prevent sensorineural hearing loss.

Otitis Media
- Upper respiratory infections
- Allergies
- Barotrauma
  - Descent in an airplane
  - Underwater diving

Otosclerosis
- Hereditary

Hearing Loss
- Noise exposure
- Ototoxic medications

SUGGESTIONS FOR CLASSROOM ACTIVITIES

- Have students research the internet for information regarding visual and hearing loss risk factors.
- Using information obtained regarding risk factors for visual and hearing loss, have students look for similarities.
- Have students develop a teaching plan for the prevention of vision and hearing loss.

SUGGESTIONS FOR CLINICAL ACTIVITIES

- Have students review the medical records of clinical clients for potential risk factors for development of vision and hearing loss.
- Have students review the medication administration records of clinical clients for medication that are ototoxic. Have students develop a teaching plan for clients receiving these medications.

LEARNING OUTCOME 4

Identify diagnostic tests used for specific eye and ear disorders.

CONCEPTS FOR LECTURE
CONJUNCTIVITIS

1. Diagnostic procedures may include culture and sensitivity of exudates, fluorescein staining with slit lamp examination, and conjunctival scrapings. Additional laboratory testing includes blood counts and antibody titers.

POWERPOINT LECTURE SLIDES

Conjunctivitis
- C&S of exudates
- Fluorescein staining with slit lamp examination
- Conjunctival scrapings
- Blood counts
- Antibody titers

CORNEAL DISORDERS

2. Visual acuity is tested on all clients who present with refractory or corneal disorders.
3. Other diagnostic testing includes fluorescein stain with slit lamp examination and conjunctival or ulcer scrapings. Blood counts or antibody titers may also be ordered.

EYE TRAUMA

4. When trauma to the eye is known or suspected, a thorough examination is conducted to determine the type and extent of the injury.
5. Fluorescein staining and ophthalmoscopic examination is performed. Facial x-rays, CT scan, and ultrasonography may be ordered.
6. The immediate priority of care for clients with chemical burns is flushing the affected eye with copious amounts of fluid.

GLAUCOMA

7. Routine eye examinations are recommended for early detection. Measurements of intraocular pressure, fundoscopy to assess the optic disk, and visual field testing are used for diagnosis and monitoring of treatment effectiveness.
8. Diagnostic testing includes tonometry, fundoscopy, gonioscopy, and visual field testing.

AGE-RELATED MACULAR DEGENERATION

9. AMD is diagnosed through vision and retinal examination. The Amsler grid may be used to identify distortions of central vision.
10. Fluorescein angiograms allow detection of leaks in wet AMD.

RETINAL DETACHMENT

11. Diagnosis is established by client manifestations and examination of the ocular fundus by ophthalmoscopy.
12. Interventions are directed toward bringing the retina and choroid back into contact and reestablishing the blood and nutrient supply to the retina.

OTITIS EXTERNA

13. Diagnosis is usually based on the history and physical examination. Examination may be done using a pneumatic otoscope.
14. Diagnostic testing includes impedance audiometry, a CBC, and culture of drainage if appropriate.

ACUTE MASTOIDITIS

15. X-ray may demonstrate loss of septa between mastoid air cells.

Corneal Disorders
- Visual acuity
- Fluorescein stain with slit lamp examination
- Conjunctival or ulcer scrapings
- Blood counts
- Antibody titers

Eye Trauma
- Fluroescein staining
- Ophthalmoscopic examination
- Facial x-rays
- CT scan
- Ultrasonongraphy

Glaucoma
- Routine eye examinations
  - Early detection
- Measurements of intraocular pressure
- Fundoscopy to assess the optic disk
- Visual field testing
- Tonometry
- Fundoscopy
- Gonioscopy
- Visual field testing

Age-Related Macular Degeneration
- Vision/retinal examination
- Amsler grid
- Fluorescein angiograms

Retinal Detachment
- Fundal examination

Otitis Externa
- Pneumatic otoscope examination
- Impedance audiometry
- CBC
- Culture of drainage

Acute Mastoiditis
- X-ray

Otosclerosis
- Rinne test

Inner Ear Disorder
- Caloric testing (electronystagmography)
- Rinne
- Weber
- X-rays
- CT scans
- Glycerol testing

Hearing Loss
- Gross testing of hearing
- Rinne
- Weber
- Audiometry
- Speech audiometry
- Tympanometry
- Acoustic reflex testing

OTOSCLEROSIS

16. The Rinne test shows bone sound conduction to be equal or greater than air conduction, which is abnormal.

INNER EAR DISORDERS

17. The following diagnostic studies may be ordered: caloric testing (electronystagmography), Rinne and Weber testing, X-rays and CT scans, and glycerol testing.

HEARING LOSS

18. Hearing evaluation includes gross testing of hearing, the Rinne and Weber tests, audiometry, speech audiometry, tympanometry, and acoustic reflex testing.

SUGGESTIONS FOR CLASSROOM ACTIVITIES

- Have students identify those tests that are independent nursing functions. Have students investigate proper examination techniques. Have students practice techniques on models or student volunteers.
- Have students identify those tests that are not within the scope of nursing practice. Have students identify nursing responsibilities associated with the examinations.

SUGGESTIONS FOR CLINICAL ACTIVITIES

- Help students identify which clinical clients would be candidates for these examinations. Help students perform the examinations identified. Have students share their learning in post-conference.

LEARNING OUTCOME 5

Discuss the effects of and nursing implications for medications prescribed to treat eye and ear disorders.

CONCEPTS FOR LECTURE

CONJUNCTIVITIS

1. Conjunctivitis is treated with antibiotic, antiviral, or anti-inflammatory drugs as appropriate. Most are delivered topically, but for severe infections or cellulitis, medications may be administered by subconjunctival injection and/or intravenous infusion.
2. Frequent eye irrigations and soaking the lids with warm saline compresses may facilitate removal of crusts and exudate.

CORNEAL DISORDERS

3. Infectious processes are treated with antibiotic or antiviral therapy as appropriate. Medications are generally topical, but may be administered by subconjunctival injection and/or intravenous infusion. Corticosteroids may be prescribed for treatment of inflammatory response, but should be avoided in the presence of local infections.

DISORDERS THAT AFFECT THE EYELIDS

4. Topical antibiotics may be prescribed for the client with hordeolum or to treat infection from eyelid deformity.

POWERPOINT LECTURE SLIDES

Conjunctivitis
- Medications
  - Antibiotic
  - Antiviral
  - Anti-inflammatory
- Most delivered topically
  - Eye irrigations
  - Soaking lids with warm saline compresses
- Some by subconjunctival injection
- Some by intravenous infusion

Eye Trauma
- Narcotic analgesics
  - Morphine sulfate
- Sedation
- Antiemetics
- Antibiotics
  - IV Cefazolin
  - IV Gentamicin
- Carbonic anhydrase inhibitor
  - Acetazolamide
  - Dichlorphenamide

Uveitis
- Immunosuppressive therapy

5. Marginal blepharitis is often treated by cleansing the lid margins with a "no-tears" baby shampoo.

EYE TRAUMA

6. Pain is managed with narcotic analgesics such as morphine. The client may also require sedation and antiemetic medications.

7. Antibiotics such as intravenous cefazolin (Ancef) or gentamicin (Garamycin) are prescribed to prevent infection.

8. A carbonic anhydrase inhibitor such as acetazolamide (Diamox) or dichlorphenamide (Daranide) may be prescribed to reduce intraocular pressure.

UVEITIS

9. Immunosuppressive therapy may be used to suppress the inflammatory response.

10. Atropine may be prescribed for associated inflammation of the iris.

11. Analgesics may be necessary.

GLAUCOMA

12. The primary pharmacologic agents used to treat glaucoma are topical beta-adrenergic blocking agents, adrenergics, prostaglandin analogs, or carbonic anhydrase inhibitors. Oral carbonic anhydrase inhibitors may also be used.

13. In acute angle-closure glaucoma, diuretics may be used to achieve a rapid decrease in intraocular pressure prior to surgical intervention. Fast-acting miotic drops, such as acetylcholine, are also administered to constrict the pupil and draw the iris away from the angle and the canal of Schlemm.

AGE-RELATED MACULAR DEGENERATION

14. The progress of dry AMD can be slowed through the use of high-dose antioxidants and zinc.

HIV INFECTION

15. In addition to the general treatment of HIV infection with retroviral medications, specific therapies may be directed toward the ocular manifestations of the disease.

OTITIS EXTERNA

16. Topical antibiotics and corticosteroid may be ordered in combination to provide immediate relief of the pain, swelling, and itching.

17. Fungal infections may be treated with 1% tolnaftate solution.

OTITIS MEDIA

18. Antiinflammatory, decongestant, or antihistamine medications may be used.

- Atropine
- Analgesics

Glaucoma
- Medications
  ○ Topical
    – Beta-adrenergic blocking agents
    – Adrenergics
    – Prostaglandin analogs
    – Carbonic anhydrase inhibitors
  ○ Oral
    – Carbonic anhydrase inhibitors

Acute Angle-Closure Glaucoma
- Diuretics
- Fast-acting miotic drops
  ○ Acetylcholine

19. Acute otitis media usually is treated with antibiotic therapy.
20. Symptomatic relief may be provided by analgesics, antipyretics, and local application of heat.

ACUTE MASTOIDITIS

21. Acute mastoiditis is treated aggressively with antibiotic therapy.

CHRONIC OTITIS MEDIA

22. Systemic antibiotics are prescribed for exacerbations of purulent otitis media.

INNER EAR DISORDER

23. Scopolamine patches may be used for vertigo.
24. Diuretics, central nervous system depressants, sedatives, and antiemetic medications may be administered for inner ear disorders.
25. Intravenous fluids may be administered to maintain fluid and electrolyte balances.

SUGGESTIONS FOR CLASSROOM ACTIVITIES

- Using anatomic models, explain proper technique for instillation of eye drops and ear drops.
- Have students explain why a steroid medication would not be administered to a client with a local eye infection.
- View the animation about pilocarpine that is provided on the textbook DVD-ROM. Use the information provided as a start for discussion of medications used to treat eye disorders.

SUGGESTIONS FOR CLINICAL ACTIVITIES

- Have students review client medication administration records for medications being given for eye or ear disorders. Have students develop medication information sheets for these drugs, including indications, dosages, nursing implications, side effects, and teaching requirements.

LEARNING OUTCOME 6

Describe surgical and other invasive procedures used to treat eye and ear disorders, identifying their implications for nursing care.

CONCEPTS FOR LECTURE
CORNEAL DISORDERS

1. Laser eye surgery is commonly performed to correct refractive errors such as myopia, hyperopia, and astigmatism. A laser is used to permanently change the shape of the cornea.
2. Types of laser surgery include: laser in-situ keratomileusis (LASIK); photorefractive keratectomy (PRK); laser epithelial keratomileusis (LASEK); and laser thermokeratoplasty (LTK).
3. Postoperatively clients may experience a temporary loss of contrast sharpness, over- or under-correction of visual acuity, dry eyes, or temporarily decreased night vision.
4. Diffuse lamellar keratitis (DLK) is a rare complication of surgery that can lead to vision impairment.

POWERPOINT LECTURE SLIDES

Corneal Disorders
- Laser eye surgery
  - Permanently changes shape of the cornea
  - Used to correct refractory errors
  - Types of laser surgery
    - Laser in-situ keratomileusis (LASIK)
    - Photorefractive keratectomy (PRK)
    - Laser epithelial keratomileusis (LASEK)
    - Laser thermokeratoplasty (LTK)
  - Post-operative findings
    - Temporary loss of contrast sharpness
    - Over- or under-correction of visual acuity
    - Dry eyes
    - Temporarily decreased night vision
  - Complications
    - Diffuse lamellar keratitis (DLK)

5. Phototherapeutic keratectomy (PTK) provides an alternative to corneal transplants in treating corneal dystrophies, scars, and some infections.
6. Corneal transplant or keratoplasty is replacement of diseased cornea by healthy corneal tissue from a donor.
7. Corneal transplant may be either lamellar (superficial layer of cornea is removed and replaced with a graft) or penetrating (full thickness of cornea is removed and replaced by donor tissue).
8. Risk of transplant rejection is low.

DISORDERS THAT AFFECT THE EYELIDS

9. Excision and drainage may be necessary if hordeolum or chalazion are not cleared by application of local heat.
10. In entropion or ectropion, surgery may be performed to correct the defect.

EYE TRAUMA

11. Penetrating wounds of the eye generally require surgical intervention by an ophthalmic surgeon. Preoperatively, the nurse should be careful not to put pressure on the eye itself, but to gently cover it with sterile gauze or an eye pad.
12. Embedded objects should be immobilized and the eye protected with a shield. In addition, patching the unaffected eye decreases ocular movement.

CATARACTS

13. Surgical removal is the only treatment used at this time for cataracts. No medical treatment is available to prevent or treat them.
14. Surgical removal of the cataract and lens is indicated when the cataract has developed to the point that vision and activities of daily living are affected or when presence of the cataract causes a secondary condition such as glaucoma or uveitis.
15. Intracapsular extraction removes the entire lens and its surrounding capsule. This procedure is rarely done today.
16. Extracapsular extraction removes the anterior capsule, nucleus, and cortex of the lens, but leaves the posterior capsule intact.
17. Ultrasound vibrations may be used to break the lens material into fragments (phacoemulsification), which are then suctioned out of the eye.
18. Implantation of a polymethylmethacrylate intraocular lens is done at the time of surgery.
19. If lens implantation is not done, convex corrective glasses or contact lenses may be used to correct vision.

GLAUCOMA

20. Trabeculoplasty and trabeculectomy filtration surgery are the most commonly used procedures in the surgical management of chronic open-angle glaucoma.

- Phototherapeutic keratectomy (PTK)
  - Alternative to corneal transplants
- Corneal transplant
  - Keratoplasty
  - Types
    - Lamellar
    - Penetrating

Enucleation
- Surgical removal of an eye
  - Trauma
  - Infection
  - Glaucoma
  - Intractable pain
  - Malignancy
- Complications
  - Hemorrhage
  - Infection
- Postoperative nursing care
  - Teaching
  - Psychologic support
  - Observation for complications
- Fitting of conformer

Impacted Cerumen or Foreign Body
- Physical removal
  - Ear curet
  - Forceps
  - Right-angle hook
- Insects
  - Mineal oil or topical lidocaine
- Organic bodies
  - Do not apply water
- Suction

21. If these procedures are not effective, either photoco-agulation or cyclocryotherapy may be used to destroy portions of the ciliary body. This reduces the amount of aqueous humor produced.
22. Surgical procedures used in the treatment of acute angle-closure glaucoma include gonioplasty, laser iridotomy, and peripheral iridectomy.

AGE-RELATED MACULAR DEGENERATION

23. Wet AMD is treated with laser surgery or photody-namic therapy.

DIABETIC RETINOPATHY

24. Laser photocoagulation is used to treat both the non-proliferative and proliferative forms of diabetic retinopathy.
25. Vitrectomy may be performed if the client has severe proliferative disease.

RETINAL DETACHMENT

26. A surgical procedure called scleral buckling may be used. Cryotherapy or laser photocoagulation may be used to reattach the retina to the choroid.
27. Air may also be injected into the vitreous cavity in a procedure called pneumatic retinopexy.

RETINITIS PIGMENTOSA

28. There is no effective treatment for retinitis pigmentosa.

ENUCLEATION

29. Enucleation is the surgical removal of an eye. This procedure is necessary because of trauma, infection, glaucoma, intractable pain, or malignancy.
30. Enucleation may be performed under local or general anesthesia.
31. Hemorrhage and infection are the most commonly seen complications.
32. Postoperative nursing care includes teaching, psy-chologic support, and observation for potential complications.
33. Within 1 week of surgery a temporary prosthesis called a conformer is fitted into the empty socket.

IMPACTED CERUMEN OR FOREIGN BODY

34. Impacted wax, objects, or insects may require physi-cal removal using an ear curet, forceps, or right-angle hook inserted via an otoscope and ear speculum.
35. Mineral oil or topical lidocaine may be used to immo-bilize or kill insects.
36. Water should not be applied to organic foreign bod-ies such as beans.
37. Suction may be required to remove smooth, round objects.

OTITIS MEDIA

38. Myringotomy (an incision of the tympanic membrane) may be performed to relieve the pressure.
39. Tympanocentesis (insertion of a needle into the tympanic membrane) may be performed to allow aspiration of fluid and pus from the middle ear.
40. Myringotomy with insertion of tympanostomy tubes allows for ventilation and drainage of the middle ear during healing.

ACUTE MASTOIDITIS

41. Mastoidectomy is surgical removal of the infected mastoid air cells, bone, and pus, and inspection of the underlying dura for possible abscess.
42. A modified mastoidectomy involves removal of as little tissue as possible to avoid disrupting hearing.
43. A radical mastoidectomy involves removal of middle ear structures including the incus and malleus as well as the diseased portions of the mastoid process.
44. Tympanoplasty is the surgical reconstruction of the middle ear that can restore or preserve hearing.

CHRONIC OTITIS MEDIA

45. Tympanic membrane perforation is repaired with a tympanoplasty to restore sound conduction and the integrity of the middle ear.

OTOSCLEROSIS

46. Clients with otosclerosis may choose conservative treatment.
47. Surgical treatment involves a stapedectomy and middle ear reconstruction or stapedotomy.

INNER EAR DISORDERS

48. Surgical procedures may include endolymphatic decompression, vestibular neurectomy, or labyrinthectomy.

ACOUSTIC NEUROMA

49. Treatment of choice is surgical excision. Microsurgical techniques may preserve hearing.
50. The translabyrinthine approach provides good access to the tumor, but may destroy hearing.
51. Larger tumors may require craniotomy.

HEARING LOSS

52. Reconstructive surgeries of the middle ear, such as a stapedectomy or tympanoplasty, may help restore hearing with a conductive hearing loss.
53. For a client with sensorineural hearing loss, a cochlear implant may be the only hope for restoring sound perception.

LEARNING OUTCOME 7

Discuss the nurse's role in caring for clients with impaired vision or hearing loss.

CONCEPTS FOR LECTURE

CONJUNCTIVITIS

1. The nursing role in treating conjunctivitis is primarily one of education to prevent the disorder and its spread when it does occur.
2. Nursing diagnoses include: *Risk for Infection* and *Risk for Disturbed Sensory Perception: Visual*.

CORNEAL DISORDERS

3. Nursing care of the client with corneal disorder may involve direct care, but more often focuses on prevention and education.
4. Nursing diagnoses include: *Risk for Disturbed Sensory Perception: Visual; Acute Pain;* and *Risk for Injury.*

DISORDERS THAT AFFECT THE EYELIDS

5. The nursing role focuses on education and comfort measures.

EYE TRAUMA

6. The primary nursing diagnosis is *Impaired Tissue Integrity: Ocular.*

UVEITIS

7. Nursing care is supportive, and focuses on promotion of comfort and teaching about the disorder and its management.

CATARACTS

8. Patient advocacy, psychologic and emotional support, and teaching/learning needs are typically of high priority for these clients than physical care needs.
9. Nursing diagnoses include: *Decision Conflict: Cataract Removal and Risk for Ineffective Therapeutic Regimen Management.*

GLAUCOMA

10. Nursing diagnoses include: *Disturbed Sensory Perception: Visual; Risk for Injury;* and *Anxiety.*

POWERPOINT LECTURE SLIDES

Conjunctivitis
- Prevention education
- Nursing diagnoses
  - *Risk for Infection*
  - *Risk for Disturbed Sensory Perception: Visual*

Corneal Disorders
- Prevention education
- Nursing diagnoses
  - *Risk for Disturbed Sensory Perception: Visual*
  - *Acute Pain*
  - *Risk for Injury*

AGE-RELATED MACULAR DEGENERATION

11. Nursing care focuses on prompt recognition of manifestations and rapid referral of these clients for ophthalmologic evaluation.

12. For clients with slowly progressive manifestations, the nursing focus is on helping the client and family members adapt to the gradual decline in vision.

DIABETIC RETINOPATHY

13. The nursing care focus for diabetic retinopathy is primarily educational.

RETINAL DETACHMENT

14. The nursing focus for the client with a detached retina is on early identification and treatment.

15. Nursing diagnoses include: *Ineffective Tissue Perfusion: Renal,* and *Anxiety.*

RETINITIS PIGMENTOSA

16. Nursing care focuses on providing information about the disease and low-vision aids. Clients should be referred for genetic counseling.

OTITIS EXTERNA

17. The primary nursing diagnosis is *Impaired Tissue Integrity.*

IMPACTED CERUMEN OR FOREIGN BODY

18. Any client with evidence of a new conductive hearing loss or complaints of discomfort and fullness in one ear should be evaluated for possible obstruction.

19. Teaching is a key component of nursing care.

OTITIS MEDIA

20. The primary nursing diagnosis is *Pain.*

ACUTE MASTOIDITIS

21. Nursing care focuses on adequate, effective antibiotic therapy, communication, and safety.

CHRONIC OTITIS MEDIA

22. The priority of nursing care is prevention of chronic otitis media and cholesteratoma.

23. Teaching includes medication management and effect of surgical procedures on hearing.

OTOSCLEROSIS

24. Education and referral of the client to appropriate community agencies are important nursing care priorities.

25. Nursing diagnoses include: *Risk for Injury; Disturbed Sensory Perception: Auditory; Impaired Verbal Communication;* and *Anxiety.*

INNER EAR DISORDER

26. Nursing diagnoses include: *Risk for Trauma* and *Disturbed Sleep Pattern*.

ACOUSTIC NEUROMA

27. Nursing care for clients who have undergone surgical removal of an acoustic neuroma focuses on preserving cerebral function.

HEARING LOSS

28. The nurse should include the type and extent of hearing loss, the client's adaptation to the loss, the availability of assistive devices, and the client's ability and willingness to use assistive devices when planning and implementing care.
29. Nursing diagnoses include: *Disturbed Sensory Perception: Auditory; Impaired Verbal Communication;* and *Social Isolation.*

SUGGESTIONS FOR CLASSROOM ACTIVITIES

- Review the case study about retinal detachment that is provided on the textbook Companion Website. Use the information presented to develop a plan of care for the client.
- Have students list nursing diagnoses that are commonly appropriate for clients with eye or ear disorders. Discuss nursing interventions appropriate for each nursing diagnosis.

SUGGESTIONS FOR CLINICAL ACTIVITIES

- Assign clinical students to the care of a client with an eye or ear disorder.

CHAPTER 49
ASSESSING CLIENTS WITH REPRODUCTIVE SYSTEM AND BREAST DISORDERS

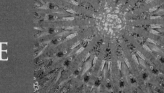

RESOURCE LIBRARY

 PRENTICE HALL NURSING MEDIALINK DVD-ROM

Audio Glossary
NCLEX-RN® Review

 COMPANION WEBSITE

Audio Glossary
NCLEX-RN® Review
Care Plan Activity: STDs
Case Studies
   Assessing Sexual Function
   Irregular Menstrual Cycle
Exercise: Sexual Function Health History
MediaLink Applications: Breast Cancer Screening
Links to Resources

📖 IMAGE LIBRARY

Figure 49.1 The male reproductive system.
Figure 49.2 Palpating the male inguinal area for bulges.
Figure 49.3 Inspecting the external urinary meatus of the male.
Figure 49.4 Structure of the female breast.
Figure 49.5 The external organs of the female reproductive system.
Figure 49.6 The internal organs of the female reproductive system.

Figure 49.7 Comparison of the ovarian and menstrual cycles.
Figure 49.8 Possible pattern for palpation of the breast.
Figure 49.9 Palpating the axillary lymph nodes.
Figure 49.10 Palpating Skene's glands.
Figure 49.11 Palpating Bartholin's glands.

LEARNING OUTCOME 1

Describe the anatomy, physiology, and functions of the male and female reproductive systems, including the breasts.

CONCEPTS FOR LECTURE
REPRODUCTIVE SYSTEM

1. The reproductive organs, in conjunction with the neuroendocrine system, produce hormones important in biologic development and sexual behavior. Functions of the reproductive organs are sexual pleasure and reproduction.

MALE REPRODUCTIVE SYSTEM

2. The male reproductive system consists of paired testes, the scrotum, ducts, glands, and the penis. The breasts are also considered part of the male reproductive system.
3. The male breast is comprised primarily of an areola and a small nipple.
4. The penis is composed of a shaft and a tip called the glans which is covered with the foreskin or prepuce. In circumcised men, the foreskin has been removed. The shaft consists of three columns of erectile tissue.

POWERPOINT LECTURE SLIDES

Reproductive System
- Purposes
  - Produce hormones
  - Sexual pleasure
  - Reproduction

Male Reproductive System
- Paired testes
- Scrotum
- Ducts
- Glands
- Penis
- Breasts

Sperm Production
- Seminiferous tubules
- Efferent ducts
- Retis testes
- Epididymis

The two outer columns are called the corpora cavernosa. The central column is the corpus spongiosum. Erection occurs when the penile masses become filled with blood in response to a parasympathetic reflex.

5. The scrotal sac consists of two layers. The outer layer is skin that is continuous with the perineum and thighs. The inner layer is muscle and fascia. The scrotum regulates the temperature of the testes, and moves closer to the body for warmth and away from the body to cool.

6. The paired testes produce sperm and testosterone. They are suspended in the scrotum by the spermatic cord and are surrounded by an inner tunica albuginea and an outer tunica vaginalis.

7. The seminiferous tubules lead into the efferent ducts and become the rete testes. The efferent ducts join the epididymis, which is a long, coiled tube that lies over the outer surface of the testes. The epididymis is the final area for the storage and maturation of sperm. During sexual excitement, the epididymis contracts and propels the sperm through the vas deferens to the ampulla, where they are stored until ejaculation.

8. Seminal fluid consists of fluids from the seminal vesicles, the epididymis, the prostate gland, and the Cowper's glands. This fluid nourishes the sperm, provides bulk, and increases its alkalinity. During ejaculation, seminal fluid mixes with sperm at the ejaculatory duct and becomes semen.

9. The prostate gland encircles the urethra just below the urinary bladder. Secretions of the prostate gland make up about one-third of the volume of the semen.

10. Spermatogenesis is the series of physiologic events that generate sperm in the seminiferous tubules. Sperm in different stages of development are stored in Sertoli's cells.

11. The events of spermatogenesis, which take 64–72 days, are: (1) development of primary spermatocytes from spermatogonia (sperm stem cells); (2) development of spermatids from smaller secondary spermatocytes formed from meiotic division of primary spermatocytes; and (3) elongation of the spermatids by the addition of a head and a tail with movement into the epididymis to mature.

FEMALE REPRODUCTIVE SYSTEM

12. The female reproductive system consists of the external genitalia or vulva (mons pubis, labia, clitoris, vaginal and urethral openings, and glands) and the internal organs (cervix, uterus, fallopian tubes, and ovaries). The breasts are also a part of the female reproductive system.

13. The breasts are made of adipose tissue, fibrous connective tissue, and glandular tissue. Cooper's ligaments support the breast and extend from the outer breast tissue to the nipple, and divide the breast into 15 to 25 lobes. Each lobe is made of alveolar glands connected by ducts that open to the nipple.

- Vas deferens
- Ampulla

Seminal Fluid
- Production
- Nourishes sperm
- Provides bulk
- Increases alkalinity
- Mixes with sperm at ejaculatory duct

Prostate Gland
- Encircles the urethra
- Just below the urinary bladder

Spermatogenesis
- Ongoing process from puberty to death
- Stored in Sertoli's cells
- Events of spermatogenesis

Female
- External genitalia or vulva
  - Mons pubis
  - Labia
  - Clitoris
  - Vaginal and urethral openings
  - Glands
- Internal organs
  - Cervix
  - Uterus
  - Fallopian tubes
  - Ovaries
- Breasts
- Development of ovum
  - Follicles stimulated
    - Follicle-stimulating hormone (FSH)
    - Luteninzing hormone (LH)
  - Ovulation
- Ovarian cycle
  - Three phases that occur cyclically
    - Follicular phase
    - Ovulatory phase
    - Luteal phase
- Menstrual cycle
  - Menstrual phase
  - Proliferative phase
  - Secretory phase

14. The mons pubis is a pad of adipose tissue covered with skin that lies anterior to the symphysis pubis. After puberty, the mons is covered with hair in a diamond-shaped distribution.

15. The labia majora begin at the base of the mons pubis and end at the anus. The labia minora are enclosed by the labia major and are located between the clitoris and base of the vagina.

16. The area between the labia is called the vestibule and contains openings for the vagina and urethra as well as for the Bartholin's glands and the Skene's glands. These glands secrete lubricating fluid during the sexual response cycle.

17. The clitoris is an erectile organ. Like the penis, it is highly sensitive and distends during sexual arousal.

18. The vaginal opening, called the introitus, is the opening between the internal and external genitals. It is surrounded by a connective tissue membrane called the hymen.

19. The vagina is a fibromuscular tube about 3–4 inches in length located posteriorly to the bladder and urethra and anterior to the rectum. The walls of the vagina form folds, called rugae; the upper end contains the uterine cervix.

20. The cervix projects into the vagina and has an internal os (side toward the uterus) and an external os (side toward the vagina). The endocervical canal joins the os and serves as a route for discharge of menstrual fluid and entrance of sperm.

21. The uterus is a hollow pear-shaped muscular organ and has three parts: the fundus, the body, and the cervix. It is supported in the abdomen by the broad ligaments, the round ligaments, the uterosacral ligaments, and the transverse cervical ligaments.

22. The uterus receives the fertilized ovum and provides a site for growth and development of the fetus.

23. The three layers of the uterine wall are the perimetrium (outer layer), the myometrium (middle layer), and the endometrium (inner layer). The outermost layer of the endometrium is shed during menstruation.

24. The fallopian tubes are thin cylindrical structures about 4 inches long and 2.5 inches in diameter. They are attached to the uterus on one end and supported by the broad ligaments. The open end is made of projections called fimbriae which pick up the ovum after it is discharged by the ovary. The movement of the cilia and contractions of the smooth muscle of the fallopian tubes move the ovum toward the uterus. Fertilization generally takes place in the outer portion of the fallopian tube.

25. The ovaries are located below the ends of the fallopian tubes and are attached to the uterus by a ligament and by the broad ligament. The ovaries store female germ cells and produce estrogen and progesterone. A woman's total number of ova is present at birth.

26. Each month several follicles on the ovary are stimulated by follicle-stimulating hormone (FSH) and luteinizing

hormone (LH) to mature. One or two of the mature follicles ejects an oocyte in a process called ovulation. The ruptured follicle then becomes a structure called the corpus luteum which produces both estrogen and progesterone.

27. The ovarian cycle has three consecutive phases that occur cyclically each 28 days. The follicular phase lasts from the 1st to the 10th day of the cycle. The ovulatory phase lasts from the 11th to the 14th day of the cycle and ends with ovulation. The luteal phase lasts from the 14th to the 28th day of the cycle.

28. During the follicular phase, the follicle develops and the oocyte matures.

29. The ovulatory phase begins when estrogen levels reach a level high enough to stimulate the anterior pituitary to produce a surge of LH. This phase ends with ovulation.

30. During the luteal phase, the ruptured follicle changes to a corpus luteum and begins producing progesterone and estrogen. This increase prevents the further growth and development of other follicles. If pregnancy does not occur, the corpus luteum begins to degenerate and its hormone development ceases. The secretion of LH and FSH is allowed to increase, and a new cycle begins.

31. The menstrual cycle begins with the menstrual phase in which the inner endometrial layer (functionalis) detaches and is expelled as menstrual fluid.

32. As the maturing follicle begins to produce estrogen, the proliferative phase begins, the functionalis layer is repaired and thickened.

33. In the secretory phase, the corpus luteum produces progesterone. The rising levels act on the endometrium, which causes increased vascularity and changes the inner layer to secretory mucosa and stimulates the secretion of glycogen into the uterine cavity. This causes the cervical mucus to become thick and block the internal os. If fertilization does not occur, hormone levels fall and the cycle begins again.

SUGGESTIONS FOR CLASSROOM ACTIVITIES

- Use anatomic models to outline the reproductive systems of both sexes.

LEARNING OUTCOME 2

Explain the functions of the male and female sex hormones.

CONCEPTS FOR LECTURE
MALE

1. The male sex hormones are called androgens and most are produced in the testes. The adrenal cortex also produces a small amount of androgens. Testosterone is the primary androgen produced by the testes.

POWERPOINT LECTURE SLIDES

Male
- Androgens
  - Most produced in testes
  - Small amount produced in adrenal cortex
  - Testosterone
    - Development/maintenance of sexual organs

2. Testosterone is essential for the development and maintenance of sexual organs and secondary sex characteristics, and for spermatogenesis.
3. Testosterone promotes metabolism, growth of muscles and bone, and libido.

FEMALE

4. The ovaries produce estrogens, progesterone, and androgens in a cyclic pattern.
5. Estrogens occur in three forms: estrone (E1), estradiol (E2), and estriol (E3). Estradiol is the most potent and is the form secreted in the greatest amounts by the ovaries.
6. Estrogens are essential for the development and maintenance of secondary sex characteristics. In conjunction with other hormones, estrogens stimulate the female reproductive organs to prepare for growth of a fetus. Estrogens also support skin and blood vessels, decrease rate of bone resorption, promote increased high-density lipoproteins, reduce cholesterol levels, and enhance blood clotting.
7. Progesterone primarily affects the development of breast glandular tissue and the endometrium.
8. Androgens are responsible for normal hair growth patterns at puberty.

- – Secondary sex characteristics
- – Spermatogenesis
- – Promotes metabolism
- – Promotes growth of muscles and bone
- – Supports libido

Female
- Ovaries
  - Cyclic pattern
    - – Estrogens
    - – Progesterone
    - – Androgens
- Estrogens
  - Three forms of estrogens
    - – Estrone (E1)
    - – Estradiol (E2)
    - – Estriol (E3)
  - Essential for secondary sex characteristics
  - Helps prepare for growth of a fetus
  - Supports skin and blood vessels
  - Decreases rate of bone reabsorption
  - Promotes increased high-density lipoproteins
  - Reduces cholesterol levels
  - Enhances blood clotting
- Progesterone
  - Development of breast glandular tissue
  - Endometrium
- Androgens
  - Responsible for hair growth patterns at puberty

SUGGESTIONS FOR CLASSROOM ACTIVITIES

- Have students list the sex hormones present in females and in males. Discuss the overlap of these lists and the implications to secondary sexual characteristics of both sexes.

LEARNING OUTCOME 3

Identify specific topics for consideration during a health history interview of the client with health problems involving the reproductive system and breast structures and/or functions.

CONCEPTS FOR LECTURE
MALE

1. Several diseases of the male reproductive system have a genetic component. It is especially important to ask about a family history of testicular or prostate cancer.
2. Ask about chronic diseases such as diabetes, chronic renal failure, cardiovascular disease, multiple sclerosis, spinal cord tumors or trauma, or thyroid disease.
3. Ask about use of antihypertensives, antidepressants, antispasmodics, tranquilizers, sedatives, or histamine2-receptor antagonists.
4. Ask whether the man's mother took diethylstilbestrol during her pregnancy with him and whether he had mumps as a child.
5. Explore the lifestyle and social history of the man including use of alcohol, cigarettes, and street drugs.

POWERPOINT LECTURE SLIDES

Health History: Male
- Family history of testicular or prostate cancer
- Chronic diseases
- Medication use
- Did mother take diethylstilbestrol during pregnancy?
- Did client have mumps as a child?
- Lifestyle
- Questions about sexuality

Health History: Female
- Family history of ovarian or breast cancer
- Menstrual history
- Obstetric history
- Sexual history
- Medication use

6. Ask about sexual preference.
7. Other questions about sexuality may include number of sexual partners, history of premature ejaculation, impotence or other sexual problems, any history of sexual trauma, use of condoms or other contraceptives, and current level of sexual satisfaction.

FEMALE

8. Several diseases of the female reproductive system have a genetic component. It is particularly important to ask about a family history of ovarian or breast cancer.
9. Ask about menstrual history, obstetric history, use of contraceptives, sexual history, use of medication, and reproductive system examinations. Assess the use of condoms.
10. Ask about presence of chronic illness such as diabetes mellitus, anemia, and thyroid or adrenal disorders.
11. Ask about history of diethylstilbestrol exposure in utero, exposure to asbestos, exposure to cigarette smoke, and history of fibrocystic disease.
12. Carefully explore any history of vaginal bleeding and vaginal discharge.
13. Questions about sexuality may include sexual preference, number of sexual partners, history of anorgasmia and dyspareunia, history of sexual trauma and contraceptive use, and current level of sexual satisfaction.

- Reproductive system examination history
- Chronic illnesses
- History of diethylstilbestrol exposure in utero
- Exposure to asbestos
- Exposure to cigarette smoke
- History of fibrocystic disease
- History of vaginal bleeding and vaginal discharge
- Questions about sexuality

SUGGESTIONS FOR CLASSROOM ACTIVITIES

- Discuss therapeutic communication techniques that are useful when interviewing clients in regard to sexual disorders or history.
- Identify the functional health pattern implications of various findings discovered in sexual history interview.

SUGGESTIONS FOR CLINICAL ACTIVITIES

- Assist students in identification of pertinent sexual history data for clinical clients.

LEARNING OUTCOME 4

Describe normal variations in assessment findings for the older adult.

CONCEPTS FOR LECTURE
MALE

1. A significant number of older men have some degree of benign prostatic hyperplasia.
2. Aging results in thinning of the epithelial tissue and mucosa of the seminal vesicles. This thinning reduces the ability of the vesicles to hold fluid.
3. Sclerosis of penile arteries and veins may occur which results in a longer time to achieve an erection and ejaculation. The client may be impotent.

FEMALE

4. Atrophy and sagging of the breast tissue occurs with aging.
5. Vaginal changes including decreased lubrication, shortening, and narrowing. These changes result in more easy

POWERPOINT LECTURE SLIDES

Male
- Benign prostatic hyperplasia
- Changes in seminal vesicles
- Penile changes
- Impotence

Female
- Breast tissue changes
- Vaginal changes
- Changes at menopause

irritation of the vagina. Lubricants are necessary for comfortable intercourse.

6. As menopause becomes complete, the uterus shrinks and the fallopian tubes shrink and shorten. Ovaries become smaller. Loss of estrogen results in weakness of the pelvic floor, loss of skin tone and growth of facial hair. The weakness of the pelvic floor may result in stress incontinence.

SUGGESTIONS FOR CLINICAL ACTIVITIES

- Have students review the assessment of older adults and help them identify assessment changes that are a part of normal aging.

LEARNING OUTCOME 5

Identify manifestations of impairment in male and female reproductive system and breast structure or function.

CONCEPTS FOR LECTURE

BREAST

1. A smooth, firm, mobile, tender disc of breast tissue behind the areola indicates gynecomastia, which is an abnormal enlargement of the breast(s) in men which requires additional investigation.
2. A hard, irregular nodule in the nipple area suggests carcinoma.
3. Enlarged axillary nodes are common with infections of the hand or arm but may be caused by cancer.
4. Enlarged supraclavicular nodes may indicate metastasis.

GROIN

5. A bulge in the inguinal or femoral area that increases with straining suggests a hernia.

PENIS

6. Phimosis may be congenital or due to recurrent balanoposthitis.
7. Narrow or inflamed foreskin can cause paraphimosis.
8. Balanitis is associated with bacterial or fungal infections.
9. Ulcers, vesicles, or warts on the penis suggest a sexually transmitted infection.
10. Nodules or sores on the penis seen in uncircumcised men may be cancer.
11. Erythema or discharge from the urinary meatus indicates inflammatory disease.
12. Excoriation or inflammation of the skin of the penis suggests lice or scabies.

SCROTUM

13. A unilateral or bilateral poorly-developed scrotum suggests cryptorchidism.
14. Swelling of the scrotum may indicate indirect inguinal hernia, hydrocele, or scrotal edema.

POWERPOINT LECTURE SLIDES

Manifestations of Impairment: Male
Breast
- Gynecomastia
- Hard, irregular nodule in nipple area
- Enlarged axillary nodes
- Enlarged supraclavicular nodes
Groin
- Bulge in inguinal/femoral area
Penis
- Phimosis
- Paraphimosis
- Balanitis
- Ulcers, vesicles, or warts
- Nodules/sores on penis
- Urinary meatus erythma or discharge
- Excoriation or inflammation of penile skin
Scrotum
- Unilateral/bilateral poorly developed scrotum
- Swelling of the scrotum
- Tender, painful scrotal swelling
- A painless testicular nodule
Prostate
- Enlargement and obliteration of median sulcus
- Enlargement with asymmetry/tenderness
- Hard irregular nodule

Manifestations of Impairment: Female
Breast
- Retractions, dimpling, abnormal contours
- Peau d'orange/unilateral venous patterns
- Redness
- Recent unilateral inversion of nipple
- Asymmetry in direction in which nipples point
- Tenderness upon breast palpation
- Nodules in tail of breast
- Hard, irregular, poorly delineated, fixed unilateral masses

15. Tender, painful scrotal swelling occurs in acute epididymitis, acute orchitis, torsion of the spermatic cord, and strangulated hernia.
16. A painless nodule in the testis is associated with testicular cancer.

PROSTATE

17. Enlargement of the prostate with obliteration of the median sulcus suggests benign prostatic hypertrophy.
18. Enlargement of the prostate with asymmetry and tenderness suggests prostatitis.
19. A hard, irregular prostatic nodule is seen in carcinoma.

FEMALE BREAST

20. Retractions, dimpling, and abnormal contours of the breast may suggest benign lesions, but may also suggest malignancy.
21. Thickened, dimpled skin on the breast with enlargement of the pores (peau d'orange) and unilateral venous patterns are associated with malignancy.
22. Redness of the breast may be seen with infection or malignancy.
23. Peau d'orange may be first noted in the areola.
24. Recent unilateral inversion of the nipple or asymmetry in the direction in which the nipples point suggests cancer.
25. Tenderness upon breast palpation may be related to premenstrual fullness, fibrocystic disease, or inflammation. Thickness may also indicate cancer.
26. Nodules in the tail of the breast may be enlarged lymph nodes.
27. Hard, irregular, fixed unilateral masses that are poorly delineated suggest carcinoma.
28. Bilateral, single or multiple, round, mobile, well-delineated masses are consistent with fibrocystic breast disease or fibroadenoma.
29. Swelling, tenderness, erythema, and heat may be seen with mastitis.
30. Loss of nipple elasticity is seen with cancer.
31. Blood or serous discharge is associated with intraductal papilloma.
32. Milky discharge not due to prior pregnancy and found on both sides suggests galactorrhea which is sometimes associated with a pituitary tumor.
33. Unilateral discharge from one or two ducts can be seen in fibrocystic breast disease, intraductal papilloma, or carcinoma.

FEMALE AXILLARY

34. Rash may be due to allergy or other causes.
35. Signs of inflammation and infections may be due to infection of the sweat glands.
36. Enlarged axillary nodes are most often due to infection of the hand or arm but can be caused by malignancy.

- Bilateral, single or multiple, round, mobile, well-delineated masses
- Swelling, tenderness, erythema, and heat
- Loss of nipple elasticity
- Blood or serous discharge
- Bilateral milky discharge not due to prior pregnancy
- Unilateral discharge from one or two ducts

Axillary
- Rash
- Signs of inflammation and infections
- Enlarged axillary nodes
- Enlarge supraclavicular nodes

External Genitalia
- Excoriation, rashes or lesions of labia
- Bulging of labia
- Varicosities
- Ulcers or vesicles on labia
- Small, firm, round cystic nodules in labia
- Wartlike lesions
- Firm, painless ulcers
- Shallow, painful ulcers
- Ulcerated or red raised lesions in older women
- Enlargement of the clitoris
- Swelling, discoloration, or lacerations of vaginal opening
- Discharge from or lesions on vaginal opening
- Fissures or fistulas associated with vaginal opening
- Discharge/tenderness of Skene's glands
- A nontender mass in posteriolateral labia majora
- Swelling, redness, or tenderness
- Bulging of the anterior vaginal wall
- Bulging of the posterior vaginal wall
- Protrusion of the cervix or uterus into vagina
- Inflammation, lesions, growths on perineum

Vagina and Cervix
- Bluish color of cervix/vaginal mucosa
- Pale cervix
- Cervix to the right or left of midline
- Projection of cervix more than 3 cm into vaginal canal
- Transverse or star-shaped cervical lacerations
- Enlarged cervix
- Small, white, or yellow raised, round areas on cervix
- Cervical polyps
- Retroverted uterus
- Retroflexed uterus
- Pain on movement of the cervix
- Objective signs of pregnancy
- Myomas
- Ovarian tumors
- Profuse menstrual bleeding
- Irregular bleeding
- Postmenopausal bleeding

37. Enlarged supraclavicular nodes are associated with lymphatic metastases from abdominal or thoracic carcinoma.

FEMALE EXTERNAL GENITALIA

38. Excoriation, rashes, or lesions of the labia suggest inflammatory or infective processes.
39. Bulging of the labia that increases with straining suggests a hernia.
40. Varicosities may be present on the labia.
41. Ulcers or vesicles on the labia may be symptoms of sexually transmitted diseases.
42. Small, firm, round cystic nodules in the labia suggest sebaceous cysts.
43. Wart-like lesions suggest condylomata accuminata.
44. Firm, painless ulcers suggest chancre of primary syphilis.
45. Shallow, painful ulcers suggest herpes infection.
46. Ulcerated or red, raised lesions in older women suggest vulvar carcinoma.
47. Enlargement of the clitoris may be a symptom of a masculinizing condition.
48. Swelling, discoloration, or lacerations of the vaginal opening may be caused by trauma.
49. Discharge from or lesions on the vaginal opening may be symptoms of infection.
50. Fissures or fistulas associated with the vaginal opening may be related to injury, infection, spreading of a malignancy, or trauma.
51. Discharge from Skene's glands and/or tenderness suggests infection.
52. A nontender mass in the posteriolateral portion of the labia majora is indicative of a Bartholin's cyst.
53. Swelling, redness, or tenderness, especially if unilateral, may indicate abscess of Bartholin's glands.
54. Bulging of the anterior vaginal wall and urinary incontinence during straining suggest a cystocele.
55. Bulging of the posterior vaginal wall during straining suggests a rectocele.
56. Protrusion of the cervix or uterus into the vagina indicates uterine prolapse.
57. Inflammation, lesions, and growths present on the perineum may be seen in infections or cancer.

VAGINA AND CERVIX

58. Bluish color of the cervix and vaginal mucosa may be a sign of pregnancy.
59. A pale cervix is associated with anemia.
60. A cervix to the right or left of midline may indicate a pelvic mass, uterine adhesions, or pregnancy.
61. Projection of the cervix more than 3 cm into the vaginal canal may indicate a pelvic or uterine mass.
62. Transverse or star-shaped cervical lacerations reflect trauma that causes tearing of the cervix.
63. An enlarged cervix is associated with infection.

64. Nabothian cysts (small, white, or yellow raised, round areas on the cervix) are considered normal but may become infected.

65. Cervical polyps may be cervical or endometrial in origin.

66. The uterus may be retroverted (tilted backward) or retroflexed (angled backward).

67. Pain on movement of the cervix during manual examination suggests pelvic inflammatory disease (PID).

68. Softening of the uterine isthmus (Hegar's sign), softening of the cervix (Goodell's sign), and uterine enlargement may be objective signs of pregnancy.

69. Firm, irregular nodules that vary greatly in size and are continuous with the uterine surface are likely to be myomas.

70. Unilateral or bilateral smooth, compressible adnexal masses are found in ovarian tumors.

71. Profuse menstrual bleeding is seen with endometrial polyps, dysfunctional uterine bleeding (DUB), and the use of an intrauterine device.

72. Irregular bleeding may be associated with endometrial polyps, DUB, uterine or cervical carcinoma, or oral contraceptives.

73. Postmenopausal bleeding is seen with endometrial hyperplasia, estrogen therapy, and endometrial cancer.

SUGGESTIONS FOR CLASSROOM ACTIVITIES

- View the case study about irregular menstrual cycle that is provided on the textbook Companion Website. Use the information in the case study as a starting point for discussion of care of the client described.

SUGGESTIONS FOR CLINICAL ACTIVITIES

- Have students review the medical records of clinical clients for indications of sexual disorders. Help students identify pertinent assessment questions, techniques, and findings.

Chapter 50
Nursing Care of Men with Reproductive System and Breast Disorders

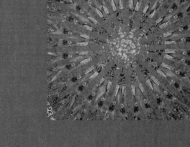

Resource Library

 Prentice Hall Nursing Medialink DVD-ROM

Audio Glossary
NCLEX-RN® Review
Animation/Video
   Testicular Self-Examination

 Companion Website

Audio Glossary
NCLEX-RN® Review
Care Plan Activity: Radical Prostatectomy
Case Studies
   Benign Prostatic Hyperplasia
   Prostatitis
Teaching Plan: ED Medication and Safety
MediaLink Applications
   Prostate Cancer Prevention
   Sleep Apnea and Erectile Dysfunction
Links to Resources

Image Library

Figure 50.1 Types of penile implants.
Figure 50.2 Common disorders of the scrotum.
Figure 50.3 Benign prostatic hyperplasia.
Figure 50.4 *A,* In a transurethral resection of the prostate, a resectoscope inserted through the

urethra is used to remove excess prostate tissue.
B, In a retropubic prostatectomy, prostate tissue is removed through an abdominal incision.
Figure 50.5 Method of operation of an artificial urinary sphincter.

Learning Outcome 1

Explain the pathophysiology, manifestations, complications, interdisciplinary care, and nursing care of disorders of the male reproductive system, including disorders of sexual function, the penis, the testes and scrotum, the prostate gland, and the breast.

Concepts for Lecture
Disorders of Sexual Function

1. Erectile dysfunction (ED) is the inability of the male to attain and maintain an erection sufficient to permit satisfactory sexual intercourse. ED may or may not be associated with loss of libido.
2. Impotence involves a total inability to achieve erection, and inconsistent ability to achieve erection, or the ability to sustain only brief erections.
3. Age-related changes in sexual function involve cellular and tissue changes in the penis, decreased sensory activity, hypogonadism, and the effects of chronic illness.
4. Diagnostic tests that may be ordered include blood chemistry, testosterone, prolactin, thyroxin, and PSA levels. Nocturnal penile tumescence and rigidity (NPTR) monitoring helps differentiate between psychogenic and organic causes. Cavernosometry and

PowerPoint Lecture Slides

Disorders of Sexual Function
- Erectile dysfunction (ED)
- Impotence
- Age-related changes
- Diagnostic tests
  - Blood chemistry
  - Hormone levels
  - PSA
  - Nocturnal penile tumescence and rigidity (NPTR)
  - Cavernosometry and cavernosography
- Treatment
  - Mechanical devices
- Common nursing diagnoses
  - Sexual dysfunction
  - Situational low self-esteem

cavernosography of the corpora are used to evaluate arterial inflow and venous outflow of the penis.

5. Mechanical devices that may be prescribed for treatment of ED include the vacuum constriction device (VCD).

6. Common nursing diagnoses include: *Sexual Dysfunction* and *Situational Low Self-Esteem.*

EJACULATORY DYSFUNCTION

7. Types of ejaculatory dysfunction include: retrograde ejaculation, premature ejaculation, and delayed ejaculation.

PENIS: PHIMOSIS, PARAPHIMOSIS, PRIAPISM

8. Phimosis is constriction of the foreskin so that it cannot be retracted over the glans penis. This disorder may be congenital or may be related to chronic infections under the foreskin. A related disorder is paraphimosis in which the foreskin is tight and constricted and is not able to cover the glans penis. The glans becomes engorged and edematous and is painful. This condition may result in ischemia of the glans.

9. Priapism is an involuntary, sustained, painful erection that is not associated with sexual arousal. This condition may result in ischemia and fibrosis of the erectile tissue with high risk of subsequent impotence. Primary priapism results from conditions such as tumors, infection, or trauma. Secondary priapism is caused by blood disorders, neurologic disorders, renal failure, and some medications.

10. Conservative treatment of priapism includes iced saline enemas, intravenous ketamin administration, and spinal anesthesia. Blood may be aspirated from the corpus through the dorsal glans, followed by catheterization and pressure dressings to maintain decompression. More aggressive surgery to create vascular shunts may be necessary.

11. Nursing care of priapism focuses on assessing the penis, monitoring urinary output, and providing pain control.

CANCER OF THE PENIS

12. Cancer of the penis is rare in North America.

13. Squamous cell carcinoma accounts for 95% of all penile cancers, and usually develops as a nodular or wart-like or red velvety lesion on the glans or foreskin. If the lesion is treated before inguinal node involvement, chances for a cure are good.

14. Diagnosis is made by biopsy of the lesion and any suspicious inguinal nodes.

15. Treatment may include radiation or chemotherapeutic intervention.

16. Education can help prevent this disease or provide early detection and cure.

- Ejaculatory dysfunction
  - Retrograde ejaculation
  - Premature ejaculation
  - Delayed ejaculation

Penis
- Phimosis
- Paraphimosis
- Priapism
  - Primary
  - Secondary
  - Conservative treatment
    - Iced saline enemas
    - Intravenous ketamin
    - Spinal anesthesia
    - Aspiration of blood from corpus
  - Aggressive treatment
    - Surgery to create vascular shunts
  - Nursing care of priapism
    - Assessment
    - Monitoring urinary output
    - Providing pain control

Cancer of the Penis
- Squamous cell carcinoma
- Diagnosis
  - Biopsy of lesion
  - Biopsy of inguinal nodes
- Treatment
  - Radiation
  - Chemotherapy
- Nursing care for penile amputation
  - Body image
  - Self-concept
  - Education of surgical effects

Testes and Scrotum
- Benign scrotal mass
  - Hydroceles
  - Spermatoceles
  - Varicoceles
  - Nursing care
    - Anxiety reduction
    - Comfort measures
- Epididymitis
  - Men under 35
    - C. trachomatis
    - N. gonorrhoeae
  - Men older than 35
    - UTI
    - Prostatitis
  - Manifestations
    - Pain
    - Edema
    - Erythema
  - Complications
    - Abscess formation
    - Infarction of the testes
    - Infertility

17. If the man has penile amputation, the nursing care focuses on body image, self-concept, and education of the effects of surgery.

BENIGN SCROTAL MASS

18. Most scrotal masses are benign. Common masses are hydroceles, spermatoceles, and varicoceles.
19. A hydrocele is a collection of fluid within the tunica vaginalis. Hydroceles may develop because of an imbalance between the production and reabsorption of fluid within the layer of the scrotum. Other factors include trauma, infection, or tumor.
20. A spermatocele is a mobile, usually painless mass that forms when efferent ducts in the epididymis dilate and form a cyst. Treatment is not usually necessary and spermatoceles are not associated with infertility.
21. A varicocele is an abnormal dilation of a vein within the spermatic cord. The dilated vein forms a soft mass that may be painful and can cause infertility.
22. Nursing care focuses on reducing anxiety and teaching about comfort measures.

EPIDIDYMITIS

23. Epididymitis is an infection or inflammation of the epididymis. In men under 35, the disorder is often caused by *C. trachomatis* or *N. gonorrhoeae*. In men older than 35, epididymitis is associated with a urinary tract infection or prostatitis and may be self-limiting with no need for treatment.
24. Manifestations of infectious epididymitis include pain and local edema that can progress to erythema and edema of the entire scrotum.
25. Complications of infectious epididymitis include abscess formation, infarction of the testes, and infertility.
26. Diagnosis is achieved by culture from a urethral swab or epididymal aspiration.
27. Nursing care involves symptomatic relief and teaching. Treatment may require weeks or months of medication.

ORCHITIS

28. Orchitis is an acute inflammation of infection of the testes.
29. It most commonly occurs as a complication of a systemic illness (such as mumps) or an extension of epididymitis. Trauma, including vasectomy and other scrotal surgeries, may cause inflammation of the testes.
30. Bed rest, scrotal support and elevation, hot or cold compresses, antibiotic therapy, and analgesics for pain are prescribed. If a hydrocele occurs, it is aspirated.

- ○ Diagnosis
  - – Urethral culture
  - – Epididymal aspiration
- ○ Nursing care
  - – Symptomatic relief
  - – Teaching
- Orchitis
  - ○ Etiology
    - – Complication of systemic illness (mumps)
    - – Extension of epididymitis
    - – Trauma
  - ○ Treatment
    - – Bed rest
    - – Scrotal support and elevation
    - – Hot or cold compresses
    - – Antibiotic therapy
    - – Analgesics
    - – Aspiration of hydrocele
- Testicular torsion
  - ○ Potentially a medical emergency
  - ○ Etiology
    - – Spontaneous
    - – Trauma
    - – Physical exertion
  - ○ Complications
    - – Vascular engorgement
    - – Ischemia
  - ○ Diagnosis
    - – History and physical
    - – Testicular scanning
    - – Prostate ultrasound
- Testicular cancer
  - ○ Types
    - – Seminoma
    - – Nonseminomas
  - ○ Manifestations
    - – Enlargement of one testicle with discomfort
    - – Abdominal ache
    - – Heaviness of the scrotum
  - ○ Dissemination
    - – Lymphatic
    - – Vascular
  - ○ Interdisciplinary care
    - – Diagnosis
    - – Elimination of the cancer
    - – Prevention or treatment of metastasis
  - ○ Diagnosis
    - – hCG and AFP
    - – LDH
  - ○ Therapy
    - – Radiation therapy
    - – Surgery
  - ○ Nursing diagnoses
    - – *Deficient Knowledge*
    - – *Ineffective Sexuality Patterns*

Testicular Torsion

31. Testicular torsion is twisting of the spermatic cord with scrotal swelling and pain and is potentially a medical emergency.
32. Testicular torsion may occur spontaneously or may follow trauma or physical exertion.
33. Complications are vascular engorgement and ischemia.
34. Diagnosis is achieved by history and physical, testicular scanning, and/or prostate ultrasound.

Testicular Cancer

35. The most common type of testicular cancer is the seminoma type and it is believed to arise from the seminiferous epithelium of the testes. Nonseminomas contain more than one cell type; they include embryonal carcinoma, teratoma, choriocarcinoma, and yolk cell carcinoma.
36. The first sign of testicular cancer may be a slight enlargement of one testicle with some discomfort. There may be an abdominal ache and a feeling of heaviness in the scrotum. Lymphatic dissemination usually leads to disease in the retroperitoneal lymph nodes; whereas vascular dissemination can lead to metastasis in the lungs, bone, or liver. Manifestations of metastasis include lower extremity edema, back pain, cough, hemoptysis, or dizziness. HCG-producing tumors may cause breast enlargement.
37. Care focuses on diagnosis, elimination of the cancer, and prevention or treatment of metastasis.
38. Diagnosis is made by serum tumor markers (hCG and AFP) and LDH analysis.
39. Radiation therapy is used for stage 1 seminoma to treat cancer in the retroperitoneal lymph nodes, the most frequent site for distant metastasis.
40. Nursing diagnoses include: *Deficient Knowledge* and *Ineffective Sexuality Patterns*.

Prostate Gland

41. Prostatitis is a term used to refer to different types of inflammatory disorders of the prostate gland. Prostatodynia is a condition in which the client experiences the symptoms of prostatitis, but shows no evidence of inflammation or infection.
42. The types of prostatitis are: acute bacterial prostatitis, chronic bacterial prostatitis, chronic prostatitis/pelvic pain syndrome, and asymptomatic inflammatory prostatitis.
43. Men with asymptomatic inflammatory prostatitis have no subjective symptoms, but are diagnosed when a biopsy or prostatic fluid examination is conducted.
44. Acute bacterial prostatitis is most often caused by an ascending infection from the urethra or reflux of infected urine into the ducts of the prostate gland.
45. Manifestations include fever, malaise, muscle and joint pain, urinary frequency and urgency, dysuria,

Prostate Gland
- Prostatitis
  - Types
    - Prostatodynia
    - Acute bacterial prostatitis
    - Chronic bacterial prostatitis
    - Chronic prostatitis/pelvic pain syndrome
    - Asymptomatic inflammatory prostatitis
  - Manifestations
    - May be absent
    - Fever
    - Malaise
    - Muscle and joint pain
    - Urinary frequency and urgency
    - Dysuria
    - Urethral discharge
    - Dull, aching pain
    - Enlargement/pain of prostate
- Chronic bacterial prostatitis
  - History of recurrent UTI
  - Manifestations
    - Urinary frequency and urgency
    - Dysuria
    - Low back pain
    - Perineal discomfort
    - Epididymitis
- Chronic prostatitis/chronic pelvic pain syndrome
  - Types
    - Inflammatory
    - Noninflammatory
  - Diagnosis
    - Urine culture
    - Prostate secretion culture
    - Xray
    - Ultrasound
  - Nursing care
    - Symptom management
- Benign prostatic hyperplasia
  - Common and age related
  - Risk factors
    - Aging
    - Family history
    - Race
    - Diet high in meats and fats
  - Necessary preconditions
    - Age of 50 or over
    - Presence of testes
  - Etiology
    - Aging prostate more sensitive to DHT
    - Relative increase in estrogen to testosterone levels
  - Pathophysiology
    - Hyperplasia
    - Hypertrophy
  - Manifestations
    - Obstruction

and urethral discharge. There may be a dull, aching pain in the perineum, rectum, or lower back. On physical examination, the prostate is enlarged and painful.

46. Men with chronic bacterial prostatitis often present with a history of recurrent UTI.

47. Manifestations are urinary frequency and urgency, dysuria, low back pain, and perineal discomfort. Epididymitis may be associated.

48. Chronic prostatitis/chronic pelvic pain syndrome is the most common and least understood of the syndromes. The two types are inflammatory and noninflammatory.

49. Inflammatory prostatitis is believed to be an autoimmune disorder, but the actual cause is unknown. Manifestations are low back pain; urinary manifestations; pain in the penis, testicles, scrotum, lower back, and rectum; decreased libido; and painful ejaculations. There are no bacteria in the urine, but there are abnormal inflammatory cells in prostatic secretions.

50. Noninflammatory prostatitis has manifestations similar to those of inflammatory prostatitis, but there is no evidence of urinary to prostatic infection or inflammation.

51. Diagnostic studies for prostatitis are urine and prostate secretion examination and cultures and x-ray or ultrasound studies.

52. Nursing care focuses on symptom management.

BENIGN PROSTATIC HYPERPLASIA

53. Benign prostatic hyperplasia (BPH) is a common age-related, nonmalignant enlargement of the prostate gland.

54. Risk factors for development of BPH include aging, family history, race, and a diet high in meat and fats.

55. Two necessary preconditions for BPH are age of 50 or over and the presence of testes.

56. The androgen that mediates prostatic growth at all ages is dihydrotestosterone (DHT). Although androgen levels decrease with aging, the aging prostate appears to become more sensitive to available DHT.

57. Increasing estrogen levels associated with aging or a relative increase in estrogen related to testosterone levels may contribute to prostatic hyperplasia.

58. The prostate enlarges through formation and growth of nodules (hyperplasia) and enlargement of glandular cells (hypertrophy).

59. Manifestations include those from obstruction (weak urinary stream, increased time to void, hesitancy, incomplete bladder emptying, and postvoid dribbling) and irritation (frequency, urgency, incontinence, nocturia, dysuria, and bladder pain). Urinary retention may become chronic.

- · Weak urinary stream
- · Increased time to void
- · Hesitancy
- · Incomplete bladder emptying
- · Postvoid dribbling
- – Irritation
  - · Frequency
  - · Urgency
  - · Incontinence
  - · Nocturia
  - · Dysuria
  - · Bladder pain
  - · Urinary retention
- ○ Complications
  - – Diverticula on bladder wall
  - – Obstruction of ureters
  - – Infection
  - – Hydroureter
  - – Hydronephrosis
  - – Renal insufficiency
- ○ Interdisciplinary care
  - – Diagnosis
  - – Correcting of minimizing urinary obstruction
  - – Preventing/treating complications
- ○ Diagnosis
  - – Physical exam
  - – Laboratory tests
- ○ International Prostate Symptom Score
- ○ Nursing diagnoses
  - – *Deficient Knowledge*
  - – *Urinary Retention*
  - – *Risk for Infection*
  - – *Risk for Imbalanced Fluid Volume*
- ● Prostate cancer
  - ○ Etiology
    - – Unknown
    - – Linked to androgens
  - ○ Pathophysiology
    - – Almost all are adenocarcinomas
    - – Develop in peripheral zones
    - – May metastasize directly
    - – May metastasize by lymph and blood
  - ○ Manifestations
    - – May be asymptomatic
    - – Pain from metastasis to bone
    - – Urinary manifestations like BPH
    - – Blood in urine or ejaculate
  - ○ Interdisciplinary care
    - – Diagnosis
    - – Elimination or containment of cancer
    - – Prevention or treatment of complications
  - ○ Diagnosis
    - – Definitively only by biopsy
    - – Nodular, fixed gland
    - – PSA levels
    - – Transrectal ultrasound
    - – Urinalysis

60. Complications include diverticula on the bladder wall, obstruction of the ureters, infection, hydroureter, hydronephrosis, and renal insufficiency.

61. Interdisciplinary care includes diagnosing the disorder, correcting or minimizing the urinary obstruction, and preventing or treating complications.

62. The diagnosis of BPH involves both physical examination and laboratory tests to not only diagnose the disease but also to differentiate it from prostate cancer.

63. Laboratory testing includes serum creatinine and urine WBCs, RBCs, and bacteria. PSA levels are obtained to rule out prostate cancer. Urinary function is assessed by measuring residual urine with ultrasonography or postvoiding catheterization and through uroflowmetry.

64. The International Prostate Symptom Score uses a scale of 0 (not at all) to 5 (almost always) to collect data about areas such as feeling as though the bladder did not empty with urinating, need to urinate within 2 hours after urinating, starting and stopping the stream several times while urinating, and straining to urinate.

65. Nursing diagnoses include: *Deficient Knowledge; Urinary Retention; Risk for Infection;* and *Risk for Imbalanced Fluid Volume.*

PROSTATE CANCER

66. The exact etiology of prostate cancer in unknown, although androgens are believed to have a role in its development.

67. Almost all primary prostate cancers are adenocarcinomas, and develop in the peripheral zones of the prostate gland.

68. The tumor may metastasize and involve the seminal vesicles or bladder by direct extension. Metastasis by lymph and venous channels is common.

69. Early stage prostate cancer is often asymptomatic. Pain from metastasis to bone may be the initial manifestation. Urinary manifestations are often like those of BPH. There may be blood in the urine or ejaculate.

70. Death usually occurs secondary to debility caused by multiple sites of skeletal metastasis.

71. Care of the man with prostate cancer focuses on diagnosis, elimination or containment of the cancer, and prevention or treatment of complications. There is no proven clinical strategy to prevent the development of prostate cancer.

72. Definitive diagnosis can be made only by biopsy. DRE will find the prostate gland nodular and fixed. PSA levels are used to diagnose and stage prostate cancer and to monitor response to treatment.

73. Transrectal ultrasonography (TRUS) may be used with DRE if abnormal or if the PSA is elevated. Other tests may include urinalysis, cystoscopy, bone scan, MRI, or CT scan.

- – Cystoscopy
- – Bone scan
- – MRI
- – CT scan
- ○ Treatment
  - – Radiation therapy
  - – Androgen deprivation therapy
- ○ Nursing diagnoses
  - – *Urinary Incontinence* (Reflex, stress, total)
  - – *Sexual Dysfunction*
  - – *Acute/Chronic Pain*

Breast
- • Gynecomastia
  - ○ Etiology
    - – High ratio of estradiol to testosterone
    - – Obesity
    - – Testicular tumors
    - – Liver disease
    - – Adrenal carcinoma
    - – TB
    - – Hodgkin's disease
    - – Injury
    - – Orchitis
    - – Some medications
  - ○ Nursing care
    - – Education about cause/treatment
    - – Emotional support
- • Breast cancer
  - ○ Etiology
    - · Unclear
    - · Hormonal
    - · Genetic
    - · Environmental
  - ○ Pathophsyiology
    - – Similar to females
    - – Lobular cancer rare in males
  - ○ Treatment
    - – Like treatment for females
      - · Surgery
      - · Radiation
      - · Chemotherapy
      - · Hormone therapy
      - · Castration
  - ○ Nursing care
    - – Essentially the same as for women
    - – Additional concerns
      - · Shame
      - · Embarassment

74. Radiation therapy may be used as a primary treatment for prostate cancer. Long-term problems with impotence and urinary incontinence may be avoided, and survival rates are often comparable. Radiation may be delivered by external beam or interstitial implants of radioactive seeds of iodine, gold, palladium, or iridium. Radiation therapy may be used palliatively for the client with metastatic prostate cancer.

75. Androgen deprivation therapy is used to treat advanced prostate cancer. Strategies to induce androgen deprivation vary from orchiectomy to oral administration of hormonal agents.

76. Nursing diagnoses include: *Urinary Incontinence* (Reflex, Stress, Total); *Sexual Dysfunction;* and *Acute/Chronic Pain.*

BREAST

77. Gynecomastia, which is the abnormal enlargement of the male breast, is thought to result from a high ratio of estradiol to testosterone. Any condition that increases estrogen activity or decreases testosterone can contribute to gynecomastia.

78. Conditions that increase estrogen activity include obesity, testicular tumors, liver disease, and adrenal carcinoma.

79. Conditions that decrease testosterone production include chronic illnesses such as TB or Hodgkin's disease, injury, and orchitis.

80. Drugs such as digitalis, opiates, and chemotherapeutic agents are also associated with gynecomastia.

81. Nursing care of the client with gynecomastia includes education about the cause and treatment of the condition, and emotional support.

82. The etiology of male breast cancer is unclear; hormonal, genetic, and perhaps environmental factors appear to be important.

83. Male breast cancer is clinically and histologically similar to female breast cancer, although lobular cancer is rare in males.

84. Treatment for male breast cancer is much like the treatment of female breast cancer. Surgery, radiation, chemotherapy, or hormonal therapy are the conventional treatments. Castration is the most successful palliative measure in men with advanced breast cancer.

85. Nursing care for the man with breast cancer is essentially the same as for the woman with breast cancer. Additional concerns may be embarrassment or shame about the condition.

SUGGESTIONS FOR CLASSROOM ACTIVITIES

- View the case study about benign prostatic hyperplasia that is provided on the textbook Companion Website. Use the information provided to develop a care plan for the client.
- View the case study about prostatitis that is provided on the textbook Companion Website. Use the information provided to develop a care plan for the client.
- Divide the class into small groups and assign each group one of the disorders presented in this chapter. Have the students outline the pathophysiology, manifestations, complications, interdisciplinary care, and nursing care of the disorder assigned. Share the information in class.
- Have the class develop a list of nursing diagnoses commonly appropriate to men who have the disorders presented in class. Discuss the nursing interventions for each nursing diagnosis.

SUGGESTIONS FOR CLINICAL ACTIVITIES

- Assign students to clients who are experiencing one of the disorders presented in this chapter. Have the students develop a plan of care for the client assigned. In post-conference, compare and contrast the care plans according to client characteristics and disease process.

LEARNING OUTCOME 2

Compare and contrast the risk factors for cancer of the penis, testes, and prostate gland.

CONCEPTS FOR LECTURE
CANCER OF THE PENIS

1. Phimosis and poor genital hygiene are risk factors, as are viral HPV and HIV infections. Ultraviolet light exposure may also play a role.

CANCER OF THE TESTES

2. The cause of testicular cancer is unknown, but both congenital and acquired factors have been associated with tumor development. Risk factors include: age, cryptorchidism, genetic predisposition, cancer of the other testicle, occupational risks, presence of multiple atypical nevi, HIV infection, cancer in situ, body size, and maternal hormone use.

CANCER OF THE PROSTATE GLAND

3. Cancer of the prostate is the most common type of cancer among men and the second leading cause of death in North America.
4. Risk factors include age, race, genetic and hereditary factors, having a vasectomy, and dietary factors such as high animal fat and excessive supplemental vitamin A.

POWERPOINT LECTURE SLIDES

Penis
- Phimosis
- Poor genital hygiene
- HPV
- HIV
- Ultraviolet light exposure

Testes
- Unknown
- Risk factors
  - Age
  - Cryptorchidism
  - Genetic predisposition
  - Cancer of the other testicle
  - Occupational risks
  - Presence of multiple atypical nevi
  - HIV infection
  - Cancer in situ
  - Body size
  - Maternal hormone use

Prostate Gland
- Risk factors
  - Age
  - Race
  - Genetic and hereditary factors
  - Having a vasectomy
  - High animal fat diet
  - Excessive supplemental vitamin A

LEARNING OUTCOME 3

Discuss the purposes, nursing implications, and health education for medications and treatments used to treat disorders of sexual function, the penis, the testes and scrotum, the prostate gland, and the breast.

CONCEPTS FOR LECTURE

SEXUAL FUNCTION

1. Erectile dysfunction (ED) can be treated with medications taken orally, injected directly into the penis, or inserted into the urethra at the tip of the penis.
2. Oral medications include sildenafil citrate (Viagra), vardenafil hydrochloride (Levitra), or tadalafil (Cialis). These medications should not be taken by men who are also taking nitrate-based drugs or alpha-blockers. Tadalafil (Cialis) should also not be taken by men also taking erythromycin or rifampicin, ketoconazole or itraconazole, or protease inhibitors.
3. Hormone replacement therapy with testosterone injections or topical patches may be used for men with documented androgen deficiency and who do not have prostate cancer.
4. Injectable medications, including papaverine and prostaglandin E injection directly into the penis, may be used. Alprostadil (Caverject) may be injected into the penis or placed in the urethra as a minisuppository.

PENIS

5. Men who use intracavernous injection therapy or Cialis for erectile dysfunction are at risk for priapism. The nurse should include information about when to seek treatment for this possible disorder.

TESTES AND SCROTUM

6. Severe epididymitis may require hospitalization and intravenous antibiotics. Less acute forms respond to outpatient antibiotic therapy. The sexual partner may also require treatment.
7. Chemotherapy for cancer of the testes may include platinum-based combinations such as BEP and EP.

PROSTATE GLAND

8. Bacterial prostatitis is treated with appropriate antibiotic therapy. NSAIDs are used for pain relief and anticholinergics may reduce voiding symptoms.

POWERPOINT LECTURE SLIDES

Sexual Function
- Oral medications
  - Not with nitrate based drugs
  - Not with alpha-blockers
    - Sildenafil citrate
    - Vardenafil hydrochloride
    - Tadalafil
  - Tadalafil not with
    - Erythromycin
    - Rifampincin
    - Ketoconazole
    - Itraconazole
    - Protease inhibitors
- Hormone replacement therapy
  - Testosterone injections
  - Topical patches
- Injectable medications
  - Papaverine
  - Prostaglandin E injection
  - Alprostadil

Testes and Scrotum
- Severe epididymitis
  - Hospitalization
  - IV antibiotics
  - Sexual partner treatment
- Cancer
  - Chemotherapy
    - Platinum-based combinations

Prostate Gland
- Bacterial prostatitis
  - Appropriate antibiotics
  - NSAIDs
  - Anticholinergics
- Prostatodynia
  - Alpha-adrenergic blocking agents
  - Muscle relaxants
- BPH, medication therapy
  - Antiandrogen agents
  - Alpha-adrenergic antagonists

9. Prostatodynia is treated symptomatically to relieve muscle tension, usually with alpha-adrenergic blocking agents or muscle relaxants.

10. For BPH, medication therapy focuses on antiandrogen agents that inhibit the conversion of testosterone to DHT and alpha-adrenergic antagonists that relieve obstruction and increase the flow of urine.

11. Phytotherapy used for BPH include saw palmetto berry, the bark of *Pygeum Africanum*, the roots of *Echinacea purpurea* and *Hypoxis rooperi,* and the leaves of the trembling poplar.

12. Toremifene (Acapodene) is being studied as a treatment for men with abnormal prostate growth to help prevent the growths from becoming malignant.

BREAST

13. In severe cases of gynecomastia, tamoxifen is given to decrease estrogen activity.

- ○ Phytotherapy
  - – Saw palmetto berry
  - – Bark of *Pygeum Africanum*
  - – Roots of *Echinacea*
  - – *Pupurea*
  - – *Hypoxis roper*
  - – Leaves of trembling poplar
- ○ Toremifene

Breast
- Gyneocomastia
  - ○ Tamoxifen

SUGGESTIONS FOR CLASSROOM ACTIVITIES

- Have students identify the risks of taking medications for erectile dysfunction along with nitrates or alpha-blockers. Identify assessment findings that would indicate an emergency situation in these clients. Have students discuss why a man who takes nitrates or alpha-blockers might be tempted to be dishonest about taking a medication for erectile dysfunction.

SUGGESTIONS FOR CLINICAL ACTIVITIES

- Have students identify medications that are used for sexual disorders in males. Have students develop medication information sheets regarding these medications. In the information, include indications, contraindications, doses, nursing implications, and teaching implications.

LEARNING OUTCOME 4

Describe the various surgical procedures used to treat disorders of the male reproductive system.

CONCEPTS FOR LECTURE

1. Surgical treatment for erectile dysfunction (ED) involves either revascularization procedures or implantation of prosthetic devices.

2. Severe phimosis or paraphimosis may require surgical circumcision, with antibiotic therapy if an infection is present.

3. In penile cancer, large lesions may require partial or total amputation of the penis.

4. Surgical treatment of testicular torsion involves detorsion of the testicle and fixation to the scrotum. If the testicle is necrotic or has sustained significant damage, an orchiectomy may be performed.

5. Surgical treatment for cancer of the testes may include radical orchiectomy with a modified retroperitoneal lymph node dissection.

6. Minimally invasive surgery for BPH includes transurethral microwave thermotherapy and transurethral needle ablation (TUNA). Both surgeries focus on destruction of enough prostatic tissue to relieve symptoms.

7. A transurethral resection of the prostate (TURP) is the surgical procedure used most often. Obstructing prostate tissue is removed using the wire loop of a

POWERPOINT LECTURE SLIDES

Erectile Dysfunction
- Revascularization procedures
- Implantation of prosthetic devices

Severe Phimosis/Paraphimosis
- Circumcision

Penile Cancer
- Large lesions
  - ○ Partial or total amputation of the penis

Testicular Torsion
- Detorsion of testicle
- Fixation to scrotum
- Orchiectomy

Cancer of the Testes
- Radical orchiectomy
- Modified retroperitoneal lymph node dissection

BPH
- Transurethral microwave thermotherapy
- Transurethral needle ablation (TUNA)
- Transurethral resection of the prostate (TURP)

resectoscope and electrocautery inserted through the urethra. No external incision is necessary. Complications include postoperative hemorrhage, clot retention, inability to void, urinary tract infection, incontinence, impotence, and retrograde ejaculation.

8. Transurethral incision of the prostate (TUIP) is a procedure in which small incisions are made in the smooth muscle where the prostate is attached to the bladder. The gland is split to reduce pressure on the urethra and no tissue is removed.

9. When the prostate gland is very large, an open prostatectomy may be performed.

10. In laser surgery for BPH, the surgeon uses a cystoscope to pass a YAG laser fiber through the urethra into the prostate and then vaporizes obstructing prostate tissue with several short bursts of energy.

11. Newer therapies include minimally invasive procedures such as balloon urethroplasty and placement of intraureteral stents.

12. Surgery for prostate cancer includes several types of prostatectomies. TURP may be used in early disease in older men.

13. Radical prostatectomy involves removal of the prostate, prostatic capsule, seminal vesicles, and a portion of the bladder neck.

14. Retropubic prostatectomy may be performed because it allows adequate control of bleeding, visualization of the prostate bed and bladder neck, and access to pelvic lymph nodes.

15. Perineal prostatectomy is often preferred for men who are poor surgical risks because it takes less time and involves less bleeding.

16. Suprapubic prostatectomy is rarely used because control of bleeding is difficult.

○ Complications
   – Postoperative hemorrhage
   – Clot retention
   – Inability to void
   – Urinary tract infection
   – Incontinence
   – Impotence
   – Retrograde ejaculation
• Transurethral incision of the prostate (TUIP)
• Open prostatectomy
• Laser surgery
• Balloon urethroplasty
   ○ Placement of intraureteral stents

Prostate Cancer
• TURP
• Radical prostatectomy
• Retropubic prostatectomy
• Perineal prostatectomy
• Suprapubic prostatectomy

SUGGESTIONS FOR CLASSROOM ACTIVITIES

• Using anatomic models, describe the surgical procedures presented in the chapter. Have students discuss the nursing implications of caring for the client preoperatively and postoperatively.

• Review the care plan activity about radical prostatectomy that is provided on the textbook Companion Website. Using the information presented, discuss the care of the client and develop a care plan.

SUGGESTIONS FOR CLINICAL ACTIVITIES

• Assign students to clinical clients who have undergone or will undergo one of the procedures presented in the chapter. Have students develop a plan of care for the assigned client. Share the care plans in post-conference.

Chapter 51
Nursing Care of Women with Reproductive System and Breast Disorders

Resource Library

 PRENTICE HALL NURSING MEDIALINK DVD-ROM

Audio Glossary
NCLEX-RN® Review
Animation
   Premenstrual Syndrome

 COMPANION WEBSITE

Audio Glossary
NCLEX-RN® Review
Care Plan Activity: Postoperative Hysterectomy Care
Case Studies
   Breast Cancer
   Endometriosis
Teaching Plans
   Breast Cancer
   Mammogram
MediaLink Applications
   Pap Smears
   Post-Menopause Dietary Recommendations
Links to Resources

IMAGE LIBRARY

Figure 51.1 Laparoscopy.
Figure 51.2 Displacements of the uterus within the uterine cavity.
Figure 51.3 Prolapse of the uterus can vary from mild to complete.
Figure 51.4 Types of uterine fibroid tumors (leiomyomas).
Figure 51.5 Conization, the surgical removal of a cone-shaped section of the cervix, is used to treat microinvasive carcinoma of the cervix.

Figure 51.6 Vulvectomy for vulvar carcinoma.
Figure 51.7 Fibrocystic breast changes.
Figure 51.8 Types of breast biopsy.
Figure 51.9 Types of mastectomy.
Figure 51.10 Types of breast reconstruction surgeries.
Figure 51.11 Postmastectomy exercises.

Learning Outcome 1

Explain the pathophysiology, manifestations, complications, interdisciplinary care, and nursing care of disorders of female sexual function, menstrual disorders, structural disorders, reproductive tissue disorders, and breast disorders.

Concepts for Lecture
Disorders of Female Sexual Function

1. Dyspareunia:
   - Dyspareunia is pain during intercourse.
   - Physical conditions that cause dyspareunia include imperforate hymen, vaginal scarring, or vaginismus.
   - Early traumatic events, such as sexual abuse, fear of men, or rape may contribute to this disorder.
2. Inhibited sexual desire:
   - Inhibition of sexual desire may result from psychogenic causes such as childhood teaching, painful experiences, or cultural or religious values.
   - Fear of pregnancy or sexually transmitted diseases and depression can also contribute to this disorder.

PowerPoint Lecture Slides

Disorders of Female Sexual Function
- Dyspareunia
- Inhibited sexual desire
- Orgasmic dysfunction
- PMS
- Dysmenorrhea
- Dysfunctional uterine bleeding
- Uterine dysplacement
- Vaginal fistula
- Cysts or polyps
- Leiomyoma
- Endometriosis
- Breast disorders

3. Orgasmic dysfunction
   - Anorgasmia is the most prevalent sexual problem among women.
   - Psychogenically-induced anorgasmia may result from unresolved conflicts about sexual activity.
   - Organic causes of anorgasmia include the presence of disease that results in general debilitation or that affects the sexual response cycle, and the use of drugs that depress the central nervous system.
   - Primary anorgasmia exists when a woman has never experienced an orgasm during the waking state.
   - Secondary anorgasmia exists when a woman who previously experienced orgasm is no longer able to do so.
4. Nursing care focuses on the type of sexual dysfunction with a thorough history. The goal of treatment is to increase self-awareness and understanding of communication and their relationship to sexual desire.

PREMENSTRUAL SYNDROME

5. Premenstrual syndrome (PMS) is a complex of manifestations that are limited to 3 to 14 days before menstruation and are relieved by the onset of menses.
6. Manifestations include mood swings, breast tenderness, fatigue, irritability, food cravings, and depression.
7. If PMS is disabling it is called by the psychiatric label premenstrual dysphoric disorder.
8. It is believed that hormonal changes associated with menstruation contribute to the problem.
9. Increased production of aldosterone results in sodium retention and edema.
10. Decreased levels of monoamine oxidase in the brain are associated with depression.
11. Reduced levels of serotonin can lead to mood swings.
12. Goals are to relieve manifestations and to help develop self-care patterns that will help the woman anticipate and cope more effectively with future episodes of PMS.
13. There are no definitive tests for PMS. The regular recurrence of manifestations preceding the onset of menses for at least 3 months leads to a diagnosis of PMS.
14. Treatment includes regular exercise, avoiding caffeine, and a diet low in simple sugars and high in lean proteins.
15. For severe symptoms, ovulation may be suppressed by use of gonadotropin-releasing hormone agonists, oral contraceptives, or danazol (Danocrine).
16. Progesterone and antiprostaglandin agents such as NSAIDs may help relieve cramping.
17. Diuretics may be prescribed to relieve bloating.
18. Selective serotonin reuptake inhibitors may be used to manage mood and some physical manifestations of PMS.
19. Alternative and complementary therapies for PMS include dietary, exercise, and relaxation and stress management strategies.
20. Herbal remedies include black cohosh, ginger, chaste tree berry, and evening primrose oil.
21. Nursing diagnoses include: *Acute Pain* and *Ineffective Coping.*

DYSMENORRHEA

22. Dysmenorrhea is pain or discomfort associated with menstruation. Primary dysmenorrhea occurs without specific pelvic pathology and is most often seen in girls who have just begun menstruating. Secondary dysmenorrhea is related to identified pelvic disease.

23. Primary dysmenorrhea may be related to excessive production of prostaglandin that causes the uterine muscle fibers to contract. This contraction results in uterine ischemia and pain. Psychologic factors may contribute.

24. Secondary dysmenorrhea is related to underlying organic conditions that involve scarring or injury to the reproductive tract.

25. Manifestations may be severe enough to disrupt activities of daily living.

26. Care of the woman with menstrual pain focuses on identifying the underlying cause, reestablishing functional capacity, and managing pain.

27. Diagnostic testing includes Pap smears, cervical and vaginal cultures, ultrasound of the pelvis and vagina, and CT scans or MRI.

28. Laboratory tests include FSH and LH levels, progesterone and estradiol levels, and thyroid function tests.

29. Surgeries include laparoscopy and dilation and curettage (D&C).

30. Medications used to treat dysmenorrhea are analgesics, prostaglandin inhibitors, or oral contraceptives.

31. Alternative and complementary therapies include regular physical exercise, supplementing the diet with zinc and calcium, and using herbal remedies. Using a heating pad on the abdomen or taking a warm bath may also help reduce pain.

32. Nursing care for primary dysmenorrhea focuses on controlling manifestations and providing education.

33. Nursing care for secondary dysmenorrhea varies according to the underlying cause.

DYSFUNCTIONAL UTERINE BLEEDING

34. Dysfunctional uterine bleeding (DUB) refers to vaginal bleeding that is usually painless but abnormal in amount, duration, or time of occurrence.

35. Types of DUB include primary and secondary amenorrhea, oligomenorrhea, menorrhagia, metrorrhagia, and postmenopausal bleeding.

36. Stress, extreme weight changes, use of oral contraceptives or intrauterine devices, and postmenopausal status can predispose a woman to DUB.

37. Pathophysiologically, DUB is generally related to a hormone imbalance or presence of a neoplasm.

38. Amenorrhea is the absence of menstruation. Primary amenorrhea is absence of menarche by age 16, or by age 14 if secondary sex characteristics fail to develop. Secondary amenorrhea is absence of menses for at least 6 months in a previously menstruating woman.

39. Oligomenorrhea is scant menses usually related to hormone imbalance.

40. Menorrhagia is excessive or prolonged menstruation.
41. Metrorrhagia is bleeding between menstrual periods. Mittleschmerz is midcycle spotting associated with ovulation and is not considered metrorrhagia.
42. Anovulation is the absence of ovulation.
43. The interdisciplinary care of a woman with DUB focuses on identifying and treating the underlying cause.
44. Diagnostic testing includes Pap smear, pelvic ultrasound, hysteroscopy, or endometrial biopsy.
45. Laboratory studies include CBC, thyroid function testing, endocrine studies, and serum progesterone levels.
46. For anovulatory DUB, oral contraceptives may be prescribed for 3 to 6 months. Progesterone or medroxyprogesterone may be prescribed to regulate uterine bleeding.
47. Ovulatory DUB may be treated with progestins. Oral iron supplements may be necessary.
48. Surgical interventions emphasize the least invasive method that proves effective. Surgeries include D&C, endometrial ablation, and hysterectomy.
49. Nursing diagnoses include: *Anxiety* and *Sexual Dysfunction*.

Uterine Displacement

50. The uterus may be displaced within the pelvic cavity or may descend into the vaginal canal.
51. Retroversion of the uterus is a backward tilting of the uterus toward the rectum.
52. Retroflexion of the uterus involves a flexing or bending of the uterine corpus backward toward the rectum.
53. Anteversion is an exaggerated forward tilting of the uterus.
54. Anteflexion is a flexing or folding of the uterine corpus upon itself.
55. Uterine prolapse is described by degree. First-degree prolapse involves a descent of less than half the uterine corpus into the vagina. Second-degree prolapse involves the descent of the entire uterus into the vagina canal. Third-degree prolapse, or procidentia, is complete prolapse of the uterus outside the body.
56. Prolapse of the uterus is often accompanied by cystocele or rectocele.
57. Displacement or prolapse of the uterus, bladder, or rectum can be congenital or acquired. Congenital tilting or flexion of the uterus is rare; the condition is usually the result of scarring or inflammation. Prolapse may be related to weakened pelvic musculature.
58. Interdisciplinary care focuses on identifying the cause of the structural disorder, correcting or minimizing the condition, relieving pain, preventing or treating infection, and supporting and educating the woman.
59. Surgical procedures depend upon the structures affected. Common surgical procedures include colporrhaphy, Marshall-Marchetti-Kranz procedure, surgical repositioning of a prolapsed uterus, and hysterectomy.

60. A pessary is a removable device that is inserted into the vagina to provide temporary support for the uterus or bladder. This device may be used when surgery is contraindicated.
61. Nursing diagnoses include: *Stress Incontinence* and *Anxiety*.

VAGINAL FISTULA

62. A vaginal fistula may be vesicovaginal or rectovaginal and may develop as a complication of childbirth, gynecologic or urologic surgery, or radiation therapy.
63. Diagnosis of vesicovaginal fistula is made by instilling dye into the urinary bladder through a catheter and observing the vagina for leakage. Dye may also be injected intravenously as it is excreted by the kidneys. Urine and vaginal cultures may be performed to rule out infection. Antibiotics are administered.
64. Nursing care is similar to that for the woman with a displacement disorder.

CYSTS OR POLYPS

65. Bartholin's gland cysts are the most common cystic disorder of the vulva and are caused by infection or obstruction of Bartholin's glands.
66. Cervical polyps develop at the vaginal end of the cervix, have a stem, and are highly vascular. These are the most common of the benign cervical lesions.
67. Endometrial cysts and polyps are caused by endometrial overgrowth and are often filled with old blood. They are the result of endometrial implants on the ovary and are associated with endometriosis.
68. Ovarian cysts can be follicular cysts or corpus luteum cysts. Follicular cysts develop as a result of failure of the mature follicle to rupture or failure of an immature follicle to reabsorb fluid after ovulation. Corpus luteum cysts develop as a result of increased hormone production.
69. Polycystic ovarian syndrome (POS) is an endocrine disorder characterized by excess androgens and a long-term lack of ovulation. Etiology is unknown. Manifestations include amenorrhea or irregular menses, hirsutism, obesity, acne, hypertension, sleep apnea, infertility, and insulin resistance. Women with POS are at increased risk for development of early-onset type II diabetes, heart disease, breast cancer, and endometrial cancer.
70. Complications include infection, rupture, infertility, hemorrhage, and recurrence.
71. Interdisciplinary care focuses on identifying and correcting the disorder and preventing a recurrence.
72. Diagnostic tests include laparoscopy, ultrasound or x-ray, pregnancy testing, LH levels, testosterone levels, and FSH levels.
73. Antibiotics and oral contraceptives are often prescribed to treat these disorders.
74. Nursing care focuses on relieving pain, implementing measures to correct the disorder, and preventing recurrence and complications.

LEIOMYOMA

75. Leiomyomas are also known as fibroid tumors. These benign tumors originate from the smooth muscle of the uterus. They are the most common form of pelvic tumor.

76. There is a strong association between fibroid growth and estrogen stimulation.

77. Intramural fibroids are the most common type and occur embedded in the myometrium.

78. Subserous fibroid tumors lie beneath the serous lining of the uterus and project into the peritoneal cavity.

79. Submucosal fibroid tumors lie beneath the endometrial lining of the uterus.

80. Fibroid tumors may be asymptomatic or can lead to pelvic pressure, pain, dysmenorrhea, menorrhagia, and fatigue. Constipation and urinary urgency and frequency may occur.

81. Treatment depends upon size and location of the tumors, severity of manifestations, client age, and childbearing status.

82. Tests used to diagnose uterine fibroids may include an ultrasound and a laparoscopy.

83. Leuprolide acetate (Lupron) is used to decrease the size of the tumor if surgery is contraindicated. Gonadotropin-releasing hormones agonists are also administered.

ENDOMETRIOSIS

84. Endometriosis is a condition in which multiple, small, usually benign implantations of endometrial tissue develop.

85. These implantations most commonly occur in the pelvic cavity, but may also be found in other areas of the body, such as in the lungs.

86. It is most common in women who postpone childbearing.

87. Risk factors include early menarche, regular periods with a cycle less than 27 days, menses that last more than 7 days, heavier flow, increased menstrual pain, and a history of the condition in first-degree female relatives.

88. The cause of endometriosis is unclear, but theories include the metaplasia theory, the retrograde menstruation theory, and the transplantation theory.

89. The abnormally-located endometrial tissue responds to cyclic ovarian hormone stimulation and bleeding occurs at the site of implantation, which results in scarring, inflammation, and adhesions.

90. The progressive scarring may interfere with the woman's ability to conceive.

91. A history of dysmenorrhea, dyspareunia, and infertility strongly suggest endometriosis.

92. Diagnostic tests include pelvic ultrasound, laparoscopy, and CBC with differential.

93. Medications include analgesics such as NSAIDs and hormone therapy.

94. Surgical interventions include laparoscopy with laser ablation or total hysterectomy.
95. Nursing care involves providing pain relief, providing education, and helping the client cope with treatment outcomes.
96. The most common nursing diagnosis is anxiety.

BREAST DISORDERS

97. Benign breast disorders occur frequently in response to hormonal, nutritional, physical, and environmental stimuli.
98. Benign breast disorders include fibrocystic breast changes, fibroadenomas, intraductal papilloma, duct ectasia, fat necrosis, and mastitis.
99. Fibrocystic changes or fibrocystic breast disease is the physiologic nodularity and breast tenderness that increases and decreases with the menstrual cycle.
100. Manifestations are bilateral or unilateral pain or tenderness in the upper, outer quadrants. Nipple discharge may occur. Multiple, mobile cysts may form.
101. Intraductal papilloma is a tiny, wart-like growth on the inside of the peripheral mammary duct that causes discharge from the nipple. Discharge may be clear and sticky or bloody. The condition is most common in women in their 30s and 40s.
102. Mammary duct ectasia is a palpable lumpiness found beneath the areola. It involves periductal inflammation, dilation of the ductal system, and accumulation of fluid and dead cells that block the involved ducts. Manifestations include sticky, thick discharge with burning and itching around the nipple, with inflammation. Nipple retraction may occur.

SUGGESTIONS FOR CLASSROOM ACTIVITIES

- Divide the students into small groups and assign each group one of the disorders presented in this chapter. Have each group develop a short discussion of the disorder, including pathophysiology, manifestations, and treatments. Have students present the material learned in a sharing session.

SUGGESTIONS FOR CLINICAL ACTIVITIES

- Assign students to care for a client who has one of the disorders presented in this chapter. Have students develop a plan of care for the client. Share the material in post-conference.

LEARNING OUTCOME 2

Describe the physiologic process of menopause.

CONCEPTS FOR LECTURE

1. Menopause is the permanent cessation of menses.
2. The climacteric, or perimenopausal, period denotes the time during which reproductive function gradually ceases. This period may last for several years.
3. In the United States, most women stop menstruating between 48 and 55 years of age.
4. Earlier menopause is associated with genetics, smoking, higher altitude, and obesity.

POWERPOINT LECTURE SLIDES

Menopause
- Permanent cessation of menses
  - Climacteric, or perimenopausal, period
  - Surgical menopause
  - Chemical menopause
  - Natural menopause

5. After menopause the risk for heart disease, osteoporosis, macular degeneration, cognitive changes, and breast cancer increases.
6. Surgical menopause occurs when the ovaries are removed in premenopausal women, which drastically reduces the production of estrogen and progesterone.
7. Chemical menopause often occurs during cancer chemotherapy, when cytotoxic drugs arrest ovarian function.
8. As ovarian function decreases, production of estradiol decreases. This hormone is ultimately replaced by estrone as the major ovarian estrogen. Estrone is produced in small amounts and has only about one-tenth of the biologic activity of estradiol. Progesterone is also markedly reduced.

SUGGESTIONS FOR CLASSROOM ACTIVITIES

- Using anatomic models, describe the physiologic process of menopause. Identify the physiologic basis for common manifestations.

LEARNING OUTCOME 3

Compare and contrast the incidence, risk factors, pathophysiology, manifestations, diagnosis, treatment and nursing care for cancer of the cervix, endometrium, ovary, vulva, and breast.

CONCEPTS FOR LECTURE
CERVICAL CANCER

1. Cancer of the cervix is the second most common cancer in women worldwide and the 16th most common cancer in women in the United States.
2. Risk factors for development of cervical cancer include infection of the external genitalia and anus with HPV, first intercourse before 16 years of age, multiple sex partners or male partners with multiple sex partners, history of sexually transmitted diseases, infection with HIV, smoking, poor nutritional status, family history of cervical cancer, and exposure to DES in utero.
3. Most cervical cancers are squamous cell cancers that begin as precancerous dysplasia or cervical intraepithelial neoplasia. Systems of grading of dysplastic changes in the cervix use the term cervical intraepithelial neoplasia or the Bethesda system. Carcinoma in situ is localized; invasive cancer spreads to deeper layers.
4. Squamous cell cancers spread by direct invasion of accessory structures, including the vaginal wall, pelvic wall, bladder, and rectum. Metastasis is most frequently confined to the pelvic area, but distant metastasis may occur through the lymphatic system.
5. Preinvasive cancer is limited to the cervix and rarely causes manifestations.
6. Invasive cancer causes vaginal bleeding after intercourse or between menstrual periods and a vaginal discharge that increases as the cancer progresses.

POWERPOINT LECTURE SLIDES

Cervical Cancer
- Second most common cancer in women worldwide
- The 16th most common cancer in women in the United States
- Risk factors
  ○ Infection of the external genitalia and anus with HPV
  ○ First intercourse before 16 years of age
  ○ Multiple sex partners
  ○ Male partners with multiple sex partners
  ○ History of sexually transmitted diseases
  ○ Infection with HIV
  ○ Smoking
  ○ Poor nutritional status
  ○ Family history of cervical cancer
  ○ Exposure to DES in utero
- Pathophysiology
  ○ Squamous cell cancers
- Diagnostic tests
  ○ Pap smear
  ○ Colposcopy
  ○ Cervical biopsy
  ○ MRI
  ○ CT
- Chemotherapy
- Radiation therapy
- Nursing diagnoses

7. Manifestations of advanced disease include referred pain in the back or thighs, hematuria, bloody stools, anemia, and weight loss.
8. The goals of interdisciplinary care are to eradicate the cancer and minimize complications and metastasis.
9. Diagnostic tests used to diagnose cervical cancer include a Pap smear and colposcopy and cervical biopsy. MRI or CT may be used to evaluate the spread of the tumor.
10. Chemotherapy is used for tumors not responsive to other therapy, tumors that cannot be removed, or as adjunct therapy if metastasis has occurred.
11. Radiation therapy is used to treat invasive cervical cancer.
12. Nursing diagnoses include *Fear* and *Impaired Tissue Integrity*.

ENDOMETRIAL CANCER

13. Endometrial cancer is the most frequently diagnosed pelvic cancer in the United States. Most endometrial cancer is diagnosed in postmenopausal women. When diagnosed and treated early in the disease, the 5-year survival rates are about 90%.
14. Risk factors for the development of endometrial cancer are prolonged estrogen stimulation, obesity, anovulatory menstrual cycles, decreasing ovarian function, estrogen-secreting tumors, and unopposed estrogen therapy. Medical conditions that increase the risk of endometrial cancer are diabetes mellitus, hypertension, and polycystic ovary disease. Tamoxifen therapy also increases risk. Family history of hereditary non-polyposis colon cancer increases risk.
15. Most endometrial malignancies are adenocarcinomas that are slow to grow and metastasize. These malignancies develop in the glandular cells or endometrial lining of the uterus. Tumor growth generally begins in the fundus, invades the myometrium, and spreads throughout the reproductive tract. Metastasis occurs by means of lymphatic spread, through the fallopian tubes to the peritoneal cavity, and to the rest of the body via the blood stream.
16. Manifestations include abnormal, painless vaginal bleeding, pelvic cramping, bleeding after intercourse, lower abdominal pressure, lymph node enlargement, pleural effusion, abdominal masses, and ascites.
17. Interdisciplinary care focuses on eradication of the cancer and minimization of complications and metastasis.
18. Tests to diagnose endometrial cancer include vaginal or transvaginal ultrasound, endometrial biopsy, and D&C.
19. Chemotherapy is less effective than with other forms of cancer. Progesterone therapy may be used for recurrent disease.
20. Treatment with internal or external radiation may be performed.
21. Nursing diagnoses include: *Acute Pain; Disturbed Body Image;* and *Ineffective Sexuality Pattern*.

- ○ *Fear*
- ○ *Impaired Tissue Integrity*

Endometrial Cancer
- Most frequently diagnosed pelvic cancer in United States
- Most endometrial cancer diagnosed postmenopausal
- Risk factors
  - ○ Prolonged estrogen stimulation
  - ○ Obesity
  - ○ Anovulatory menstrual cycles
  - ○ Decreasing ovarian function
  - ○ Estrogen-secreting tumors
  - ○ Unopposed estrogen therapy
  - ○ Some medical conditions
  - ○ Tamoxifen
  - ○ Family history of hereditary nonpolyposis
- Pathophysiology
  - ○ Most are adenocarcinomas
  - ○ Develop in the glandular cells or endometrial lining
  - ○ Metastasis
- Manifestations
  - ○ Abnormal, painless vaginal bleeding
  - ○ Pelvic cramping
  - ○ Bleeding after intercourse
  - ○ Lower abdominal pressure
  - ○ Lymph node enlargement
  - ○ Pleural effusion
  - ○ Abdominal masses
  - ○ Ascites
- Diagnostic testing
  - ○ Vaginal or transvaginal ultrasound
  - ○ Endometrial biopsy
  - ○ D&C
- Chemotherapy
  - ○ Less effective
- Progesterone therapy
- Internal or external radiation
- Nursing diagnoses
  - ○ *Acute Pain*
  - ○ *Disturbed Body Image*
  - ○ *Ineffective Sexuality Pattern*

Ovarian Cancer
- Fourth most common gynecologic cancer in United States
- Risk factors
  - ○ Family history of ovarian cancer
  - ○ Having no children or giving birth after age 35
  - ○ Exposure to talc or asbestos
  - ○ Endometriosis
  - ○ Pelvic inflammatory disease
  - ○ Living in a western civilized country
- Pathophysiology
  - ○ Most are epithelial tumors
  - ○ Spreads by local shedding of cancer cells

OVARIAN CANCER

22. Ovarian cancer is the fourth most common gynecologic cancer in the United States.
23. Risk factors include family history of ovarian cancer, having no children or giving birth after age 35, exposure to talc or asbestos, endometriosis, pelvic inflammatory disease, and living in a western civilized country.
24. Protective factors include long-term contraceptive use, having a child before age 25, tubal ligation, breastfeeding, and hysterectomy.
25. Most ovarian cancers are epithelial tumors, and originate from the surface of the epithelium of the ovary.
26. Ovarian cancer usually spreads by local shedding of cancer cells into the peritoneal cavity and by direct invasion of the bowel and bladder. Tumor cells also spread through the lymph and blood. Staging for ovarian cancer is based on surgical and histologic evaluation.
27. Manifestations of ovarian cancer include indigestion, urinary frequency, abdominal bloating, and constipation. Pelvic pain sometimes occurs.
28. Interdisciplinary care of ovarian cancer focuses on removal of as much tumor as possible.
29. Tests used to diagnose ovarian cancer include transvaginal or abdominal ultrasounds and CT scans. The CA-125 antigen level blood test is also useful.
30. Combination chemotherapy regimens using cyclophosphamide and cisplatin or other agents may be employed.
31. Nursing care for women with ovarian cancer is similar to the nursing care for women with other gynecologic surgeries.

CANCER OF THE VULVA

32. Cancer of the vulva occurs most often in women over 50 years of age.
33. The cause of this cancer is unknown, but there is evidence to associate it with sexually transmitted diseases, particularly HPV. Herpes simplex type 2 infection has also been associated with vulvar cancer. Other risk factors include advanced age, diabetes, and a history of leukoplakia.
34. Most vulvar cancers are epidermoid or squamous cell. The primary site is usually the labia majora. Metastasis occurs by direct extension into the vagina, perineal skin, anus, and urethra. The cancer also spreads through the lymphatic system.
35. Manifestations include exophytic lesions (proliferating outward), endophytic lesions (proliferating inwardly), ulcerative lesions, or verrucous lesions (resembling a wart). Pruritus, perineal pain and bleeding, and dysuria may occur.
36. Interdisciplinary care focuses on eradicating the lesion and reducing risk of recurrence.
37. Diagnosis is based on results of an excisional biopsy of the lesions.
38. Surgery is the most common treatment.

- ○ Spreads by direct invasion
- ○ Can also spread through lymph and blood
- Manifestations
  - ○ Indigestion
  - ○ Urinary frequency
  - ○ Abdominal bloating
  - ○ Constipation
  - ○ Pelvic pain
- Tests
  - ○ Transvaginal or abdominal ultrasounds
  - ○ CT scans
  - ○ CA-125 antigen level
- Treatment
  - ○ Combination chemotherapy
- Nursing care
  - ○ Similar to that for gynecologic surgeries

Cancer of the Vulva
- Occurs most often after age 50
- Pathophysiology
  - ○ Epidermoid or squamous cell
  - ○ Primary site usually labia majora
  - ○ Metastasis direct extension
  - ○ Also spreads through lymphatic system
- Manifestations
  - ○ Exophytic lesions
  - ○ Endophytic lesions
  - ○ Ulcerative lesions
  - ○ Verrucous lesions
  - ○ Pruritus
  - ○ Perineal pain and bleeding
  - ○ Dysuria
- Diagnosis
  - ○ Excisional biopsy of lesions
- Surgery
- Nursing diagnoses
  - ○ *Impaired Tissue Integrity*

Breast Cancer
- Unregulated growth of abnormal cells
- Most commonly occurring cancer in women
- Risk factors
  - ○ Age and gender
  - ○ Genetic risk factors
  - ○ Family history of breast cancer
  - ○ Personal history of breast cancer
  - ○ Previous breast biopsy
  - ○ Previous breast irradiation
  - ○ Menstruation before 12/menopause after 50
- Lifestyle related factors
  - ○ Using oral contraceptives
  - ○ Not having children
  - ○ Having children only after 30
  - ○ Using HRT for over 5 years
  - ○ Not breast feeding
  - ○ Drinking alcohol
  - ○ Obesity
  - ○ High-fat diets

39. Nursing care is similar to that of women with endometrial cancer. Nursing diagnoses include *Impaired Tissue Integrity*.

BREAST CANCER

40. Breast cancer is the unregulated growth of abnormal cells in breast tissue.
41. It is the most commonly-occurring cancer in women.
42. Risk factors for the development of breast cancer include: (1) age and gender; (2) genetic risk factors; (3) family history of breast cancer; (4) personal history of breast cancer; (5) previous breast biopsy; (6) previous breast irradiation; and (7) menstruation before age 12 or menopause after age 50.
43. Lifestyle-related factors include using oral contraceptives, not having children or having them after age 30, using HRT for over 5 years, not breastfeeding, drinking alcohol, obesity, high-fat diets, physical inactivity, and environmental pollution.
44. Two breast cancer susceptibility genes have been identified: BRCA1 on chromosome 17 and BRAC2 on chromosome 13.
45. Cancers of the breast are classified as noninvasive (in situ) or invasive.
46. Breast cancer may also be classified as carcinoma of the mammary ducts, carcinoma of mammary lobules, or sarcoma of the breast. The most common type is infiltrating ductal carcinoma.
47. Breast cancer can metastasize to other sites through the blood stream or lymphatic system. Common sites of metastasis are bone, brain, lung, liver, skin, and lymph nodes.
48. Manifestations include a nontender lump in the breast, abnormal nipple discharge, a rash around the nipple area, nipple retraction, dimpling of the skin, or a change in position of the nipple. Breast cancer is usually painless.
49. Diagnosis of breast cancer begins with detection. Treatment depends upon stage of the cancer, the age of the woman, and the woman's preferences.
50. Tests include mammography, percutaneous needle biopsy, and breast biopsy.
51. Tamoxifen citrate (Nolvadex) is an oral medication that interferes with estrogen activity and is used to treat advanced breast cancer, as an adjuvant for early stage breast cancer, and as a preventive treatment for women at high risk for developing breast cancer.
52. Other pharmaceutical treatments for breast cancer include immunotherapy and chemotherapy. Chemotherapy is often accompanied by other drugs such as Avastin and Femara.
53. Radiation therapy is typically used following breast cancer surgery to destroy any remaining cancer cells that could cause a recurrence or metastasis.
54. A new radiation treatment is intraoperative radiotherapy.
55. Nursing diagnoses include: *Anxiety; Decisional Conflict; Anticipatory Grieving; Risk for Infection; Risk for Injury;* and *Disturbed Body Image*.

- ○ Physical inactivity
- ○ Environmental pollution
- Breast cancer genes
- Manifestations
  - ○ Nontender lump in the breast
  - ○ Abnormal nipple discharge
  - ○ Rash around the nipple area
  - ○ Nipple retraction
  - ○ Dimpling of the skin
  - ○ Change in position of nipple
  - ○ Usually painless
- Diagnosis
  - ○ Begins with detection
- Medications
  - ○ Tamoxifen citrate
  - ○ Immunotherapy
  - ○ Chemotherapy
- Radiation therapy
- Nursing diagnoses
  - ○ *Anxiety*
  - ○ *Decisional Conflict*
  - ○ *Anticipatory Grieving*
  - ○ *Risk for Infection*
  - ○ *Risk for Injury*
  - ○ *Disturbed Body Image*

LEARNING OUTCOME 4

Discuss the purposes, nursing implications, and health education for clients and their families for cancer screening, medications, and treatments for women with disorders of the reproductive system and breast.

CONCEPTS FOR LECTURE

1. The American Cancer Society recommends a cancer-related checkup every year after the age of 40. This checkup includes examination for cancers of the thyroid, ovaries, lymph nodes, oral cavity, and skin. It includes screening for cervical, breast, and colorectal cancer.
2. Nursing diagnoses include: *Deficient Knowledge; Ineffective Sexuality Pattern; Situational Low Self-Esteem;* and *Disturbed Body Image.*

CERVICAL CANCER

3. The American Cancer Society recommends that women should begin annual screening for cervical cancer with the Pap test about 3 years after beginning to have vaginal intercourse. These screenings should begin no later than age 21.
4. At or after age 30, after three consecutive normal Pap tests, screening can be performed every 2–3 years.
5. Women 70 years of age or older who have had three or more normal Pap smears in the last 10 years may choose to stop cervical cancer screening.

ENDOMETRIAL CANCER

6. All perimenopausal and postmenopausal women need annual pelvic examinations. Women should be taught to report any unexpected bleeding or spotting.

BREAST DISORDERS

7. Mammography can detect breast tumors 2 years before they are palpable.
8. The American Cancer Society recommends annual mammograms beginning at age 40 and clinical breast exams every 3 years for women in their 20s and 30s.

MEDICATIONS

9. Hormone replacement therapy (HRT) is controversial, but may be prescribed to alleviate severe manifestations of menopause. HRT should be used for a limited time only and only after the woman has been educated about known risks.
10. HRT may include estrogen alone or a combination of estrogen and progestin.

POWERPOINT LECTURE SLIDES

- Cancer-related checkup
  - Every year after the age of 40
    - Thyroid
    - Ovaries
    - Lymph nodes
    - Oral cavity
    - Skin
  - Screening
    - Cervical
    - Breast
    - Colorectal
- Nursing diagnoses
  - *Deficient Knowledge*
  - *Ineffective Sexuality Pattern*
  - *Situational Low Self-Esteem*
  - *Disturbed Body Image*

Cervical Cancer
- Annual screening for cervical cancer
  - Pap test about 3 years after beginning intercourse
  - No later that age 21
- After three consecutive normal Pap tests
  - Every 2–3 years
- 70 years of age or older
  - 3 or more normal Pap smears in 10 years
    - May choose to stop cervical cancer screening

Endometrial Cancer
- Annual pelvic examinations
  - Report any unexpected bleeding or spotting

Breast Disorders
- Annual mammograms beginning at age 40
- Clinical breast exams every 3 years
  - 20s and 30s

Medications
- Hormone replacement therapy (HRT)
- Selective estrogen receptor modulators (SERMs)
- Tamoxifen and toremifene

11. Long-term HRT increases the risk for breast cancer, ovarian cancer, asthma, urinary incontinence, and venous thrombosis.
12. Selective estrogen receptor modulators (SERMs) bind to estrogen receptors and exert site-specific effects.
13. Tamoxifen and toremifene have a beneficial effect on bone mineral density and serum lipids and decrease risk of invasive breast cancer in women at high risk.

SUGGESTIONS FOR CLASSROOM ACTIVITIES

• Have students develop a chart that outlines the cancer screening recommended by the American Cancer Society.

SUGGESTIONS FOR CLINICAL ACTIVITIES

• Have students develop and implement a teaching plan regarding cancer screening for clinical clients.
• Have students identify the nursing implications of administering chemotherapeutic medications.

LEARNING OUTCOME 5

Discuss alternative and complementary therapies used by women to relieve manifestations associated with menopause and menstrual disorders.

CONCEPTS FOR LECTURE

1. Alternative and complementary therapies include acupuncture, biofeedback, massage, herbals, vitamin supplements, meditation, and yoga.
2. Herbs thought to be useful in the treatment of menopausal symptoms include: black cohosh, vitex, agnue castii, ginseng, Chinese tonic of He Shou Wu, cong quai, golden seal, flaxseed, and evening primrose.
3. Supplements used in the treatment of menopausal symptoms include: vitamin E and soy protein.

POWERPOINT LECTURE SLIDES

Menopause Therapy
  • Alternative and complementary therapies
    ○ Acupuncture
    ○ Biofeedback
    ○ Massage
    ○ Herbals
    ○ Vitamin supplements
    ○ Meditation
    ○ Yoga

SUGGESTIONS FOR CLASSROOM ACTIVITIES

• Have students research the internet for websites associated with alternative and complementary therapies for menopausal and menstrual disorders. Discuss the validity of the sites. Discuss the nursing implications of this information.

SUGGESTIONS FOR CLINICAL ACTIVITIES

• Discuss assessment techniques and communication strategies to encourage client disclosure of use of alternative and complementary therapies.

LEARNING OUTCOME 6

Describe the surgical procedures used to treat female reproductive system and breast disorders.

CONCEPTS FOR LECTURE
THERAPEUTIC D&C

1. The cervical canal is dilated and the uterine wall is scraped. This procedure is used to diagnose and treat DUB and other disorders.
2. D&C is contraindicated in women who have been taking anticoagulant drugs.

POWERPOINT LECTURE SLIDES

Hysterectomy
  • Removal of uterus
  • Premenopausal women
    ○ Ovaries are generally left in place
  • Postmenopausal women
    ○ Complete hysterectomy
  • Abdominal hysterectomy
    ○ Preexisting abdominal scar is present
    ○ Adhesions are thought to be present

ENDOMETRIAL ABLATION

3. The endometrial layer of the uterus is permanently destroyed using laser surgery or electrosurgical resection.
4. This procedure is performed in women who do not respond to pharmacological management or D&C and ends both menstruation and reproduction.

HYSTERECTOMY

5. The removal of the uterus may be performed when medical management of bleeding disorders is unsuccessful or malignancy is present.
6. In premenopausal women, the ovaries are generally left in place; in postmenopausal women, a complete hysterectomy is usually performed.
7. Abdominal hysterectomy is performed when a preexisting abdominal scar is present, when adhesions are thought to be present, or when a large operating field is necessary. The surgical incision may be either longitudinal or a Pfannenstiel (bikini cut).
8. Vaginal hysterectomy is removal of the uterus through the vagina. This approach is desirable when the uterus has descended into the vagina or if the urinary bladder or rectum have prolapsed into the vagina. There is no visible abdominal scar.

COLPORRHAPHY

9. Colporrhaphy is repair of a cystocele.
10. The pelvic muscles are shortened, which provides tighter support for the bladder.

MARSHAL-MARCHETTI-KRANTZ PROCEDURE

11. This procedure involves resuspension of the urinary bladder.

SURGICAL PROCEDURES FOR POLYPS AND CYSTS

12. Surgical procedures for these disorders include polyp removal through a vaginal speculum or transcervically. Incision and drainage of surface cysts is common. Uterine cysts may be punctured through laser surgery or a wedge resection of the ovary may be necessary. Rarely, oophorectomy is performed.

FIBROID TUMORS

13. Myomectomy is removal of the tumor without removing the entire uterus. This procedure may be performed by laparoscopic laser.
14. Hysterectomy is performed if tumors are large, and if bleeding or other problems continue in postmenopausal women.
15. Uterine fibroid embolization is a procedure in which a catheter is guided through the femoral artery to the uterus and the artery that supplies the fibroid is embolized with tiny particles.

- ○ Large operating field is necessary
- ○ Surgical incision
  - – Longitudinal
  - – Pfannenstiel (bikini cut)
- Vaginal hysterectomy
- ○ Uterus has descended into the vagina
- ○ Urinary bladder or rectum prolapsed into vagina
- ○ No visible abdominal scar

Surgical Procedures for Polyps and Cysts
- Removal
- ○ Through vaginal speculum
- ○ Transcervically
- Surface cysts
- ○ Incision and drainage
- Uterine cysts
- ○ Laser surgery
- ○ Wedge resection
- ○ Oophorectomy

Cancer of the Cervix
- Loop diathermy
- Laser surgery with colposcopy
- Cryosurgery
- Conization
- Hysterectomy or radical hysterectomy
- Pelvic exenteration
  - ○ Anterior exenteration
  - ○ Posterior exenteration

Breast Cancer
- Mastectomy
  - ○ Radical mastectomy
  - ○ Simple mastectomy
  - ○ Segmental mastectomy
  - ○ Lumpectomy
  - ○ Modified radical mastectomy
- Axillary node dissection
- Sentinel node biopsy
- Breast reconstruction
  - ○ Placement of a submuscular implant
  - ○ Use of a tissue expander followed by an implant
  - ○ Transposition of muscle and blood supply from the abdomen and back
  - ○ Tranverse rectus abdominis myocutaneous (TRAM) free tissue flap

CANCER OF THE CERVIX

16. Loop diathermy is a technique in which a wire is used to both cut and coagulate during excision of the dysplastic region of the cervix.
17. Laser surgery is used along with colposcopy provided that the cancer is limited to the cervical epithelium. Cryosurgery may also be used for noninvasive lesions.
18. Conization is performed to treat microinvasive carcinoma when colposcopy cannot define the limits of invasion.
19. Hysterectomy or radical hysterectomy is performed for invasive lesion.
20. Pelvic exenteration, which is the removal of all pelvic contents, is done if cancer recurs without involvement of the lymph system.
21. An anterior exenteration is removal of the uterus, ovaries, fallopian tubes, vagina, bladder, urethra, and lymphatic vessels and nodes. An ileal conduit is created for excretion of urine.
22. A posterior exenteration is removal of the uterus, ovaries, uterine tubes, bowel, and rectum. A colostomy is created for excretion of feces.

ENDOMETRIAL CANCER

23. Total abdominal hysterectomy and bilateral salpingo-oophorectomy is performed.

OVARIAN CANCER

24. Treatment may be limited to removal of one ovary, but total hysterectomy with bilateral salpingo-oophorectomy and removal of the omentum is usually performed.

CANCER OF THE VULVA

25. Early, noninvasive lesions may be treated with laser surgery, cryosurgery, or electrocautery.
26. Simple vulvectomy involves removal of the vulva, labia majora and minora, clitoris, and prepuce.
27. Radical vulvectomy involves removal of all the tissue in a simple vulvectomy and the subcutaneous tissue and regional lymph node.

BREAST CANCER

28. Mastectomy is the surgical procedure done to treat breast cancer. Types of mastectomy include: radical mastectomy, simple mastectomy, segmental mastectomy or lumpectomy, and modified radical mastectomy. Axillary node dissection is generally performed during surgery for all invasive breast cancers.
29. Nonsurgical methods of detecting lymph node involvement include sentinel node biopsy.
30. Lumpectomy is defined as excision of the primary tumor and adjacent breast tissue followed by radiation therapy.

31. Breast reconstruction may be performed at the time of the mastectomy or at any time thereafter. Procedures include placement of a submuscular implant, the use of a tissue expander followed by an implant, transposition of muscle and blood supply from the abdomen and back, or a transverse rectus abdominis myocutaneous (TRAM) free tissue flap.

SUGGESTIONS FOR CLASSROOM ACTIVITIES

- Review the care plan activity about postoperative hysterectomy care that is provided on the textbook Companion Website. Use the information presented to discuss the plan of care for clients undergoing reproductive surgeries.

SUGGESTIONS FOR CLINICAL ACTIVITIES

- Assign students to care for clients who are undergoing reproductive surgeries. Have students investigate the psychosocial response to the surgery and develop a plan of care to help the client cope with their physical changes. Share the information learned in post-conference.

CHAPTER 52
NURSING CARE OF CLIENTS WITH SEXUALLY TRANSMITTED INFECTIONS

RESOURCE LIBRARY

⊙ PRENTICE HALL NURSING MEDIALINK DVD-ROM

Audio Glossary
NCLEX-RN® Review
Animation
   Gonorrhea

COMPANION WEBSITE

Audio Glossary
NCLEX-RN® Review
Care Plan Activity: Gonorrhea
Case Studies
   Pelvic Inflammatory Disease
   Syphilis
Teaching Plans
   Risk of Cancer with HPV
   Singles and Safer Sex
MediaLink Applications
   HPV
   HPV Prevention
Links to Resources

📖 IMAGE LIBRARY

Figure 52.1 Genital herpes blisters as they appear on the labia.
Figure 52.2 Genital warts (condyloma acuminatum) on the *A,* vulva and *B,* penis.

Figure 52.3 Yeast infection on female genitalia.
Figure 52.4 Chancre of primary syphilis on the penis.

LEARNING OUTCOME 1

Explain the incidence, prevalence, characteristics, and prevention/control of sexually transmitted infections (STIs).

CONCEPTS FOR LECTURE

1. Sexually transmitted infections are transmitted by vaginal, oral, and anal intimate contact and intercourse. STIs also include systemic diseases such as TB, hepatitis, and HIV/AIDS that can be transmitted from an infected person to a partner.
2. Sexually transmitted infections are caused by bacteria, chlamydiae, viruses, fungi, protozoa, and parasites.
3. STIs occur in more than half of all people at some point in their life and are the most frequent infections encountered by reproductive health professionals.
4. Women and infants are disproportionately affected by STIs.
5. Introduction of oral contraceptives as a primary source of birth control decreased the use of condoms. Oral contraceptives do not protect against STIs.
6. The incidence of STIs is highest in young adults ages 15 to 24.
7. An "epidemiologic synergy" exists among all STIs. Individuals who are infected with STIs are at a greater risk of acquiring HIV if they are exposed to the virus.

POWERPOINT LECTURE SLIDES

Sexually Transmitted Infections
- Transmission
  - Intimate contact
    - Vaginal
    - Oral
    - Anal
  - Intercourse
- Systemic disease
  - TB
  - Hepatitis
  - HIV/AIDS
- Etiology
  - Bacteria
  - Chlamydiae
  - Viruses
  - Fungi
  - Protozoa
  - Parasites

8. Characteristics of STIs include: (1) most can be prevented by the use of latex condoms; (2) they can be transmitted during both heterosexual and homosexual activities, including nonpenetrating intimate exposure; (3) for treatment to be effective, sexual partners of the infected persons must also be treated; (4) two or more STIs frequently coexist in the same client.

9. Complications of STIs include: pelvic inflammatory disease, ectopic pregnancy, infertility, chronic pelvic pain, neonatal illness and death, and genital cancer.

10. Prevention and control of STIs is based on the principles of education, detection, effective diagnosis, and treatment of infected persons; and evaluation, treatment, and counseling of sex partners of people who are infected.

11. The most effective way to prevent sexual transmission of HIV and other STIs is to avoid sexual intercourse with an infected partner.

12. Gonorrhea, syphilis, and AIDS are reportable diseases in every state, and chlamydial infections are reportable in most states.

- Prevalence
  - Occur in over 50% of people at some point
  - Women/infants disproportionately affected
  - Highest in ages 15–24
- Risk factors
  - Decreased use of condoms
- Epidemiologic synergy
- Characteristics
  - Most can be prevented by use of latex condoms
  - Heterosexual/homosexual activities
    - Includes nonpenetrating intimate exposure
  - Sexual partners must be treated
  - Two or more STIs frequently coexist
- Complications
  - Pelvic inflammatory disease
  - Ectopic pregnancy
  - Infertility
  - Chronic pelvic pain
  - Neonatal illness and death
  - Genital cancer
- Prevention and control
  - Education
  - Detection
  - Effective diagnosis
  - Treatment of infected persons
  - Evaluation, treatment, counseling of sex partners
- Reportable disorders
  - All states
    - Gonorrhea
    - Syphilis
    - AIDS
  - Most states
    - Chlamydial infections

SUGGESTIONS FOR CLASSROOM ACTIVITIES

- Divide students into small groups and assign one of the disorders presented in this chapter to each group. Have the groups research the prevalence of the disorder assigned on a global, national, state, and county level. Discuss particular prevention/control techniques being used locally. Discuss education to the public.

LEARNING OUTCOME 2

Compare and contrast the pathophysiology, manifestations, interdisciplinary care, and nursing care of genital herpes, genital warts, vaginitis, chlamydia, gonorrhea, syphilis, and pelvic inflammatory disease.

CONCEPTS FOR LECTURE
GENITAL HERPES

1. Genital herpes are caused by the herpes simplex viruses HSV-1 and HSV-2.

2. There is no cure for genital herpes and treatments are primarily symptomatic.

3. HSV-1 is associated with cold sores, but may be transmitted to the genital area by oral intercourse or by self-inoculation through poor hand washing practices.

POWERPOINT LECTURE SLIDES

Genital Herpes
- Herpes simplex viruses HSV-1 and HSV-2
- No cure
- HSV-1 associated with cold sores
- HSV-2 causes genital herpes
- Pathophysiology
  - Neurotropic viruses
  - Ascend peripheral nerves to dorsal root ganglia
  - Reactivation, return to nerve root of skin

4. HSV-2 is transmitted by sexual activity or during childbirth from an infected woman. HSV-2 is the virus that causes genital herpes.

5. HSV viruses are neurotropic viruses, and grow in neurons and maintain their disease potential even when there are no manifestations. The virus ascends through the peripheral nerves to the dorsal root ganglia, where it remains dormant. The virus is impervious to treatment while dormant. For unknown reasons, the virus may reactivate and return to the nerve root of the skin and cause lesions.

6. Initial manifestations include painful red papules in the genital area. These papules then form small, painful blisters filled with clear fluid that contains virus particles. The blisters break, which sheds the highly infectious virus and creates patches of painful ulcers.

7. Average duration of the first episode infection is 12 days.

8. Recurrent infections have an average length of 4–5 days. The period of time between episodes is called latency.

9. Prodromal symptoms of recurrent outbreaks include burning, itching, tingling, or throbbing at sites where lesions generally appear. Pain may also be present in the legs, groin, or buttocks.

10. Definitive diagnosis requires isolation of the virus in tissue culture.

11. Nursing diagnoses include: *Acute Pain; Sexual Dysfunction;* and *Anxiety.*

GENITAL WARTS

12. Genital warts (condylomata acuminata) are caused by the human papilloma virus (HSV). The incubation period is 6 weeks to 8 months.

13. HPV infection may be asymptomatic. When manifestations are present, they include: characteristic lesions that are single or multiple, painless, soft, moist, pink, or flesh-colored. The four types of genital warts are condyloma acuminata, keratotic warts, papular warts, and flat warts.

14. Treatment is directed at removal of the warts, relief of symptoms, and health teaching.

15. Treatments include medications, wart removal by cryotherapy, electrocautery, laser vaporization, or surgical excision. Carbon dioxide laser surgery may be used.

16. Nursing diagnoses include: *Deficient Knowledge* and *Fear.*

VAGINAL INFECTIONS

17. Bacterial vaginosis or nonspecific vaginitis is the most common cause of vaginal infection in women of reproductive age.

18. Primary manifestation is a thin, grayish-white discharge with a foul, fishy odor.

19. Candidiasis is a moniliasis or yeast infection caused by *Candida albicans*, a normal vaginal flora.

- Initial manifestations
  - Painful red papules in genital area
  - Small, painful blisters
  - Blisters rupture
  - Patches of painful ulcers
- Progression
  - First episode 12 days
  - Recurrent infections 4–5 days
  - Between episodes: latency
- Prodromal symptoms
  - Burning
  - Itching, tingling
  - Throbbing
  - Pain in legs, groin, buttocks
- Definitive diagnosis
  - Isolation of virus in tissue culture
- Nursing diagnoses
  - *Acute Pain*
  - *Sexual Dysfunction*
  - *Anxiety*

Genital Warts
- Condylomata acuminata
- Caused by human papilloma virus
- Manifestations
  - May be asymptomatic
  - Characteristic lesions
- Treatments
  - Medications
  - Wart removal
- Nursing diagnoses
  - *Deficient Knowledge*
  - *Fear*

Vaginal Infections
- Bacterial vaginosis or nonspecific vaginitis
  - Primary manifestation
    - Thin, grayish-white discharge
    - Foul, fishy odor
- Candidiasis
  - Moniliasis or yeast infection
  - *Candida albicans*
  - Manifestations
    - Odorless, thick, cheesy discharge
    - Itching/irritation of vulva
    - Vaginadysuria
    - Dyspareunia
- Trichomoniasis
  - *Trichomonas vaginalis*
  - Manifestations
    - Men
      - Asymptomatic
      - Dysuria
      - Urethral discomfort
    - Women
      - Frothy, green-yellow vaginal discharge
      - Strong fishy odor
      - Itching and irritation

20. Manifestations include an odorless, thick, cheesy vaginal discharge accompanied by itching and irritation of the vulva, vaginadysuria, and dyspareunia.
21. Trichomoniasis is caused by *Trichomonas vaginalis* which is a protozoan parasite.
22. Symptoms usually appear in 5–28 days of exposure and most commonly affect the vagina in women and the urethra in men.
23. Most men are asymptomatic, but may experience dysuria and urethral discomfort.
24. Women have a frothy, green-yellow vaginal discharge with a strong fishy odor, often accompanied by itching and irritation of the genitalia.
25. Diagnosis is made by cervical culture or examination of discharge.
26. Nursing diagnoses for women with vaginal infections include: *Deficient Knowledge* and *Acute Pain.*

CHLAMYDIA

27. Chlamydia is a group of sexually-transmitted infections caused by *Chlamydia trachomatis.*
28. Infections caused by chlamydia include acute urethral syndrome, nongonococcal urethritis, mucopurulent cervicitis, and pelvic inflammatory disease.
29. The organism that causes chlamydia resembles both a virus and a bacteria. It enters the body as an elementary body, enters the cells, and changes into a reticulate body. This reticulate body divides within the cell, then bursts the cell and infects adjoining cells.
30. Incubation is from 1–3 weeks, but the organism may be present for months or years without producing symptoms in women. Manifestations are dysuria, frequency, and discharge.
31. Diagnostic testing includes gram stain of discharge, direct fluorescent antibody tests, enzyme-linked immunosorbent assays, ligase tests, or nucleic acid amplification tests.
32. Nursing care includes eradication of the infection, prevention of future infections, and management of any chronic complications.

GONORRHEA

33. Gonorrhea is caused by *Neisseria gonorrhoeae* and is the most common reportable communicable disease in the United States.
34. Portal of entry can be the genitourinary tract, eyes, oropharynx, anorectum, or skin. Without treatment the disease rapidly disseminates to other organs.
35. In men, manifestations are a serous, milky, or purulent discharge from the penis. Regional lymphadenopathy may occur.
36. Many women remain asymptomatic. In symptomatic women, manifestations are dysuria, urinary frequency, abnormal menses, increased vaginal discharge, and dyspareunia.

- Diagnosis
  - Cervical culture
  - Examination of discharge
- Nursing diagnoses
  - *Deficient Knowledge*
  - *Acute Pain*

Chlamydia
- Caused by *Chlamydia trachomatis*
- Pathophysiology
  - Organism resembles both virus and bacteria
  - Enters body as an elementary body
  - Changes to reticulate body
  - Reticulate body divides in cell
- Manifestations
  - May be asymptomatic for years
  - Dysuria, frequency, and discharge
- Diagnostic testing
  - Gram stain of discharge
  - Direct fluorescent antibody tests
  - Enzyme-linked immunosorbent assays
  - Ligase tests
  - Nucleic acid amplification tests
- Nursing care
  - Eradication of infection
  - Prevention of future infections
  - Management of chronic complications

Gonorrhea
- *Neisseria gonorrhoeae*
- Portal of entry
  - Genitourinary tract
  - Eyes
  - Ooropharynx
  - Anorectum
  - Skin
  - Rapidly dissemination to other organs
- Manifestations
  - Male
    - Serous, milky, or purulent discharge
    - Regional lymphadenopathy
  - Women
    - May remain asymptomatic
    - Dysuria, urinary frequency
    - Abnormal menses
    - Increased vaginal discharge
    - Dysparenuia
- Anorectal gonorrhea
  - Most often seen in homosexual men
  - Manifestations
    - Pruritus
    - Mucopurulent rectal discharge
    - Rectal bleeding and pain
    - Constipation
- Gonococcal pharyngitis
  - Oral sexual contact with infected partner
  - Manifestations
    - Fever

37. Anorectal gonorrhea is most often seen in homosexual men. Manifestations include pruritus, mucopurulent rectal discharge, rectal bleeding and pain, and constipation.

38. Gonococcal pharyngitis occurs primary after oral sexual contact with an infected partner. Manifestations are fever, sore throat, and enlarged lymph glands.

39. Diagnosis is based on cultures from infected mucous membranes, examination of urine, and gram stain. Testing for concurrent STIs is recommended.

40. Nursing diagnoses include: *Noncompliance* and *Impaired Social Interaction*.

SYPHILIS

41. Syphilis is a complex systemic STI caused by *Treponema pallidum* and is transmitted from open lesions during any sexual contact. The organism can survive for days in fluids. Incubation is 10–90 days.

42. The infective agent can enter the body through any break in the skin or mucous membrane. Once in the body, the infection is spread through the blood and lymph. Congenital syphilis is transferred to the fetus through the placental circulation.

43. Three clinical stage of syphilis are primary, secondary, and tertiary. A latency period when no signs of disease are evident may occur.

44. Primary stage is characterized by the appearance of a chancre and by regional enlargement of lymph nodes.

45. Manifestations of secondary syphilis may appear 2 weeks to 6 months after the initial chancre disappears. Manifestations include a skin rash; sore throat; generalized lymphadenopathy; condyloma lata on the labia, anus, or corner of the mouth; flulike symptoms; and alopecia. These manifestations generally disappear in 2–6 weeks.

46. The disease may become latent for up to 50 years. It cannot be transmitted sexually, but can be transmitted by blood.

47. Benign late syphilis is characterized by localized development of infiltrating tumors in the skin, bones, and liver that generally responds promptly to treatment.

48. Diffuse inflammatory syphilis involves the central nervous system and cardiovascular system. Much of the damage is irreversible.

49. Diagnosis is complex and includes a careful history and physical and laboratory evaluation of lesions and blood. Laboratory tests include VDRL, RPR, FTA-ABS, immunofluorescent staining of early lesions or lymph node aspiration, and darkfield microscopy of a specimen from a chancre.

50. Nursing diagnoses include: *Risk for Injury; Anxiety;* and *Low Self-Esteem*.

PELVIC INFLAMMATORY DISEASE

51. Pelvic inflammatory disease (PID) is a term used to describe infections of the pelvic organs.

- – Sore throat
- – Enlarged lymph glands
- ○ Diagnosis
  - – Cultures from infected mucous membranes
  - – Examination of urine
  - – Gram stain
  - – Testing for concurrent STIs recommended
- • Nursing diagnoses
  - ○ *Noncompliance*
  - ○ *Impaired Social Interaction*

Syphilis
- • *Treponema pallidum*
- • Pathophysiology
  - ○ Enters body through break in skin/mucous membrane
  - ○ Spreads through blood and lymph
  - ○ Congenital syphilis transfers through placental circulation
- • Primary stage
  - ○ Chancre
  - ○ Regional lymph node enlargement
- • Secondary stage
  - ○ Skin rash
  - ○ Sore throat
  - ○ Generalized lymphadenopathy
  - ○ Condyloma lata
  - ○ Flulike symptoms
  - ○ Alopecia
- • Latency
  - ○ Up to 50 years
  - ○ Cannot be transmitted sexually
  - ○ Can be transmitted by blood
- • Benign late syphilis
  - ○ Localized development of infiltrating tumors
- • Diffuse inflammatory syphilis
  - ○ Involves CNS and CV system
- • Diagnosis
  - ○ Careful history and physical
  - ○ VDRL
  - ○ RPR
  - ○ FTA-ABS
  - ○ Immunofluorescent staining
  - ○ Darkfield microscopy
- • Nursing diagnoses
  - ○ *Risk for Injury*
  - ○ *Anxiety*
  - ○ *Low Self-Esteem*

Pelvic Inflammatory Disease
- • Infections of the pelvic organs
- • Types of PID
  - ○ Salpingitis (fallopian tube infection)
  - ○ Oophoritis (ovarian infection)
  - ○ Cervicitis (cervical infection)
  - ○ Endometritis (endometrial infection)
  - ○ Infections of pelvic peritoneum
  - ○ Infections of pelvic vascular system

52. Types of PID are salpingitis (fallopian tube infection), oophoritis (ovarian infection), cervicitis (cervical infection), endometritis (endometrial infection), and infections of the pelvic peritoneum and the pelvic vascular system.
53. PID is caused by one of a number of infectious agents and may represent dual infection.
54. PID results from the entry of pathogenic microorganisms into the vagina. These microbes then move into the uterus and ascend from the endocervical canal to the fallopian tubes and ovaries.
55. Manifestations of PID include fever, purulent vaginal discharge, severe lower abdominal pain, and pain on cervical movement. PID may be only mildly symptomatic.
56. Tests to diagnose PID include CBC with differential, laparoscopy, or laparotomy.
57. Surgery for PID may include drainage of abscess, removal of adhesions, or surgical removal of uterus, fallopian tubes, and ovaries.
58. Nursing diagnoses include: *Risk for Injury* and *Deficient Knowledge.*

- Etiology
  - One of a number of agents
  - Dual infection
- Pathophysiology
  - Entry of pathogenic microorganisms into vagina
  - Microbes then move into the uterus
  - Ascend from the endocervical canal
- Manifestations
  - Fever
  - Purulent vaginal discharge
  - Severe lower abdominal pain
  - Pain on cervical movement
  - May be only mildly symptomatic
- Diagnosis
  - CBC with differential
  - Laparoscopy
  - Laparotomy
- Surgery
  - Drainage of abscess
  - Removal of adhesions
  - Surgical removal of organs
- Nursing diagnoses
  - *Risk for Injury*
  - *Deficient Knowledge*

SUGGESTIONS FOR CLASSROOM ACTIVITIES

- Complete the case studies about pelvic inflammatory disease and syphilis that are provided on the textbook Companion Website. Use the information presented to discuss the care of these clients.

SUGGESTIONS FOR CLINICAL ACTIVITIES

- Have students review the medical records of clinical clients for risk of development of STIs. Discuss preventative measures and education. Discuss therapeutic communication techniques useful in discussing sensitive topics.

LEARNING OUTCOME 3

Explain the risk factors for and complications of STIs.

CONCEPTS FOR LECTURE
GENITAL WARTS

1. Women are at greater risk for genital infections because they have a larger mucosal surface area exposed in the genital area.
2. Women who are infected with HPV are at increased risk of cervical cancer.

VAGINAL INFECTION

3. Women with bacterial vaginosis are at risk for pelvic inflammatory disease, preterm labor, premature rupture of membranes, and postpartum endometritis.
4. Risk factors for the development of candidiasis infection are increased estrogen levels, antibiotics, diabetes mellitus, and fecal contamination.

POWERPOINT LECTURE SLIDES

Genital Warts
- Women are at greater risk
- Women infected with HPV have higher risk of cervical cancer

Vaginal Infection
- Risks
  - Pelvic inflammatory disease
  - Preterm labor
  - Premature rupture of membranes
  - Postpartum endometritis

Candidiasis Infection
- Risk factors
  - Increased estrogen levels
  - Antibiotic use
  - Diabetes mellitus
  - Fecal contamination

Chlamydia

5. Chlamydia can ascend into the female reproductive tract and cause PID, endometritis, and salpingitis. These infections are a major cause of infertility and ectopic pregnancy.
6. Male complications of chlamydia infection are epididymitis, prostatitis, sterility, and Reiter's syndrome.
7. Chlamydia is the leading cause of preventable blindness in the newborn.

Gonorrhea

8. Gonorrhea rates for African Americans are 30% higher than for non-Hispanic whites.
9. Risk factors for development of gonorrhea are residence in large urban areas, being transients, early onset of sexual activity, multiple serial or consecutive sex partners, drug use, prostitution, and previous gonorrheal or concurrent STI infections.
10. In men, gonorrhea can cause acute, painful inflammation of the prostate, epididymis, and periurethral glands and can lead to sterility.
11. In women, it can cause pelvic inflammatory disease, endometritis, salpingitis, and pelvic peritonitis.
12. In the neonate, gonorrhea can cause ophthalmia neonatorum, rhinitis, infection of joints, lethal blood infections, or anorectal infection.
13. Gonorrhea can spread to the blood and joints and increases susceptibility to and transmission of HIV.

Syphilis

14. The infection rate decreased with invention of penicillin. Syphilis continues to be a significant problem in some urban centers. Specific populations, such as African Americans, transients, drug users, and the homeless have high rates of infection.
15. Rates of syphilis among men who have sex with men is increasing.

Pelvic Inflammatory Disease

16. Sexually active women ages 16–24 are most at risk. Risk factors include history of STIs, bacterial vaginosis, multiple sexual partners, douching, and previous PID.
17. Complications of PID include pelvic abscess, infertility, ectopic pregnancy, chronic pelvic pain, pelvic adhesions, dyspareunia, and chronic pelvic pain. Abscess formation is common.

Chlamydia
- Female complications
  - PID
  - Endometritis
  - Salpingitis
  - Infertility
  - Ectopic pregnancy
- Male complications
  - Epididymitis
  - Prostatitis
  - Sterility
  - Reiter's syndrome
- Newborn complications
  - Blindness

Gonorrhea
- Risks
  - Race
  - Residence in large urban areas
  - Being transient
  - Early onset of sexual activity
  - Multiple serial or consecutive sex partners
  - Drug use
  - Prostitution
  - Previous gonorrhea
  - Concurrent STI infections
- Male complications
  - Inflammation
    - Prostate
    - Epididymis
    - Periurethral glands
  - Sterility
- Female complications
  - PID
  - Endometritis
  - Salpingitis
  - Pelvic peritonitis
- Newborn complications
  - Ophthalmia neonatorum
  - Rhinitis
  - Infection of joints
  - Lethal blood infections
  - Anorectal infection
- Generic complications
  - Can spread to blood and joints
  - Increases susceptibility to HIV
  - Increases transmission of HIV

Syphilis
- Rate decreased with invention of penicillin
- Risk population
  - African Americans
  - Transients
  - Drug users
  - Homeless
  - Men having sex with men

Pelvic Inflammatory Disease
- Risk population
  - ○ Sexually active women ages 16–24
- Risk factors
  - ○ History of STIs
  - ○ Bacterial vaginosis
  - ○ Multiple sexual partners
  - ○ Douching
  - ○ Previous PID
- Complications
  - ○ Pelvic abscess
  - ○ Infertility
  - ○ Ectopic pregnancy
  - ○ Chronic pelvic pain
  - ○ Pelvic adhesions
  - ○ Dyspareunia

SUGGESTIONS FOR CLASSROOM ACTIVITIES

- Review the care plan activity about college women and risk of cancer with HPV that is provided on the textbook Companion Website. Complete the activity and lead a discussion of risk management for this client.
- Review the care plan activity about single older adults and safer sex that is provided on the textbook Companion Website. Complete the activity and lead a discussion of risk management for this client.

SUGGESTIONS FOR CLINICAL ACTIVITIES

- Have students investigate the facility policy and procedure regarding use of antibiotic eye drops in the eyes of newborns. Discuss why this procedure is necessary.

LEARNING OUTCOME 4

Discuss the effects and nursing implications of medications and treatments used to treat STIs.

CONCEPTS FOR LECTURE

GENITAL HERPES

1. Acyclovir (Zovirax) helps reduce the length and severity of the first episode and is the treatment of choice.
2. In cases that are resistant to acyclovir, foscarnet (Foscavir) may be used.
3. Other medications are valacyclovir (Valtrex) and famcyclovir (Famvir).

GENITAL WARTS

4. Topical agents such as podofilox and imiquimod, or podiphyllin and trichloroacetic acid are used.
5. Vaccines for various types of HPV are being developed.

VAGINAL INFECTIONS

6. Pharmacologic treatment varies with the organism. Self-medication with an incorrect agent may occur.

POWERPOINT LECTURE SLIDES

Genital Herpes
- Acyclovir
- Foscarnet
- Valacyclovir
- Penciclovir
- Famcyclovir

Genital Warts
- Topical agents
  - ○ Podofilox and iminquimod
  - ○ Podiphyllin and trichloracetic
- Vaccines

Vaginal Infections
- Varies with the organism
- Self-medication

Chlamydia
- Azithromycin
- Doxycycline
- Erythromycin
- Both partners treated concurrently

CHLAMYDIA

7. Medications for chlamydial infections include azithromycin, doxycycline, or erythromycin. Both partners must be treated at the same time.

GONORRHEA

8. Ciprofloxacin, ofloxacin, levofloxan, and ceftriaxone are used to treat gonorrhea.
9. Azithromycin or doxycycline may be added to treat any coexisting chlamydial infection.
10. Newborns are routinely treated with an antibacterial agent eye drop to the conjunctiva within one hour of birth.

SYPHILIS

11. Treatment of choice for primary and secondary syphilis is benzathine penicillin G. Oral doxycycline or erythromycin is given to those who are allergic to penicillin.
12. Jarisch-Herxheimer reaction may occur as a result of treatment.

PELVIC INFLAMMATORY DISEASE

13. Combination antibiotic therapy with at least two broad-spectrum antibiotics is the typical treatment for PID. Commonly prescribed antibiotics include doxycycline, cefoxitin, clindamycin, gentamicin, ofloxacin, and ceftriaxone. The antiprotozoal agent, metronidazole may also be administered.
14. Analgesics are administered for pain.

Gonorrhea
- Ciproflaxacin
- Ofloxacin
- Levofloxan
- Ceftriaxone
- Azithromycin or doxycycline for coexisting chlamydia
- Antibacterial eyedrops for newborns

Syphilis
- Benzathine penicillin G
- Doxycycline
- Erythromycin
- Jarisch-Herxheimer reaction

Pelvic Inflammatory Disease
- Combination antibiotic therapy
- Doxycycline
- Cefoxitin
- Clindamycin
- Gentamicin
- Ofloxacin
- Ceftrixone
- Metronidazole
- Analgesics

SUGGESTIONS FOR CLASSROOM ACTIVITIES

- Have students group the medications commonly given for STIs according to mechanism of action. Discuss nursing implications of giving these medications.
- Discuss the statement, "self-medication with an incorrect agent may occur" as it applies to care of the woman with a vaginal infection. Discuss management and education of this client.

SUGGESTIONS FOR CLINICAL ACTIVITIES

- Have students review the medication administration records of clinical clients who are being treated for STIs. Once students identify these medications, have them create medication information sheets including dosages, nursing implications, and teaching implications of the medications.

UNIT 1
DIMENSIONS OF MEDICAL-SURGICAL NURSING

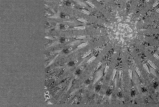

FUNCTIONAL HEALTH PATTERN

Health Perception-Health Management

CONCEPTS FOR LECTURE

1. The medical diagnoses related to altered Health Perception-Health Management Functional Health Pattern include: hypertension, diabetes mellitus, cancer, chronic obstructive pulmonary disease, stroke, and alcoholism.
2. The Health Perception-Health Management Functional Health Pattern includes healthcare behaviors.
3. Preventive healthcare measures include performing routine examinations, making dietary changes, and making lifestyle changes to maintain a healthier body.
4. Health Perception-Health Management is affected by healthcare behaviors such as health promotion, illness prevention, medical treatment, and follow-up care.
5. Health Perception-Health Management is affected by modifiable and nonmodifiable factors that influence health care.
6. Improper health management affects the body's ability to maintain itself, which leads to clinical manifestations such as vomiting, bleeding, and pain.
7. Priority nursing diagnoses for Health Perception-Health Management Functional Health Pattern include: *Health-Seeking Behaviors, Deficient Knowledge, Ineffective Health Maintenance,* and *Risk for Injury.*
8. Other nursing diagnoses applicable to clients with deficits in health perception or health management include: *Self-Care Deficit* and *Low Self-Esteem.*

LECTURE OUTLINE IN POWERPOINT

Unit 1: Dimensions of Medical-Surgical Nursing
Health Perception and Health Management
Functional Health Pattern
- Medical diagnoses
  ○ Hypertension, diabetes mellitus
  ○ Cancer, chronic obstructive pulmonary disease
  ○ Stroke, alcoholism
Health Perception and Health Management
- Healthcare behaviors
  ○ Have yearly physical examination
  ○ Have routine eye examinations
  ○ Keep up-to-date immunizations
Health Perception and Health Management
- Health preventative measures
  ○ Perform breast self-examinations
  ○ Perform testicular examinations
  ○ Use sunscreen
  ○ Make dietary changes for well-balanced diet
  ○ Decrease alcohol intake
Health Perception and Health Management
- Health preventative measures
  ○ Stop smoking
  ○ Begin regular exercise
  ○ Practice safe sex
  ○ Use stress reduction activities
Health Perception and Health Management
- Healthcare behaviors
  ○ Health promotion
  ○ Illness prevention activities
  ○ Medical treatments
  ○ Follow-up care
Factors That Can Be Altered
- Diet
- Substance abuse, smoking
- Socioeconomic status
- Occupational exposure
Factors That Cannot Be Altered
- Genetics
- Age
- Race
Improper Health Management
- Manifestations
  ○ Vomiting
  ○ Bleeding
  ○ Pain

Priority Nursing Diagnoses
- *Health-Seeking Behaviors*
- *Deficient Knowledge*
- *Ineffective Health Maintenance*
- *Risk for Injury*

Nursing Diagnoses from Other Functional Health Patterns
- *Self-Care Deficit*
- *Low Self-Esteem*

SUGGESTIONS FOR CLASSROOM ACTIVITIES

- Compare modifiable and nonmodifiable healthcare factors.
- Have students obtain an immunization schedule from the internet and research new immunizations being developed. Discuss which clients should or should not obtain immunizations.
- Divide students into 10 groups. Assign an end-of-unit question to each group. Have them answer the questions and give a rationale for the answer they choose. Discuss why the other answers are incorrect.

SUGGESTIONS FOR CLINICAL ACTIVITIES

- Arrange for students to participate in a health fair. Have them take blood pressures, discuss breast self-examinations or testicular examinations, discuss a well-balanced nutrition plan, and explain the benefits of an exercise program or smoking cessation program.
- Have students develop a teaching tool on preventive health measures. Use the teaching tool to hand out to clients.
- Arrange for students to administer immunizations at a clinic or flu vaccines in a nursing home. Discuss why immunizations and vaccinations are important in health prevention.

CLINICAL SCENARIOS

See End-of-Unit Summary for Unit 1 in Textbook

CONCEPTS FOR LECTURE

1. Client care is prioritized according to the seriousness of their condition.
2. Prioritized nursing diagnoses assist the nurse in developing a plan of care for the client.

LECTURE OUTLINE IN POWERPOINT

Prioritize Clients in Order of Visit
- Cora Clark with prolapsed uterus
- Tom Smith with osteomyelitis
- Marguerite Garcia with Type II diabetes, CHF
- Sebastian Huian with stroke

Priority Nursing Diagnoses for Cora Clark
- *Risk for Infection*
- *Self-Care Deficit*

Priority Nursing Diagnoses for Tom Smith
- *Ineffective Bone Tissue Perfusion*
- *Impaired Skin Integrity*

Priority Nursing Diagnoses for Marguerite Garcia
- *Decreased Cardiac Output*
- *Ineffective Health Maintenance*

Priority Nursing Diagnoses for Sebastian Huian
- *Self-Care Deficit*
- *Impaired Verbal Communication*

SUGGESTIONS FOR CLASSROOM ACTIVITIES

- Have students read clinical scenarios and prioritize the clients in the order they should be seen. Discuss why the clients should be seen in priority order.
- Have students choose two priority nursing diagnoses for each clinical scenario client. Explain the rationale for each nursing diagnosis.

SUGGESTIONS FOR CLINICAL ACTIVITIES

- Assign students to provide nursing care for more than one client. Have them prioritize the order in which to provide care for the clients and discuss their rationale.
- Have students develop priority nursing diagnoses for the clients to whom they are providing nursing care.

CASE STUDY

See End-of-Unit Summary for Unit 1 in Textbook

CONCEPTS FOR LECTURE

1. Nursing diagnoses are developed based on the medical diagnosis, physical assessment, the client's health history, and pathophysiology of the disease process.
2. The nursing process is used as a guide to develop a plan of care.

LECTURE OUTLINE IN POWERPOINT

Client with Deficient Knowledge
- Based on
  - Medical diagnosis
    - Pelvic inflammatory disease
  - Manifestations
  - Health history
  - Pathophysiology of disease process

Nursing Process
- Assessment
- Plan
- Nursing diagnosis
- Implementation
- Expected outcomes, evaluation

Nursing Diagnoses
- *Acute Pain*
- *Ineffective Health Maintenance*
- *Risk for Injury*

SUGGESTIONS FOR CLASSROOM ACTIVITIES

- Read the case study from the End-of-Unit Summary for Unit 1 in class. Review the concept map from the End-of-Unit Summary to develop a plan of care for the client.

SUGGESTIONS FOR CLINICAL ACTIVITIES

- Have students develop a concept map for clients to whom they provide nursing care in a healthcare setting.

Unit 2
Alterations in Patterns of Health

Functional Health Pattern

Health Perception-Health Management

Concepts for Lecture

1. The medical diagnoses related to altered Health Perception-Health Management Functional Health Pattern include: surgery, terminal illness, impending death, alcoholism or other substance abuse, or victim of multiple or mass casualty incident.
2. The Health Perception-Health Management Functional Health Pattern includes factors that influence health-care behaviors.
3. The Health Perception-Health Management Functional Health Pattern includes the ability or inability to change healthcare practices.
4. Health Perception-Health Management is affected by factors that interfere with health care.
5. Health Perception-Health Management is affected by factors that interfere with the level of wellness.
6. Impaired health management affects the body's ability to maintain itself, which leads to clinical manifestations such as: anxiety, grief, and death.
7. Priority nursing diagnoses for Health Perception-Health Management Functional Health Pattern include: *Impaired Skin Integrity, Risk for Injury, Ineffective Therapeutic Regimen Management,* and *Powerlessness.*
8. Other nursing diagnoses applicable to clients with deficits in health management include: *Impaired Verbal Communication* and *Ineffective Individual Coping.*

Lecture Outline in PowerPoint

Unit 2: Alterations in Patterns of Health
Health Perception and Health Management
Functional Health Pattern
- Medical diagnoses
  - Surgery
  - Terminal illness, impending death
  - Alcoholism, substance abuse
  - Victim of multiple or mass casualty incident

Health Perception and Health Management
- Factors influencing healthcare behaviors
  - Had previous surgery, complications with surgery
  - Problems with anesthesia
  - Current prescribed medications
  - Taking over-the-counter medications

Health Perception and Health Management
- Factors influencing healthcare behaviors
  - Amount of alcohol intake
  - Types of substances abused
  - Influence of substance abuse on family
  - Exposure to environmental hazards

Health Perception and Health Management
- Factors influencing healthcare behaviors
  - Any sensory deficits
  - Any sight or speech impairments, language spoken
  - Have a living will, Do-Not-Resuscitate orders
  - Have a power of attorney, religious considerations
  - End-of-life issues discussed with family

Health Perception and Health Management
- Healthcare behaviors
  - Ability to change healthcare practices
  - Inability to change healthcare practices

Factors That Interfere with Health Care
- Lack of understanding of health practices
  - Altered cognition, altered coping
- Inability to take responsibility for health needs
  - Alcoholism, substance abuse
- Lack of communication skills
  - Non-English speaking, illiterate

Factors That Interfere with Wellness
- Inability to change declining health
  - Cancer, kidney failure, impending death

- Need for treatment
  - Surgery
- Catastrophic events
  - MVA, weather-related event injuries, burns

Impaired Health Management
- Manifestations
  - Anxiety
  - Grief
  - Death

Priority Nursing Diagnoses
- *Impaired Skin Integrity*
- *Risk for Injury*
- *Ineffective Therapeutic Regimen Management*
- *Powerlessness*

Nursing Diagnoses from Other Functional Health Patterns
- *Impaired Verbal Communication*
- *Ineffective Individual Coping*

SUGGESTIONS FOR CLASSROOM ACTIVITIES

- Discuss the end-of-unit questions in class as a group. Assist students to choose the correct answer and discuss the rationale for the correct answer. Review why the other answers are incorrect.
- Invite a nurse legal consultant or nurse lawyer to speak to the class about the legalities of a living will, do-not-resuscitate orders, and power of attorney.
- In class, discuss cultural and religious beliefs regarding the health care of clients from various ethnic groups.

SUGGESTIONS FOR CLINICAL ACTIVITIES

- Assign students to provide nursing care to non-English speaking clients or clients with sight or speech impairments. In post-conference, have students discuss how they communicated with the clients and what problems they encountered.
- Assign students to interview clients who are scheduled for surgery. Have them address if the client understands the surgery, has had previous surgery, any complications with previous surgery, and their feelings about anesthesia.
- Have students attend an Alcoholics Anonymous, Narcotics Anonymous, or other substance abuse meeting and write a paper about their observations.
- If possible, assign students to clients with impending death. In post-conference, have students discuss the clinical manifestations observed and whether family was involved or not. Discuss the procedures for care after death.

CLINICAL SCENARIOS

See End-of-Unit Summary for Unit 2 in Textbook

CONCEPTS FOR LECTURE

1. Client care is prioritized according to the seriousness of their condition.
2. Prioritized nursing diagnoses assist the nurse in developing a plan of care for the client.

LECTURE OUTLINE IN POWERPOINT

Prioritize Clients in Order of Visit
- Peter Black
- Mary Black
- Paul Goetz
- John Linzer

Priority Nursing Diagnoses for Peter Black
- *Risk for Peripheral Neurovascular Dysfunction*
- *Impaired Skin Integrity*

Priority Nursing Diagnoses for Mary Black
- *Acute Pain*
- *Fear*

Priority Nursing Diagnoses for Paul Goetz
- *Powerlessness*
- *Ineffective Family Coping*

Priority Nursing Diagnoses for John Linzer
- *Disturbed Sensory Perception*
- *Anxiety*

SUGGESTIONS FOR CLASSROOM ACTIVITIES	SUGGESTIONS FOR CLINICAL ACTIVITIES
• Have students read clinical scenarios and prioritize the clients in the order they should be seen. Discuss why the clients should be seen in the priority order. • Have students choose two priority nursing diagnoses for each clinical scenario client. Explain the rationale for each nursing diagnosis.	• Assign students to provide nursing care for more than one client. Have them prioritize which client should receive care first and discuss their rationale. • Have students develop priority nursing diagnoses for the clients to whom they are providing nursing care.

CASE STUDY

See End-of-Unit Summary for Unit 2 in Textbook

CONCEPTS FOR LECTURE

1. Nursing diagnoses are developed based on the medical diagnosis, physical assessment, the client's health history, and pathophysiology of the disease process.
2. The nursing process is used as a guide to develop a plan of care.

LECTURE OUTLINE IN POWERPOINT

Client with Anxiety
- Based on
  - Medical diagnosis
    - Severe comminuted left leg fracture
    - Lacerated spleen, bruising
  - Physical assessment, health history
  - Pathophysiology of disease process

Nursing Process
- Assessment
- Plan
- Nursing diagnosis
- Implementation, expected outcomes
- Evaluation

Nursing Diagnoses
- *Acute Pain*
- *Risk for Infection*
- *Disturbed Body Image*

SUGGESTIONS FOR CLASSROOM ACTIVITIES	SUGGESTIONS FOR CLINICAL ACTIVITIES
• Read the case study from the End-of-Unit Summary for Unit 2 in class. Review the concept map from the End-of-Unit Summary. Have students work together in groups to develop a plan of care for the client.	• Have students develop a concept map for clients to whom they provide nursing care in a healthcare setting.

UNIT 3
PATHOPHYSIOLOGY AND PATTERNS OF HEALTH

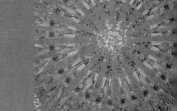

FUNCTIONAL HEALTH PATTERN

Health Perception-Health Management

CONCEPTS FOR LECTURE

1. The medical diagnoses related to altered Health Perception-Health Management Functional Health Pattern include: Down syndrome, cystic fibrosis, sickle cell anemia, Huntington disease, hemophilia, Alzheimer's disease, chronic pain, dehydration, electrolyte imbalance, metabolic or respiratory acidosis, metabolic or respiratory alkalosis, shock, traumatic injury, bacterial infection, viral infection, sepsis, chronic inflammation, HIV/AIDS, rheumatoid arthritis, systemic lupus erythematosus, multiple sclerosis, anaphylaxis, tissue transplant, and cancer.
2. The Health Perception-Health Management Functional Health Pattern includes healthcare behaviors that interfere with health.
3. The Health Perception-Health Management Functional Health Pattern includes early intervention and health promotion-focused care.
4. Health Perception-Health Management is affected by factors that change or disrupt genes or genetic structure.
5. Health Perception-Health Management is affected by factors that change or disrupt cells in the body.
6. Alterations in health management may affect the body's ability to maintain itself, which leads to clinical manifestations such as: rapid weight loss, tachycardia, and tachypnea.
7. Priority nursing diagnoses for Health Perception-Health Management Functional Health Pattern include: *Risk for Infection, Acute Pain, Disturbed Body Image,* and *Risk for Violence.*
8. Other nursing diagnoses applicable to clients with deficits in health perception or health management include: *Impaired Tissue Integrity* and *Risk for Post-trauma Syndrome.*

LECTURE OUTLINE IN POWERPOINT

Unit 3: Pathophysiology and Patterns of Health
Health Perception and Health Management
Functional Health Pattern
- Medical diagnoses
  - Down syndrome, cystic fibrosis, hemophilia
  - Sickle cell anemia, Huntington disease, dehydration
  - Alzheimer's disease, chronic pain, electrolyte imbalance
  - Metabolic or respiratory acidosis
  - Metabolic or respiratory alkalosis
Health Perception and Health Management
- Medical diagnoses
  - Shock, traumatic injury, HIV/AIDS
  - Bacterial infection, viral infection, sepsis
  - Chronic inflammation, rheumatoid arthritis
  - Systemic lupus erythmatosus, multiple sclerosis
  - Anaphylaxis, cancer
Health Perception and Health Management
- Healthcare behaviors interfere with health
  - Have genetic disorder
  - Have family history of genetic disorder
  - Complaints of pain
  - Have significant body fluid loss
  - Have body fluid edema
Health Perception and Health Management
- Healthcare behaviors interfere with health
  - Complains of cardiac arrhythmias
  - Complains of muscle weakness or spasms
  - Complains of numbness or tingling
  - Changes in respiratory patterns
  - Have personality changes or confusion
Health Perception and Health Management
- Healthcare behaviors interfere with health
  - Had any seizures activity, traumatic injuries
  - Had a blood transfusion
  - Treated for shock, infection
  - Problems with wound healing, allergies
  - Have any autoimmune disorders
Health Perception and Health Management
- Healthcare behaviors
  - Early intervention
  - Health promotion-focused care

Factors That Change or Disrupt Genes
- Genetic alterations
  - Down syndrome, chronic myelogenous leukemia
- Autosomal dominant inheritance patterns
  - Breast and ovarian cancer, Huntington disease
- Autosomal inheritance recessive inheritance
  - Cystic fibrosis, sickle cell anemia

Factors That Change or Disrupt Genes
- X-linked recessive inheritance
  - Hemophilia
- Monogenic inheritance
  - Prader-Willi syndrome

Factors That Change or Disrupt Cells
- Altered immune response
  - Hypersensitivity, rheumatoid arthritis, HIV/AIDS
- Inflammation
  - Osteoarthritis, *mycobacterium* tuberculosis
- Infection
  - Influenza, meningitis

Factors That Change or Disrupt Cells
- Cancer
  - Leukemia, lymphoma, sarcoma
- Trauma
  - Rape, burns, fractures, gunshot wounds
- Shock
  - Hypovolemic, septic, anaphylactic

Factors That Change or Disrupt Cells
- Fluid volume alterations
  - Dehydration, edema
- Electrolyte imbalance
  - Hyponatremia, hypernatremia, hypokalemia, hyperkalemia, hypocalcemia
- Acid-base imbalance
  - Respiratory or metabolic acidosis, respiratory or metabolic alkalosis

Alteration in Health Management
- Manifestations
  - Rapid weight loss
  - Tachycardia
  - Tachypnea

Priority Nursing Diagnoses
- *Risk for Infection*
- *Acute Pain*
- *Disturbed Body Image*
- *Risk for Violence*

Nursing Diagnoses from Other Functional Health Patterns
- *Impaired Tissue Integrity*
- *Risk for Post-Trauma Syndrome Post Traumatic*

SUGGESTIONS FOR CLASSROOM ACTIVITIES

- Administer the end-of-unit questions as a quiz. After completing the quiz, discuss the answers to the questions and give the rationale for the answers. Discuss why the other answers are incorrect.

SUGGESTIONS FOR CLINICAL ACTIVITIES

- Assign students to the emergency department or a trauma intensive care unit to observe nursing care of trauma clients. Have them develop a concept map or nursing care plan for a client they observed.

Suggestions for Classroom Activities *continued*

- Review disease processes or disorders caused by changes or disruptions in cells, such as fluid volume changes, electrolyte imbalances, cancers, infections, and trauma. Discuss the role of the nurse in health prevention and health management with clients with these disorders.
- Review disease processes or disorders caused by genetic factors, such as inheritance of disorders such as Down syndrome, cystic fibrosis, and sickle cell anemia. Discuss the nurse's role in genetic counseling and the impact of the results on the client and family.
- Compare the manifestations and laboratory studies of a bacterial infection with a viral infection. Discuss the similarities and differences in medical treatment and nursing care. Discuss ways to prevent infections and have students develop a teaching tool to teach clients ways to prevent infections.
- Electrolyte imbalances may be prevented by teaching clients about proper nutrition. Have students identify foods that contain electrolytes, such as sodium, potassium, calcium, and so on.

Suggestions for Clinical Activities *continued*

- Have students shadow a respiratory therapist on client rounds. Have students look at arterial blood gas reports on the client's medical records. Have them determine which type of acidosis or alkalosis the client has. Discuss with the respiratory therapist the appropriate treatment.
- Have students visit a hospice treatment facility or spend a day with a hospice nurse to observe the health maintenance plan for clients with cancer disorders or end-of-life disorders.

CLINICAL SCENARIOS

See End-of-Unit Summary for Unit 3 in Textbook

Concepts for Lecture

1. Client care is prioritized according to the seriousness of the client's condition.
2. Prioritized nursing diagnoses assist the nurse in developing a plan of care for the client.
3. Strategies for prioritizing clients are based on the ABCs, Maslow's hierarchy of needs, developmental considerations, or crisis intervention.

Lecture Outline in PowerPoint

Prioritize Clients in Order of Visit
- Tamra Sanders with sickle cell crisis
- Allen Barber with an inflammation of incision site
- Mia Windham with maculopapular rash
- Harry Anderson with AIDS

Strategies for Prioritizing Client Care
- ABCs
- Maslow's hierarchy of needs
- Developmental considerations
- Crisis intervention

Suggestions for Classroom Activities

- Have students read the clinical scenarios and prioritize the clients in the order they should be seen. Discuss the rationale for the priority order.
- Have students choose two priority nursing diagnoses for each clinical scenario client. Explain the rationale for each nursing diagnosis.
- The ABCs of client care are airway, bleeding, and circulation. Shortness of breath is a priority problem because the airway is being compromised. Tamra Sanders is in a sickle cell crisis with shortness of breath and severe chest pain. The shortness of breath can be treated with oxygenation but the severe chest pain needs to be relieved as well. Maslow's hierarchy

Suggestions for Clinical Activities

- Assign students to provide nursing care for more than one client. Have them prioritize the order of care for the clients and discuss their rationale.
- Have students listen to the nurse's report at the beginning of the shift. Discuss prioritizing nursing care for all the clients. Discuss which activities can be delegated to a nurse's aide, an LPN, and RN.

of needs classifies pain relief or bodily comfort as a physiologic need; therefore, pain relief for a pain scale of 10/10 is also a high priority for nursing care of this client.

CASE STUDY

See End-of-Unit Summary for Unit 3 in Textbook

CONCEPTS FOR LECTURE

1. Nursing diagnoses are developed based on the medical diagnosis, physical assessment, the client's health history, and the pathophysiology of the disease process.
2. The nursing process is used as a guide to develop a plan of care for the client.

LECTURE OUTLINE IN POWERPOINT

Client with Ineffective Breathing Pattern
- Based on
  - Medical diagnosis
    - Lung cancer
  - Physical assessment
  - Health history
  - Pathophysiology of disease process

Nursing Process
- Assessment
- Plan
- Nursing diagnosis
- Implementation, expected outcomes
- Evaluation

Nursing Diagnoses
- *Activity Intolerance*
- *Altered Nutrition: Less Than Body Requirements*
- *Chronic Pain*
- *Deficient Knowledge*

SUGGESTIONS FOR CLASSROOM ACTIVITIES

- Read the case study from the End-of-Unit Summary for Unit 3 in class. Review the concept map from the End-of-Unit Summary to develop a plan of care for the client.

SUGGESTIONS FOR CLINICAL ACTIVITIES

- Have students develop concept maps for clients they provide nursing care for in the acute or chronic healthcare setting.

UNIT 4
RESPONSES TO ALTERED INTEGUMENTARY STRUCTURE AND FUNCTION

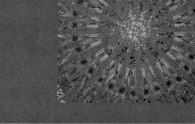

FUNCTIONAL HEALTH PATTERN

Nutritional-Metabolic

CONCEPTS FOR LECTURE

1. The medical diagnoses related to altered Nutritional-Metabolic Functional Health Pattern include: psoriasis, cysts, folliculitis, cellulitis, candidiasis, pediculosis, herpes zoster, seborrheic dermatitis, acne vulgaris, nonmelanoma skin cancer, malignant melanoma, basal cell carcinoma, pressure ulcers, hirsutism, alopecia, paronychia, or burn trauma.
2. The Nutritional-Metabolic Functional Health Pattern includes healthcare behaviors that interfere with nutrition and metabolism.
3. The Nutritional-Metabolic Functional Health Pattern includes food and fluid consumption to maintain nutritional and metabolic needs of the body, to provide protection against the environment, and to promote maintenance and repair of body tissues.
4. Factors that affect the integumentary system are lack of nutrients that lower the body's resistance, exposure to extreme temperatures, adverse effects from medications, and heredity.
5. Affects of improper nutrition include: inability to maintain protection of the body, inability to regulate body temperature, inability to regulate fluid and electrolyte balance, breakdown of protective mechanisms, and sensory function interference.
6. Alterations in nutrition and metabolism may affect the body's ability to maintain itself, which leads to clinical manifestations such as: skin ulcerations, infection, and alopecia.
7. Priority nursing diagnoses for Nutritional-Metabolism Functional Health Pattern include: *Impaired Skin Integrity, Risk for Infection, Deficient Fluid Volume,* and *Disturbed Body Image.*
8. Other nursing diagnoses applicable to clients with alterations in nutrition and metabolism include: *Acute Pain* and *Ineffective Protection.*

LECTURE OUTLINE IN POWERPOINT

Unit 4: Responses to Altered Integumentary Structure and Function
Nutritional-Metabolic Functional Health Patterns
- Medical diagnoses
  - Psoriasis, cysts, folliculitis, cellulitis, candidiasis, pediculosis
  - Herpes zoster, seborrheic dermatitis, acne vulgaris
  - Nonmelanoma skin cancer, malignant melanoma
  - Basil cell carcinoma, pressure ulcers, hirsutism
  - Alopecia, paronychia, burn trauma
Nutritional-Metabolic
- Healthcare behaviors which interfere with nutrition
  - Monitor intake of food or fluids
  - Complaining of gaining or losing weight
  - Taking medications or supplements
  - Evaluate condition of skin, hair, nails
  - Complaints of itching, rashes, bruising
Nutritional-Metabolic
- Healthcare behaviors interfere with nutrition
  - Changes in moles or warts
  - Have pressure areas on sacrum, hips, ankles
  - Have any skin disorders
  - Use protection against temperature extremes
Nutritional-Metabolic
- Food and fluid consumption
  - To maintain nutrition and metabolic needs
  - To supply nutrients to integumentary system
  - To increase protection against environment
  - To promote maintenance and repair
Factors Affecting Integumentary System
- Lack of nutrients lower's body resistance
  - Infection
    - Bacterial or viral
  - Skin breakdown
    - Pressure ulcers
Factors Affecting Integumentary System
- Exposure to temperature extremes
  - Frostbite
  - Burn trauma
- Medication adverse effects
  - Hirsutism
  - Alopecia

Affects of Improper Nutrition
- Inability to maintain protection
- Inability to regulate body temperature
- Inability to maintain fluid and electrolyte balance
- Breakdown of protective mechanisms
- Interferes with sensory function

Improper Nutrition-Metabolism
- Manifestations
  ○ Skin ulcerations
  ○ Infection
  ○ Alopecia

Priority Nursing Diagnoses
- *Impaired Skin Integrity*
- *Risk for Infection*
- *Deficient Fluid Volume*
- *Disturbed Body Image*

Nursing Diagnoses from Other Functional Patterns
- *Acute Pain*
- *Ineffective Protection*

SUGGESTIONS FOR CLASSROOM ACTIVITIES

- Divide students into 10 groups. Assign an end-of-unit question to each group. Have them answer the questions and give a rationale for the answer they chose. Discuss why the other answers are incorrect.
- A diet high in protein and calories is needed for repair of injured tissue, such as burn trauma and pressure ulcers. Bring in a variety of children's play foods and have students select meal plans that are high in protein and calories.
- Show pictures of the manifestations of inflammatory and infectious conditions of the skin. Have students identify the condition, treatment, and nursing care for each condition.
- Discuss how the body's metabolic functioning affects the maintenance or breakdown of the skin. Identify how body temperature, fluids and electrolytes, and nutrition affect the skin.

SUGGESTIONS FOR CLINICAL ACTIVITIES

- Have students perform skin assessments on clients. Identify risk factors for pressure ulcers and perform a risk assessment. Discuss interventions for the stages of pressure sores and measures for pressure sore prevention.
- Arrange for students to make rounds with a wound specialist nurse. Identify products used for wound care. Discuss how nutrition plays a role in healing skin wounds.
- Arrange for students to assist a school nurse with performing examinations for head lice (pediculosis). Discuss the medications used for lice treatment. Have students develop a teaching plan for the parents of children with head lice, including care of clothing, bedding, hair brushes and combs, and stuffed animals.

CLINICAL SCENARIOS

See End-of-Unit Summary for Unit 4 in Textbook

CONCEPTS FOR LECTURE

1. Client care is prioritized according to the seriousness of the client's condition.
2. Prioritized nursing diagnoses assist the nurse in developing a plan of care for the client.
3. Strategies for prioritizing clients are based on the ABCs, Maslow's hierarchy of needs, developmental considerations, or crisis intervention.

LECTURE OUTLINE IN POWERPOINT

Prioritize Clients in Order of Visit
- Mrs. Carter with cellulitis in right calf
- Mr. Jenkins with herpes zoster
- Mr. Johnson with elbow contractures
- Mr. Ugandi with toxic epidermal necrolysis

Strategies for Prioritizing Client Care
- ABCs
- Maslow's hierarchy of needs
- Developmental considerations
- Crisis intervention

SUGGESTIONS FOR CLASSROOM ACTIVITIES

- Have students read the clinical scenarios and prioritize the clients in the order they should be seen. Discuss the rationale for the priority order.
- Have students choose two priority nursing diagnoses for each clinical scenario client. Explain the rationale for each nursing diagnosis.
- According to Maslow's hierarchy of needs, basic needs of water, nourishment, and comfort must be met before higher levels of needs can be met. Mr. Ugandi is being treated for toxic epidermal necrolysis, possibly related to AIDS. Until his skin is completely healed, fluids and electrolytes are lost through the open areas, temperature control and the skin's protective mechanisms are compromised, and comfort is difficult to attain.

SUGGESTIONS FOR CLINICAL ACTIVITIES

- Assign students to provide nursing care for more than one client. Have them prioritize the order of nursing care for the clients and discuss their rationale.
- Have students develop priority nursing diagnoses for the clients to which they are providing nursing care in the acute or chronic healthcare setting.

CASE STUDY

See End-of-Unit Summary for Unit 4 in Textbook

CONCEPTS FOR LECTURE

1. Nursing diagnoses are developed based on the medical diagnosis, physical assessment, the client's health history, and the pathophysiology of the disease process.
2. The nursing process is used as a guide to develop a plan of care for the client.

LECTURE OUTLINE IN POWERPOINT

Client with Impaired Skin Integrity
- Based on
  - Medical diagnosis
    - First and second degree burns
  - Physical assessment
  - Health history
  - Pathophysiology of disease process
Nursing Process
- Assessment
- Plan
- Nursing diagnosis
- Implementation, expected outcomes
- Evaluation
Nursing Diagnosis
- *Acute Pain*
- *Risk for Infection*
- *Impaired Mobility*

SUGGESTIONS FOR CLASSROOM ACTIVITIES

- Read the case study from the End-of-Unit Summary for Unit 4 in class and review the concept map from the End-of-Unit Summary. Divide students into groups to develop a plan of care for the client. Assign each group a different topic to address, such as nutrition, pharmacology, wound treatment, and laboratory studies.

SUGGESTIONS FOR CLINICAL ACTIVITIES

- Have students develop concept maps for clients to which they provide nursing care in an acute or chronic healthcare setting.

UNIT 5
RESPONSES TO ALTERED ENDOCRINE FUNCTION

FUNCTIONAL HEALTH PATTERN

Nutritional-Metabolic

CONCEPTS FOR LECTURE

1. The medical diagnoses related to altered Nutritional-Metabolic Functional Health Pattern include: Graves' disease, myxedema coma, cancer of the thyroid, hyperparathyroidism, hypoparathyroidism, Cushing's syndrome, Addison's disease, pheochromocytoma, gigantism, syndrome of inappropriate antidiuretic hormone secretion, diabetes insipidus, and diabetes mellitus.
2. The Nutritional-Metabolic Functional Health Pattern includes endocrine problems that interfere with nutrition and metabolism.
3. The Nutritional-Metabolic Functional Health Pattern includes endocrine gland function that produces and releases hormones, regulates metabolism, distributes nutrients after digestion, regulates growth and reproduction, regulates gender differentiation, and regulates fluid and electrolyte balance.
4. Factors that affect the functions of the endocrine system are lack of hormones or excess hormones.
5. Endocrine gland function is regulated by a negative or positive feedback system that regulates functioning of organs to maintain homeostasis of the internal environment.
6. Alterations in nutrition and metabolism may affect the body's ability to maintain itself, which leads to clinical manifestations such as: weight loss, blurred vision, and increased urination.
7. Priority nursing diagnoses for Nutritional-Metabolism Functional Health Pattern include: *Imbalanced Nutrition: Less than Body Requirements, Deficient Fluid Volume, Hyperthermia*, and *Impaired Skin Integrity*.
8. Other nursing diagnoses applicable to clients with alterations in nutrition and metabolism include: *Disturbed Body Image* and *Ineffective Therapeutic Regimen Management*.

LECTURE OUTLINE IN POWERPOINT

Unit 5: Responses to Altered Endocrine Function
Nutritional-Metabolic Functional Health Patterns
- Medical diagnoses
  - Graves' disease, myexedema coma, thyroid cancer
  - Hyperparathyroidism, hypoparathyroidism, gigantism
  - Cushing's syndrome, Addison's disease, pheochromocytoma
  - Syndrome of inappropriate antidiuretic hormone secretion
  - Diabetes insipidus, diabetes mellitus
Nutritional-Metabolic
- Endocrine problems interfere with nutritional status
  - On a prescribed diet
  - Monitor daily intake of foods and fluids
  - Increased appetite with loss of weight
  - Noticed edema of hands and feet
  - Have difficulty swallowing or swelling of neck
Nutritional-Metabolic
- Endocrine problems interfere with nutritional status
  - Increase or decrease in urination
  - Changes in energy levels
  - Visual changes
  - Complains of sleep disturbances
Nutritional-Metabolic
- Endocrine problems interfere with nutritional status
  - Notice changes in hair distribution, skin texture
  - Note change in memory or ability to concentrate
  - Use hormones or steroids
  - Have family history of endocrine disorders
Nutritional-Metabolic
- Endocrine system
  - Produces and releases hormones
  - Regulates metabolism – biochemical processes
  - Distributes nutrients after digestion
  - Regulates growth, reproduction, gender differentiation
  - Regulates fluid and electrolyte balance
Lack of Hormones
- Disorders of thyroid gland
  - Hypothyroidism
- Disorders of parathyroid gland
  - Hypoparathyroidism

- Disorders of adrenal gland
  - ○ Chronic adrenocortical insufficiency

Lack of Hormones
- Disorders of pituitary gland
  - ○ Hypopituitarism, diabetes insipidus
- Disorders of pancreas
  - ○ Hypoglycemia

Excess Hormones
- Disorders of thyroid gland
  - ○ Hyperthyroidism
- Disorders of parathyroid gland
  - ○ Hyperparathyroidism
- Disorders of adrenal gland
  - ○ Hypercortisolism

Excess Hormones
- Disorders of pituitary gland
  - ○ Hyperpituitarism, SIADH
- Disorders of pancreas
  - ○ Hyperglycemia

Nutritional-Metabolic
- Endocrine glands
  - ○ Secrete hormones which bind to receptors
  - ○ Initiate or regulate function of organ
  - ○ Regulated by negative feedback system
  - ○ Regulated by positive feedback system
  - ○ Maintain homeostasis of internal environment

Imbalance of Nutrition – Metabolism
- Manifestations
  - ○ Weight loss
  - ○ Blurred vision
  - ○ Increased urination

Priority Nursing Diagnoses
- *Imbalanced Nutrition: Less than Body Requirements*
- *Deficient Fluid Volume*
- *Hyperthermia*
- *Impaired Skin Integrity*

Nursing Diagnoses from Other Functional Health Patterns
- *Disturbed Body Image*
- *Ineffective Therapeutic Regimen Management*

SUGGESTIONS FOR CLASSROOM ACTIVITIES

- Divide students into 10 groups. Assign an end-of-unit question to each group. Have them answer the questions and give a rationale for the answer they chose. Discuss why the other answers are incorrect.
- Divide students into groups of two. Assign one student to be an endocrine organ. Have the student identify the purpose of the assigned organ and the hormone(s) released by the endocrine organ. Assign the other students to be the hormone(s). Have the student identify the effects of the hormone(s) on target tissues in the body. Review negative and positive feedback systems.

SUGGESTIONS FOR CLINICAL ACTIVITIES

- Assign students to provide nursing care to clients with an endocrine disorder or who have had surgery for an endocrine disorder. Have them develop a concept map or nursing care plan for the client.
- Have students provide a diabetic luncheon for the nursing unit staff. Have students plan the menu and have each student bring a dish from the menu. Each student is responsible for knowing what food group the dish is from and the diabetic exchange value of the food.

Suggestions for Classroom Activities *continued*

- Develop a matching quiz with the endocrine organs listed on one side and the hormones listed on the other side. Give a reward to the student who can match them correctly in the shortest amount of time.
- Arrange for a diabetic educator to speak to the students during post-conference regarding nursing care for clients with type I and type II diabetes mellitus. Discuss medications, nutrition, exercise, complications, and sick day management.
- Compare hypothyroidism with hyperthyroidism, and hypoadrenal disease with hyperadrenal disease. Discuss manifestations, nutrition, laboratory studies, and pharmacologic treatment for each condition.

Suggestions for Clinical Activities *continued*

- Have students develop a poster on the pharmacologic treatment for diabetes mellitus, including types of insulin medication, how to draw up insulin properly, and how to administer insulin correctly.

CLINICAL SCENARIOS

See End-of-Unit Summary for Unit 5 in Textbook

Concepts for Lecture

1. Client care should be prioritized according to the seriousness of the client's condition.
2. Prioritized nursing diagnoses assist the nurse in developing a plan of care for the client.
3. Strategies for prioritizing clients are based on the ABCs, Maslow's hierarchy of needs, developmental considerations, or crisis intervention.

Lecture Outline in PowerPoint

Prioritize Clients in Order of Visit
- Mrs. Rant with renal calculi
- Mr. Blew with hyperglycemia
- Mr. Rite with head injury
- Mrs. Fox with hypoglycemia

Strategies for Prioritizing Client Care
- ABCs
- Maslow's hierarchy of needs
- Developmental considerations
- Crisis intervention

Suggestions for Classroom Activities

- Have students read the clinical scenarios and prioritize the clients in the order they should be seen. Discuss the rationale for the priority order.
- Have students choose two priority nursing diagnoses for each clinical scenario client. Explain the rationale for each nursing diagnosis.
- In developmental considerations, cognitive development increases the ability to recognize and solve problems. In the elderly client, cognitive abilities decline, which decreases the ability to problem-solve; short-term memory also decreases. Mrs. Fox, who is 86 years old, was found by her daughter in a comatose state due to a blood sugar reading of 45 and her heart rate was 50. Due to her age, Mrs. Fox may not have been taking her prescribed medications properly, which resulted in her symptoms and a comatose state. The case manager will interview the client and her daughter to investigate the home situation and determine the need for changes.

Suggestions for Clinical Activities

- Assign students to provide nursing care for more than one client. Have them prioritize the order to provide nursing care for the clients and discuss their rationale.
- Have students develop priority nursing diagnoses for the clients to whom they are providing nursing care in the acute or chronic healthcare setting.

CASE STUDY

See End-of-Unit Summary for Unit 5 in Textbook

CONCEPTS FOR LECTURE

1. Nursing diagnoses are developed based on the medical diagnosis, physical assessment, the client's health history, and the pathophysiology of the disease process.
2. The nursing process is used as a guide to develop a plan of care for the client.

LECTURE OUTLINE IN POWERPOINT

Client with *Imbalanced Nutrition: More Than Body Requirements*
- Based on
  - Medical diagnosis
    - Type II diabetes mellitus
  - Physical assessment
  - Health history
  - Pathophysiology of disease process

Nursing Process
- Assessment
- Plan
- Nursing diagnosis
- Implementation, expected outcomes
- Evaluation

Nursing Diagnoses
- *Impaired Tissue Perfusion*
- *Risk for Injury*
- *Deficient Knowledge*

SUGGESTIONS FOR CLASSROOM ACTIVITIES

- Read the case study from the End-of-Unit Summary for Unit 5 in class. Review the concept map from the End-of-Unit Summary to develop a plan of care for the client.

SUGGESTIONS FOR CLINICAL ACTIVITIES

- Have students develop concept maps for clients to whom they provide nursing care in the acute or chronic healthcare setting.

UNIT 6
RESPONSES TO ALTERED NUTRITION

FUNCTIONAL HEALTH PATTERN

Nutritional-Metabolic

CONCEPTS FOR LECTURE

1. The medical diagnoses related to altered Nutritional-Metabolic Functional Health Pattern include: gastroesophageal reflux disease, cholelithiasis and cholecystitis, hepatitis, and pancreatitis.
2. The Nutritional-Metabolic Functional Health Pattern includes healthcare behaviors that interfere with nutritional status.
3. The Nutritional-Metabolic Functional Health Pattern includes nutrition as the process by which the body ingests, absorbs, transports, uses, and eliminates food to provide energy to maintain life.
4. Lack of proper nutrients may lead to nutritional disorders, inflammatory responses, or eating disorders.
5. Excess intake of nutrients may lead to obesity, nutritional disorders, and inflammatory responses.
6. Nutrients are used by the body to promote growth, maintenance, and repair.
7. Alterations in nutrition and metabolism may affect the body's ability to maintain itself, which leads to clinical manifestations such as: nausea, heartburn, and pain.
8. Priority nursing diagnoses for Nutritional-Metabolism Functional Health Pattern include: *Imbalanced Nutrition: Less than Body Requirements, Deficient Fluid Volume, Nausea,* and *Impaired Skin Integrity.*
9. Other nursing diagnoses applicable to clients with alterations in nutrition and metabolism include: *Acute Pain and Diarrhea.*

LECTURE OUTLINE IN POWERPOINT

Unit 6: Responses to Altered Nutrition
Nutritional-Metabolic Functional Health Pattern
- Medical diagnoses
  - Gastroesophageal reflux disease
  - Cholelithiasis, cholecystitis
  - Hepatitis, pancreatitis
Nutritional-Metabolic
- Healthcare behaviors interfere with nutritional status
  - Changes in appetite
  - On a prescribed diet, medications
  - Monitor daily intake of food and fluid
  - Adds salt or eats processed foods
Nutritional-Metabolic
- Healthcare behaviors interfere with nutritional status
  - Types of fluids consumed
  - Use of dietary supplements
  - Difficulty chewing or swallowing
  - Gaining or losing weight
Nutritional-Metabolic
- Nutrition of foods
  - Ingestion, absorption
  - Transport, use
  - Elimination
  - Determined by daily consumption of food, fluid okay
  - Provides energy to maintain life
Lack of Proper Nutrients
- Nutritional disorders
  - Dehydration, malnutrition
- Inflammatory responses
  - Gastritis, hepatitis
- Eating disorders
  - Anorexia nervosa, bulimia nervosa
Excess Intake of Nutrients
- Nutritional disorders
  - Obesity, alcoholic cirrhosis, cholelithiasis, elevated serum triglycerides
- Inflammatory responses
  - Acute pancreatitis
Body's Use of Nutrients
- Promote growth
- Promote maintenance
- Promote repair

Improper Intake of Nutrition
- Manifestations
  - Nausea
  - Heartburn
  - Pain

Priority Nursing Diagnoses
- *Imbalanced Nutrition: Less than Body Requirements*
- *Deficient Fluid Volume*
- *Nausea*
- *Impaired Skin Integrity*

Nursing Diagnoses from Other Functional Health Patterns
- *Acute Pain*
- *Diarrhea*

SUGGESTIONS FOR CLASSROOM ACTIVITIES

- Divide students into 10 groups. Assign an end-of-unit question to each group. Instruct the student groups to answer the questions and give a rationale for the answer they chose. Discuss why the other answers are incorrect.
- Using a model of the gastrointestinal system, trace food as it would move through the body from the mouth to the anus. Discuss the digestive processes of ingestion, absorption, transport, use, and elimination.
- Compare anorexia nervosa with bulimia nervosa, or cirrhosis with hepatitis. Discuss the similarities and differences in populations affected, and nursing interventions between the two nutritional disorders.
- Identify causes and types of dehydration. Review manifestations and complications. Discuss treatment options and nursing interventions.
- Develop a Bingo game; the categories across the top are types of diets and the six rows below each category are types of foods. For example, under the high potassium diet category, the foods listed may be orange juice, bananas, mushrooms, and so on; under the high calcium diet category, the foods listed may be milk, ice cream, cheese, yogurt, and so on. The instructor calls out the food product and the student who marks six in a row wins the game.

SUGGESTIONS FOR CLINICAL ACTIVITIES

- Assign students to provide nursing care to clients with gastrointestinal or nutritional disorders. Instruct them to develop a teaching plan for a client to instruct about a well-balanced diet based on the client's prescribed diet, that is, low-fat diet, low-salt diet, high-protein diet, and so on.
- Assign students to make rounds with a dietician or nutritionist. Have students identify specialized diets for clients with gastrointestinal disorders, nutritional disorders, or eating disorders.
- Have students make cards for the most common medications prescribed for gastrointestinal disorders. Include the drug classification, use, dosage, adverse effects, and desired response for each medication.

CLINICAL SCENARIOS

See End-of-Unit Summary for Unit 6 in Textbook

CONCEPTS FOR LECTURE

1. Client care should be prioritized according to the seriousness of the client's condition.
2. Prioritized nursing diagnoses assist the nurse in developing a plan of care for the client.
3. Strategies for prioritizing clients are based on the ABCs, Maslow's hierarchy of needs, developmental considerations, or crisis intervention.

LECTURE OUTLINE IN POWERPOINT

Prioritize Clients in Order of Visit
- Thomas Jones with cirrhosis of the liver
- Joseph Brown with acute gastritis
- Ruth Green with cholelithiasis and cholecystitis
- Tonya Cooper with dehydration r/t anorexia nervosa

Strategies for Prioritizing Client Care
- ABCs
- Maslow's hierarchy of needs
- Developmental considerations
- Crisis intervention

SUGGESTIONS FOR CLASSROOM ACTIVITIES

- Assign clinical scenarios to students. Instruct them to prioritize the clients in the order they should be seen. Discuss the rationale for the priority order.
- Have students choose two priority nursing diagnoses for each clinical scenario. Explain the rationale for each nursing diagnosis.
- Crisis intervention is composed of precipitating events, the client's perception of the events, and the client's usual coping methods. In the clinical scenario about Tonya Cooper, she is admitted with dehydration, weakness, and fainting related to anorexia nervosa. Her weight is below the ideal body weight for her height. Clients with anorexia nervosa perceive themselves as having excess body weight and develop patterns for weight loss. They become so absorbed with weight loss that they become malnourished. Treatment consists of changing the client's perception of their body image, strategies to improve self-esteem, and monitoring eating patterns to restore appropriate nutritional intake and weight gain.

SUGGESTIONS FOR CLINICAL ACTIVITIES

- Assign students to provide nursing care for more than one client. Have them prioritize the order in which to provide nursing care for the clients and discuss their rationale.
- Ask students to develop priority nursing diagnoses for the clients to whom they are providing nursing care in the acute or chronic healthcare setting.

CASE STUDY

See End-of-Unit Summary for Unit 6 in Textbook

CONCEPTS FOR LECTURE

1. Nursing diagnoses are developed based on the medical diagnosis, physical assessment, the client's health history, and the pathophysiology of the disease process.
2. The nursing process is used as a guide to develop a plan of care for the client.

LECTURE OUTLINE IN POWERPOINT

Client with Imbalanced Nutrition: Less Than Body Requirements
- Based on
  - Medical diagnosis
    - Acute gastritis
  - Physical assessment
  - Health history
  - Pathophysiology of disease process
Nursing Process
- Assessment
- Plan
- Nursing diagnosis
- Implementation, expected outcomes
- Evaluation
Nursing Diagnoses
- *Nausea*
- *Diarrhea*
- *Deficient Fluid Volume*

SUGGESTIONS FOR CLASSROOM ACTIVITIES

- Read the case study from the End-of-Unit Summary for Unit 6 in class. Review the concept map from the End-of-Unit Summary to develop a plan of care for the client.

SUGGESTIONS FOR CLINICAL ACTIVITIES

- Instruct students to develop a concept map for the clients to whom they are assigned to provide nursing care in the acute or chronic healthcare setting.

UNIT 7
RESPONSES TO ALTERED BOWEL ELIMINATION

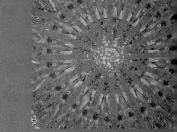

FUNCTIONAL HEALTH PATTERN

Elimination

CONCEPTS FOR LECTURE

1. The medical diagnoses related to altered Elimination Functional Health Pattern include: diarrhea, constipation, irritable bowel syndrome, fecal incontinence, appendicitis, peritonitis, gastroenteritis, protozoal bowel infection, helminthic disorder, inflammatory bowel disorder, sprue, lactose deficiency, short bowel syndrome, polyps, colorectal cancer, hernia, intestinal obstruction, diverticular disease, hemorrhoids, or anorectal lesions.
2. The Elimination Functional Health Pattern includes healthcare behaviors that interfere with the client's bowel elimination status.
3. The Elimination Functional Health Pattern includes bowel function, which can be affected by inflammation, infection, tumors, obstructions, or changes in structure.
4. Direct factors that affect consistency of stool include: food and fluid intake, food poisoning, bacterial population, surgical procedures, medical conditions, medication intake, and herbal preparation intake.
5. Indirect factors that affect consistency of stool include: psychologic stress, depression, voluntary postponement of defecation, or decreased exercise activity.
6. Bowel elimination is the end product of digestion.
7. Alterations in bowel elimination may affect the body's ability to maintain itself, which leads to clinical manifestations such as: diarrhea, constipation, and flatus.
8. Priority nursing diagnoses for bowel Elimination Functional Health Pattern include: *Bowel Incontinence, Diarrhea, Constipation,* and *Deficient Fluid Volume.*
9. Other nursing diagnoses applicable to clients with alterations in bowel elimination include: *Acute Pain* and *Imbalanced Nutrition: Less Than Body Requirements.*

LECTURE OUTLINE IN POWERPOINT

Unit 7: Responses to Altered Bowel Elimination
Elimination Functional Health Pattern
- Medical diagnoses
  - Diarrhea, constipation, irritable bowel syndrome
  - Fecal incontinence, appendicitis, peritonitis, gastroenteritis
  - Protozoal bowel infection, helminthic disorder, sprue
Elimination Functional Health Pattern
- Medical diagnoses
  - Inflammatory bowel disorder, lactose deficiency, hernia
  - Short bowel syndrome, polyps, colorectal cancer
  - Intestinal obstruction, diverticular disease
  - Hemorrhoids, anorectal lesions
Elimination
- Healthcare behaviors interfere with elimination
  - Bowel movement pattern
  - Changes in bowel routine
  - Changes in color and consistency of stool
  - Loose bowel movements
  - Strain excessively with bowel movements
Elimination
- Healthcare behaviors interfere with elimination
  - Use of laxatives
  - Causes of bleeding with bowel movement
  - Causes of cramping or abdominal pain
  - Taking medications that affect bowel movement
Elimination
- Healthcare behaviors interfere with elimination
  - Illnesses or surgery that affect bowel movements
  - Any food intolerances or on special diet
  - Had a colonoscopy or other diagnostic tests
  - Have an ostomy and care of ostomy
Elimination
- Bowel function affected by
  - Inflammation
  - Infection
  - Tumors, obstructions
  - Change in intestinal structure
Direct Factors That Affect Consistency of Stool
- Food and fluid intake
  - Constipation, diarrhea
- Food poisoning
  - Diarrhea

- Bacterial population
  - Diarrhea

Direct Factors That Affect Consistency of Stool
- Surgical procedures
  - Constipation
- Medical conditions
  - Constipation

Direct Factors That Affect Consistency of Stool
- Medications
  - Constipation
  - Diarrhea
- Herbal preparations
  - Diarrhea
  - Constipation

Indirect Factors That Affect Consistency of Stool
- Psychological stress
  - Diarrhea
- Depression
  - Constipation

Indirect Factors That Affect Consistency of Stool
- Voluntary postponement of defecation
  - Constipation
  - Abdominal pain
- Decreased exercise activity
  - Constipation

Bowel Elimination
- Absorption of nutrients during digestion
- Elimination of indigestible materials

Improper Bowel Elimination
- Manifestations
  - Diarrhea
  - Constipation
  - Flatus

Priority Nursing Diagnoses
- *Bowel Incontinence*
- *Diarrhea*
- *Constipation*
- *Deficient Fluid Volume*

Nursing Diagnoses from Other Functional Health Patterns
- *Acute Pain*
- *Imbalanced Nutrition: Less Than Body Requirements*

SUGGESTIONS FOR CLASSROOM ACTIVITIES

- Divide students into 10 groups. Assign an end-of-unit question to each group. Instruct students to answer the questions and give a rationale for the answer selected. Discuss why the other answers are incorrect.
- Review disease processes or disorders caused by health behaviors that interfere with elimination such as overuse of laxatives, and medications and diet. Discuss teaching that may be done by the nurse to treat or prevent these disease processes or disorders.

SUGGESTIONS FOR CLINICAL ACTIVITIES

- Assign students to provide nursing care to clients with gastrointestinal disorders. Have them provide ostomy care when available. Have them discuss the nursing care provided in post-conference and complete a concept map or nursing care plan that utilizes the nursing process.
- Arrange for students to observe in the endoscopy unit. Have students follow a client from admission to the outpatient unit, to the endoscopy lab to observe a colonscopy examination, and to follow the client to

- Using a model of the gastrointestinal system, review the formation and passage of bowel contents through the system. Discuss absorption of nutrients and the importance of nutrition in clients who have short gut syndrome.
- Divide students into small groups and have them develop an NCLEX®-style question related to bowel elimination that includes the rationale for the answer. Instruct students to include information concerning the portion of the nursing process utilized in the question development. Share the questions and answers at the end of the class.

the recovery area and discharge. Assign the students a process paper that involves their observations, the role of the nurse, preprocedure medication administered, how the procedure was performed, and the discharge criteria.
- Have students complete a gastrointestinal scenario on a human simulator model in the clinical laboratory, such as an open appendectomy postoperative client with peritonitis from a ruptured appendix. Have students perform dressing changes and administer intravenous fluids with piggyback antibiotics. Have the model develop an allergic reaction to the antibiotic to test students' knowledge of the appropriate interventions.

CLINICAL SCENARIOS

See End-of-Unit Summary for Unit 7 in Textbook

CONCEPTS FOR LECTURE

1. Client care should be prioritized according to the seriousness of the client's condition.
2. Prioritized nursing diagnoses assist the nurse in developing a plan of care for the client.
3. Strategies for prioritizing clients are based on the ABCs, Maslow's hierarchy of needs, developmental considerations, or crisis intervention.

LECTURE OUTLINE IN POWERPOINT

Prioritize Clients in Order of Visit
- Jason Phillips with right lower quadrant pain
- Mary Joslin with diarrhea and abdominal cramping
- Grace Freeman with a colostomy
- Paul Bruner with an abdominal mass

Strategies for Prioritizing Client Care
- ABCs
- Maslow's hierarchy of needs
- Developmental considerations
- Crisis intervention

SUGGESTIONS FOR CLASSROOM ACTIVITIES

- Instruct students to read the clinical scenarios and prioritize the clients in the order they should be seen. Discuss the rationale for the priority order.
- Instruct students to choose two priority nursing diagnoses for each clinical scenario client. Explain the rationale for each nursing diagnosis.
- Maslow's hierarchy of needs includes pain relief as a physiological need. Jason Phillips is admitted with right lower quadrant pain, low grade fever, tachycardia, and nausea. A sudden relief of pain may indicate a ruptured appendix. The physician needs to be notified for further evaluation and the possibility of surgery. A ruptured appendix may result in peritonitis.

SUGGESTIONS FOR CLINICAL ACTIVITIES

- Assign students to provide nursing care for more than one client. Instruct them to prioritize the order in which to provide nursing care for the clients and discuss the rationale.
- Instruct students to develop priority nursing diagnoses for the clients to whom they are providing nursing care in the acute or chronic healthcare setting.

CASE STUDY

See End-of-Unit Summary for Unit 1 in Textbook

CONCEPTS FOR LECTURE

1. Nursing diagnoses are developed based on the medical diagnosis, physical assessment, the client's health history, and the pathophysiology of the disease process.
2. The nursing process is used as a guide to develop a plan of care for the client.

LECTURE OUTLINE IN POWERPOINT

Client with Diarrhea
- Based on
  - Medical diagnosis
    - Ulcerative colitis
  - Physical assessment
  - Health history
  - Pathophysiology of disease process

Nursing Process
- Assessment
- Plan
- Nursing diagnosis
- Implementation, expected outcomes
- Evaluation

Nursing Diagnoses
- *Disturbed Body Image*
- *Risk for Deficient Fluid Volume*
- *Pain*

SUGGESTIONS FOR CLASSROOM ACTIVITIES

- Read the case study from the End-of-Unit Summary for Unit 7 in class. Review the concept map from the End-of-Unit Summary to develop a plan of care for the client.

SUGGESTIONS FOR CLINICAL ACTIVITIES

- Instruct students to develop a concept map for clients to whom they provide nursing care in the acute or chronic healthcare setting.

UNIT 8
RESPONSES TO ALTERED URINARY ELIMINATION

FUNCTIONAL HEALTH PATTERN

Elimination

CONCEPTS FOR LECTURE

1. The medical diagnoses related to altered Elimination Functional Health Pattern include: urinary tract infection, urinary calculi, urinary tract tumor, urinary retention, neurogenic bladder, urinary incontinence, congenital kidney malformation, polycystic kidneys, glomerular disease, vascular kidney disease, kidney trauma, renal tumor, acute renal failure, or chronic renal failure.

2. The Elimination Functional Health Pattern includes healthcare behaviors that interfere with the client's urinary elimination status.

3. The urinary system includes the kidneys, ureters, urinary bladder, and urethra. Disorders of these organs affect urine production and waste elimination.

4. Disorders may affect urinary elimination with too little or too much urinary output.

5. Functions of the urinary system are to: regulate body fluids, filter metabolic wastes from bloodstream, absorb needed substances and water into bloodstream, and eliminate metabolic wastes and water as urine.

6. Alterations in urinary elimination may affect the body's ability to maintain itself, which leads to clinical manifestations such as: hematuria, proteinuria, and pyuria.

7. Priority nursing diagnoses for urinary Elimination Functional Health Pattern include: *Urinary Retention, Stress Urinary Incontinence, Impaired Urinary Elimination,* and *Urge Urinary Incontinence.*

8. Other nursing diagnoses applicable to clients with alterations in urinary elimination include: *Ineffective Health Maintenance* and *Acute Pain.*

LECTURE OUTLINE IN POWERPOINT

Unit 8: Responses to Altered Urinary Elimination
Elimination Functional Health Pattern
- Medical diagnoses
  - Urinary tract infection, urinary calculi
  - Urinary tract tumor, urinary retention,
  - Neurogenic bladder, urinary incontinence
  - Congenital kidney malformation, polycystic kidneys

Elimination Functional Health Pattern
- Medical diagnoses
  - Glomerular disease, vascular kidney disease
  - Kidney trauma, renal tumor
  - Acute renal failure, chronic renal failure

Elimination
- Health behaviors interfere with elimination
  - Times per day to urinate
  - Times during night to urinate
  - Emptying bladder with urination
  - Burning or pain upon urination
  - Strong urge to urinate, blood in urine

Elimination
- Health behaviors interfere with elimination
  - Change in amount, color, odor of urine
  - Difficulty stopping or starting urination
  - Problems with incontinence of urine
  - Pain in back or costovertebral angle

Elimination
- Health behaviors interfere with elimination
  - Amount and type of fluid intake
  - Surgery or other treatment for bladder/kidney disease
  - Taking medication for urinary problems
  - Wear an external catheter, indwelling catheter

Elimination
- Urinary system
  - Kidneys, ureters, urinary bladder, urethra
  - Disorders affect urine production, waste elimination

Disorders with Too Little Urinary Output
- Obstruction
  - Tumors
- Disease
  - Glomerulonephritis, pyelonephritis, renal calculi, renal failure
- Medications, trauma
  - Urinary retention

Disorders with Too Much Urinary Output
- Disease
  - Diabetes mellitus
- Infection
  - Urinary tract infection

Functions of Urinary System
- Regulate body fluids
- Filter metabolic wastes
- Absorb needed substances and water
- Eliminate metabolic wastes and water

Alterations in Urinary Elimination
- Manifestations
  - Hematuria
  - Proteinuria
  - Pyuria

Priority Nursing Diagnoses
- *Urinary Retention*
- *Stress Urinary Incontinence*
- *Impaired Urinary Elimination*
- *Urge Urinary Incontinence*

Nursing Diagnoses from Other Functional Health Patterns
- *Ineffective Health Maintenance*
- *Acute Pain*

SUGGESTIONS FOR CLASSROOM ACTIVITIES

- Divide students into 10 groups. Assign an end-of-unit question to each group. Have them answer the questions and give a rationale for the answer they chose. Discuss why the other answers are incorrect.
- Using a model of the urinary tract system, explain functioning of the kidney, how urine is produced, and the path of urinary excretion from the body.
- Review health behaviors that interfere with urinary elimination such as incontinence, pain, urgency, medications, and fluid intake. Discuss disease processes or disorders that result from these behaviors and teaching that may be done by the nurse to treat or prevent these disease processes or disorders.
- Obtain paint chips from a hardware or paint store to demonstrate different colors of urine: straw color for normal urine, dark yellow for concentrated urine, red for fresh bloody urine, tea-colored for old bloody urine, dark yellow-green for bilirubin in urine, and blue or green for medications in urine.

SUGGESTIONS FOR CLINICAL ACTIVITIES

- Assign students to provide nursing care to clients with kidney disorders or diseases. Have them develop a concept map or nursing care plan for the client that utilizes the nursing process.
- Arrange for students to observe at a dialysis center. Have them write a paper about their observations at the dialysis center and have them compare hemodialysis with peritoneal dialysis.
- Have students complete a genitourinary scenario on a human simulator model in the clinical laboratory, such as a postoperative nephrectomy client. Have the model develop a hemorrhage that necessitates a return to surgery. Upon return from surgery, have students perform dressing changes with a J-P drain, indwelling urinary catheter care, administer intravenous fluids, and administer antibiotics and pain medication.

CLINICAL SCENARIOS

See End-of-Unit Summary for Unit 8 in Textbook

CONCEPTS FOR LECTURE

1. Client care should be prioritized according to the seriousness of the client's condition.
2. Prioritized nursing diagnoses assist the nurse in developing a plan of care for the client.

LECTURE OUTLINE IN POWERPOINT

Prioritize Clients in Order of Visit
- Phillip Jones with a bruised right kidney
- Agnes Smith with urinary tract infection
- Joseph Rouse with kidney stones
- Angela Baldwin with glomerulonephritis

3. Strategies for prioritizing clients are based on the ABCs, Maslow's hierarchy of needs, developmental considerations, or crisis intervention.

Strategies for Prioritizing Client Care
- ABCs
- Maslow's hierarchy of needs
- Developmental considerations
- Crisis intervention

SUGGESTIONS FOR CLASSROOM ACTIVITIES

- Have students read the clinical scenarios and prioritize the clients in the order they should be seen. Discuss the rationale for the priority order.
- Have students choose two priority nursing diagnoses for each clinical scenario client. Explain the rationale for each nursing diagnosis.
- In the ABCs, C stands for circulation. Joseph Rouse is pale, cool, and clammy due to severe left-sided flank pain. Acute pain initiates the "flight or fight" response which increases cardiac contractility and results in an increase in heart rate, increase in respiratory rate, sweating, pallor, and anxiety. Renal spasms cause a vasovagal response that results in decreased blood pressure and syncope. Medicating for pain and renal spasms should help to relieve some of the symptoms he is experiencing.

SUGGESTIONS FOR CLINICAL ACTIVITIES

- Assign students to provide nursing care for more than one client. Have them prioritize the order in which to provide nursing care for the clients and discuss their rationale.
- Have students develop priority nursing diagnoses for the clients to whom they are providing nursing care in the acute or chronic healthcare setting.

CASE STUDY

See End-of-Unit Summary for Unit 8 in Textbook

CONCEPTS FOR LECTURE

1. Nursing diagnoses are developed based on the medical diagnosis, physical assessment, the client's health history, and the pathophysiology of the disease process.
2. The nursing process is used as a guide to develop a plan of care for the client.

LECTURE OUTLINE IN POWERPOINT

Nursing Diagnosis
- Based on Impaired Urinary Elimination
  - Medical diagnosis
    - Chronic renal failure
  - Physical assessment
  - Health history
  - Pathophysiology of disease process
Nursing Process
- Assessment
- Plan
- Nursing diagnosis
- Implementation, expected outcomes
- Evaluation
Nursing Diagnoses
- *Ineffective Therapeutic Regimen*
- *Imbalanced Nutrition: More than Body Requirements*
- *Ineffective Health Maintenance*

SUGGESTIONS FOR CLASSROOM ACTIVITIES

- Read the case study from the End-of-Unit Summary for Unit 8 in class. Review the concept map from the End-of-Unit Summary to develop a plan of care for the client.

SUGGESTIONS FOR CLINICAL ACTIVITIES

- Have students develop a concept map for clients to whom they provide nursing care in the acute or chronic healthcare setting.

UNIT 9
RESPONSES TO ALTERED CARDIAC FUNCTION

FUNCTIONAL HEALTH PATTERN

Activity-Exercise

CONCEPTS FOR LECTURE

1. The medical diagnoses related to altered Activity-Exercise Functional Health Pattern include: myocardial infarction, heart failure, and valvular heart disease.
2. The Activity-Exercise Functional Health Pattern includes healthcare behaviors that interfere with the client's cardiac function.
3. The Activity-Exercise Functional Health Pattern includes activities of daily living and patterns of exercise and activity. The heart delivers fuel that provides energy production to the cells in order to accomplish these activities.
4. The heart's pumping ability is affected by damage to the heart muscle caused by ischemic processes, inflammatory responses, and cardiac muscle disorders.
5. The heart's pumping ability is affected by excessive cardiac workload caused by hypertension, valve disorders, and congenital defects.
6. When the heart fails to pump effectively, less fuel is delivered to cells, energy production fails, and activity decreases.
7. Alterations in cardiac function may affect the body's ability to maintain itself, which leads to clinical manifestations such as: fatigue, shortness of breath, dyspnea, and tachycardia.
8. Priority nursing diagnoses for the Activity-Exercise Functional Health Pattern include: *Decreased Cardiac Output, Activity Intolerance, Fatigue,* and *Ineffective Tissue Perfusion.*
9. Other nursing diagnoses applicable to clients with alterations in cardiac function include: *Acute Pain* and *Anxiety.*

LECTURE OUTLINE IN POWERPOINT

Unit 9: Responses to Altered Cardiac Function
Activity-Exercise Functional Health Pattern
- Medical diagnoses
  - Myocardial infarction
  - Heart failure
  - Valvular heart disease
Activity-Exercise
- Response to activity
- Heart rate increases or decreases
- Respiratory rate and effort
- Become lightheaded during activity
- Have chest pain during activity
- Oxygen saturation stable or drop with activity
Activity-Exercise
- Heart pumps to deliver fuel to cells
- Energy production results from fuel
- Expenditure of energy for activities of daily living, exercise
Damage to Heart Muscle
- Ischemic processes
  - Coronary heart disease
- Inflammatory responses
  - Rheumatic carditis, endocarditis
- Primary cardiac muscle disorder
  - Cardiomyopathy
Excessive Cardiac Work
- Excessive workload
  - Hypertension, valve disorder, congenital defects
Decreased Cardiac Function
- Decreased pumping ability
- Less fuel delivered to cells
- Energy production fails
- Decreased activity abilities
Impaired Cardiac Function
- Manifestations
  - Fatigue
  - Shortness of breath, dyspnea
  - Tachycardia
Priority Nursing Diagnoses
- *Decreased Cardiac Output*
- *Activity Intolerance*
- *Fatigue*
- *Ineffective Tissue Perfusion*
Nursing Diagnoses from Other Functional Patterns
- *Acute Pain*
- *Anxiety*

SUGGESTIONS FOR CLASSROOM ACTIVITIES

- Divide students into 10 groups. Assign an end-of-unit question to each group. Have them answer the questions and give a rationale for the answer they chose. Discuss why the other answers are incorrect.
- Using a model of the cardiac system, trace a drop of blood throughout the system. Discuss cardiac terminology such as preload, afterload, cardiac output, murmurs, thrills, and so on. Review how the heart responds to activity and exercise.
- Review disease processes or disorders that damage heart muscle, increase the workload of the heart, and decrease heart function. Discuss teaching that may be done by the nurse to assist the client to increase activity levels and to decrease further cardiac compromise.
- Have students listen to heart sounds on a computer. Websites such as http://www.blaufuss.org have various heart sounds. Have the student hold a stethoscope to the computer speaker and listen to the heart sounds through a stethoscope.

SUGGESTIONS FOR CLINICAL ACTIVITIES

- Assign students to provide nursing care to clients with cardiac disorders. Have them discuss the nursing care provided in post-conference and complete a concept map or nursing care plan that utilizes the nursing process.
- Arrange for students to observe at a cardiac rehabilitation program. Identify the cardiac exercise programs set up for the clients. Discuss the role of a cardiac rehabilitation nurse.
- Have students complete a cardiovascular scenario on a human simulator model in the clinical laboratory, such as a client with congestive heart failure who goes into cardiac arrest. Have students demonstrate a cardiovascular assessment, CPR, and administer medications and intravenous fluids.

CLINICAL SCENARIOS

See End-of-Unit Summary for Unit 9 in Textbook

CONCEPTS FOR LECTURE

1. Client care should be prioritized according to the seriousness of the client's condition.
2. Prioritized nursing diagnoses assist the nurse in developing a plan of care for the client.
3. Strategies for prioritizing clients are based on the ABCs, Maslow's hierarchy of needs, developmental considerations, or crisis intervention.

LECTURE OUTLINE IN POWERPOINT

Prioritize Clients in Order of Visit
- Betty Williams with anterior myocardial infarction
- Arnold Markus with acute heart failure
- Sandra Thomas with mitral regurgitation
- Randall Stevens with infective endocarditis

Strategies for Prioritizing Client Care
- ABCs
- Maslow's hierarchy of needs
- Developmental considerations
- Crisis intervention

SUGGESTIONS FOR CLASSROOM ACTIVITIES

- Have students read the clinical scenarios and prioritize the clients in the order they should be seen. Discuss the rationale for the priority order.
- Have students choose two priority nursing diagnoses for each clinical scenario patient. Explain the rationale for each nursing diagnosis.
- In the ABCs, C stands for circulation. Betty Williams is admitted with an acute anterior myocardial infarction. Myocardial infarction is caused by an obstruction in a coronary artery that results in decreased circulation to heart muscle. Necrosis of a portion of cardiac muscle results. In Betty Williams' case, the interruption of blood circulation is in an anterior portion of her heart. She is treated successfully with nitroglycerine and thrombolytic therapy.

SUGGESTIONS FOR CLINICAL ACTIVITIES

- Assign students to provide nursing care for more than one client. Have them prioritize the order in which to provide nursing care for the clients and discuss their rationale.
- Have students develop priority nursing diagnoses for the clients to whom they are providing nursing care in the acute or chronic healthcare setting.

CASE STUDY

See End-of-Unit Summary for Unit 9 in Textbook

CONCEPTS FOR LECTURE

1. Nursing diagnoses are developed based on the medical diagnosis, physical assessment, the client's health history, and the pathophysiology of the disease process.
2. The nursing process is used as a guide to develop a plan of care.

LECTURE OUTLINE IN POWERPOINT

Client with Decreased Cardiac Output
- Based on
  - Medical diagnosis
    - Acute heart failure
  - Physical assessment
  - Health history
  - Pathophysiology of disease process

Nursing Process
- Assessment
- Plan
- Nursing diagnosis
- Implementation, expected outcomes
- Evaluation

Nursing Diagnoses
- *Excess Fluid Volume*
- *Activity Intolerance*
- *Fatigue*

SUGGESTIONS FOR CLASSROOM ACTIVITIES

- Read the case study from the End-of-Unit Summary for Unit 9 in class. Review the concept map from the End-of-Unit Summary to develop a plan of care for the client.

SUGGESTIONS FOR CLINICAL ACTIVITIES

- Have students develop a concept map for clients to whom they provide nursing care in the acute or chronic healthcare setting.

UNIT 10
RESPONSES TO ALTERED PERIPHERAL PERFUSION

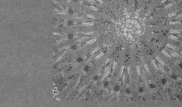

FUNCTIONAL HEALTH PATTERN

Activity-Exercise

CONCEPTS FOR LECTURE

1. The medical diagnoses related to altered Activity-Exercise Functional Health Pattern include: anemia, polycythemia, leukemia, malignant lymphoma, multiple myeloma, neutropenia, infectious mononucleosis, thrombocytopenia, hemophilia, disseminated intravascular coagulation, hypertension, aneurysm, and peripheral vascular disease.

2. The Activity-Exercise Functional Health Pattern includes healthcare behaviors that interfere with peripheral tissue perfusion.

3. The Activity-Exercise Functional Health Pattern includes alterations in the functions of blood: transporting oxygen, nutrients, hormones, and metabolic wastes; protecting against invasion of pathogens; maintaining blood coagulation; and regulating fluids, electrolytes, acids, bases, and body temperature.

4. The Activity-Exercise Functional Health Pattern includes alterations in the function of the lymphatic system which helps to maintain sufficient blood volume.

5. Disorders that interfere with the functioning of the blood and lymphatic systems, including constriction, obstruction, inflammation, and vasospasm, result in insufficient physiologic energy to carry out activities of daily living.

6. Factors affected by too few blood cells: anemia, leucopenia, and thrombocytopenia.

7. Factors affected by too many blood cells: polycythemia, leukocytosis, and lymphocytosis.

8. Disorders of peripheral tissue perfusion lead to problems with blood pressure regulation, decreased peripheral artery function, problems with aortic structure, decreased venous circulation, and decreased lymphatic circulation.

9. Alterations in peripheral tissue perfusion may affect the body's ability to maintain itself, leading to clinical manifestations such as: fatigue, edema, and bleeding.

10. Priority nursing diagnoses for Activity-Exercise Functional Health Pattern are: *Ineffective Tissue Perfusion, Decreased Cardiac Output, Risk for Peripheral Neurovascular Dysfunction,* and *Activity Intolerance.*

11. Other nursing diagnoses applicable to clients with alterations in peripheral tissue perfusion are: *Impaired Tissue Integrity* and *Effective Therapeutic Regimen Maintenance.*

LECTURE OUTLINE IN POWERPOINT

Unit 10: Responses to Altered Peripheral Tissue Perfusion

Activity-Exercise Functional Health Pattern
- Medical diagnoses
  - Anemia, polycythemia, leukemia, malignant lymphoma
  - Multiple myeloma, neutropenia, infectious mononucleosis
  - Thrombocytopenia, hemophilia, disseminated intravascular coagulation
  - Hypertension, aneurysm, peripheral vascular disease

Activity-Exercise Functional Health Pattern
- Medical diagnoses
  - Thromboangitis obliterans, Raynaud's disease
  - Acute arterial occlusion, venous thrombosis, varicose veins
  - Chronic venous insufficiency, lymphadenopathy, lymphedema

Activity-Exercise
- Interferes with peripheral tissue perfusion
  - Exercise regularly
  - Have leg pain with activity or at rest
  - Swelling of ankles end of day, at night, while sitting
  - Have leg cramps at night

Activity-Exercise
- Interferes with peripheral tissue perfusion
  - Temperature or position affect symptoms
  - Have pain, burning, numbness, tingling
  - Changes in skin color, temperature, hair texture
  - Interferes with peripheral tissue perfusion

Activity-Exercise
- Interferes with peripheral tissue perfusion
  - Changes in ulcers or skin irritations, varicose veins
  - Swelling of neck glands after infection
  - Increased fatigue or weakness
  - History of illness, surgery, environmental exposure
  - Take medications, drink alcohol or smoke

Activity-Exercise
- Functions of blood
  - Transporting oxygen, nutrients, hormones, metabolic waste

---

- Protecting against invasion of pathogens
- Maintaining blood coagulation
- Regulating fluid, electrolytes, acids, bases, temperature

Activity-Exercise
- Functions of lymphatic system
  - Maintain sufficient blood volume

Activity-Exercise
- Disorders interfering with blood and lymph
  - Constriction, obstruction
  - Inflammation, vasospasm
  - Insufficient physiologic energy for ADLs

Factors Affected by Too Few Blood Cells
- Anemia
  - Blood loss, nutritional, hemolytic
- Leukopenia
  - Neutropenia, autoimmune disorders
- Thrombocytopenia
  - Aplastic anemia, thrombocytopenia purpura, DIC

Factors Affected by Too Many Blood Cells
- Polycythemia
  - Polycythemia vera, secondary polycythemia
- Leukocytosis
  - Leukemia
- Lymphocytosis
  - Malignant lymphoma, multiple myeloma

Peripheral Tissue Perfusion
- Disorders lead to
  - Blood pressure regulation problems
  - Decreased peripheral artery function
  - Problems with aortic structure
  - Decreased venous circulation, lymphatic circulation

Impaired Peripheral Tissue Perfusion
- Manifestations
  - Fatigue
  - Edema
  - Bleeding

Priority Nursing Diagnoses
- *Ineffective Tissue Perfusion*
- *Decreased Cardiac Output*
- *Risk for Peripheral Neurovascular Dysfunction*
- *Activity Intolerance*

Nursing Diagnoses from Other Functional Health Patterns
- *Impaired Tissue Integrity*
- *Effective Therapeutic Regimen Maintenance*

SUGGESTIONS FOR CLASSROOM ACTIVITIES

- Divide students into 10 groups. Assign an end-of-unit question to each group. Have them answer the questions and give a rationale for the answer they chose. Discuss why the other answers are incorrect.
- Using a model of the lymphatic system, trace movement of lymph throughout the body. Discuss the function of the lymphatic system.

SUGGESTIONS FOR CLINICAL ACTIVITIES

- Assign students to provide nursing care to clients with alterations in peripheral tissue perfusion. Have them discuss the nursing care provided in post-conference and complete a concept map or nursing care plan that utilizes the nursing process.

SUGGESTIONS FOR CLASSROOM ACTIVITIES *continued*

- Review disease processes or disorders that interfere with peripheral tissue perfusion. Discuss teaching that may be done by the nurse to assist the client to increase activity levels and to decrease further cardiac compromise.
- Compare heparin and the new low molecular weight heparins with warfarin (Coumadin). Review bleeding precautions, laboratory studies, diet, antidotes, and use of a Medic-Alert bracelet.

SUGGESTIONS FOR CLINICAL ACTIVITIES *continued*

- Arrange for students to observe a nurse practitioner in a cardiovascular office. Have them write a paper about the role of the nurse practitioner and the teaching by the nurse practitioner, including activity, diet, and medications.
- Arrange for students to work with a school nurse to take blood pressures on children in the school system or with an industrial nurse to take blood pressures on adults in a factory. Have students identify normal and abnormal blood pressures in children and adults.
- Have students complete a cardiovascular scenario on a human simulator model in the clinical laboratory, such as a client with deep vein thrombosis. Have students demonstrate a cardiovascular assessment, discuss laboratory studies, administer subcutaneous anticoagulant medications, and wean to oral anticoagulant medications.

CLINICAL SCENARIOS

See End-of-Unit Summary for Unit 10 in Textbook

CONCEPTS FOR LECTURE

1. Client care should be prioritized according to the seriousness of the client's condition.
2. Prioritized nursing diagnoses assist the nurse in developing a plan of care for the client.
3. Strategies for prioritizing clients are based on the ABCs, Maslow's hierarchy of needs, developmental considerations, or crisis intervention.

LECTURE OUTLINE IN POWERPOINT

Prioritize Clients in Order of Visit
- Theresa Cartwright with a deep vein thrombosis
- Bessie Gregg with delirium tremens
- Scott Jacoby with leukemia
- Robert Tucker with abdominal aortic aneurysm

Strategies for Prioritizing Client Care
- ABCs
- Maslow's hierarchy of needs
- Developmental considerations
- Crisis intervention

SUGGESTIONS FOR CLASSROOM ACTIVITIES

- Have students read the clinical scenarios and prioritize the clients in the order they should be seen. Discuss the rationale for the priority order.
- Have students choose two priority nursing diagnoses for each clinical scenario client. Explain the rationale for each nursing diagnosis.
- In the ABCs, C stands for circulation. Theresa Cartwright is admitted with a deep vein thrombosis, or blood clot, in a calf. A thrombosis interrupts blood circulation by narrowing or completely occluding a blood vessel. Immediate treatment is essential because a blood clot may dislodge, travel to the pulmonary artery, and cause a pulmonary embolism that may be fatal. Mrs. Cartwright is being treated with heparin to prevent further blood clots from forming.

SUGGESTIONS FOR CLINICAL ACTIVITIES

- Assign students to provide nursing care for more than one client. Have them prioritize the order of nursing care for the clients and discuss their rationale.
- Have students develop priority nursing diagnoses for the clients to whom they are providing nursing care in the acute or chronic healthcare setting.

CASE STUDY

See End-of-Unit Summary for Unit 10 in Textbook

CONCEPTS FOR LECTURE

1. Nursing diagnoses are developed based on the medical diagnosis, physical assessment, the client's health history, and the pathophysiology of the disease process.
2. The nursing process is used as a guide to develop a plan of care for the client.

LECTURE OUTLINE IN POWERPOINT

Nursing Diagnosis
- Based on Ineffective Therapeutic Regimen Management
  - Medical diagnosis
    - Hypertension
  - Physical assessment
  - Health history
  - Pathophysiology of disease process
Nursing Process
- Assessment
- Plan
- Nursing diagnosis
- Implementation, expected outcomes
- Evaluation
Nursing Diagnoses
- *Imbalanced Nutrition: More Than Body Requirements*
- *Ineffective Health Maintenance*

SUGGESTIONS FOR CLASSROOM ACTIVITIES

- Read the case study from the End-of-Unit Summary for Unit 10 in class. Review the concept map from the End-of-Unit Summary to develop a plan of care for the client.

SUGGESTIONS FOR CLINICAL ACTIVITIES

- Have students develop a concept map for clients to whom they provide nursing care in the acute or chronic healthcare setting.

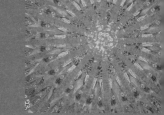

FUNCTIONAL HEALTH PATTERN

Activity-Exercise

CONCEPTS FOR LECTURE

1. The medical diagnoses related to altered Activity-Exercise Functional Health Pattern include: viral respiratory infection, sinusitis, pharyngitis, laryngeal infection, diphtheria, pertussis, respiratory trauma or obstruction, epistaxis, obstructive sleep apnea, upper respiratory tumors, bacterial respiratory infection, severe acute respiratory syndrome, lung abscess, tuberculosis, inhalation anthrax, fungal infections, lung cancer, pleuritis, pleural effusion, pneumothorax, hemothorax, inhalation injury, asthma, COPD, cystic fibrosis, atelectasis, occupational lung disease, sarcoidosis, pulmonary embolism, pulmonary hypertension, and respiratory failure.

2. The Activity-Exercise Functional Health Pattern includes healthcare behaviors that interfere with respiratory function.

3. The Activity-Exercise Functional Health Pattern includes disorders that result in insufficient physiologic energy to carry out activities of daily living. The respiratory system is a gas exchange system that provides cells with oxygen and eliminates carbon dioxide with each respiration.

4. The amount of gas exchange in the respiratory system is affected by factors that impact respirations, such as infection or inflammatory disorders, respiratory trauma or obstruction, or tumors.

5. The amount of gas exchange in the respiratory system is affected by factors that impact ventilation, such as infections or inflammatory disorders, pleural disorders, trauma, inhalation injury, obstructive disorders, pulmonary vascular disorders, and respiratory failure.

6. The upper respiratory system functions to maintain breathing through a patent airway and to allow communication.

7. The lower respiratory system functions to move air in and out of the lungs (ventilation), and to perform gas exchange across the alveolar-capillary membrane (respiration).

8. Alterations in respiratory function may affect the body's ability to maintain itself, which leads to clinical manifestations such as: rhinorrhea, cyanosis, and wheezing.

9. Priority nursing diagnoses for Activity–Exercise Functional Health Pattern include: *Ineffective Breathing*

LECTURE OUTLINE IN POWERPOINT

Unit 11: Responses to Altered Respiratory Function
Activity-Exercise Functional Health Pattern
- Medical diagnoses
  - Viral respiratory infection, sinusitis, pharyngitis
  - Laryngeal infection, diphtheria, pertussis, epistaxis
  - Respiratory trauma or obstruction, lung abscess
  - Obstructive sleep apnea, upper respiratory tumors

Activity-Exercise Functional Health Pattern
- Medical diagnoses
  - Bacterial respiratory infection, tuberculosis, fungal infection
  - Acute respiratory syndrome, inhalation anthrax
  - Lung cancer, pleuritis, pleural effusion, pneumothorax
  - Hemothorax, inhalation injury, asthma, cystic fibrosis

Activity-Exercise Functional Health Pattern
- Medical diagnoses
  - Chronic obstructive pulmonary disease, atelectasis
  - Occupational lung disease, sarcoidosis, pulmonary embolism
  - Pulmonary hypertension, respiratory failure

Activity-Exercise
- Respiratory patterns interfere with health status
  - Any difficulty breathing or shortness of breath
  - Use pillows at night to sleep
  - Complains of painful breathing
  - Has productive or nonproductive cough
  - Color and odor of sputum

Activity-Exercise
- Respiratory patterns interfere with health status
  - Smoke, exposed to second-hand smoke, chemicals
  - Medical history respiratory disorders
  - Taking medications for respiratory problems
  - Use oxygen, had chest-x-ray, TB skin test

Activity-Exercise
- Insufficient physiologic energy
- Gas exchange system

Factors Affecting Respiration
- Infectious or inflammatory disorders
  - Influenza, sinusitis, laryngitis, pertussis

Pattern, Ineffective Airway Clearance, Impaired Spontaneous Ventilation, and *Impaired Gas Exchange.*

10. Other nursing diagnoses applicable to clients with alterations in respiratory function include: *Disturbed Sleep Pattern* and *Ineffective Therapeutic Regimen Management.*

- Respiratory trauma or obstruction
  - Epistaxis, obstructive sleep apnea
- Tumors
  - Nasal polyps, cancer

Factors Affecting Ventilation
- Infections or inflammatory disorders
  - Bronchitis, pneumonia, tuberculosis
  - Acute respiratory syndrome
- Pleural disorders
  - Pleural effusion, pneumothorax

Factors Affecting Ventilation
- Trauma
  - Flail chest, pulmonary contusion
- Inhalation injury
  - Smoke inhalation, near-drowning
- Obstructive disorders
  - Asthma, COPD, cystic fibrosis

Factors Affecting Ventilation
- Pulmonary vascular disorders
  - Pulmonary embolism
- Respiratory failure
  - Acute respiratory distress syndrome

Upper Respiratory System
- Maintain breathing
- Allow communication

Lower Respiratory System
- Ventilation
- Respiration

Impaired Respiratory Function
- Manifestations
  - Rhinorrhea
  - Cyanosis
  - Wheezing

Priority Nursing Diagnoses
- *Ineffective Breathing Pattern*
- *Ineffective Airway Clearance*
- *Impaired Spontaneous Ventilation*
- *Impaired Gas Exchange*

Nursing Diagnoses from Other Functional Health Patterns
- *Disturbed Sleep Pattern*
- *Ineffective Therapeutic Regimen Management*

SUGGESTIONS FOR CLASSROOM ACTIVITIES

- Administer the end-of-unit questions as a quiz. After completing the quiz, discuss the answers to the questions and give the rationale for the answers. Discuss why the other answers are incorrect.
- Have students breathe through a straw with their nose plugged for 30 seconds. Then have students try to blow up a balloon through a straw to demonstrate breathing through a compromised airway, such as with emphysema or asthma.
- Assign small groups of students to do presentations about respiratory medications in post-conference.

SUGGESTIONS FOR CLINICAL ACTIVITIES

- Assign students to provide nursing care to clients with respiratory disorders. Have students perform suctioning and tracheostomy care when available. Have them discuss the nursing care provided in post-conference and complete a concept map or nursing care plan that utilizes the nursing process.
- Arrange for students to discuss asthma teaching at a health fair. Have them develop a teaching tool to instruct clients about risk factors and treatment. Have them demonstrate peak flow meter monitoring, use of inhalers, and use of spacers.

- Assign each group a different class of medications to present, such as bronchodilators, methylxanthines, antiinflammatories, leukotriene antagonists, mast cell stabilizers, and monoclonal antibodies.
- Have students listen to lung sounds on a computer. Websites such as http://www.rale.ca include various lung sounds. Have the student hold a stethoscope to the computer speaker and listen to the lung sounds through a stethoscope.

- Arrange for students to observe pulmonary function testing in the respiratory laboratory. Have them write a paper about client preparation for testing, how tests are performed, and results of the testing.
- Have students complete a respiratory scenario on a human simulator model in the clinical laboratory, such as a client with a severe asthma attack. Have students demonstrate a respiratory assessment, administration of oxygen, administration of medications and intravenous fluids, perform chest physiotherapy, and discuss client teaching.

CLINICAL SCENARIOS

See End-of-Unit Summary for Unit 11 in Textbook

CONCEPTS FOR LECTURE

1. Client care should be prioritized according to the seriousness of the client's condition.
2. Prioritized nursing diagnoses assist the nurse in developing a plan of care for the client.
3. Strategies for prioritizing clients are based on the ABCs, Maslow's hierarchy of needs, developmental considerations, or crisis intervention.

LECTURE OUTLINE IN POWERPOINT

Prioritize Clients in Order of Visit
- Jack Holt with bacterial pneumonia
- Maggie Sawyer with COPD and DVT
- James Mohr with head, chest, neck injuries
- Amy Campbell with asthma attack

Strategies for Prioritizing Client Care
- ABCs
- Maslow's hierarchy of needs
- Developmental considerations
- Crisis intervention

SUGGESTIONS FOR CLASSROOM ACTIVITIES

- Have students read the clinical scenarios and prioritize the clients in the order they should be seen. Discuss the rationale for the priority order.
- Have students choose two priority nursing diagnoses for each clinical scenario client. Explain the rationale for each nursing diagnosis.
- In the ABCs, A stands for airway. James Mohr is being treated for head, neck, and chest injuries due to a MVA. A tracheostomy has been placed to maintain a patent airway, which is necessary for life. He begins coughing, which is an indication that he needs to be suctioned to maintain the patency of the tracheostomy. As healing of his injuries takes place, the tracheostomy may be capped for weaning. When he is able to tolerate 24 hours of capping, the tracheostomy may be discontinued.

SUGGESTIONS FOR CLINICAL ACTIVITIES

- Assign students to provide nursing care for more than one client. Have them prioritize the order of nursing care for the clients and discuss their rationale.
- Have students develop priority nursing diagnoses for the clients to whom they are providing nursing care in the acute or chronic healthcare setting.

CASE STUDY

See End-of-Unit Summary for Unit 11 in Textbook

CONCEPTS FOR LECTURE

1. Nursing diagnoses are developed based on the medical diagnosis, physical assessment, the client's health history, and the pathophysiology of the disease process.
2. The nursing process is used as a guide to develop a plan of care for the client.

LECTURE OUTLINE IN POWERPOINT

Client with Impaired Gas Exchange
- Based on
  - Medical diagnosis
    - COPD
  - Physical assessment
  - Health history
  - Pathophysiology of disease process

Nursing Process
- Assessment
- Plan
- Nursing diagnosis
- Implementation, expected outcomes
- Evaluation

Nursing Diagnoses
- *Ineffective Airway Clearance*
- *Risk for Impaired Spontaneous Ventilation*

SUGGESTIONS FOR CLASSROOM ACTIVITIES

- Read the case study from the End-of-Unit Summary for Unit 11 in class. Review the concept map from the End-of-Unit Summary to develop a plan of care for the client.

SUGGESTIONS FOR CLINICAL ACTIVITIES

- Have students develop a concept map for clients to whom they provide nursing care in the acute or chronic healthcare setting.

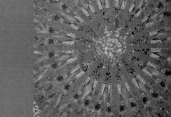

FUNCTIONAL HEALTH PATTERN

Activity–Exercise

CONCEPTS FOR LECTURE

1. The medical diagnoses related to altered Activity-Exercise Functional Health Pattern include: strain, sprain, joint dislocation, fracture, amputation, carpal tunnel syndrome, osteoporosis, Paget's disease, gout, osteomalacia, osteoarthritis, muscular dystrophy, rheumatoid arthritis, ankylosing spondylitis, reactive arthritis, systemic lupus erythematosus, polymyositis, Lyme disease, osteomyelitis, bone tumors, systemic sclerosis, scoliosis, low back pain, and hammertoe.

2. The Activity-Exercise Functional Health Pattern includes healthcare behaviors that interfere with musculoskeletal function.

3. The Activity-Exercise Functional Health Pattern includes disorders that result in insufficient physiologic movement to carry out activities of daily living. The bones serve as the framework for the body and for the attachment of the muscles, tendons, and ligaments. Innervaton by the nervous system permits contraction and relaxation of muscle.

4. Movement is affected by factors that result from excessive external force to tissues, tendons, ligaments, and bones.

5. Movement is affected by factors that result from internal disorders or deformities to joints, bones, and muscles.

6. Musculoskeletal functions include support, protection, movement, mineral storage, and hematopoiesis.

7. Alterations in musculoskeletal function may affect the body's ability to maintain itself, which leads to clinical manifestations such as: pain, limited mobility, and swelling.

8. Priority nursing diagnoses for Activity-Exercise Functional Health Pattern include: *Risk for Disuse Syndrome, Risk for Falls, Impaired Physical Mobility,* and *Risk for Peripheral Neurovascular Dysfunction.*

9. Other nursing diagnoses applicable to clients with alterations in musculoskeletal function include: *Impaired Skin Integrity* and *Risk for Disturbed Sensory Perception–Tactile.*

LECTURE OUTLINE IN POWERPOINT

Unit 12: Responses to Altered Musculoskeletal Function
Activity-Exercise Functional Health Pattern
- Medical diagnoses
  - Strain, sprain, joint dislocation, fracture, amputation
  - Carpal tunnel syndrome, osteoporosis, Paget's disease
  - Gout, osteomalacia, osteoarthritis, muscular dystrophy
  - Rheumatoid arthritis, ankylosing spondylitis, reactive arthritis

Activity-Exercise Functional Health Pattern
- Medical diagnoses
  - Systemic lupus erythematosus, polymyositis, Lyme disease
  - Osteomyelitis, bone tumors, systemic sclerosis
  - Scoliosis, low back pain, hammertoe

Activity-Exercise
- Interferes with musculoskeletal function
  - Increased pain with movement
  - Have muscle weakness or cramps
  - Have redness or swelling of joints
  - Have muscle or bone diseases or injuries

Activity-Exercise
- Interferes with musculoskeletal function
  - Had surgery or physical therapy
  - Taking medications, calcium, herbal supplements
  - Exercise regularly or heavy lifting
  - Use assistive devises for ambulation

Musculoskeletal System
- Bones
  - Framework for body
  - Attachment for muscles, tendons, ligaments
- Innervation
  - Permits muscle contraction and relaxation

Factors Resulting from Excessive External Force
- Tissues
  - Contusion
- Tendons
  - Strain, epicondylitis

Factors Resulting from Excessive External Force
- Ligaments
  - Sprain
- Bones
  - Dislocation, fracture, amputation

Factors Result from Internal Disorders or Deformities
- Joints
  - Arthritis, gout, hammertoe
- Bones
  - Osteoporosis, Paget's disease, osteomalacia
  - Osteomyelitis, tumors, scoliosis

Factors Result from Internal Disorders or Deformities
- Muscles
  - Muscular dystrophy, polymyositis

Musculoskeletal Functions
- Support
- Protection
- Movement
- Mineral storage
- Hematopoiesis

Impaired Musculoskeletal Function
- Manifestations
  - Pain
  - Limited Mobility
  - Swelling

Priority Nursing Diagnoses
- *Risk for Disuse Syndrome*
- *Risk for Falls*
- *Impaired Physical Mobility*
- *Risk for Peripheral Neurovascular Dysfunction*

Nursing Diagnoses with Deficits in Musculoskeletal Function
- *Impaired Skin Integrity*
- *Risk for Disturbed Sensory Perception-Tactile*

SUGGESTIONS FOR CLASSROOM ACTIVITIES

- Divide students into 10 groups. Assign an end-of-unit question to each group. Have them answer the questions and give a rationale for the answer they chose. Discuss why the other answers are incorrect.
- Using a model of the musculoskeletal system, review the functions of the musculoskeletal system. Discuss changes that occur with aging. Review how activity and exercise affect the aging process.
- Review disease processes or disorders that impair musculoskeletal function. Discuss teaching that may be done by the nurse to assist the client to decrease further movement disabilities and to prevent complications of immobility.
- Have students walk with crutches, a cane, and a walker to develop an understanding of client teaching with these devices. Have them maneuver in a wheelchair and practice performing wheelchair transfers to learn the safety measures involved in wheelchair transfers.
- Have students wear a pair of wool or leather gloves and try to tie their shoes to demonstrate the decreased manual dexterity of a client with arthritis or other deforming disorder of the hands. Discuss how to help a client with hand and feet deformities or disorders to complete activities of daily living.

SUGGESTIONS FOR CLINICAL ACTIVITIES

- Assign students to provide nursing care to clients with musculoskeletal disorders on the orthopedic unit. Have them discuss the nursing care provided in post-conference and complete a concept map or nursing care plan that utilizes the nursing process.
- Arrange for students to practice setting up traction. Discuss types of traction and the uses of each type. Review nursing care of a client in traction.
- Arrange for students to observe in a rehabilitation unit. Have them spend time with a physical therapist who works with clients recovering from injuries, musculoskeletal surgeries, or are amputees. Have them review the use of assistive devices.
- Have students complete a musculoskeletal scenario on a human simulator model in the clinical laboratory, such as a client with postoperative repair of hip and femur fractures. Have students demonstrate musculoskeletal and neurovascular assessments, traction care, wound care, morphine PCA administration, antibiotic administration, and intravenous fluids. Discuss possible complications, such as fat embolism, infections, constipation, and compartment syndrome. Review client teaching needs for discharge.

CLINICAL SCENARIOS

See End-of-Unit Summary for Unit 12 in Textbook

CONCEPTS FOR LECTURE

1. Client care should be prioritized according to the seriousness of the client's condition.
2. Prioritized nursing diagnoses assist the nurse in developing a plan of care for the client.
3. Strategies for prioritizing clients are based on the ABCs, Maslow's hierarchy of needs, developmental considerations, or crisis intervention.

LECTURE OUTLINE IN POWERPOINT

Prioritize Clients in Order of Visit
- Jesse Drummond with bilateral below-the-knee amputations
- Joyce Stevens with hip replacement surgery
- José Rivera with osteomyelitis
- Kim Wong with systemic lupus erythmatosus

Strategies for Prioritizing Client Care
- ABCs
- Maslow's hierarchy of needs
- Developmental considerations
- Crisis intervention

SUGGESTIONS FOR CLASSROOM ACTIVITIES

- Have students read the clinical scenarios and prioritize the clients in the order they should be seen. Discuss the rationale for the priority order.
- Have students choose two priority nursing diagnoses for each clinical scenario client. Explain the rationale for each nursing diagnosis.
- In development considerations, aging causes degeneration and loss of cartilage in one or more joints. Decreases in bone density predispose a person to fractures and decreases in activity and exercise result in muscle atrophy and decreased muscle strength. Joyce Stevens, who is 84 years old, is hospitalized for hip replacement surgery. With the use of anticoagulants, the client needs to be observed for signs of internal bleeding and thrombocytopenia. Due to immobility and compromised circulation from surgery, the client is at risk for pneumonia, atelectasis, or pulmonary embolism. Shortness of breath needs to be evaluated and reported to the healthcare provider immediately. Due to anesthesia and surgery, the elderly client is often disoriented and confused for several days after surgery.

SUGGESTIONS FOR CLINICAL ACTIVITIES

- Assign students to provide nursing care for more than one client. Have them prioritize the order of nursing care for the clients and discuss their rationale.
- Have students develop priority nursing diagnoses for the clients to whom they are providing nursing care in the acute or chronic healthcare setting.

CASE STUDY

See End-of-Unit Summary for Unit 12 in Textbook

CONCEPTS FOR LECTURE

1. Nursing diagnoses are developed based on the medical diagnosis, physical assessment, the client's health history, and the pathophysiology of the disease process.
2. The nursing process is used as a guide to develop a plan of care for the client.

LECTURE OUTLINE IN POWERPOINT

Client with Impaired Physical Mobility
- Based on
  - Medical diagnosis
    - Compound fracture of left femur
  - Physical assessment
  - Health history
  - Pathophysiology of disease process

Nursing Process
- Assessment
- Plan
- Nursing diagnosis
- Implementation, expected outcomes
- Evaluation

Nursing Diagnoses
- *Risk for Peripheral Neurovascular Dysfunction*
- *Acute Pain*
- *Risk for Infection*

SUGGESTIONS FOR CLASSROOM ACTIVITIES

- Read the case study from the End-of-Unit Summary for Unit 12 in class. Review the concept map from the End-of-Unit Summary to develop a plan of care for the client.

SUGGESTIONS FOR CLINICAL ACTIVITIES

- Have students develop a concept map for clients to whom they provide nursing care in the acute or chronic healthcare setting.

UNIT 13

RESPONSES TO ALTERED NEUROLOGIC FUNCTION

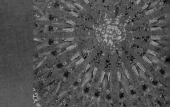

FUNCTIONAL HEALTH PATTERN

Cognitive-Perceptual

CONCEPTS FOR LECTURE

1. The medical diagnoses related to altered Cognitive-Perceptual Functional Health Pattern include: traumatic brain injury, spinal cord injury, cerebral vascular accident (CVA), and aneurysm.

2. The Cognitive-Perceptual Functional Health Pattern includes healthcare behaviors that interfere with neurologic function.

3. The Cognitive-Perceptual Functional Health Pattern includes the regulation and integration of body functions, mental abilities, and emotions. The neurologic system, which controls these functions, is made up of the central nervous system and peripheral nervous system.

4. Factors that affect cognition and perception are: decreased blood flow to neurons, injury to neurologic tissue, alterations in electrical activity, infections, and degeneration or alteration of neurons and neurotransmitters.

5. The Cognitive-Perceptual Functional Pattern includes the neurologic functional abilities of language, memory, judgment, decision-making, and sensation.

6. Alterations in neurologic function may affect the body's ability to maintain itself, which leads to clinical manifestations such as: altered level of consciousness, aphasia or dysphagia, and seizures.

7. Priority nursing diagnoses for Cognitive-Perceptual Functional Health Pattern include: *Altered Cerebral Tissue Perfusion, Impaired Verbal Communication, Powerlessness,* and *Acute Confusion.*

8. Other nursing diagnoses applicable to clients with alterations in neurologic function include: *Impaired Swallowing* and *Impaired Physical Mobility.*

LECTURE OUTLINE IN POWERPOINT

Unit 13: Responses to Altered Neurologic Function
Cognitive-Perceptual Functional Health Pattern
- Medical diagnoses
  - Traumatic brain injury, spinal cord injury
  - Cerebral vascular accident (CVA), aneurysm
Cognitive-Perceptual
- Interferes with neurologic function
  - Have difficulty with memory
  - Is speech affected (aphasia)
  - Difficulty finding words in conversation
  - Understand but unable to respond
Cognitive-Perceptual
- Regulation and integration
  - All body functions
  - Mental abilities
  - Emotions
- Central and peripheral nervous systems
Factors Affecting Cognition and Perception
- Decreased blood flow to neurons
  - Stroke, ruptured aneurysm, arteriovenous malformation
  - Spinal cord injury, increased intracranial pressure
- Alterations in electrical activity
  - Seizures
Factors Affecting Cognition and Perception
- Injury to neurologic tissue
  - Traumatic brain injury, skull fractures
  - Spinal cord injury, herniated vertebral disk
  - Brain or spinal cord tumors
Factors Affecting Cognition and Perception
- Infections
  - Meningitis, encephalitis, rabies, tetanus, botulism
- Degeneration or alteration of neurons and neurotransmitters.
  - Alzheimer's disease, Parkinson's disease, Huntington's disease
  - Multiple sclerosis, myasthenia gravis, Guillian-Barré
Neurologic function
- Language
- Memory
- Judgment
- Decision-making
- Sensation

Impaired Cognitive–Perceptual Patterns
- Manifestations
  - Altered level of consciousness
  - Aphasia or dysphagia
  - Seizures

Priority Nursing Diagnoses
- *Altered Cerebral Tissue Perfusion*
- *Impaired Verbal Communication*
- *Powerlessness*
- *Acute Confusion*

Nursing Diagnoses from Other Functional Health Patterns
- *Impaired Swallowing*
- *Impaired Physical Mobility*

SUGGESTIONS FOR CLASSROOM ACTIVITIES

- Divide students into 10 groups. Assign an end-of-unit question to each group. Have them answer the questions and give a rationale for the answer they choose. Discuss why the other answers are incorrect.
- Using a model of the neurologic system, trace movement of cerebral spinal fluid throughout the brain and spine. Discuss the functions of the neurologic system.
- Review disease processes or disorders that interfere with neurologic function. Discuss teaching that may be done by the nurse to assist the client to increase activity levels and to decrease further neurologic compromise.
- Develop a self-learning module about the care of clients with seizure disorders. Identify types of seizures. Describe nursing care during a seizure and in the postictal state. Discuss medications used to control seizure disorders, including dosages, side effects, and nursing considerations. Explain the use of a ketogenic diet and surgical management to control seizures. Develop an NCLEX®-style quiz as a pretest and posttest to evaluate student learning.

SUGGESTIONS FOR CLINICAL ACTIVITIES

- Assign students to provide nursing care to clients with alterations in neurologic function. Have them discuss the nursing care provided in post-conference and complete a concept map or nursing care plan that utilizes the nursing process.
- Arrange for students to observe an occupational therapist assist the client with rehabilitation needs and with activities of daily living. Have them write a paper about the role of the nurse in the rehabilitation of clients.
- Have students complete a neurovascular scenario on a human simulator model in the clinical laboratory, such as a client with a spinal cord injury. Have students demonstrate a neurologic assessment, demonstrate positioning and turning of the client, discuss laboratory and diagnostic studies, administer medications, discuss nutritional status including appropriate diet and calorie counts, use therapeutic communication to assess psychological status, and provide care of complications due to immobility and autonomic dysreflexia.

CLINICAL SCENARIOS

See End-of-Unit Summary for Unit 13 in Textbook

CONCEPTS FOR LECTURE

1. Client care should be prioritized according to the seriousness of the client's condition.
2. Prioritized nursing diagnoses assist the nurse in developing a plan of care for the client.
3. Strategies for prioritizing clients are based on the ABCs, Maslow's hierarchy of needs, developmental considerations, or crisis intervention.

LECTURE OUTLINE IN POWERPOINT

Prioritize Clients in Order of Visit
- Jose Hernandez with cerebrovascular accident
- Jane Thomas with lumbar laminectomy
- Cesar Phillips with stroke and hypertension
- Tonya Walton with subdural hematoma

Strategies for Prioritizing Client Care
- ABCs
- Maslow's hierarchy of needs
- Developmental considerations
- Crisis intervention

Suggestions for Classroom Activities

- Have students read the clinical scenarios and prioritize the clients in the order they should be seen. Discuss the rationale for the priority order.
- Have students choose two priority nursing diagnoses for each clinical scenario client. Explain the rationale for each nursing diagnosis.
- The ACT crisis intervention model stands for assessment or appraisal of immediate medical needs, implementing crisis intervention, and trauma treatment plans. Jose Hernandez is found alone at home, and is unable to speak to move the right side of his body. Appraisal of the situation indicates an immediate need for medical intervention. A transfer to a health facility is implemented. Mr. Hernandez is undergoing medical treatment for a CVA (stroke) which has left him with a continuing inability to speak, paralysis on the right side of his body, and respiratory difficulties. Interdisciplinary discharge planning will be needed due to Mr. Hernandez's inability to care for himself or to live alone.

Suggestions for Clinical Activities

- Assign students to provide nursing care for more than one client. Have them prioritize the order in which to provide nursing care for the clients and discuss their rationale.
- Have students develop priority nursing diagnoses for the clients to whom they are providing nursing care in the acute or chronic healthcare setting.

Case Study

See End-of-Unit Summary for Unit 13 in Textbook

Concepts for Lecture

1. Nursing diagnoses are developed based on the medical diagnosis, physical assessment, the client's health history, and the pathophysiology of the disease process.
2. The nursing process is used as a guide to develop a plan of care for the client.

Lecture Outline in PowerPoint

Client with Altered Tissue Perfusion: Cerebral
- Based on
  - Medical diagnosis
    - CVA
  - Physical assessment
  - Health history
  - Pathophysiology of disease process
Nursing Process
- Assessment
- Plan
- Nursing diagnosis
- Implementation, expected outcomes
- Evaluation
Nursing Diagnoses
- *Impaired Verbal Communication*
- *Self-Care Deficit*
- *Impaired Physical Mobility*
- *Risk for Impaired Swallowing*

Suggestions for Classroom Activities

- Read the case study from the End-of-Unit Summary for Unit 13 in class. Review the concept map from the End-of-Unit Summary to develop a plan of care for the client.

Suggestions for Clinical Activities

- Have students develop a concept map for clients to whom they provide nursing care in the acute or chronic healthcare setting.

UNIT 14
RESPONSES TO ALTERED VISUAL AND AUDITORY FUNCTION

FUNCTIONAL HEALTH PATTERN

Cognitive-Perceptual

CONCEPTS FOR LECTURE

1. The medical diagnoses related to altered Cognitive-Perceptual Functional Health Pattern include: conjunctivitis, keratitis, corneal abrasion, cataracts, glaucoma, macular degeneration, diabetic retinopathy, retinal detachment, retinitis pigmentosa, otitis media, impacted cerumen, acute mastoiditis, otosclerosis, Ménière's disease, acoustic neuroma, and hearing loss.

2. The Cognitive-Perceptual Functional Health Pattern includes healthcare behaviors that interfere with visual and auditory function.

3. The Cognitive-Perceptual Functional Health Pattern includes the pathways for visual and auditory stimuli to the brain and for the maintenance of position sense and equilibrium. Deficits in vision and hearing can limit self-care, mobility, independence, communication, and relationships with others.

4. Factors that affect cognition and perception of the eye are: infection, inflammation, trauma, refractive errors, and visual deficits.

5. Factors that affect cognition and perception of the ear are: infection, inflammation, hearing deficits, and inner ear disorders.

6. The Cognitive-Perceptual Functional Pattern includes visual and auditory function abilities to receive and organize information, to communicate, to gain access to information, and to derive pleasure from sights and sounds.

7. Alterations in visual and auditory function may affect the body's ability to maintain itself, which leads to clinical manifestations such as: presbyopia, pain, and vertigo.

8. Priority nursing diagnoses for the Cognitive-Perceptual Functional Health Pattern include: *Disturbed Sensory Perception, Impaired Verbal Communication, Impaired Environmental Interpretation Syndrome*, and *Decisional Conflict*.

9. Other nursing diagnoses applicable to clients with alterations in visual and auditory function include: *Anxiety* and *Ineffective Health Maintenance*.

LECTURE OUTLINE IN POWERPOINT

Unit 14: Responses to Altered Visual and Auditory Function
Cognitive-Perceptual Functional Health Pattern
- Medical diagnoses
  - Conjunctivitis, keratitis, corneal abrasion, cataracts, glaucoma
  - Macular degeneration, diabetic retinopathy, retinal detachment
  - Otitis media, impacted cerumen, acute mastoiditis
  - Otosclerosis, Ménière's disease, acoustic neuroma
Cognitive-Perceptual
- Interferes with perceptual function
  - Complain if changes in vision
  - See rings of color or halos around lights
  - See flashes of light or floaters
  - Difficulty reading fine print
Cognitive-Perceptual
- Interferes with perceptual function
  - Wears corrective eyewear
  - Have pain in eyes or ears
  - Had eye trauma, surgery, or infections
  - Use eye or ear medications
Cognitive-Perceptual
- Interferes with perceptual function
  - Have family history, or eye or ear disorders
  - Difference in hearing between ears
  - Difficulty hearing sounds, conversations
  - Complain of hearing buzzing, ringing, crackling noises
Cognitive-Perceptual
- Interferes with perceptual function
  - Had ear surgery
  - Have swelling, tenderness, drainage in ears
  - Complain of dizziness
  - Wear hearing aid, use protective earplugs
Cognitive-Perceptual
- Eyes
  - Pathway for visual stimuli to brain
- Ears
  - Pathway for auditory stimuli to brain
  - Maintains position sense and equilibrium
Cognitive-Perceptual
- Deficits in vision and hearing
  - Limit self-care, mobility

- ○ Limit independence
- ○ Limit communication
- ○ Limit relationships with others

Factors Affecting Structure and Function of Eyes
- Infection and inflammation
  - ○ Conjunctivitis, keratitis, corneal ulcer
- Trauma
  - ○ Corneal abrasion

Factors Affecting Structure and Function of Eyes
- Refractive errors
  - ○ Myopia, hyperopia, presbyopia
- Visual deficits
  - ○ Cataracts, glaucoma, retinal detachment
  - ○ Macular degeneration, diabetic retinopathy

Factors Affecting Structures and Function of Ears
- Infection and inflammation
  - ○ Otitis media, external otitis, mastoiditis
- Hearing deficits
  - ○ Impacted cerumen, otosclerosis, presbycusis
  - ○ Hearing loss

Factors Affecting Structures and Function of Ears
- Inner ear disorders
  - ○ Labyrinthitis, Ménière's disease, vertigo

Auditory and Visual Function
- Ability to receive and organize information
- Ability to communicate
- Gain access to information
- Derive pleasure from sights and sounds

Impaired Cognitive–Perceptual Patterns
- Manifestations
  - ○ Presbyopia
  - ○ Pain
  - ○ Vertigo

Priority Nursing Diagnoses
- *Disturbed Sensory Perception*
- *Impaired Verbal Communication*
- *Impaired Environmental Interpretation Syndrome*
- *Decisional Conflict*

Nursing Diagnoses from Other Functional Health Patterns
- *Anxiety*
- *Ineffective Health Maintenance*

SUGGESTIONS FOR CLASSROOM ACTIVITIES

- Divide students into 10 groups. Assign an end-of-unit question to each group. Have them answer the questions and give a rationale for the answer they choose. Discuss why the other answers are incorrect.
- Using a model of the eye and ear systems, trace movement of light from the eye to the brain and movement of sound waves from the ear to the brain. Discuss the functions of the visual and auditory systems.
- Review disease processes or disorders that interfere with visual and auditory function. Discuss how to communicate with and to perform nursing care on the client who has cognitive and perceptual deficits.

SUGGESTIONS FOR CLINICAL ACTIVITIES

- Assign students to provide nursing care to clients with alterations in visual and auditory function. Have them discuss the nursing care provided in post-conference and complete a concept map or nursing care plan that utilizes the nursing process.
- Arrange for students to spend a day at an outpatient eye surgery center to observe eye surgery such as cataract and laser surgeries. Have students identify the roles of the nurse in preoperative, operative, and postoperative nursing care of clients with eye surgery.
- Have students complete a cognitive-perceptual scenario on a human simulator model in the clinical

- Have students perform a task wearing a blindfold to develop an understanding of the client who is unable to see. Discuss how to do discharge teaching to a client with visual deficits. Then, give a brief lecture in a quiet voice while having students wear ear plugs to develop an understanding of the client who is unable to hear. Discuss how to do discharge teaching to a client with hearing deficits.

laboratory, such as a client with retinal detachment after being hit in the eye by a baseball. Have students demonstrate an assessment of the eye injury, prepare the client for surgery, administer medication, provide postoperative nursing care, and instruct discharge teaching.

CLINICAL SCENARIOS

See End-of-Unit Summary for Unit 14 in Textbook

CONCEPTS FOR LECTURE

1. Client care should be prioritized according to the seriousness of the client's condition.
2. Prioritized nursing diagnoses assist the nurse in developing a plan of care for the client.
3. Strategies for prioritizing clients are based on the ABCs, Maslow's hierarchy of needs, developmental considerations, or crisis intervention.

LECTURE OUTLINE IN POWERPOINT

Prioritize Clients in Order of Visit
- Andrew Hardy with diabetic retinopathy and retinal detachment
- Gladys Harvey with right eye cataract
- Georgia Stanley with Ménière's disease
- Kenneth Koch with right ear tympanoplasty

Strategies for Prioritizing Client Care
- ABCs
- Maslow's hierarchy of needs
- Developmental considerations
- Crisis intervention

SUGGESTIONS FOR CLASSROOM ACTIVITIES

- Have students read the clinical scenarios and prioritize the clients in the order they should be seen. Discuss the rationale for the priority order.
- Have students choose two priority nursing diagnoses for each clinical scenario client. Explain the rationale for each nursing diagnosis.
- In the ABCs, C stands for circulation. Andrew Hardy is admitted with hyperglycemia. He has a history of type I diabetes. Upon assessment, the eye symptoms he is having indicate diabetic retinopathy with a retinal detachment. With diabetic retinopathy, cells of the retinal vessels die and leak fluid into the eye. Fragile capillaries bleed easily, which cause hemorrhages in the retina and result in seeing black spots and blurred vision. With retinal detachment, fluid collects under the retina, which results in a separation of the retina from the epithelium that causes flashes of light. Mr. Hardy needs immediate treatment to decrease his blood glucose to a normal level, to surgically repair the retinal detachment, and to seal the leaking blood vessels with laser surgery in order to prevent blindness.

SUGGESTIONS FOR CLINICAL ACTIVITIES

- Assign students to provide nursing care for more than one client. Have them prioritize the order in which to provide nursing care for the clients and discuss their rationale.
- Have students develop priority nursing diagnoses for the clients to whom they are providing nursing care in the acute or chronic healthcare setting.

CASE STUDY

See End-of-Unit Summary for Unit 14 in Textbook

CONCEPTS FOR LECTURE

1. Nursing diagnoses are developed based on the medical diagnosis, physical assessment, the client's health history, and the pathophysiology of the disease process.
2. The nursing process is used as a guide to develop a plan of care for the client.

LECTURE OUTLINE IN POWERPOINT

Client with Disturbed Sensory Perception: Visual
- Based on
  - Medical diagnosis
    - Open angle glaucoma
  - Physical assessment
  - Health history
  - Pathophysiology of disease process

Nursing Process
- Assessment
- Plan
- Nursing diagnosis
- Implementation, expected outcomes
- Evaluation

Nursing Diagnoses
- *Risk for Injury*
- *Impaired Home Maintenance*
- *Anxiety*

SUGGESTIONS FOR CLASSROOM ACTIVITIES

- Read the case study from the End-of-Unit Summary for Unit 14 in class. Review the concept map from the End-of-Unit Summary to develop a plan of care for the client.

SUGGESTIONS FOR CLINICAL ACTIVITIES

- Have students develop a concept map for clients to whom they provide nursing care in the acute or chronic healthcare setting.

UNIT 15
RESPONSES TO ALTERED REPRODUCTIVE FUNCTION

FUNCTIONAL HEALTH PATTERN

Sexuality-Reproductive

CONCEPTS FOR LECTURE

1. The medical diagnoses related to altered Sexuality-Reproductive Functional Health Pattern include: erectile dysfunction, ejaculatory dysfunction, phimosis, priapism, cancer of penis or testicles, epididymitis, prostatitis, menopause, premenstrual syndrome, dysmenorrhea, uterine displacement, endometriosis, cervical or endometrial cancer, ovarian or vulva cancer, breast cancer, genital herpes, genital warts, chlamydia, gonorrhea, syphilis, and pelvic inflammatory disease.

2. The Sexuality-Reproductive Functional Health Pattern includes healthcare behaviors that interfere with reproductive function.

3. The Sexuality-Reproductive Functional Health Pattern includes satisfaction with sexuality and sexual relationships, reproductive patterns, male prostate history, and female menstrual and menopausal history.

4. Factors that interfere with sexual function in males are: sexual dysfunction, penis disorders, disorders of testis and scrotum, disorders of prostate gland, and infection.

5. Factors that interfere with sexual function in females are: sexual dysfunction, menopause, menstrual disorders, structural disorders, disorders of reproductive tissue, and infection.

6. Reproductive function in males may be affected by disorders that pose risk to fertility, sexual function, and urinary function.

7. Reproductive function in females may be affected by disorders that pose risk to reproduction, sexual function, menstrual function, and sense of well-being.

8. Alterations in reproductive function may affect the body's ability to maintain itself, which leads to clinical manifestations such as: phimosis, erectile dysfunction, dysmenorrhea, and premenstrual dysfunction.

9. Priority nursing diagnoses for Sexuality-Reproductive Functional Health Pattern include: *Sexual Dysfunction, Ineffective Sexuality Patterns,* and *Rape-Trauma Syndrome.*

10. Other nursing diagnoses applicable to clients with alterations in reproductive function include: *Disturbed Body Image* and *Powerlessness.*

LECTURE OUTLINE IN POWERPOINT

Unit 15: Responses to Altered Reproductive Function
Sexuality–Reproductive Functional Health Pattern
- Medical diagnoses
  - Erectile dysfunction, ejaculatory dysfunction, phimosis
  - Cancer of penis or testicles, epididymitis, prostatitis
  - Benign prostatic hyperplasia, priapism

Sexuality-Reproductive Functional Health Pattern
- Medical diagnoses
  - Menopause, premenstrual syndrome, dysmenorrhea
  - Uterine displacement, endometriosis, cervical cancer
  - Endometrial, ovarian or vulva cancer, breast cancer
  - Genital herpes, genital warts, pelvic inflammatory disease

Sexuality-Reproductive
- Interferes with reproductive function
  - Have changes in urination
  - Ability to achieve or maintain an erection
  - Take medication to facilitate sexual ability
  - Have discharge or bleeding from penis

Sexuality-Reproductive
- Interferes with reproductive function
  - Complain of pain in groin area
  - Family history of testicular or prostate cancer
  - Have more than one sexual partner
  - Use contraceptives

Sexuality-Reproductive
- Interferes with reproductive function
  - Have history of sexual abuse or trauma
  - Had sexually transmitted diseases
  - Had surgery on reproductive organs
  - Perform self-breast or prostate examinations

Sexuality-Reproductive
- Interferes with reproductive function
  - Age at start or end of menstrual periods
  - Complain of menstrual difficulties
  - Complain of vaginal itching, discharge, bleeding
  - Ever been pregnant, miscarry

Sexuality-Reproductive
- Interferes with reproductive function
  - Take medication or herbals for menopause
  - Family history reproductive cancers

- Date of last mammogram or gynecologic examination
- Have cultural practices or beliefs

Sexuality-Reproductive
- Sexuality and sexual relationships
- Reproductive patterns
- Male prostate history
- Female menstrual and menopause history

Factors Interfering with Sexual Function
- Sexual dysfunction
  - Erectile dysfunction, ejaculatory dysfunction
- Penis disorders
  - Priapism, phimosis, cancer
- Disorders of testis and scrotum
  - Epididymitis, orchitis, cancer
- Disorders of prostate gland
  - Prostatitis, benign prostatic hyperplasia, cancer
- Infection
  - Gonorrhea, syphilis

Factors Interfering with Sexual Function
- Sexual dysfunction
  - Dyspareunia
- Menopause
- Menstrual disorders
  - Premenstrual syndrome, dysmenorrhea
  - Dysfunctional uterine bleeding
- Structural disorders
  - Uterine displacement, vaginal fistula
- Disorders of reproductive tissue
  - Uterine polyps, endometriosis, cancer
- Infection
  - Genital herpes, genital warts, chlamydia, PID

Reproductive Function in Males
- Affects
  - Fertility
  - Sexual function
  - Urinary function

Reproductive Function in Females
- Affects
  - Reproduction
  - Sexual function
  - Menstrual function
  - Sense of well-being

Impaired Sexuality-Reproductive Patterns
- Manifestations
  - Phimosis
  - Erectile dysfunction
  - Dysmenorrhea
  - Premenstrual dysfunction

Priority Nursing Diagnoses
- *Sexual Dysfunction*
- *Ineffective Sexuality Patterns*
- *Rape-Trauma Syndrome*

Nursing Diagnoses from Other Functional Health Patterns
- *Disturbed Body Image*
- *Powerlessness*

SUGGESTIONS FOR CLASSROOM ACTIVITIES

- Assign an end-of-unit question to students as they enter the classroom. As the instructor is discussing a topic, call on the students who have the question about the topic being discussed. Have them answer the question and give a rationale for the answer chosen. Discuss why the other answers are incorrect.
- Using a model of the male reproductive system, trace movement of sperm and semen through the reproductive organs. Discuss the functions and hormones of the male reproductive system.
- Using a model of the female reproductive system, trace movement of the egg through the reproductive organs. Review the menstrual cycle and menopause. Discuss the functions and hormones of the female reproductive system.
- Review disease processes or disorders that interfere with reproductive and sexual function. Discuss teaching that may be done by the nurse to assist the client with understanding sexuality and reproductive disorders.
- Have a panel of male and female clients who have experienced cancer of the reproductive system talk to the students about their experiences with the disease, including the manifestations leading to the diagnosis, laboratory and diagnostic studies they had, treatments, complications, and how having cancer has affected their lives.

SUGGESTIONS FOR CLINICAL ACTIVITIES

- Assign students to provide nursing care to clients with alterations in reproductive function. Have them discuss the nursing care provided in post-conference and complete a concept map or nursing care plan that utilizes the nursing process.
- Arrange for students to present a class about sexually transmitted diseases and contraception to a group of young adults. Have them include ways to prevent sexually transmitted diseases and the complications that may result from these diseases. Have the students demonstrate the different types of birth control and how to apply condoms correctly (apply a condom over a banana).
- Have students complete a reproductive scenario on a human simulator model in the clinical laboratory, such as a client with benign prostatic hyperplasia. Have students demonstrate a urinary assessment and assist the healthcare provider with a prostate assessment, discuss laboratory and diagnostic studies, prepare the client for surgery, perform postoperative care including bladder irrigation and indwelling urinary catheter care, administer medications, and complete discharge health teaching.

CLINICAL SCENARIOS

See End-of-Unit Summary for Unit 15 in Textbook

CONCEPTS FOR LECTURE

1. Client care should be prioritized according to the seriousness of the client's condition.
2. Prioritized nursing diagnoses assist the nurse in developing a plan of care for the client.
3. Strategies for prioritizing clients are based on the ABCs, Maslow's hierarchy of needs, developmental considerations, or crisis intervention.

LECTURE OUTLINE IN POWERPOINT

Prioritize Clients in Order of Visit
- Daryl Foster with sickle cell crisis
- Barney Green with transurethral resection of prostate
- Tara Morris with pelvic inflammatory disease
- Regina Perkins with uterine fibroids

Strategies for Prioritizing Client Care
- ABCs
- Maslow's hierarchy of needs
- Developmental considerations
- Crisis intervention

SUGGESTIONS FOR CLASSROOM ACTIVITIES

- Have students read the clinical scenarios and prioritize the clients in the order they should be seen. Discuss the rationale for the priority order.
- Have students choose two priority nursing diagnoses for each clinical scenario client. Explain the rationale for each nursing diagnosis.

SUGGESTIONS FOR CLINICAL ACTIVITIES

- Assign students to provide nursing care for more than one client. Have them prioritize the order in which to provide nursing care for the clients and discuss their rationale.
- Have students develop priority nursing diagnoses for the clients to whom they are providing nursing care in the acute or chronic healthcare setting.

- In developmental considerations, Piaget's formal operational stage of cognitive development is the increase in the ability to think abstractly, the ability to use planning to think ahead, and the ability to recognize and solve problems. Tara Morris is a 21-year-old admitted with pelvic inflammatory disease (PID). She has the cognitive ability to understand that PID may be the result of sexual intercourse and complications may result in an increased risk for ectopic pregnancy, infertility, and chronic pelvic pain. Ms. Morris needs to be allowed time to express her feelings about having PID, and to understand the use of contraception and lifestyle factors to prevent contacting PID again.

CASE STUDY

See End-of-Unit Summary for Unit 15 in Textbook

CONCEPTS FOR LECTURE

1. Nursing diagnoses are developed based on the medical diagnosis, physical assessment, the client's health history, and the pathophysiology of the disease process.
2. The nursing process is used as a guide to develop a plan of care for the client.

LECTURE OUTLINE IN POWERPOINT

Impaired Tissue Integrity
- Based on
  - Medical diagnosis
    - Breast cancer
  - Physical assessment
  - Health history
  - Pathophysiology of disease process

Nursing Process
- Assessment
- Plan
- Nursing diagnosis
- Implementation, expected outcomes
- Evaluation

Nursing Diagnoses
- *Ineffective Tissue Perfusion*
- *Risk for Infection*
- *Acute Pain*
- *Disturbed Body Image*

SUGGESTIONS FOR CLASSROOM ACTIVITIES

- Read the case study from the End-of-Unit Summary for Unit 15 in class. Review the concept map from the End-of-Unit Summary to develop a plan of care for the client.

SUGGESTIONS FOR CLINICAL ACTIVITIES

- Have students develop a concept map for clients to whom they provide nursing care in the acute or chronic healthcare setting.

NCLEX-RN® Test Questions

The following questions are similar to those that may appear on the NCLEX-RN® exam. Some questions may have one or more correct response. During this review you should select the best response(s).

CHAPTER 1

1.1 The new nurse is studying the five core competencies for healthcare providers. Which of the following are a part of these core competencies? (Select all that apply.)
1. Use primary nursing to deliver care.
2. Use informatics to deliver care.
3. Work in interdisciplinary teams.
4. Replace quality improvement initiatives with work redesign methods.
5. Use evidence-based practice.

Answer: 2, 3, 4
Rationale: The National Academy of Sciences proposed a set of five core competencies that all healthcare professionals should possess to meet the needs of the 21st-century health system. These core competencies are patient-centered care, interdisciplinary teams, evidence-based practice, quality improvement, and informatics. Primary care is a method of providing client care.
Evaluation
Comprehension
Safe, Effective Care Environment

1.2 The nurse is using a specific process to plan smoking cessation activities for a client. Which of the following is this nurse most likely using to plan the care for this client?
1. critical pathways
2. evidence-based practice
3. nursing process
4. variance analysis

Answer: 3
Rationale: The nursing process is a series of critical thinking activities that nurses use to provide care to clients. The purpose of care may be to promote wellness, restore health, or facilitate coping with a disability or death. The use of critical pathways and evidence-based practice are primarily used to manage disease conditions. The use of variance analysis implies the use of statistical-based research.
Planning
Application
Safe, Effective Care Environment

1.3 Which of the following best demonstrates a nurse using critical thinking when providing client care?
1. A nurse checks a laboratory manual before providing care.
2. A nurse lists alternative interventions available to provide client care.
3. A nurse is confused when the only planned intervention fails to help a client.
4. A nurse checks every intervention with the charge nurse before providing care.

Answer: 2
Rationale: Critical thinking is thinking about *one's own* thinking. It is self-directed thinking that involves attitudes and skills. The purpose of the thinking, level of knowledge, prejudices, information sources, option identification, and personal values should all be considered with critical thinking. Although the nurse may use a laboratory manual when planning or providing care, it is not the best selection. The nurse who is unable to make independent decisions or employ alternative interventions lacks some of the basic characteristics associated with critical thinking.
Evaluation
Analysis
Safe, Effective Care Environment

1.4 A new nurse tells her mentor "you always seem so poised when you interact with the client. It is as if you always know what to do. Can you teach me how to do that?" What characteristic does this mentor possess in relation to critical thinking?
1. self-confidence
2. independent thinking
3. empathy
4. discipline

Answer: 1
Rationale: Confidence in one's own decisions is gained through the use of critical thinking. Independent thinking is demonstrated by the ability to make decisions with minimal input from others. Empathy involves being able to relate in an understanding manner with others. Discipline involves self-control.
Assessment
Analysis
Safe, Effective Care Environment

1.5 The nurse stops to think about a previous client care situation before providing care to a current client. This nurse is using what critical thinking skill?

Answer: 4
Rationale: Reflection occurs when time is taken to think about a situation and compare it to other similar situations. Divergent thinking involves thinking about multiple items simultaneously. Reasoning allows the nurse to use the powers of deduction. Clarifying is the use of thinking skills to enhance clarity and reduce confusion.

1. divergent thinking 2. reasoning 3. clarifying 4. reflection	Evaluation Application Safe, Effective Care Environment

1.6 The nurse working on a quality improvement study wants to evaluate a client care process. Which of the following can the nurse use to evaluate this process?
    1. critical pathway
    2. nursing process
    3. variance analysis
    4. evidence-based practice
	Answer: 2
	Rationale: The nursing process can serve as a framework for the evaluation of quality care. The use of critical pathways, variance analysis, and evidence-based practice would not provide the best, recommended means to evaluate a client care process.
	Implementation
	Application
	Safe, Effective Care Environment

1.7 The nurse is reviewing the outcome of client care that was provided. Which of the following nursing process steps should the nurse use next?
    1. assessment
    2. planning
    3. evaluation
    4. implementation
	Answer: 3
	Rationale: The data gained during the evaluation of provided client care serves as the assessment. The nurse can then proceed to create a nursing diagnosis based upon this information. The steps in the nursing process are interrelated, interdependent, and used cyclically. During the assessment phase, the nurse is actively collecting data. Implementation is the phase of the nursing process during which the nurse performs interventions. Determining the needs of the client and devising a plan of action take place during the planning phase.
	Evaluation
	Application
	Safe, Effective Care Environment

1.8 A client tells the nurse, "I have pain in my leg when I stand too long." This information would be considered:
    1. evaluative data.
    2. objective data.
    3. qualitative data.
    4. subjective data.
	Answer: 4
	Rationale: Information that is perceived only by the person experiencing it is called subjective data. Evaluative data is used to assess responses to care that are delivered. Qualitative data refers to the presence or absence of a factor. Objective data can be measured by someone or something other than the client.
	Assessment
	Application
	Safe, Effective Care Environment

1.9 While providing care to a client, the nurse stops to assess a new client problem. The assessment in this situation would be:
    1. an initial assessment.
    2. an objective assessment.
    3. a focused assessment.
    4. a subjective assessment.
	Answer: 3
	Rationale: Focused assessments enable the nurse to monitor the status of an actual or potential problem that was previously identified. The initial assessment refers to the first interaction. Subjective and objective assessments are not indicated in this scenario.
	Assessment
	Application
	Safe, Effective Care Environment

1.10 At the completion of an assessment, the nurse chooses a nursing diagnosis that best defines the client's health problems. Which type of clinical judgment will this nurse use?
    1. diagnostic reasoning
    2. evidence-based practice
    3. critical pathway
    4. nursing process
	Answer: 1
	Rationale: Diagnostic reasoning is a form of clinical judgment used to make decisions about which diagnostic label best describes the patterns of client data. Evidence-based practice refers to the implementation of care initiatives which have been supported by research. A critical pathway is a healthcare plan developed to provide care with a multidisciplinary, managed action focus. The nursing process is a systematic method of critically thinking used to promote wellness, maintain health, restore health or facilitate coping with disability and death.
	Diagnosis
	Application
	Safe, Effective Care Environment

1.11 The nurse is creating outcome criteria for the nursing diagnoses for a client. Which of the following should the nurse include when creating the criteria? 1. They should be written as nursing goals.	Answer: 4 Rationale: Outcome criteria for nursing diagnoses are client-centered, time-specific, and measurable. They are classified into three domains: cognitive, affective, and psychomotor. The focus of the outcome criteria is the client not upon the nurse. While the outcome criteria are often written as statements, this option does not encompass all of the criteria the way the correct answer does.

2. They should be written as statements. 3. They should be written as psychomotor only. 4. They should be written to address the client, and be time-specific and measurable.	Outcome criteria are not limited to psychomotor skills they may also be cognitive or affective. Planning Application Safe, Effective Care Environment
1.12 The nurse is implementing a plan of care for a client. After providing care, what should the nurse do as the final step in the process? 　1. nothing 　2. give the charge nurse a report. 　3. Document 　4. Reassess the client.	Answer: 3 Rationale: Documenting interventions is the final component of implementation as well as being a legal requirement. Ongoing assessment of the client is an essential component of implementation but it is not the final step. Nursing action is required after the completion of care. Providing report is an ongoing process and not necessarily completed after implementing the plan of care. Planning Application Safe, Effective Care Environment
1.13 A client care issue has been raised about the actions taken by a nurse who was asked to provide care to a client whose healthcare decisions were considered controversial. The unit's nurse manager is concerned that care was not appropriately provided. Which of the following should be consulted to protect the client and to evaluate the care in question? 　1. hospital quality improvement guidelines 　2. nursing code of ethics 　3. nurse practice act 　4. critical pathway	Answer: 2 Rationale: An established code of ethics is one criterion that defines a profession. Ethics are principles of conduct. Codes of ethics for nurses provide a frame of reference for ideal nursing behaviors that are congruent with the principles expressed in the Code for Nurses. Quality improvement efforts are used to assess and ensure care is provided and as a means to identify needed changes in care practices. The nurse practice act provides the standards for an individual state's stance on the nurse's scope of practice. A critical pathway is a healthcare plan developed to provide care with a multidisciplinary, managed action focus. Planning Analysis Safe, Effective Care Environment
1.14 A client tells the nurse, "I have an advance directive that I want you to follow." Which of the following will this document provide for the nurse? 　1. the client's preferences for health care should the client become mentally incapacitated 　2. a complete plan of care for the client 　3. the answers to any care dilemmas for the client 　4. directions regarding when to use universal precautions for the client	Answer: 1 Rationale: An advance directive, or living will, is a document in which a client formally states preferences for health care in the event that he or she later becomes mentally incapacitated. The client's care plan and information regarding the use of universal precautions are hospital-based sources of information. Client care dilemmas will be decided on a case-by-case basis and do not relate to the information in this question. Evaluation Application Safe, Effective Care Environment
1.15 The nurse is preparing a client to go home. Which of the following skills are the most important for the nurse to adequately prepare this client? 　1. the ability to follow written orders 　2. the ability to use critical thinking 　3. familiarity with adult learning principles 　4. the ability to support client decision making	Answer: 3 Rationale: The nurse will function as an educator when preparing a client for discharge. In order to do this adequately, the nurse will need to have some level of familiarity of adult learning principles to effectively provide and evaluate the outcome of client education. Following written orders and using critical thinking would be considered basic caregiver skills. The ability to support client decision making relates to the role of client advocate. Planning Application Safe, Effective Care Environment

1.16 The nurse is preparing to provide client care information to a group of unlicensed assistive personnel. Which type of care delivery system is this nurse most likely using to provide client care?
1. functional nursing
2. team nursing
3. primary nursing
4. case management

Answer: 2
Rationale: Team nursing is practiced by teams of healthcare providers with various levels of education, including unlicensed assistive personnel. Functional nursing is not a recognized term. The concept of team nursing utilizes variously educated healthcare team members. The team works together and provides the care for which they are individually trained. In primary nursing, total nursing care is provided by the assigned nurse. The needs and care of a group of clients in which the goal is maximized outcomes and cost containment is the focus of case management.
Evaluation
Application
Safe, Effective Care Environment

1.17 A nurse has delegated the collection of vital signs, including blood pressure readings, to two unlicensed assistive personnel. The delegation of this work means the nurse is:
1. not responsible for these vital signs.
2. not accountable for these vital signs.
3. responsible to re-measure all of the vital signs.
4. accountable for the care that was delegated.

Answer: 4
Rationale: When the nurse delegates nursing care activities to another person, that person is authorized to act in the place of the nurse, while the nurse retains the accountability for the activities performed. The nurse retains responsibility/ accountability for the vital signs. The nurse is accountable for reviewing the data collected and ensuring it is done appropriately. The purpose of delegation is to share tasks as appropriate not to increase the work load of the primary nurse.
Implementation
Application
Safe, Effective Care Environment

1.18 The nurse is consulting a critical pathway to help make client care decisions. Which type of care delivery model is this nurse most likely using to provide client care?
1. primary nursing
2. case management
3. functional nursing
4. team nursing

Answer: 2
Rationale: Critical pathways are often used in conjunction with case management models and/or quality improvement efforts. Both critical pathways and case management involve providing care or overseeing care to a group of clients having similar diagnoses. Primary nursing refers to the provision of all nursing care by a single assigned nurse. In team nursing, the care is provided based upon the education level of the team members.
Implementation
Application
Safe, Effective Care Environment

1.19 Client chart audits provide the nurses with information that impacts the future outcomes of client care. What should the nurses do with this information?
1. Nothing.
2. Submit it to the agency's accrediting body.
3. Place it in a file to compare with the next set of audits.
4. Use the information to create an action plan to address any negative findings.

Answer: 4
Rationale: Data from chart audits or the result of quality assurance audits can be used to develop a plan of action to resolve differences or issues with client care. The nurses are expected to use the information if it will have a positive impact on the nursing practice. Obtaining information and then failing to use it has no useful purpose. While the accrediting body of an institution may encourage quality improvement activities, there is no reason to provide the chart audit results.
Planning
Application
Safe, Effective Care Environment

1.20 A graduate nurse is attending a seminar regarding the role of the nurse as a client advocate. After the session, the students engage in a discussion. Which of the following statements by the graduate nurse indicates the need for further education?
1. "Being a client advocate entails making efforts to improve client outcomes."

Answer: 3
Rationale: The nurse who serves as a client advocate, the nurse may assist and support the client in decision making. The nurse cannot make decisions for the client. The remaining answer choices are elements of being a successful client advocate.
Evaluation
Analysis
Safe, Effective Care Environment

2. "Providing education to the client and family is a key way to be a positive client advocate."
3. "Client advocates have the authority to make decisions for the client."
4. "Communicating client needs to the members of the healthcare team is a role of the client advocate."

CHAPTER 2

2.1 A client asks the nurse, "What's the difference between having good health and being well?" Which of the following could the nurse say in response?
1. "There isn't a difference."
2. "Good health maximizes individual potential."
3. "Wellness is a passive state of freedom from illness."
4. "Wellness maximizes individual potential."

Answer: 4
Rationale: Wellness is an integrated method of functioning that is oriented toward maximizing the potential of the individual's capabilities within the environment in which the client is functioning. The concepts are related but not the same. The process of wellness is active. Good health is relatively static. Since the state is passive, the individual does nothing to move toward their maximum potential.
Implementation
Application
Health Promotion and Maintenance

2.2 A client tells the nurse, "Everyone in my family holds extra weight around their hips and legs." The nurse realizes this client is describing which of the following health risk factors?
1. genetic makeup
2. cognitive ability
3. cultural background
4. developmental level

Answer: 1
Rationale: Genetic makeup affects personality, temperament, body structure, intellectual potential, and susceptibility to the development of hereditary alterations in health. Cognition refers to the intellectual aspects. Culture refers to individuals who share customs and beliefs. There may or may not be a common family involved. The developmental level of an individual refers to their position within a series of stages which are identified by similar traits or tasks.
Implementation
Application
Health Promotion and Maintenance

2.3 An African-American client comes into the clinic for a routine check-up. The nurse realizes this client is most prone to developing which of the following health conditions?
1. tuberculosis
2. hypertension
3. diabetes mellitus
4. glaucoma

Answer: 2
Rationale: Certain diseases occur at a higher rate in some races and ethnic groups than others. In the United States, hypertension is more common in African Americans.
Assessment
Application
Health Promotion and Maintenance

2.4 The nurse is caring for a male client with heart disease. Which of the following would be considered the health promotion behavior with the greatest impact for this client?
1. Perform breast self-examinations.
2. Have a tetanus booster every ten years.
3. Cease smoking.
4. Perform foot self-examinations daily.

Answer: 3
Rationale: The client in this scenario has a history of heart disease with is directly impacted by smoking. To reduce or stop smoking could promote an elevated level of wellness for this client. Teaching health-promoting behaviors is a component of medical-surgical nursing. Breast self-examination is typically for females. Tetanus boosters are necessary but not necessarily critical for this client. Performing a foot self-examination is not indicated for this client's health problem.
Planning
Application
Health Promotion and Maintenance

2.5 The client asks the nurse for information about healthy living. Which of the

Answer: 1, 3, 4
Rationale: Healthy living includes three balanced meals, moderate/regular exercise, sleeping seven to eight hours per day, limit alcohol but favor small

following topics should the nurse review with this client? (Select all that apply.)
   1. Eat three balanced meals per day.
   2. Incorporate mild exercise into a daily routine.
   3. Sleep seven to eight hours per day.
   4. Cease smoking.
   5. Avoid red wine.
	amounts of red wine, eliminate smoking, and keep sun exposure to a minimum.
	Implementation
	Application
	Health Promotion and Maintenance

2.6 A client is admitted with an alteration in pancreatic functioning. The nurse realizes this client is experiencing which of the following causes of disease?
   1. mechanical
   2. biologic
   3. psychological
   4. normative
	Answer: 2
	Rationale: Diseases may have mechanical, biologic, or normative causes. Biologic causes of disease affect body function and are the result of genetic defects, the effects of aging, infestation and infection, alterations in the immune system, and alterations in normal organ secretions. In this client scenario, an alteration in pancreatic functioning is the result of a biologic cause. Mechanical causes of disease result in damage to the structure of the body and are the result of trauma or extremes of temperature. Normative causes of disease are psychological but involve a mind-body interaction, so that physical manifestations occur in response to the psychological disturbance.
	Diagnosis
	Application
	Physiological Integrity

2.7 A client with an acute illness asks, "How long will I be sick? I need to get back to work." The nurse realizes this client's statement will:
   1. adversely affect the recovery phase.
   2. have no impact on the recovery phase.
   3. cause the client to have a relapse.
   4. most likely cause the client to adhere to the treatment plan.
	Answer: 4
	Rationale: The degree of severity of the illness and the method of treatment both affect the length of time required, as do the person's compliance with treatment plans and motivation to return to normal health. There is no information available to indicate the client will suffer a relapse or have an incomplete recovery.
	Evaluation
	Application
	Physiological Integrity

2.8 A client with a chronic illness says, "I must be getting better because I don't have any of the symptoms I used to have." The nurse realizes this client is demonstrating:
   1. remission.
   2. exacerbation.
   3. denial.
   4. cure.
	Answer: 1
	Rationale: During periods of remission, the client does not demonstrate symptoms even though, clinically, the disease is still present. Exacerbation refers to an increase in clinical manifestations. Denial refers to the refusal of the illness condition. Cure refers to the disease being completely gone, and there is no indication of that in this scenario.
	Evaluation
	Application
	Physiological Integrity

2.9 The nurse is planning a primary prevention program for a group of clients. Which of the following topics could be included in this program?
   1. the purpose of diabetes mellitus detection screenings
   2. the need for annual tuberculosis tests
   3. the goals of cardiac rehabilitation
   4. seat belt safety
	Answer: 4
	Rationale: Primary prevention programs include those that prevent or delay the onset of disease. Examples include genetic counseling, smoking and alcohol prevention, protection against environmental risks, nutritious foods, industrial hazard prevention, immunizations, safe sexual practice, and seat belt safety. Secondary prevention activities are used to manage acute healthcare issues. The goals of cardiac rehabilitation, diabetes screening, and tuberculosis testing are types of tertiary prevention. Tertiary prevention is employed to manage chronic conditions.
	Planning
	Application
	Health Promotion and Maintenance

2.10 A 22-year-old client says, "I have no reason to keep going. I have no job, no home, and no family." The nurse realizes this client is at risk for: 1. onset of disease.	Answer: 3 Rationale: Intentional self-harm is the third leading cause of death in young adults. The client's comments concerning the lack of a reason to live may indicate a suicide potential. The comments being made are not normal behaviors for young adults. Once such comments have been made it would be a grave error to do nothing. The question does not address any unsafe sexual practices.

2. nothing. This is normal young adult behavior. 3. suicide. 4. unsafe sexual practices.	Assessment Analysis Health Promotion and Maintenance
2.11 A female client says, "I seem to be gaining weight ever since I turned 40." Which statement by the nurse is most therapeutic? 1. "You aren't as young as you used to be." 2. "You must be overeating." 3. "There isn't anything you can do about it." 4. "The metabolic rate change that occurs with age and less physical activity could be the cause."	Answer: 4 Rationale: Weight gain in middle adulthood is the result of a decrease in physical activity, and a decline in metabolic rate. Making assumptions or discouraging remarks as in option 1 and 2 are not appropriate. There is not adequate information to determine if the client's dietary intake is excessive. Diet and exercise may be indicated and there is no reason to assume these interventions would not be effective. Implementation Analysis Health Promotion and Maintenance
2.12 A 47-year-old female client says, "I worry about my parents everyday and my job is overwhelming." The nurse realizes this client is most at risk for: 1. psychosocial stress. 2. developing cancer. 3. a divorce. 4. committing suicide.	Answer: 1 Rationale: The middle adult years can be filled with stress related to employment, family changes, and aging parents. There is inadequate information presented to make any assumptions about the potential for cancer, divorce, or suicide. Evaluation Analysis Health Promotion and Maintenance
2.13 The middle-aged adult client says, "I want to spend more time volunteering at the local food bank." The nurse identifies this statement as being: 1. a desire to be around food. 2. a potential weight management problem for the client. 3. of no significance. 4. an achievement of a significant developmental task.	Answer: 4 Rationale: The achievement of significant developmental tasks in the middle adult include acceptance of the aging body, respect of oneself, freedom to be independent, accepting the changes in the family role, enjoying success from work and family, and pursuing charitable and altruistic activities. The client's desire is appropriate for their developmental age. This is a factor of significance to this client. No information is presented to support the concerns about a desire to be around food or weight management issues. Evaluation Analysis Health Promotion and Maintenance
2.14 A middle-aged adult is asking questions about avoiding the onset of heart disease. Which of the following would be an appropriate intervention for this client? 1. Tell the client that heart disease is not a concern at their age. 2. Ask the client the reasons for concern. 3. Suggest that the client attend a one-day seminar about ways to prevent or reduce heart disease. 4. Sign them up to learn CPR.	Answer: 3 Rationale: Programs to instruct the client about heart disease means the client accepts responsibility for his or her own health. This type of instruction can be one-on-one or in a seminar format. Advising the client that heart disease is not a concern is incorrect. The opportunity for learning is available. Asking the client about the need for concern is not the most therapeutic response. CPR is not a preventative activity. Planning Application Health Promotion and Maintenance
2.15 A 79-year-old male comes into the clinic for prescription renewals. The nurse realizes this client would be categorized as being: 1. middle-aged. 2. young-old. 3. middle-old. 4. old-old.	Answer: 3 Rationale: The older adult period begins at age 65 and can be divided into three periods: young-old (age 65 to 74), middle-old (age 75 to 84), and old-old (over age 85). Assessment Knowledge Health Promotion and Maintenance

2.16 A middle-old client says, "I wish I didn't have high blood pressure and this arthritis is killing me." The most therapeutic response by the nurse would be:
1. "These illnesses are an unfortunate occurrence associated with aging."
2. "Be glad you don't have cancer."
3. "I would think you would be happy just to be alive."
4. "I don't expect to see your age myself."

Answer: 1
Rationale: Most older adults have one chronic health problem, while many have multiple illnesses. So the most therapeutic response is that these illnesses are an unfortunate occurrence associated with aging. The remaining responses are not therapeutic and are degrading to the client.
Implementation
Application
Health Promotion and Maintenance

2.17 An old-old client tells the nurse, "I hate all of those throw rugs my daughter has on the floor." Which of the following is the most significant risk factor for this client?
1. pneumonia
2. falls
3. urinary tract infection
4. obesity

Answer: 2
Rationale: The three major causes of injury in the elderly are from falls, fire, and motor vehicle accidents. Falls with the resulting hip fractures are the most significant in terms of long-term disability and death. Obesity is not necessarily a risk factor for this client. The risk of infection does increase with aging but is not the most significant risk factor for this client.
Assessment
Comprehension
Health Promotion and Maintenance

2.18 A middle-old client is not recovering as anticipated from an acute respiratory infection. Which statement by the nurse can provide the most useful assessment information?
1. "Have you been able to purchase the antibiotics the doctor prescribed?"
2. "Are you drinking enough fluids?"
3. "Are you sleeping at least seven hours per night?"
4. "Are you eating at least five servings of fruits and vegetables per day?"

Answer: 1
Rationale: The older adult who lives on a fixed income might have to make a choice between food and medication, which results in under-medication and under-treatment of an illness. The other statements do have importance but do not provide the most useful information.
Assessment
Analysis
Physiological Integrity

2.19 An elderly client says, "I can't ask my daughter to do too much for me during the day because she has to go to work." The nurse realizes this client is describing which of the following family features?
1. interdependence
2. maintaining boundaries
3. adapting to change
4. performing family tasks

Answer: 2
Rationale: The family creates boundaries that guide its members, and provides a unique and distinct family culture. This culture provides values. Interdependence refers to the behaviors of individual family members which are constantly influenced by the other members of the family. Adaptation to change refers to the alteration of the family as members are added and others leave. Within each family there are assigned tasks. The focus of this question does not involve family task assignment.
Diagnosis
Analysis
Health Promotion and Maintenance

2.20 A family unit that consists of two middle-aged adults has no children who live at home. Which of the following developmental tasks is important for this family to accomplish?
1. Reestablish their relationship.
2. Close the family home.
3. Balance freedom with independence.
4. Promote joint decision making with adults and children.

Answer: 1
Rationale: The family with middle adults and children who are no longer at home has as one developmental task the reestablishment of the relationship. There is no need to close the family home. Balancing freedom and decision making are not the most important developmental tasks for this family unit.
Evaluation
Analysis
Health Promotion and Maintenance

2.21 The parent of two preschool children voices concerns to the nurse about feeling "stressed" lately and being worried about the limited amount of time to devote to the marriage. Based upon knowledge of the stages of family development, what are the primary tasks for the family during this time?
1. Encourage the educational achievement of the children in the family.
2. Adjust to increased financial responsibilities.
3. Accept mortality of older friends and family members.
4. Reestablish the marital relationship after expansion of the family.

Answer: 2
Rationale: The family with young preschool children is beginning to face the financial and emotional burdens of having a growing family. There is limited time for the couple to spend time on their own relationship. The family with school-aged children is faced with promoting the educational achievement of the family's children. Accepting the mortality of loved ones and reestablishing the marital relationships are tasks of the family with middle and older adults.
Assessment
Application
Psychosocial Integrity

CHAPTER 3

3.1 A 79-year-old client is planning to have a laminectomy. In which of the following healthcare settings is this client most likely going to have this procedure?
1. a skilled nursing facility
2. an acute care hospital
3. an ambulatory care center
4. an outpatient clinic

Answer: 2
Rationale: Today, hospitals are primarily acute care providers; hospital services are focused on highly technical care for severely ill or injured people or for people having major surgery. A skilled nursing facility would be utilized to deliver curative or restorative therapies. These therapies are not emergent in need. The ambulatory care facility is used to provide care to nonemergent/non-acute medical conditions. Outpatient services are provided for those requiring medical intervention but who are able to return to home after their treatments.
Planning
Analysis
Physiological Integrity

3.2 The nurse is teaching a group of clients at a senior center about ways to reduce their blood pressure through exercise and recreation. What type of care is this nurse providing?
1. community-based
2. community health
3. skilled nursing
4. ambulatory

Answer: 1
Rationale: Community-based care centers on individual and family healthcare needs. Care is provided directly to individuals to manage acute or chronic health problems and to promote self-care. Nursing is provided for clients wherever they are. Community health in general is provided to nonspecific groups. Skilled nursing is the provision of care focused on restorative or curative in nature. Ambulatory care is provided to clients who have nonemergent health concerns.
Implementation
Application
Health Promotion and Maintenance

3.3 The nurse is considering working as a community-based nurse. The nurse knows this is a role that may have many contributing factors for providing care. Which of the following factors may affect the health of a community? (Select all that apply.)
1. social support systems
2. political affiliations
3. community healthcare structure
4. environmental factors
5. economic resources

Answer: 1, 3, 4, 5
Rationale: The health in a community is influenced by many factors. These factors include social support systems, community healthcare structure, environment, and economic resources. Political affiliations should not be a factor that affects the nurse's ability to provide health to a community.
Evaluation
Analysis
Health Promotion and Maintenance

3.4 The home care nurse is planning to visit a client who is on Medicare. The nurse realizes that care can be provided if:
1. the home meets safety standards.
2. the client can use a wheelchair.

Answer: 3
Rationale: Coverage for care at home continues only as long as skilled providers are needed and the client is considered homebound. The use of a wheelchair and assistance from others to leave the home does not constitute homebound. The presence of other individuals in the home does not affect inclusion for Medicare.

3. the client is considered homebound. 4. the client lives alone.	Planning Application Health Promotion and Maintenance

3.5 After mass on Sunday the nurse is measuring blood pressures in the church greeting room. This nurse is most likely practicing:
    1. a Sunday day care program.
    2. scheduling parishioners for Meals-on-Wheels.
    3. the first steps to a healthcare clinic.
    4. parish nursing.
	Answer: 4
	Rationale: Parish nursing is a nontraditional community-based way of providing health promotion and health restoration nursing interventions to specific groups of people. The nurse works with the pastor and staff of a faith-based community to promote health through counseling, referrals, teaching, and assessment of healthcare needs. A Sunday day care program would involve activities more of a social nature. Meals-on-Wheels is a program which brings meals to homes. There is no information which indicates these are the initial steps to the development of a healthcare clinic.
	Implementation
	Application
	Health Promotion and Maintenance

3.6 The client is in need of home care, is on oxygen therapy, weak from surgery, has a small surgical incision, and needs to increase activity to gain independence. Which of the following home care providers will the nurse most likely suggest for this client?
    1. physical therapy
    2. speech therapy
    3. social worker
    4. occupational therapy
	Answer: 1
	Rationale: Clients receiving home care services are usually under the care of a physician with the focus of care on treatment or rehabilitation. Home care services are both professional and technical. Based upon this client's presentation and need to increase activity and gain independence, the healthcare provider most likely needed for this client will be the physical therapist. Speech therapy would be used to improve a client's speech. The social worker works with clients to locate appropriate resources after the discharge. Occupational therapy focuses on the client's abilities in performing activities of daily living.
	Planning
	Analysis
	Health Promotion and Maintenance

3.7 Upon discharge from an acute care facility, the client is referred to the hospital's home healthcare agency. This client will be receiving services from which of the following types of agencies?
    1. public
    2. voluntary
    3. private
    4. institution-based
	Answer: 4
	Rationale: An institution-based agency operates under a parent organization such as a hospital. Often, the majority of home care referrals come from the parent organization. Public agencies are open to all who desire their services and are not developed to provide home care services. Private or voluntary agencies are available to a selective populations.
	Assessment
	Application
	Safe, Effective Care Environment

3.8 During the admission of a home care client, the nurse learns the client is married, has no pets, a mother who is homebound and in the home, and has two daughters who do not reside with the client. Which of the following would the nurse consider as the client's family?
    1. the husband and daughters
    2. the husband only
    3. the husband and mother
    4. no one
	Answer: 1
	Rationale: A client's family is not limited to persons related by birth, adoption, or marriage. A person's family is anyone who gives the client support or on whom they rely for any type of need. The person does not need to be living in the same home. The client may even express that they include a pet as a family member.
	Assessment
	Application
	Safe, Effective Care Environment

3.9 A client who is being prepared for discharged from the hospital is identified as needing more care. The family is refusing a transfer to a skilled nursing facility. Which of the following can the nurse do to help this client?
    1. Nothing.
    2. Suggest home care.
    3. Contact protective services because the client is at risk.
    4. Ignore the family and schedule the client for transfer.
	Answer: 2
	Rationale: If the family believes that no help is needed and the nurse believes otherwise, the nurse may ask the family to consider an evaluative home care visit to assess the client at home. It is not unusual for one family client to think that no additional help is necessary and for another to feel differently. It would be inappropriate for the nurse to ignore the concerns being voiced by the client's family. A report to protective services is not indicated as there is no evidence the client is in any danger.
	Planning
	Analysis
	Safe, Effective Care Environment

3.10 The nurse is completing the home health admission for a client. Which one of the following initial actions should the nurse take with the plan of care created from the admission information?
1. Place it in the client's medical record.
2. Keep it during every visit.
3. Send it to the physician for review and approval.
4. Keep it in the client's home.

Answer: 3
Rationale: Once formulated, the nurse sends the plan of care back to the physician for review and approval. Once this approval is given, the nurse should check the plan with each visit, discuss the plan with the client and family, and possibly place a copy in the client's home, if desired. Although the nurse may carry the form during the visits, it is not required and thus is not the most correct answer. The plan of care may be placed in the medical record after discharge from services but that will be based upon agency policy.
Implementation
Analysis
Physiological Integrity

3.11 During the first home care visit, the nurse reviews with the client all of the information about privacy and informed consent. Which of the following documents should the nurse include in this review?
1. Bill of Rights
2. ANA standards for home health nursing
3. ANA standards for community health nursing
4. HIPAA standards

Answer: 1
Rationale: The NAHC Bill of Rights is a federal requirement for all home care agencies. The law requires its concepts to be addressed with all home care clients on the initial visit. Standards of nursing and HIPAA standards are only necessary for the nurse to know, not the client.
Implementation
Application
Safe, Effective Care Environment

3.12 During a phone call to coordinate a time for the first home care visit, the nurse learns the client is on home oxygen therapy, uses a walker for ambulation, and has minimal strength in her lower extremities. This information will be used:
1. to arrange transportation for the client.
2. to schedule a physical therapy evaluation.
3. to evaluate how well the client is doing since arriving home.
4. to plan nursing diagnoses.

Answer: 4
Rationale: Assessment begins when the nurse calls the client to arrange a visit. This information can then be used to plan nursing diagnoses that are appropriate for the client. The home nurse will visit the client in the home, so no transportation is needed. The nurse cannot comprehensively evaluate the client over the phone to determine progress. A physician's order is needed for a physical therapy evaluation.
Assessment
Analysis
Physiological Integrity

3.13 After the initial assessment of a home care client, the nurse identifies areas in which the client can improve their health status. What should the nurse do with this information? (Select all that apply.)
1. Work with the client to set goals.
2. Contract with the client to meet the goals.
3. Write this information in the plan of care.
4. Discuss with the family what to do with the information.

Answer: 1, 3
Rationale: Once significant issues and needs are identified, the nurse and client should set mutually agreed-upon goals. The new information should be added to the assessment section of the plan of care. The information would then be used to develop the rest of the plan. A contract-oriented discussion would take place after the goals are developed together. Involvement of the family may or may not be indicated. The most correct responses revolve around the client.
Planning
Application
Safe, Effective Care Environment

3.14 The home care nurse sees that a family member is not adhering to the client's prescribed plan of care and reviews the plan with this family member. The nurse is functioning in which capacity with the family?

Answer: 3
Rationale: When the family's desires differ from the client's, advocacy can be a challenge. In the event of conflict, the nurse must remain the client's primary advocate. Direct care involves the provision of interventions to the client. When in the role of educator, the nurse provides teaching to the client and family. The coordinator of services is utilized to ensure resources are being used appropriately and without conflict.

1. provider of direct care 2. educator 3. advocate 4. coordinator of services	Implementation Application Safe, Effective Care Environment

3.15 During the home care visit, the nurse learns the client cannot remember what they were taught about bathing and wound care. The nurse realizes this client:
    1. is cognitively challenged.
    2. is hard of hearing.
    3. cannot read.
    4. forgot what was taught.
	Answer: 4
	Rationale: Clients generally forget about one-third of what is said to them and their recall of specific instructions and advice is less than 50%. Forgetting what has been taught is not a sign the client has an auditory or cognitive impairment. Written instructions and review may be necessary. There is not adequate information to assume the client cannot read. When detailed teaching is done, it may be helpful to have another family member present.
	Evaluation
	Application
	Safe, Effective Care Environment

3.16 The home care nurse sees that the client uses a walker and oxygen. During the home assessment, the nurse finds several safety issues. Which of the following should the nurse be most concerned about in the client's home?
    1. grab bars in the bathroom
    2. throw rugs everywhere in the home
    3. large spaces between the furniture in the living room
    4. light switches at arms' length
	Answer: 2
	Rationale: The nurse must be alert to identifying unsafe and hazardous home conditions. The only unsafe condition for the client would be throw rugs everywhere in the home. This may cause the client to slip and fall. The placement of the furniture, grab bars, and light switches do not present a significant safety hazard.
	Evaluation
	Application
	Safe, Effective Care Environment

3.17 The nurse learns that the family has been throwing dirty dressings in with the family's regular trash. Which of the following would be appropriate for the nurse to instruct the family about this practice?
    1. No instruction is necessary, because this is what the family was taught.
    2. Make sure they are wearing sterile gloves when throwing the dressing away.
    3. Bag the dressing so as not to cause infection of other family members with the soiled dressing.
    4. Store the used dressings in a bag in the client's room.
	Answer: 3
	Rationale: Infection control in the home focuses on protecting clients, caregivers, and the community from the spread of disease. Clients need to know the importance of effective hand washing, the use of gloves, and the appropriate disposal of wastes and soiled dressings. It is the responsibility of the nurse to intervene when inappropriate actions are noted. The dressings are already soiled when removed from the client. There is no need for sterile gloves. The dressings must be discarded so storing them in the client's room would hinder that process.
	Implementation
	Application
	Safe, Effective Care Environment

CHAPTER 4

4.1 A client is being transferred from the operating room to the recovery room. The nurse in the recovery room will be providing which phase of nursing care?
    1. preoperative
    2. intraoperative
    3. postoperative
    4. restorative
	Answer: 3
	Rationale: The postoperative phase begins when the client is admitted to the recovery room and ends with the client's recovery from the surgical intervention. The preoperative phase is prior to surgery. The intraoperative phase occurs during the surgery. Restorative is not a phase of the surgical experience.
	Implementation
	Knowledge
	Physiological Integrity

4.2 A client is signing a surgical consent. Afterward the nurse also signs the form. What is the meaning of the nursing signature?	Answer: 1 Rationale: The nurse also signs the form to indicate that the correct person is signing the form and that the client was alert and aware of what was being

1. It means the client was alert and aware of what was being signed.
2. It means the client understood the procedure as described by the nurse.
3. It means the surgeon was too busy to wait for the client to sign the form.
4. It means there is a likelihood of a successful outcome.

signed. Providing a description of the surgical procedure is not the responsibility of the nurse. It is the responsibility of the physician. Obtaining the consent form is a nursing function. The physician's schedule is not a factor. Success of the outcome is not dependent upon the completion of the consent form.
Implementation
Analysis
Safe, Effective Care Environment

4.3 An elderly client is being prepared for orthopedic surgery. The nurse realizes this client is at risk for which of the following?
1. prolonged effects of anesthesia because of herbal supplements
2. decreased tolerance of general anesthesia
3. wound dehiscence
4. increased hypotensive effects of anesthesia

Answer: 2
Rationale: Older adults have age-related changes that affect physiologic, cognitive, and psychosocial responses to the stress of surgery in addition to decreased tolerance of general anesthesia and postoperative medications and delayed wound healing. There is not information provided to indicate the use of herbal supplements. Despite delayed wound healing, there is no information to support the increased risk for wound dehiscence. There is no data to support concerns with hypotension related to anesthesia.
Assessment
Analysis
Physiological Integrity

4.4 An elderly client is completing preoperative diagnostic testing. The nurse notes that the client's carbon dioxide level is elevated. Which of the following nursing interventions would be indicated for this client?
1. Monitor respiratory status and arterial blood gases.
2. Monitor serum potassium level.
3. Monitor serum sodium level.
4. Monitor intake and output.

Answer: 1
Rationale: A client with an altered carbon dioxide level could have a history of emphysema, chronic bronchitis, asthma, pneumonia, or respiratory acidosis, or it could be caused by vomiting or nasogastric suctioning. The best nursing intervention for this client would be to monitor the client's respiratory status and arterial blood gases. A review of the potassium, sodium levels, and intake and output are not the most beneficial to this client at this time.
Planning
Application
Physiological Integrity

4.5 An elderly postoperative client is given an antiemetic for nausea. Which of the following signs would indicate this client is experiencing a possible reaction to the medication?
1. confusion
2. dry mouth
3. involuntary muscle movements
4. breakthrough vomiting

Answer: 3
Rationale: Antiemetics, such as metoclopramide (Reglan) and droperidol (Inapsine) can have tranquilizing effects as well as causing an extrapyramidal reaction. The client would demonstrate involuntary muscle movements, muscle tone changes, and abnormal posturing. Elderly clients may also experience drowsiness which reduces orientation after begin given antiemetics. A dry mouth may be experienced as a result of having been, or currently being unable to have oral intake. This is not an indication of an adverse reaction.
Evaluation
Analysis
Physiological Integrity

4.6 A client's endotracheal tube is being removed after the surgical procedure. The intra-operative nurse realizes this client is in which phase of the general anesthesia process?
1. induction
2. reduction
3. maintenance
4. emergence

Answer: 4
Rationale: The final phase of anesthesia is the client's emergence from the anesthetic agents. As the client begins to awaken, the endotracheal tube is removed, which means the client is able to reestablish voluntary breathing. During the induction phase, anesthesia is administered. Reduction is not a phase of general anesthesia. In the maintenance phase, the client is positioned, the skin is prepared and surgery is performed.
Evaluation
Application
Physiological Integrity

4.7 A client has received conscious sedation for a surgical procedure. The nurse realizes this client will most likely:

Answer: 3
Rationale: Conscious sedation provides analgesia, amnesia, and moderate sedation. Conscious sedation allows the client to independently maintain an open airway and respond to verbal and physical stimulation. Endotracheal intubation is

1. not respond to any stimuli. 2. need an endotracheal tube inserted. 3. respond to physical and verbal stimuli. 4. need blood product replacements.	not done during conscious sedation. The need for blood replacement products is not indicated by the information provided in this scenario. Planning Analysis Physiological Integrity
4.8 A client is prescribed patient-controlled analgesia for postoperative pain. Which of the following should the nurse instruct the client about this analgesia? 1. "Use this analgesia regularly." 2. "Avoid the use of this because of the risk of addiction." 3. "Use this analgesia only when the pain is extremely severe." 4. "Use this analgesia every hour on the hour."	Answer: 1 Rationale: Clients using patient-controlled analgesia in the postoperative period need to be taught the importance of using the allowed dosages regularly to prevent increasing pain levels. The risk of addiction to narcotics is limited when prescribed for short-term post operative use. Allowing the pain to become severe before using the analgesic is counterproductive. Advising the client of a schedule to administer the medication is inappropriate as it is in direct opposition to the principles of patient-controlled analgesia. Implementation Application Physiological Integrity
4.9 A client is in the recovery room. Which of the following members of the healthcare team should the nurse contact regarding the client's level of pain control? 1. the surgeon 2. the anesthesiologist 3. the circulating nurse 4. the scrub nurse	Answer: 2 Rationale: The anesthesiologist or certified registered nurse anesthetist (CRNA) evaluates the client preoperatively and supervises the client's recovery in the post-anesthesia care unit (PACU). The surgeon will manage the client after discharge from the recovery room. The circulating and scrub nurses do not prescribe analgesics. Implementation Application Safe, Effective Care Environment
4.10 A recovery room nurse is consulting with a circulating nurse about a client who is having a surgical procedure. These nurses are most likely in which zone of the surgical department? 1. unrestricted 2. semi-restricted 3. restricted 4. banned	Answer: 1 Rationale: The unrestricted zone permits access by those in hospital uniforms or street clothes. The unrestricted area is often used for communication between the surgical personnel. In the semi-restricted zone there is limited access. In the restricted zone only personnel involved in the operative phase of the procedure are permitted. Banned areas do not exist. Evaluation Analysis Safe, Effective Care Environment
4.11 A client is being positioned for a hip replacement procedure. In which of the following positions will this client most likely be placed? 1. dorsal recumbent 2. semi-sitting 3. lateral chest 4. prone	Answer: 3 Rationale: The lateral chest position is used for some thoracic surgeries as well as hip replacements. The dorsal recumbent, semi-sitting, and prone positions would not allow access to the area of the body involved in the procedure. Planning Analysis Physiological Integrity
4.12 A postoperative client tells the nurse, "A book I read said that I should not eat after surgery for at least a week." Which of the following statements would be an appropriate nursing response? 1. "That's true." 2. "That's not true. You could get an infection in your stomach." 3. "I'll be giving you intravenous feedings anyway." 4. "You don't need any food to heal anyway."	Answer: 2 Rationale: Failure to use the gastrointestinal tract for more than four or five days allows the intestinal mucosa to atrophy, and puts the client at risk for infection. Although the client's statements are not supported by research, the nurse must approach the client in a therapeutic, nonthreatening manner. The administration of intravenous fluids does not replace the need for the client to begin oral intake in a timely manner. Food provides nutrients to the body and thus is needed to promote healing. Implementation Application Physiological Integrity

4.13 A client is being scheduled for surgery. Which of the following should be included in the preoperative teaching provided by the nurse?

1. information concerning the surgical procedure which will be performed by the surgeon
2. the credentials of the anesthesiologist
3. cost of the procedure
4. planned length of stay at the hospital

Answer: 4

Rationale: Client teaching should begin as soon as the client learns about the upcoming surgery. Teaching should include diagnostic tests, time of surgery, preparation for the day of surgery, including taking medications and avoiding meals and postoperative care. Providing an explanation concerning the actual procedure which will be performed is the responsibility of the physician. Discussing the credentials of the anesthesiologist is not the responsibility of the nurse. Providing information concerning the cost of the medical care is not within the scope of responsibility of the nurse.

Planning

Application

Physiological Integrity

4.14 A client has just arrived in the recovery room. How often should the nurse assess the client?

1. Every 15 minutes for the first hour.
2. Every 15 minutes for 30 minutes and then every one hour afterwards.
3. Every hour.
4. Every two hours.

Answer: 1

Rationale: The nurse generally assesses the client every 15 minutes during the first hour and if stable, every 30 minutes for the next two hours, and then every hour during the next four hours. The client is assessed every four hours afterward.

Assessment

Application

Physiological Integrity

4.15 A client is demonstrating signs of postoperative hemorrhage. Which of the following would be an appropriate nursing intervention at this time?

1. Support the client's physiologic mechanism for dissolving clots.
2. Apply sterile pads and a snug pressure dressing to the area.
3. Slow the intravenous fluid administration rate.
4. Raise the head of the client's bed.

Answer: 2

Rationale: Care of the client who is hemorrhaging focuses on stopping the bleeding and replenishing the circulating blood volume. Nursing care includes applying sterile gauze pads and a snug pressure dressing to the area. Supporting the client's physiologic mechanism for dissolving clots, slowing the intravenous fluid administration rate and raising the head of the bed would be dangerous for this client and are contraindicated.

Implementation

Application

Physiological Integrity

4.16 The nurse is assisting a post-operative client in using an incentive spirometer. Which of the following postoperative complications is this nurse attempting to avoid with this client?

1. deep vein thrombosis
2. hemorrhage
3. atelectasis
4. pulmonary embolism

Answer: 3

Rationale: Promoting lung expansion and systemic oxygenation of tissues is a goal in preventing atelectasis. Nursing care includes assisting with incentive spirometry. Deep vein thrombosis, hemorrhage, and pulmonary embolism are not related to incentive spirometer use.

Implementation

Application

Physiological Integrity

4.17 A client is in his fifth postoperative day and has sanguineous drainage with a thick, reddish appearance. The nurse realizes this client's wound is in which stage of healing?

1. stage I
2. stage II
3. stage III
4. stage IV

Answer: 2

Rationale: Stage II of wound healing occurs between days three through 14 following surgery. Sanguineous drainage with a thick, reddish appearance is the most common type of drainage from a noncomplicated surgical wound. Stage I occurs from the time of surgery through day 2. Stage III refers to the period of day 3 through 14 following surgery. The wound will exhibit granulation tissues with the onset of healing established. Stage IV takes place several months to a year following surgery. The scar becomes flat, smaller, and white.

Evaluation

Analysis

Physiological Integrity

4.18 A client who is recovering from abdominal surgery has a penrose drain. Which of the following should the nurse include in the care of this client?

Answer: 1

Rationale: Penrose drains need a safety pin at the exposed end to prevent the drain from slipping down into the wound. Unless full or assessing for a potential problem, there is no need to empty the drain until the end of the shift. There is

1. Make sure there is a safety pin on the end of the drain. 2. Empty the drain every 30 minutes. 3. Clean the wound with normal saline every two hours. 4. Remove the drain four hours postoperatively.	no need to clean the wound with saline. Removal of the drain requires a physician's order. Implementation Application Physiological Integrity
4.19 During the assessment of a postoperative client's bowel sounds, the nurse auscultates high-pitched sounds over all four abdominal quadrants. The nurse realizes this finding could indicate: 1. normal bowel function. 2. paralytic ileus. 3. the onset of flatus. 4. the onset of stool.	Answer: 2 Rationale: A distended abdomen with absent or high-pitched bowel sounds may indicate paralytic ileus. Normal bowel sounds are low in pitch. The onset or presence of flatus and stool is not accompanied by high pitched bowel sounds. Assessment Analysis Physiological Integrity
4.20 A client is scheduled for removal of a cataract. The nurse realizes this client's procedure is classified as being: 1. minor diagnostic. 2. minor elective. 3. major constructive. 4. major elective.	Answer: 2 Rationale: Surgical procedures are classified according to purpose, risk factor, and urgency. Cataract removal would be considered as minor elective surgery. Minor procedures carry minimal risk and minimal physical assault. Major procedures require extensive physical assault and/or serious risk. A diagnostic surgery is used to determine or confirm a condition. Elective procedures are suggested to the client by the physician but there is little risk if they are not performed. Constructive procedures are used to build tissue/organs which are absent. Evaluation Analysis Safe, Effective Care Environment
4.21 A client who is being admitted for surgery asks the nurse why information is being collected about the client's use of herbal and natural supplements. Which of the following statements is an appropriate nursing response? 1. "Herbal remedies may cause pain relievers to be ineffective." 2. "Herbal supplements may interact with anesthesia agents." 3. "The physician is in charge of medications." 4. "There is no need to take these preparations."	Answer: 2 Rationale: The use of herbal supplements must be documented prior to surgery. It is possible for these elements to interact with medications prescribed by the physician. Herbal remedies have not been shown to render analgesics ineffective. Stating that the physician is in charge of medications and that there is no need to take these prescriptions does not adequately respond to the client's inquiry. Implementation Application Physiological Integrity
4.22 A client is complaining of discomfort after a surgical procedure. The client voices fear of addition with taking analgesics as prescribed. What information should be provided to the client regarding these concerns? (Select all that apply.) 1. "Addiction to opioid analgesics is rare when used for short-term postoperative pain management." 2. "Psychological tolerance is not commonly experienced by clients who take narcotic analgesics during the postoperative experience."	Answer: 1, 2, 4 Rationale: The pain management needs of clients will vary and should be managed individually. The use of opioid analgesics during the postoperative period is rarely associated with physical or psychological dependency concerns. Screening is not routinely recommended for surgical clients. Implementation Analysis Physiological Integrity

3. "Clients should be screened for addiction potential prior to being given narcotics."
4. "Pain tolerance and the need for opioid analgesics is individualized."

4.23 The client who is preparing for surgery asks the nurse to keep their glasses and hearing aid in place until they are under anesthesia. Which of the following statements by the nurse demonstrates accurate, therapeutic communication?
1. "You cannot keep those in."
2. "The policies in the surgery unit will not allow it."
3. "I will contact the surgery department to discuss your requests."
4. "Certainly, you can keep them for that time."

Answer: 3
Rationale: Communication will be enhanced if the client can keep glasses and hearing aids for as long as possible. The nurse will need to check with the surgical department first before granting the client's wish. As a client advocate, the nurse is responsible for making an inquiry. The nurse does not have the authority to make the decision on behalf of the surgical department.
Implementation
Analysis
Safe, Effective Care Environment

CHAPTER 5

5.1 The nurse has accepted a change in employment and is found crying in the staff lounge. This nurse is demonstrating:
1. ambivalence.
2. relief.
3. grief.
4. stress.

Answer: 3
Rationale: Changing jobs can trigger a grief response as intense as those seen in the end of the life cycle. The job has been accepted, so the nurse may now be grieving the job that is being left. Ambivalence refers to feelings of uncertainty. Feelings of relief are manifested by a reduction in anxiety or distress concerning a situation. Stress is an emotion related to anxiety.
Assessment
Application
Psychosocial Integrity

5.2 The widow of a client is seen wearing dark clothing, dark glasses, and carrying her late husband's coffee container. The nurse realizes that this client is demonstrating:
1. morbid fixation.
2. a healthy response to a loss.
3. exaggerated grief response.
4. joy.

Answer: 2
Rationale: Grieving and mourning are healthy responses to loss. These behaviors are typical of this process, especially with married couples when one spouse has died. Morbid fixation is a reaction in which the onset of grief is delayed and dysfunctional. The client's response is not excessive or exaggerated. The client's actions are indicative of sadness not joy.
Assessment
Application
Psychosocial Integrity

5.3 A client who had a below-the-knee amputation two months ago is seen walking with a new limb prosthesis and returning to work. The nurse realizes that this client:
1. has completed the work of mourning the loss of his leg.
2. is having difficulty with grief.
3. is in denial.
4. is forgetting about the disease that caused the loss of his limb.

Answer: 1
Rationale: In one theory of the process of loss, the person gradually withdraws attachment to the lost object or person. The period of mourning, or work of mourning, ends and the person reaches a state of completion. This is the time when the client may be ready to move on and make a change such as the prosthesis or return to activities they were involved in before the loss. The client's actions indicate a positive adaptation and do not support an inability to manage their grief. Denial is manifested by behaviors or statements in which the client cannot believe the event has occurred. There is inadequate information provided to infer the client has forgotten about the disease which caused the loss of his limb. Further, forgetting an event of this magnitude is extremely unlikely.
Evaluation
Analysis
Psychosocial Integrity

5.4 A client who has just lost her spouse asks the nurse how long it will be until she feels like living again. The nurse realizes this client has to work through which of the phases of the grieving process according to Bowlby? (Select all that apply.)
1. denial
2. despair
3. detachment
4. protest

Answer: 2, 3, 4
Rationale: The theorist Bowlby believes that a person needs to work through the three phases of grief before being able to move beyond the grief process. These three phases are protest, despair, and detachment. The client's responses indicate she has acknowledged the event. Denial is associated with feelings of disbelief.
Assessment
Analysis
Psychosocial Integrity

5.5 The spouse of a former client tells the nurse that he has joined a support group to help with the loss of his wife. The nurse realizes this client is in which phase of Engel's grief process?
1. acute
2. restitution
3. long-term
4. resolution

Answer: 2
Rationale: According to Engel, there are three phases of the grief process: acute, restitution, and long-term. It is during restitution where the surviving spouse might join a support group to help cope with the loss. The acute phase is initiated by shock and disbelief, manifested by denial. During the long-term phase, the individual begins to come to terms with the loss and renew activities. Resolution is associated with the acceptance of the loss but is not one of the phases in Engel's grief process.
Assessment
Analysis
Psychosocial Integrity

5.6 A client tells the nurse, "I dread going on after the divorce is final. I have no idea how I am going to manage financially or emotionally." The nurse realizes this client is demonstrating which aspect of Caplan's stress and loss theory?
1. living without the assets and guidance
2. psychic pain
3. reduced problem-solving ability
4. emotional turmoil

Answer: 1
Rationale: According to Caplan's theory of stress and loss, there are three factors that influence a person's ability to deal with a loss. This client is demonstrating the factor of "living without the assets and guidance of the lost person or resource." Psychic pain encompasses the loss of the bond and the pain associated with coming to terms with the loss. The client is not demonstrating an inability to handle their problems by the data provided. Emotional turmoil is not a specific factor cited in Caplan's theory.
Assessment
Application
Psychosocial Integrity

5.7 The brother of a terminally ill client states, "I'll donate money to the hospital that cures my brother." The nurse realizes this statement is indicative of which phase of Kubler-Ross's loss stages?
1. denial
2. anger
3. bargaining
4. acceptance

Answer: 3
Rationale: Bargaining is an attempt to postpone the reality of the loss. Often, the family or friend of the dying client tries to make a bargain with someone to gain time or a change in the outcome. In the denial phase, there is a lack of acknowledgment and acceptance of the impending loss. During the anger phase, the individual resists the loss and expresses fury. Acceptance refers to the individual's coming to terms with the loss.
Assessment
Application
Psychosocial Integrity

5.8 A client who is a recent widow states, "I wanted to ask him for a divorce and then he died." The nurse realizes this client is at risk for:
1. accelerated grief reaction.
2. a dysfunctional grief reaction.
3. a typical grief reaction process.
4. psychosomatic disorders.

Answer: 2
Rationale: Factors that can interfere with a successful grieving reaction include ambivalent relationships prior to the loss. This does not necessarily indicate that the process will be dysfunctional or lead to a psychosomatic disorder. The client's intentions may prevent a typical grief reaction.
Diagnosis
Analysis
Psychosocial Integrity

5.9 A client tells the nurse, "My husband left me to be with God." The nurse realizes this client is demonstrating:
1. coping.
2. denial.

Answer: 3
Rationale: Regional differences in the way death is expressed in the United States include "passed away," "went to be with God," and "passed from this life." This client statement does not indicate coping, denial, or a cultural rite.
Evaluation
Application
Psychosocial Integrity

3. a regional difference in which death is expressed. 4. a cultural rite related to death.	

5.10 The nurse is assessing a dying client's spiritual beliefs about death. Which of the following acronyms may be utilized as a method to help the nurse with this assessment process?
   1. ABC
   2. FICA
   3. DABDA
   4. RACE
	Answer: 2
	Rationale: Faith, influence, community, and address form the acronym FICA. This can help the nurse move through the spiritual assessment process with a client. ABC represents airway, breathing, and circulation, and is not related to assessing a dying client's spiritual beliefs about death. DABDA represents denial, anger, bargaining, despair, and acceptance and are Kubler-Ross's stages of grieving. RACE represents the emergency evacuation procedure during a fire: remove, activate, confine, and extinguish, and are not related to this situation.
	Implementation
	Application
	Psychosocial Integrity

5.11 The nurse is having difficulty with the spouse of a dying client. Later, it is determined the reason for the difficulty is because the nurse's spouse died suddenly two year prior. Which of the following would best help this client, the spouse, and the nurse?
   1. Change the nurse's assignment.
   2. Discharge the client to be cared for at home by the spouse.
   3. Nothing. This is normal.
   4. Suggest that the nurse access websites to help with the inability to be supportive of the client's and spouse's needs at this time.
	Answer: 1
	Rationale: Nurses need to take time to analyze their own feelings and values related to loss and the expression of grief. It may be difficult for the nurse to assist others if they have not worked through their own grief situation that is similar. Suggesting access to websites may be helpful to the nurse, but is not the best choice for all involved in this situation. Discharging the client to improve the psychological comfort of the nurse is inappropriate and would not be in the best interests of the client. The nurse's responses are not normal two years after the event and warrant investigation.
	Planning
	Analysis
	Psychosocial Integrity

5.12 The client states, "My husband is the person you should talk with if I am not able to make decisions about my care." The nurse realizes the spouse has been identified as:
   1. the person who has the client's living will.
   2. the healthcare surrogate.
   3. the person with the durable power of attorney.
   4. nothing more than the spouse.
	Answer: 2
	Rationale: A healthcare surrogate is the person selected to make medical decisions when a person is no longer able to make them for him or herself. The client would have been asked to provide a copy of a living will or documentation of any legal designations, such as a durable power of attorney for health care. A durable power of attorney does not have any decision-making power related to health. This needs to specifically be a health care power of attorney.
	Evaluation
	Application
	Psychosocial Integrity

5.13 The youngest child of a client who passed away continues to receive communication and telephone calls from the hospice organization during the six months after the death. The nurse realizes this child is receiving:
   1. bereavement care.
   2. unnecessary phone calls.
   3. constant reminders of his loss that should stop.
   4. actions requested by the mother before death.
	Answer: 1
	Rationale: Hospice services end up to one year after the death of the client and are called bereavement care for the family. The services would cease at the request of family members. So soon after the loss of the child it is appropriate for this contact to continue. The phone calls are not unnecessary. The loss of the child is in the mind of the client despite the phone calls and is not an adequate reason for them to be discontinued. There is inadequate information to determine what the mother's requests were.
	Assessment
	Analysis
	Psychosocial Integrity

5.14 The family of a dying client wants to help with progressive dyspnea. Which of the following can the nurse instruct the family to provide for the client? 1. Lower the head of the bed.	Answer: 2 Rationale: Nursing care to improve respirations includes raising, not lowering, the head of the bed. Suctioning and chest physiotherapy would be considered advanced care measures and were not indicated in the scenario.

	Implementation
2. Raise the head of the bed.	Application
3. Suction the client as much as possible.	Physiological Integrity
4. Perform chest physiotherapy.	

5.15 The family of a dying client states, "She has to be in pain because all she does is moan." The nurse realizes the family is:
1. overreacting.
2. asking for more pain medication for the client.
3. not understanding that moaning can be agitation in the client.
4. considering this to be a sign the client is recovering.

Answer: 3
Rationale: Moaning, groaning, and grimacing often accompany agitation and may be misinterpreted as pain. The family thinks she is in pain, so this does not indicate an improvement in status. The responses by the family are typical and do not reflect excessive concern. There in no indication from the information provided that the family is requesting pain medication.
Evaluation
Application
Physiological Integrity

5.16 A dying client tells the nurse, "Don't let my family leave me." The nurse realizes this client is demonstrating:
1. fear of dying alone.
2. the anticipation of improving in health.
3. the need for the family to see them improve.
4. the desire to prolong life.

Answer: 1
Rationale: Family members are often afraid to be present at the time of death, yet dying alone is the greatest fear expressed by clients. There is no information provided to indicate there will be a recovery or improvement in the client's condition. While the client may wish to live longer, these behaviors are consistent with a fear of dying alone.
Evaluation
Analysis
Psychosocial Integrity

5.17 The nurse who provided care to a terminally ill client does not want to spend any time with the grieving family and begins to provide care to another client. This nurse is demonstrating:
1. empathy.
2. apathy.
3. over-emotionality.
4. blunting.

Answer: 4
Rationale: Blunting is a problem often experienced by nurses who provide care to the terminally ill. The nurse may not be able to handle the emotions appropriately right after the death and this is a coping mechanism. Empathy refers to the provision of emotional support which promotes a feeling of acceptance to the client. Apathy is an emotion characterized by a lack of concern and involvement. Over-emotionality is not a recognized term.
Evaluation
Analysis
Psychosocial Integrity

5.18 A client who has recently lost his spouse states, "I just can't cry." The nurse realizes this client is at risk for developing:
1. psychological issues.
2. depression.
3. over-emotionality.
4. somatic symptoms.

Answer: 4
Rationale: The inability to express grief can lead to the onset of somatic, or physical and emotional symptoms. Crying is considered a typical and expected part of the grief reaction in most grief theories. There is no indication this client will face an increased risk for the development of psychological issues or depression.
Evaluation
Analysis
Psychosocial Integrity

5.19 A preoperative client says to the nurse, "I hope I wake up after surgery. I don't know what my family would do if I didn't." The nurse realizes this client is demonstrating which nursing diagnosis?
1. coping
2. chronic sorrow
3. anticipatory grieving
4. death anxiety

Answer: 3
Rationale: Anticipatory grieving is a combination of intellectual and emotional responses and behavior by which people adjust their self-concept in the face of a potential loss. Chronic sorrow and death anxiety are not nursing diagnoses. This client is expressing a feeling, not demonstrating coping.
Diagnosis
Analysis
Psychosocial Integrity

6.1 A client tells the nurse, "I seem to need one more drink each night after work, just to unwind." The nurse realizes this client is describing:
1. withdrawal symptoms.
2. substance abuse.
3. tolerance.
4. intolerance.

Answer: 3
Rationale: Tolerance is a cumulative state in which a particular dose of the chemical elicits a smaller response than before. With increasing tolerance, the individual needs higher and higher doses to obtain the desired effects. Withdrawal is characterized by tremors, diaphoresis, anxiety, high blood pressure, tachycardia, and possibly convulsions. Substance abuse is the misuse of a substance characterized by dependence on the substance. Intolerance refers to the inability of the body to handle a substance.
Assessment
Application
Psychosocial Integrity

6.2 A nurse calls off from work periodically and has a known history of using alcohol. This nurse is most likely demonstrating:
1. substance abuse.
2. substance dependence.
3. tolerance.
4. withdrawal.

Answer: 1
Rationale: Substance abuse is characterized as the failure to fulfill major role obligations at work, home, or school. Substance dependence does not cause this level of failure with obligations. Tolerance refers to needing more of a substance to gain the same effect. Withdrawal occurs when a client stops using a substance.
Diagnosis
Application
Psychosocial Integrity

6.3 A client who was sexually abused as a child tells the nurse, "I just like to try different drugs recreationally." The nurse realizes this client:
1. has an addictive personality.
2. has low self-esteem and difficulty expressing emotions.
3. has a mental illness.
4. wants to fit into his peer group.

Answer: 2
Rationale: Many substance abusers have experienced sexual or physical abuse in their childhood and as a result, have low self-esteem and difficulty expressing emotion. The client did not indicate an addiction to any one substance. The peer group was not mentioned. The client has psychological needs, but it is not determined if they are to the point of mental illness.
Evaluation
Analysis
Psychosocial Integrity

6.4 The nurse manager has been alerted to an unusually high number of "wasted" narcotics in the care area. Which of the following should the nurse do about this finding?
1. Nothing. This could be a normal occurrence.
2. Have an educational program provided to all staff about narcotic use.
3. Review the records to see which clients were prescribed the wasted narcotics and interview them.
4. Realize that a substance abuse problem may be occurring with a staff member and begin closer observation.

Answer: 4
Rationale: One warning sign of an impaired nurse in the workplace is excessive "wasting" of narcotics. This nurse manager needs to realize that a substance abuse problem is occurring with a staff member and begin closer observation of the staff. Providing an educational program and interviewing clients may be part of the close observation, but it is not the most important activity by the nurse manager initially. Monitoring for and taking action for potential problems on the unit is a key role of the nurse manager. Taking no action for the excessive wasting of narcotics is inappropriate.
Implementation
Analysis
Psychosocial Integrity

6.5 A client has been diagnosed with alcoholism which is causing him to be depressed. The nurse realizes these diagnoses are indicative of:
1. sexual abuse as a child.
2. a dual disorder.
3. tolerance.
4. withdrawal.

Answer: 2
Rationale: Dual disorder is the coexistence of substance abuse and a psychiatric disorder in the same individual. One disorder can be an indication of the other. No information is presented to suspect sexual abuse. Tolerance refers to the ability to handle increasing amounts of a substance. Withdrawal symptoms typically do not include depression.
Diagnosis
Application
Psychosocial Integrity

6.6 A pregnant client continues to smoke so that she "doesn't gain a lot of weight." Which of the following can the nurse instruct this client about smoking while pregnant? 1. "It doesn't prevent weight gain." 2. "It will prevent some weight gain." 3. "It can cause low birth weight in the infant." 4. "It will not harm the infant."	Answer: 3 Rationale: Smoking while pregnant can cause infant low birth weight, spontaneous abortions, perinatal mortality, and sudden infant death. Smoking may or may not prevent weight gain in the mother. Implementation Application Health Promotion and Maintenance
6.7 A 76-year-old male who used to run a bar and restaurant comes into the clinic with progressive numbness and tingling of all four extremities. For which of the following should this client be evaluated? 1. detoxification 2. psychological dependence 3. tolerance 4. Korsakoff's psychosis	Answer: 4 Rationale: Korsakoff's psychosis is a dementia caused by a vitamin B_1 deficiency from chronic alcohol use. Besides the progressive dementia, symptoms include peripheral neuropathy characterized by numbness and tingling of the hands and feet. With this client's employment history, evaluation of this client for this psychosis would be indicated. Detoxification refers to the process of taking the client off of a substance. Psychological dependence results when a client believes they need to take or use a substance. Tolerance is the need for an ever increasing amount of a substance to achieve a certain feeling. Planning Analysis Physiological Integrity
6.8 A 48-year-old male with a history of chronic marijuana use tells the nurse that his wife cannot get pregnant and wants to have fertility testing done. Which of the following would be an appropriate response for the nurse to make to this client? 1. "Marijuana adversely affects the sperm and testosterone levels in men." 2. "It wouldn't hurt to see which partner has the fertility issues." 3. "Having a baby at his age might not be a good idea." 4. "Children would cost money and maybe he would have to reduce his marijuana use."	Answer: 1 Rationale: The reproductive system is affected by marijuana by decreasing spermatogenesis and testosterone levels in men. Fertility testing may not be necessary if the drug use stops. Answers 3 and 4 are judgment statements and should be avoided. Implementation Analysis Health Promotion and Maintenance
6.9 A 35-year-old client with a history of barbiturate abuse tells the nurse that she "likes to have a few drinks with friends." The nurse realizes this client is at risk for: 1. withdrawal symptoms. 2. dual disorders. 3. cross-tolerance. 4. psychotic illness.	Answer: 3 Rationale: With barbiturate abuse, cross-tolerance can develop to alcohol and general anesthetics. The coexistence of substance abuse/dependence and a psychiatric disorder in a single individual is known as a dual disorder. Withdrawal symptoms may include tremors, diaphoresis, anxiety, high blood pressure, tachycardia, and possibly convulsions. Assessment Application Psychosocial Integrity
6.10 A client with a crystal methamphetamine addiction is withdrawing from the drug. The family phones the clinic concerned about the client's symptoms, which include excessive fatigue, sleeping, and a voracious appetite. Which of the following can the nurse instruct this family about the client's symptoms?	Answer: 4 Rationale: Withdrawal from amphetamines produces dysphoria and craving with fatigue, prolonged sleep, excessive eating, and depression. There is no need to limit food or sleep during this phase. Implementation Analysis Psychosocial Integrity

1. Prevent the client from eating.
2. Try to keep the client awake and take to an emergency room if sleeping continues.
3. Give the client hot black coffee to keep them awake.
4. This is completely normal while withdrawing from this drug.

6.11 The nurse sees a client with excessive lacrimation, rhinorrhea, yawning, and diaphoresis despite the cool temperature in the waiting room. Which of the following do these assessment findings suggest to the nurse?
1. nicotine withdrawal
2. heroin withdrawal
3. amphetamine withdrawal
4. marijuana withdrawal

Answer: 2
Rationale: Initial withdrawal symptoms from heroin include drug craving, lacrimation, rhinorrhea, yawning, and diaphoresis which last up to ten days since the last dose of the drug. Signs of nicotine withdrawal include craving, nervousness, restlessness, increased irritability, increased appetite, and weight gain. Amphetamine and marijuana use are associated with psychological dependence.
Assessment
Analysis
Psychosocial Integrity

6.12 A client tells the nurse that she recalls "feeling funny" after taking a few sips of her drink at a night club and later remembers that she was raped. The nurse suspects that this client had been given:
1. heroin.
2. amphetamines.
3. barbiturates.
4. ecstasy.

Answer: 4
Rationale: Ecstasy has a history of being a popular rave drug and has reappeared in recent years as a date or rape drug. This drug affects impulse control and can lead to uninhibited sexual responses in women. Heroin is associated with a "rush" followed by a sense of euphoria. Amphetamines are associated with arousal and an elevation in mood. Barbiturates cause feelings of sedation.
Assessment
Application
Psychosocial Integrity

6.13 The nurse learns that there are multiple ways for organic inhalants to gain entry into the body. What are they? (Select all that apply.)
1. bagging
2. injecting
3. huffing
4. sniffing

Answers: 1, 3, 4
Rationale: Bagging involves pouring the solvent into a plastic bag and inhaling the vapor. Huffing refers to pouring the solvent on a cloth towel and inhaling the vapors. Sniffing refers to inhaling the solvent directly from the container. Injecting would not be an inhalant route.
Evaluation
Application
Psychosocial Integrity

6.14 A client tells the nurse that the new medication he is taking will cause him to be physically ill if he drinks with it. The nurse realizes this client has been prescribed:
1. disulfiram (Antabuse).
2. naltrexone (ReVia).
3. fluoxetine (Prozac).
4. magnesium sulfate.

Answer: 1
Rationale: Disulfiram (Antabuse) is a form of aversion therapy that prevents the breakdown of alcohol, and causes intense vomiting if taken while drinking alcohol. Naltrexone (ReVia) is prescribed to reduce the craving for alcohol. It blocks the brain from feeling pleasure when alcohol or other narcotics are used. Prozac is administered to stabilize mode and diminish anxiety. Magnesium is administered to reduce the incidence of postwithdrawal seizures.
Assessment
Application
Psychosocial Integrity

6.15 The nurse is interviewing a client who denies having a longstanding history of alcohol and drug use. Which of the following should the nurse do to gain information and direct care?
1. Confront the client.
2. Refer to a psychologist.
3. Utilize the CAGE questionnaire.
4. Request an inpatient evaluation.

Answer: 3
Rationale: The CAGE questionnaire is useful for individuals who deny or do not want to admit that they have an alcohol or drug use problem. It is usually self-administered. Two or more positive answers signify a problem that might need treatment. The CAGE acronym represents: cut, annoyed, guilty, and eye-opener. Direct confrontation with the client may hinder the establishment of a therapeutic environment of open communication. Initiating a referral to another medical professional and requesting an inpatient evaluation are beyond the scope of the nurse.
Evaluation
Analysis
Psychosocial Integrity

6.16 A client withdrawing from a drug is experiencing hallucinations. Which of the following nursing diagnoses would be appropriate for this client? 　1. disturbed thought processes 　2. low self-esteem 　3. deficient knowledge 　4. imbalanced nutrition	Answer: 1 Rationale: Disturbed thought processes would support the client who is demonstrating an alteration in the perception of reality, as in hallucinations. The nurse should not argue that the hallucination is not true. Nutrition and self-esteem are not related to hallucinations. Diagnosis Application Psychosocial Integrity
6.17 The nurse in the emergency department is providing care to a client with a cocaine addiction. Which of the following terms are often used for cocaine? (Select all that apply.) 　1. snow 　2. sugar 　3. purple hearts 　4. white cloud	Answer: 1, 2, 4 Rationale: Cocaine has a variety of street names, which include: bernice, bernies, big C, blow, charlie, coke, dust, girl, heaven, jay, lady, nose candy, nose powder, snow, sugar, white lady. Street names for crack, a derivative of cocaine, include: conan, freebase, rock, toke, white cloud, and white tornado. Implementation Application Psychosocial Integrity

CHAPTER 7

7.1 The nurse is planning to attend a program to learn how to respond to mass casualty incidents. There are core competencies within this program. The nurse knows that these competencies are: (Select all that apply.) 　1. critical thinking. 　2. nursing process. 　3. technical skills. 　4. communication. 　5. assessment.	Answer: 1, 3, 4, 5 Rationale: The publication "Educational Competencies for Registered Nurses Responding to Mass Casualty Incidents" lists four core competencies: critical thinking, assessment, technical skills, and communication. Nursing process is a systematic tool for nurses to utilize to manage client care. Planning Analysis Safe, Effective Care Environment
7.2 The hospital has been notified of a subway derailment with approximately 250 passengers. Many of the passengers are reported to be injured. This situation would be classified as being: 　1. a natural disaster. 　2. a multiple casualty incident. 　3. a mass casualty incident. 　4. an accidental disaster.	Answer: 3 Rationale: A mass casualty incident is one in which there are greater than 100 casualties involved. Natural disasters are caused by acts of nature or emerging diseases. A multiple casualty incident indicates the presence of greater than 1 victim. An accidental disaster is man-made. Evaluation Application Safe, Effective Care Environment
7.3 The care area has been alerted to a possible illness associated with the tainting of a popular over-the-counter pain reliever. The nurse realizes the tainting of this pain reliever could be classified as being: 　1. a nonconventional terrorist attack. 　2. a conventional terrorist attack. 　3. an accidental disaster. 　4. a natural disaster.	Answer: 1 Rationale: Nonconventional terrorism uses chemical, biological, and nuclear means to release a toxin, contaminate a food source, or contaminate some other product. This would not be classified as a disaster and is not a conventional type of terrorist attack. Assessment Application Safe, Effective Care Environment
7.4 The emergency room nurses are noting an usually high number of clients coming into the department with complaints of nausea, vomiting, and severe headache. What should be done with this information?	Answer: 2 Rationale: Healthcare providers must be alert when there is a change in the trend of symptoms within clients. The infection control nurse should be contacted. Laboratory medicine will run tests on specimens that would otherwise be discarded. The public health department is also contacted with this information. Closing the emergency room would not be necessary. Staffing may need to be adjusted based on number or acuity of clients, not just a trend in symptoms.

1. No further action is needed at this time. 2. Contact the Infection Control Department and Laboratory Medicine. 3. Close the emergency room. 4. Call for more staffing to handle all of the clients.	Implementation Application Safe, Effective Care Environment
7.5 A client comes into the clinic with the onset of itching after opening a letter received about a week ago that contained "quite a bit of white powder." It is suspected that this client has had an anthrax exposure. Which medication can the nurse anticipate that this client will most likely be prescribed? 1. normal saline solution flush to the skin 2. penicillin 3. acetaminophen 4. solumedrol	Answer: 2 Rationale: Anthrax incubation is typically one to seven days. Treatment includes the administration of penicillin, doxycycline, and fluoroquinolones. The exposure has already taken place. There is no purpose for cleaning the skin with normal saline. Acetaminophen is used as an antipyretic and analgesic. Solumedrol is used to manage allergic reactions and respiratory conditions. Planning Application Safe, Effective Care Environment
7.6 A client says to the nurse, "I'm scared about a terrorist attack since I live so close to the airport." Which of the following would be an appropriate response for the nurse to make to this client? 1. "Have you thought about moving?" 2. "That's silly to be so worried." 3. "What do you have in your home to help you in the event of a terrorist attack?" 4. "I would be concerned too."	Answer: 3 Rationale: The general public looks to nurses for information and trusts that what the nurse advises is true and accurate. The nurse should ask the client what they have prepared in their home should there be a terrorist attack. The nurse should not discount the client's fears or compound their fears. Moving because of this fear is not realistic and does little to assist the client at this time. Assessment Analysis Safe, Effective Care Environment
7.7 The nursing staff is planning to attend a disaster prevention presentation. The purpose of this education is: 1. to learn the organization's disaster plan. 2. to have the nurses participate in the plan for handling a disaster. 3. to educate the nurses about recognizing possible terrorists. 4. to learn how the nurse will participate in mitigation.	Answer: 4 Rationale: Mitigation is the action taken to prevent or reduce the harmful effects of a disaster on human health or property. A key nursing activity related to mitigation is the active participation in learning activities to be able to teach the general public. The staff should already be familiar with the organization's disaster plan. The focus of the program is prevention. Option 2 discusses management of a disaster which has already taken place. Recognition of terrorists is not the focus of the nursing team. Planning Analysis Safe, Effective Care Environment
7.8 The community is holding a memorial service to honor those members whose lives were lost in the flood one year ago. In which stage of the disaster recovery process is this community? 1. restoration 2. reconstitution 3. mitigation 4. disaster reflection	Answer: 2 Rationale: Reconstitution occurs when the life of the community returns to a "new" normal. Restoration is a recovery stage in which rebuilding takes place. Mitigation activities focus on prevention or reduction of harmful effects of a disaster. Disaster reflection is a recall of the events which have taken place. Assessment Application Safe, Effective Care Environment

7.9 During the disaster preparedness presentation, the nurse learns about the harmful effects of a dirty bomb. Which of the following treatments will preserve life in the event of this disaster?
 	
  1. support of client who will develop radiation sickness
  2. heart-lung transplant
  3. liver transplant
  4. bone marrow transplant
	Answer: 4
	Rationale: Radiation sickness results from exposure to a dirty bomb. While this condition can be deadly, it is survivable with bone marrow transplantation. While the provision of support is important for clients who have developed radiation sickness, it does not directly preserve life. Transplantation of a heart, lung, or liver will not reduce the damage caused by the radiation exposure of a dirty bomb.
	Evaluation
	Analysis
	Safe, Effective Care Environment

7.10 A client who was exposed to a thermal nuclear blast is experiencing blindness. Which of the following can the nurse instruct this client about the eye injury?
 	
  1. The blindness is permanent.
  2. The blindness will last for several years.
  3. The blindness will resolve in time. The intense light from the blast caused the temporary blindness.
  4. The blindness will resolve somewhat in time; however, the client will always have vision changes afterward.
	Answer: 3
	Rationale: Eye burn injuries are associated with the bright light flash of nuclear detonation. The intense light might blind the client momentarily. The effects will disappear with time.
	Implementation
	Application
	Safe, Effective Care Environment

7.11 A client is brought into the emergency room with chemical burns. Which of the following should the nurse do to help this client?
 	
  1. Check to see if all of the clothing has been removed and begin flushing the client's skin with water.
  2. Begin flushing the client's clothes and skin with warm water.
  3. Do not remove any jewelry.
  4. Keep the client's contact lenses in place and flush only with warm water.
	Answer: 1
	Rationale: After the chemical exposure, the client's clothing and jewelry should be removed. The chemical should then be flushed from the skin with copious amounts of cool running water. Jewelry should be removed. Contact lenses should be removed.
	Implementation
	Application
	Safe, Effective Care Environment

7.12 The National Weather Service has announced the likelihood of a large snow event in a major metropolitan area. Which of the following is most likely to occur with this weather event?
 	
  1. stress-related injuries
  2. crushing injuries
  3. myocardial infarctions
  4. burns
	Answer: 3
	Rationale: Overexertion and exhaustion are major problems during the snow shoveling following a major snowstorm. The exertion required to shovel heavy snow in the extreme cold can cause a myocardial infarction. Stress-related injuries would result in a situation which promoted anxiety. A snow event would not fulfill those criteria. Crushing injuries would result from something falling on individuals. Snow will not meet those criteria. Burn injuries will not accompany snow fall.
	Planning
	Analysis
	Physiological Integrity

7.13 The emergency response team is setting up an area to triage victims of a building blast in a major metropolitan	Answer: 3 Rationale: The cold zone is considered as the safe zone. It is the area in which a more in-depth triage of victims can occur. The hot zone is closest to the site of

area. Which of the following areas can be used to set up this triage location?
1. hot zone
2. warm zone
3. cold zone
4. clean zone

the disaster. Decontamination takes place in the hot zone. It would not provide the needed safety to perform in-depth triage activities. The warm zone is next to the hot zone. The warm zone also serves as a location for decontamination of victims. Personal protective equipment is needed. It is not a safe location for the in-depth triage.
Planning
Application
Safe, Effective Care Environment

7.14 The nurse is planning the coding for a triage disaster plan. What are the colors most associated with triage? (Select all that apply.)
1. white
2. red
3. yellow
4. black
5. green

Answer: 2, 3, 4, 5
Rationale: The four basic colors used in triage systems are red, yellow, green, and black. Red is considered critical, yellow is stable but still needs attention at a hospital, green is minor injuries, and black means they have died. The color white is not used in triage systems.
Planning
Application
Safe, Effective Care Environment

7.15 A community client arrives to the site of a disaster, hysterically crying because she was in the building that had collapsed just minutes before the disaster. Which of the following should be done with this client?
1. Advise her to go home with her family.
2. Triage this client and transport to the hospital.
3. Have a nurse talk with the client.
4. Ask psychiatric service personnel to talk with this client.

Answer: 4
Rationale: Social services personnel or psychiatric service personnel should be available to assist the "worried well" in coping with the trauma they have just experienced, witnessed, or heard about through the media. The client is very upset and should not be sent away without any intervention. The client escaped the building before it collapsed. She experienced no injuries. The triage services need to be preserved for those who suffered injuries.
Implementation
Application
Safe, Effective Care Environment

7.16 An elderly client asks the nurse, "What can we do to be prepared if there's a disaster in our community?" Which of the following can the nurse respond to this client?
1. "There is not really much we can do to be prepared."
2. "Plan to evacuate your home at a moment's notice."
3. "Make sure all of your important papers, health information, medication information, and next-of-kin information is in one place."
4. "Make sure you can call your family to come and pick you up if this happens."

Answer: 3
Rationale: The nurse should suggest this client be prepared. One step in preparation is to have a current list of medications, doses, and times of administration that should be kept in an easily-accessible, secure place. The names and phone numbers of significant persons, relatives, those with power of attorney, healthcare providers, or any others to be notified in case of emergency should also be kept in an easily-accessible place. Planning can significantly reduce the outcome in the event of a disaster. Not all disasters will require immediate evacuation from the home. Phone communication may not be possible during the initial phases of a disaster. This is not the best answer.
Planning
Application
Safe, Effective Care Environment

8.1 A client tells the nurse that her mother has type 2 diabetes and heart problems. The nurse realizes that this information:

1. means that the client will probably not change her health habits.
2. can help predict the client's future health problems.
3. helps predict the future health of the client's children.
4. means that the client keeps in touch with her parents.

Answer: 2
Rationale: Even though most individuals do not know their genetic makeup, the nurse can help plan strategies to promote and maintain health for the client. There is no evidence that the client would not change any health habits. Although the family health history is significant it will not provide a direct prediction for the client's children and is not the best answer. There is not enough information to determine the relationship between the client and her family.
Assessment
Application
Health Promotion and Maintenance

8.2 The physician has ordered chromosomal analysis for a newborn baby. Based upon your knowledge, which of the following tests has been ordered?

1. karyotype
2. newborn screen
3. carrier testing
4. preimplantation genetic diagnosis

Answer: 1
Rationale: The karyotype provides an analysis of the number and structure of the chromosomes. Newborn screening is performed shortly after birth. It seeks to identify inborn errors of metabolism. Carrier testing is completed on asymptomatic individuals who may be carriers of one copy of a gene alteration that can be transmitted to future children in an autosomal recessive or X-linked pattern of inheritance. Preimplantation genetic testing involves the detection of disease causing gene alterations in human embryos just after in vitro fertilization and before implantation in the uterus.
Assessment
Application
Health Promotion and Maintenance

8.3 A 42-year-old pregnant client asks the nurse if the baby will be born with Down syndrome. The nurse realizes that, in this chromosome abnormality, the baby has:

1. 23 pairs of chromosomes.
2. 26 pairs of chromosomes.
3. one member of a chromosome pair missing.
4. one extra member of a chromosome pair.

Answer: 4
Rationale: A zygote that is trisomic, or one that has three chromosomes instead of the usual 2, can produce the condition called Trisomy 21 or Down syndrome. The specific chromosome involved with this disorder is number 21.
Assessment
Application
Health Promotion and Maintenance

8.4 A client tells the nurse that her husband has chronic myelogenous leukemia and is concerned that any of their children will inherit the same genetic disorder. Which of the following is an appropriate nursing response?

1. "The genetic makeup that created the chronic myelogenous leukemia in your husband is not inheritable."
2. "I would be concerned, too."
3. "Maybe you should re-think having children."
4. "It could cause the same disorder, but it's a decision that you will have to make."

Answer: 1
Rationale: The chromosome translocation that is responsible for chronic myelogenous leukemia occurs in somatic cells, not germ cells, and therefore is not inheritable. All other responses are offering advice, which is not in the best interest of the client and his family and is not considered therapeutic communication.
Implementation
Application
Health Promotion and Maintenance

8.5 A client has a history of a genetic disorder and is concerned that this same disorder will be passed to his children. What information should the nurse provide to this client?

Answer: 2
Rationale: Mitochondrial genes and any diseases due to DNA alterations on those genes are transmitted through the mother in a matrilineal pattern. An affected female will pass the metabolism DNA mutation to all of her children. An affected male will not pass the metabolism DNA mutation to any of his children. It is

1. All genetic disorders are passed to future children.
2. If the genetic disorder is a disorder of metabolism, it will most likely not be passed to any children.
3. The best possible plan for this problem is to avoid children.
4. The children will inherit the disorder only if the disorder is on chromosomes 13, 18, and 21.

inappropriate for the nurse to recommend the client not have children. This recommendation steps beyond the scope of practice. Inherited disorders exist beyond those involving chromosomes 13, 18, and 21.
Implementation
Analysis
Health Promotion and Maintenance

8.6 A pregnant client tells the nurse, "I hope the baby has his father's eye color and my hair." The nurse realizes that the chances of the baby being born with this criteria are:
1. 0%
2. 25%
3. 50%
4. 75%

Answer: 3
Rationale: All genes are paired. Only one gene of a pair is transmitted to an offspring. One copy of each gene in an offspring comes from the mother and the other comes from the father. Therefore, the baby has a 50% chance of being born with the characteristics the mother is hoping for.
Evaluation
Analysis
Health Promotion and Maintenance

8.7 A baby is born with a genetic disorder that did not affect either of the parents. The nurse realizes that:
1. the mother is the carrier of the disorder.
2. the father is the carrier of the disorder.
3. the father is not the "biological father" of the baby.
4. both parents are carriers of the disorder.

Answer: 4
Rationale: A child born with a recessive condition has inherited one altered gene from their mother and one from their father. In most cases, neither of the parents is affected and therefore, each of the parents must have a single gene alteration on one chromosome of a pair and the normal, wild-type, or unaltered, form of the gene on the other chromosome. These parents would be known as carriers of the condition and they do not usually exhibit any signs and symptoms of the condition. If only one parent was affected, the child would not be born with the disorder but simply be a carrier as well. There is no evidence to support the fact the father is not the biological father.
Assessment
Analysis
Health Promotion and Maintenance

8.8 A baby is born with a genetic disorder. Neither parent has a history of this disorder. The nurse realizes that the cause of this disorder can be explained as being:
1. de novo.
2. penetrance.
3. an X-linked dominant condition.
4. evidence to justify the need for a paternity test.

Answer: 1
Rationale: When there is no previous history of a condition, including even subtle signs and symptoms of the disease, in any other immediate or distant family member, the disease may be caused by a spontaneous new mutation. This is called "de novo." Penetrance is the probability that a gene will be expressed phenotypically. X-linked conditions are recessive in nature. The need for a paternity test is not influenced by genetic conditions.
Intervention
Analysis
Health Promotion and Maintenance

8.9 Upon the completion of genetic testing, a client is happy to learn that she has a negative test result. The nurse realizes that this client needs to understand that:
1. she will never experience a genetically-caused disease.
2. any children she has will be free from genetic diseases.
3. her children might develop disease from genetic misplacement of chromosomes.
4. this is not a guarantee.

Answer: 4
Rationale: A negative test result cannot guarantee that the disease or condition might not develop in the future. The client's children may experience random chromosomal abnormalities which are seen in the rest of the population.
Evaluation
Analysis
Health Promotion and Maintenance

8.10 A client and her future husband completed genetic testing through a laboratory that they found on the internet. The client is upset because the results determined that they are at risk for having children with congenital abnormalities. Which of the following is an appropriate nursing response?

1. "Not all genetic testing laboratories are the same. It might be beneficial to validate those results with another lab."
2. "The decision for children has been made for you."
3. "Are you concerned that your future husband won't want to get married now?"
4. "I wouldn't worry about those results."

Answer: 1

Rationale: Genetic tests are often offered by laboratories before the tests have been proven safe, effective, and practical. Because the majority of genetic conditions are rare, there is often only one laboratory that offers a particular genetic test. Recently there has been much concern about "direct-to-consumer" genetic testing, which are offered at walk-in locations and also via the internet. These tests offer individuals genetic testing results in private without a physician's order and fear of discrimination, but also without education about the implications of the test results. The other nursing responses are offering advice, which is not considered therapeutic communication.

Evaluation

Application

Health Promotion and Maintenance

8.11 A client tells the nurse that her teenage son, who has a congenital abnormality, is demonstrating increasing anger and animosity toward her and her husband. The nurse realizes that the son might be:

1. behaving as a normal teenager.
2. confused.
3. fostering resentment toward his parents.
4. demonstrating disease from the congenital abnormality.

Answer: 3

Rationale: The individual who has inherited an altered disease-producing gene may foster deep resentment toward the parent who carries the altered gene. There is no evidence that these behaviors are related to disease process. Normal teens do not have to manage the implications associated with the occurrence of a congenital abnormality. The client is not confused. There is no information provided to support this assumption.

Assessment

Analysis

Health Promotion and Maintenance

8.12 The nurse is assessing a family for all diseases and conditions that exist with both living and deceased family members. This nurse is most likely creating a

Fill in the Blank: _____

Answer: Pedigree

Rationale: A pedigree is a pictorial representation or diagram of the medical history of a family. The finished pedigree presents a family's medical data and biological relationship information at a glance.

Assessment

Application

Health Promotion and Maintenance

8.13 At the conclusion of a genetic counseling session, a family member says to the nurse, "There's got to be something that you aren't telling us." The nurse realizes that this individual is:

1. feeling guilty because of the outcome of the testing.
2. demonstrating signs of a congenital abnormality.
3. angry with the findings from the testing.
4. uncomfortable with the non-directive approach taken by the genetic healthcare providers.

Answer: 4

Rationale: Many clients are accustomed to practitioners and nurses who provide decision-making direction and guidance, so clients may be uncomfortable when the nurse takes the opposite approach. They may believe that the nurse or healthcare provider is withholding very bad news. The nurse should discuss the positives and negatives of each decision and present as many options as possible through the use of therapeutic listening and communication skills. Feelings of guilt and anger are not manifested by the demeanor demonstrated by the client. There is no information provided concerning the genetic disorder being evaluated. There is an inadequate amount of data presented to link the behaviors with the disorder.

Evaluation

Analysis

Health Promotion and Maintenance

8.14 A baby with Down syndrome has been born to a mother. The mother refuses to allow any family members to

Answer: 3

Rationale: Nurses must also provide care to help alleviate any client anxiety or guilt. Anxiety of the unknown is common when awaiting diagnosis or test results, but individuals also experience anxiety from not understanding the

visit her or the newborn. The nurse realizes that this client is demonstrating:

1. postpartum depression.
2. denial.
3. anxiety and guilt.
4. poor bonding.

future implications of a confirmed genetic disease. Guilt may be associated with knowledge of the existence of a genetic condition being in a family. The nurse must support clients as they contemplate telling extended family members, friends, and neighbors about a confirmed diagnosis. Clients often do not want to tell extended family members until they are ready. The nurse should encourage open discussion and expressing fears and concerns. Guilt and shame are very common as a client deals with the loss of the expectation and dream of a healthy child. There is no evidence that the mother is in denial or has poor bonding with the infant. Postpartum depression is not an immediate response.
Assessment
Analysis
Psychosocial Integrity

8.15 A client is upset to hear the nurse say that the results of genetic testing revealed "wild-type" genes. The nurse realizes that the client does not understand that wild-type genes are:

1. normal.
2. abnormal with limitations.
3. defective.
4. unexpected.

Answer: 1
Rationale: The nurse must incorporate a "person-first" philosophy and use genetic terminology that is sensitive to the maintenance of an individual's positive self image. This can be accomplished by saying "unaltered" or "wild-type" gene instead of "normal" gene, and "altered gene," "altered, disease producing gene," or "gene alteration" instead of the terms "mutated" or "abnormal" gene when communicating genetic concerns to clients, families, other healthcare providers, or the public.
Assessment
Application
Psychosocial Integrity

8.16 A client, who is pregnant reports a family history of cystic fibrosis, asks about the risks for transmission to her child. Which of the following concepts should be included in the discussion?

1. There is less risk for transmission to male children.
2. The condition does not skip generations.
3. Male and female children are equally affected.
4. The parents must both be affected with this disorder for transmission to occur.

Answer: 3
Rationale: Cystic fibrosis is an autosomal recessive disorder. Autosomal recessive disorders are transmitted equally between male and female children. The disorder may appear to skip a generation. The parents of this disorder may be carriers but not affected.
Implementation
Application
Physiological Integrity

8.17 A newborn has just been diagnosed with a negative result from genetic testing. The nurse realizes that this finding means:

1. No further follow-up is needed.
2. There is no clinical explanation for the symptoms that are seen.
3. The baby is likely a carrier of a genetic abnormality.
4. The baby will develop symptoms of a genetic abnormality later in life.

Answer: 1
Rationale: If the purpose of a genetic test was for newborn screening and the result is negative, this means that the newborn is not expected to be tested for the condition and no follow-up is needed. There is no information provided to indicate what manifestations are present. The test results indicate the baby does not have a genetic disorder. There is no way to predict the baby's future health status.
Evaluation
Analysis
Health Promotion and Maintenance

CHAPTER 9

9.1 The nurse is assessing a client's vital signs. Which of the following should be assessed during this time?

1. peripheral pulses
2. pain

Answer: 2
Rationale: Pain is increasingly being referred to as the "fifth vital sign" with recommendations to assess for pain with every vital signs assessment. Assessment of peripheral pulses is done to check for presence and strength; it is not routinely used to assess a pulse rate. The other answers are not considered to be vital signs.

3. ability to ambulate 4. urine output	Assessment Application Physiological Integrity

9.2 The client complaining of pain has been waiting for medication to relieve the pain. Which of the following should the nurse realize about this client?
  1. The client's pain is real.
  2. The client just wants medication.
  3. The client wants attention.
  4. The client is demanding.
	Answer: 1
	Rationale: If the client says he or she has pain, the client is in pain. All pain is real. Nurses should not be judgmental when responding to a client's report of pain. This is a common bias and is a barrier to effective pain management of clients. The other responses would be a bias of the nurse's interpretation.
	Diagnosis
	Application
	Physiological Integrity

9.3 A client is complaining of muscle pain. The nurse realizes that the transmission of this pain is:
  1. over the A-delta fibers.
  2. over the B nerve fibers.
  3. over the C nerve fibers.
  4. over the D nerve fibers.
	Answer: 3
	Rationale: The pain from deep body structures such as muscle and viscera is primarily transmitted by C fibers producing burning and aching sensations. A-delta fibers are associated with acute pain such as cuts or electric burns. There are no B or D fibers involved in pain transmission.
	Diagnosis
	Application
	Physiological Integrity

9.4 A client with a history of chronic pain tells the nurse, "I do a variety of things to make my body produce its own pain reliever." The nurse realizes that this client is describing:
  1. a theory of denial.
  2. a belief in alternative methods.
  3. one reason to reduce the amount of pain medication prescribed.
  4. the body's ability to make endorphins.
	Answer: 4
	Rationale: There is a pain inhibitory center within the dorsal horns of the spinal cord. The exact nature of this inhibitory mechanism is unknown. However, the most clearly-defined chemical inhibitory mechanism is fueled by endorphins (endogenous morphines), which are naturally-occurring opioid peptides that are present in neurons in the brain, spinal cord, and gastrointestinal tract. Endorphins work by binding with opiate receptors on the neurons to inhibit pain impulse transmission. The client did not deny the pain. Alternative methods have not been employed. There was no discussion of pain medication amounts.
	Diagnosis
	Analysis
	Physiological Integrity

9.5 The nurse is providing medication to a client with acute pain. Which of the following are types of acute pain? (Select all that apply.)
  1. psychogenic
  2. somatic
  3. visceral
  4. referred
	Answer: 2, 3, 4
	Rationale: The three types of acute pain are: somatic, which arises from nerve receptors that originate in the skin or close to the surface of the body; visceral, which arises from body organs; and referred, which is perceived in an area distant from the body part that is the source of the pain. Psychogenic pain is diagnosed when no physiological source is found for the pain and exists for a long period of time.
	Assessment
	Analysis
	Physiological Integrity

9.6 A 47-year-old female client has a history of scoliosis and back pain. Which of the following types of pain does the nurse realize this client most likely is experiencing?
  1. recurrent acute pain
  2. ongoing time-limited pain
  3. chronic nonmalignant pain
  4. chronic intractable nonmalignant pain syndrome
	Answer: 3
	Rationale: Chronic nonmalignant pain is non–life-threatening pain that nevertheless persists beyond the expected time for healing. Chronic lower back pain falls into this category. No mention was made of malignancy being a cause of the pain. Back pain is typically categorized as chronic pain. Recurrent acute pain is characterized by relatively well-defined episodes of pain interspersed with pain-free episodes.
	Diagnosis
	Analysis
	Physiological Integrity

9.7 A client with a history of lumbar spinal cord nerve compression continues to complain of burning pain. The nurse realizes that this client is experiencing:	Answer: 1 Rationale: Complex regional pain syndrome is a neuropathic pain that results from nerve damage. It is characterized by continuous severe, burning pain. These conditions follow peripheral nerve damage and present the symptoms of pain, vasospasm, muscle wasting, and vasomotor changes. This pain was not

1. complex regional pain syndrome. 2. myofascial pain syndrome. 3. chronic post-operative pain. 4. phantom limb pain.	described as chronic and no limb was amputated to indicate phantom limb pain. Myofascial pain syndrome is a condition marked by injury or disease of muscle and fascial tissue. Diagnosis Analysis Physiological Integrity
9.8 A client learns that he has no physical cause for the ongoing back pain he experiences. The nurse realizes this client might be experiencing: 1. central pain. 2. phantom pain. 3. chronic postoperative pain. 4. psychogenic pain.	Answer: 4 Rationale: Psychogenic pain is experienced in the absence of any diagnosed physiologic cause or event and involves a long history of severe pain. Psychogenic pain is real, and may in turn lead to physiologic changes, such as muscle tension, that may produce further pain. Phantom pain involves an amputation. No mention was made of a surgical situation. Central pain is the result of a lesion in the brain. Diagnosis Analysis Physiological Integrity
9.9 A client with a long history of pain rarely appears to be in pain and often forgoes the use of pain medication. The nurse realizes that this client: 1. has a high pain tolerance. 2. has a low pain tolerance. 3. is addicted to pain medication. 4. does not really have pain.	Answer: 1 Rationale: Pain tolerance is the amount of pain a person can tolerate before outwardly responding to it. A client having a high tolerance to pain would rarely report pain or need analgesic management. With a low tolerance, the client would be verbalizing pain and requesting medication. If the client were addicted, their body would eventually need more medication, not less, to manage the pain. There is inadequate information to support the reports the client is not in pain. Diagnosis Analysis Physiological Integrity
9.10 A client with chronic pain tells the nurse that he "rarely sleeps more than 3 hours a night." The nurse realizes that this client is at risk for developing: 1. chronic insomnia. 2. depression. 3. high pain tolerance. 4. adult attention deficit disorder.	Answer: 2 Rationale: Depression is clearly linked to pain: serotonin, a neurotransmitter, is involved in the modulation of pain in the central nervous system. In clinically-depressed people, serotonin is decreased, which leads to an increase in pain sensations. Fatigue, the lack of sleep and pain are interrelated concepts. The focus of this question is the client's chronic pain history. There is no information available to support the onset of chronic insomnia, inferences concerning pain tolerance, or the presence of adult attention deficit disorder. Diagnosis Analysis Physiological Integrity
9.11 A client with chronic pain is desperately searching for something to relieve the pain. Which of the following would be helpful for this client to consider? 1. A thorough analysis of the pain to determine if it is truly pain. 2. Avoid the use of narcotics. 3. Evaluation by a psychiatrist to determine if the client is really depressed. 4. Develop a pain medication schedule to help avoid the onset of pain.	Answer: 4 Rationale: It is now widely accepted that anticipating pain has a noticeable effect on the amount of pain a client experiences. Offering pain relief before a pain event is well on its way can lessen the pain. The pain has already been identified as being real and chronic in nature. There is no mention of a depressed state, only the client's need to address the pain. Avoidance of narcotics may not meet the immediate needs of the client. Planning Application Physiological Integrity
9.12 A client has periodic severe nerve pain that is not being well-controlled with pain medication. The nurse thinks that this client might benefit from:	Answer: 3 Rationale: Antidepressants within the tricyclic and related chemical groups act on the production and retention of serotonin in the CNS, thus inhibiting pain sensation. They also promote normal sleeping patterns, which further alleviates the suffering of the client in pain. They are useful with neuropathic pain. Other

1. a nonsteroidal anti-inflammatory drug (NSAID).
2. a narcotic.
3. an antidepressant.
4. a local anesthetic.

medications are prescribed before introducing narcotics. The NSAID group can have serious side effects, including bleeding tendencies, and would not be appropriate in a long-term situation. A local anesthetic would not be appropriate for long-term pain management.
Planning
Analysis
Physiological Integrity

9.13 A client who is receiving pain medication around the clock complains of an acute exacerbation of pain. What should the nurse do to help this client?
1. Provide the medication ordered for breakthrough pain.
2. Talk the client through the pain.
3. Encourage the client to ignore the pain.
4. Give the client a nonsteroidal anti-inflammatory drug (NSAID).

Answer: 1
Rationale: Breakthrough pain (BTP) occurs in clients who are receiving long-acting analgesics for chronic pain. It is a transitory experience of moderate to severe pain that is often precipitated by coughing or movement but may occur spontaneously. Dosing with short-acting opioids for this type of pain should be administered as needed in addition to the ATC dose for chronic, persistent pain. The pain must be addressed; it is not appropriate to talk the client through the pain or encourage the client to ignore the pain. NSAIDs could only be given with the physician's order.
Implementation
Application
Physiological Integrity

9.14 A client with chronic pain is being started on a "patch." Which of the following should be included when instructing the client about this pain-relieving delivery system?
1. It will not work as well as oral pain medications.
2. Dosing will start with a lower dose.
3. The client will never experience breakthrough pain.
4. The client will never overdose with this delivery method.

Answer: 2
Rationale: The transdermal, or "patch," form of medication is increasingly being used because it is simple, painless, and delivers a continuous level of medication. The continuous dosage is an advantage over oral medications. Transdermal medications are easy to store and apply, and reapplication every 72 hours enhances compliance. Dosages for the "patch" start low and are increased as deemed necessary by the physician. Additional short-acting medication is often needed for breakthrough pain. Overdosage can occur with this route.
Implementation
Application
Physiological Integrity

9.15 The nurse is helping a client in pain by gently massaging the painful area. The nurse is utilizing which form of pain control with the client?
1. acupuncture
2. biofeedback
3. guided imagery
4. cutaneous stimulation

Answer: 4
Rationale: It is believed that stimulation of the skin is effective in relieving pain because it prompts closure of the gate in the substantia gelatinosa. Cutaneous stimulation may be accomplished by massage, vibration, application of heat and cold, and therapeutic touch. Touch was used, so biofeedback and guided imagery are not correct. There is no mention of the use of acupuncture needles.
Implementation
Application
Physiological Integrity

9.16 The nurse is assessing a client's pain perception. Which of the following methods of assessment would be useful for this?
1. FACES scale
2. psychological evaluation tool
3. PQRST guide
4. biofeedback rating

Answer: 3
Rationale: A client's pain perception can be assessed by using the PQRST technique: P = What precipitated (triggered, stimulated) the pain? Has anything relieved the pain? What is the pattern of the pain?; Q = What is the quality and quantity of the pain? Is it sharp, stabbing, aching, burning, stinging, deep, crushing, viselike, or gnawing?; R = What is the region (location) of the pain? Does the pain radiate to other areas of the body?; S = What is the severity of the pain?; and T = What is the timing of the pain? When does it begin, how long does it last, and how is it related to other events in the client's life? The FACES scale is a pain rating tool. Use of a psychological evaluation tool is not indicated. A biofeedback rating would not address all areas of a pain assessment.
Assessment
Application
Physiological Integrity

9.17 A client is seen talking and laughing in the clinic's waiting room yet complains of excruciating pain. The nurse realizes this client is most likely demonstrating:

1. the desire for narcotics.
2. denial.
3. fake pain.
4. inconsistent behavioral response to pain.

Answer: 4

Rationale: Behavioral responses to pain may or may not coincide with the client's report of pain and are not very reliable cues to the pain experience. The nurse needs to manage the pain if the client verbalizes that it is present, even if the nonverbal signs are not congruent. The nurse cannot decide if the client's pain is real. No mention was made of the client requesting narcotics.

Diagnosis

Analysis

Psychosocial Integrity

CHAPTER 10

10.1 A client is prescribed 20 mEq of potassium chloride. The nurse realizes that the client is receiving this replacement:

1. to sustain respiratory function.
2. to help regulate acid–base balance.
3. to keep a vein open.
4. to encourage urine output.

Answer: 2

Rationale: Electrolytes have many functions. They assist in regulating water balance, help regulate and maintain acid–base balance, contribute to enzyme reactions, and are essential for neuromuscular activity. Potassium does not sustain respiratory function. Intravenous fluids are used to keep venous access not potassium. Urinary output is impacted by intake not potassium.

Evaluation

Analysis

Physiological Integrity

10.2 An elderly client does not complain of thirst. What should the nurse do to assess that this client is not dehydrated?

1. Ask the physician for an order to begin intravenous fluid replacement.
2. Ask the physician to order a chest x-ray.
3. Assess the urine for osmolality.
4. Ask the physician for an order for a brain scan.

Answer: 3

Rationale: The thirst mechanism declines with aging, which makes older adults more vulnerable to dehydration and hyperosmolality. The nurse should check the client's urine for osmolality as a first step in determining hydration status before other detailed and invasive testing is done. It is inappropriate to seek an IV at this stage. There is no indication the client is experiencing pulmonary complications thus a chest x-ray is not indicated. There is no data to support the need for a brain scan.

Planning

Analysis

Physiological Integrity

10.3 An elderly client who is being medicated for pain had an episode of incontinence. The nurse realizes that this client is at risk for developing:

1. dehydration.
2. over-hydration.
3. fecal incontinence.
4. a stroke.

Answer: 1

Rationale: Functional changes of aging also affect fluid balance. Fear of incontinence can lead to self-limiting of fluid intake. Older adults who have self-care deficits, or who are confused, depressed, tube-fed, on bed rest, or taking medications (such as sedatives, tranquilizers, diuretics, and laxatives) are at greatest risk for fluid volume imbalance. There is inadequate information to support the risk of over-hydration, fecal incontinence, or a stroke.

Diagnosis

Analysis

Physiological Integrity

10.4 The nurse assesses a client's weight loss as being 22 lbs. How many liters of fluid did this client lose?

Fill in the blank: _____

Answer: 10 liters

Rationale: Each liter of body fluid weighs 1 kg or 2.2 lbs. This client has lost 10 liters of fluid.

Diagnosis

Analysis

Physiological Integrity

10.5 A postoperative client with a fluid volume deficit is prescribed progressive ambulation yet is weak from an inadequate fluid status. What can the nurse do to help this client?

1. Assist the client to maintain a standing position for several minutes.

Answer: 3

Rationale: The client needs to be taught how to avoid orthostatic hypotension which would include assisting and teaching the client how to move from one position to another in stages. The client should avoid prolonged standing. Bed rest can promote skin breakdown. A physician referral is needed for physical therapy intervention and is not indicated in this situation.

Implementation

Application

Physiological Integrity

2. This client should be on bed rest. 3. Assist the client to move into different positions in stages. 4. Contact physical therapy to provide a walker.	

10.6 A postoperative client is diagnosed with fluid volume overload. Which of the following should the nurse assess in this client?
  1. poor skin turgor
  2. decreased urine output
  3. distended neck veins
  4. concentrated hemoglobin and hematocrit levels
	Answer: 3
	Rationale: Circulatory overload causes manifestations such as a full, bounding pulse; distended neck and peripheral veins; increased central venous pressure; cough; dyspnea; orthopnea; rales in the lungs; pulmonary edema; polyuria; ascites; peripheral edema, or if severe, anasarca, in which dilution of plasma by excess fluid causes a decreased hematocrit and blood urea nitrogen (BUN); and possible cerebral edema. The other answers indicate a fluid volume deficit.
	Assessment
	Application
	Physiological Integrity

10.7 An elderly client is at home after being diagnosed with fluid volume overload. Which of the following should the home care nurse instruct this client to do?
  1. Wear support hose.
  2. Keep legs in a dependent position.
  3. Avoid wearing shoes while in the home.
  4. Try to sleep without extra pillows.
	Answer: 1
	Rationale: The home care nurse should instruct this client about ways to decrease dependent edema, which include wearing support hose, elevating feet when in a sitting position, and resting in a recliner or bed with extra pillows. As long as the shoes are well fitting, there is no reason to avoid wearing them.
	Planning
	Application
	Physiological Integrity

10.8 A client with fluid retention related to renal problems is admitted to the hospital. The nurse realizes that this client could possibly have which of the following electrolyte imbalances?
  1. hypokalemia
  2. hypernatremia
  3. carbon dioxide
  4. magnesium
	Answer: 2
	Rationale: The kidney is the primary regulator of sodium in the body. Fluid retention is associated with hypernatremia. The kidneys are the principal organs involved in the elimination of potassium. Renal failure is often associated with elevations of potassium levels. Carbon dioxide and magnesium abnormalities are not anticipated for this client.
	Planning
	Application
	Physiological Integrity

10.9 An elderly client comes into the clinic with the complaint of watery diarrhea for several days with abdominal and muscle cramping. The nurse realizes that this client is demonstrating:
  1. hypernatremia.
  2. hyponatremia.
  3. fluid volume excess.
  4. hyperkalemia.
	Answer: 2
	Rationale: This elderly client has watery diarrhea, which contributes to the loss of sodium. The abdominal and muscle cramps are manifestations of a low serum sodium level. Hypernatremia is associated with fluid retention and overload. Fluid volume excess is associated with hypernatremia. Hyperkalemia is associated with cardiac dysrthythmias.
	Diagnosis
	Analysis
	Physiological Integrity

10.10 A client is admitted with hypernatremia caused by being stranded on a boat in the Atlantic Ocean for five days without a fresh water source. Which of the following is this client at risk for developing?
  1. pulmonary edema
  2. atrial dysrhythmias
	Answer: 3
	Rationale: The brain experiences the most serious effects of cellular dehydration. As brain cells contract, the brain shrinks, which puts mechanical traction on cerebral vessels. These vessels may tear, bleed, and lead to cerebral vascular bleeding. The client in question would face dehydration. Pulmonary edema is not associated with dehydration. Arterial dysrhythmias are not a factor for this client. There have been no activities to support the development or occurrence of stress fractures.

3. cerebral bleeding 4. stress fractures	Diagnosis Analysis Physiological Integrity
10.11 The nurse is admitting a client who was diagnosed with acute renal failure. Which of the following electrolytes will be most affected with this disorder? 1. calcium 2. magnesium 3. phosphorous 4. potassium	Answer: 4 Rationale: Because the kidneys are the principal organs involved in the elimination of potassium, renal failure can lead to potentially serious elevations of serum potassium levels. Imbalances in calcium, magnesium, and phosphorus are less likely. Planning Analysis Physiological Integrity
10.12 A client who is taking digoxin (Lanoxin) is admitted with possible hypokalemia. Which of the following does the nurse realize might occur with this client? 1. digoxin toxicity 2. A higher dose of digoxin (Lanoxin) may be needed. 3. A diuretic may be needed. 4. fluid volume deficit	Answer: 1 Rationale: Hypokalemia increases the risk of digitalis toxicity in clients who receive this drug for heart failure. A diuretic may cause further fluid loss. More digoxin is not needed. There is inadequate information to assess for concerns related to fluid volume deficits. Planning Analysis Physiological Integrity
10.13 A client is prescribed 40 mEq potassium as a replacement. The nurse realizes that this replacement should be administered: 1. directly into the venous access line. 2. mixed in the prescribed intravenous fluid. 3. via a rectal suppository. 4. via intramuscular injection.	Answer: 2 Rationale: The intravenous route is the recommended route for undiluted potassium. Never administer undiluted potassium directly into a vein. Implementation Application Physiological Integrity
10.14 An elderly client with a history of sodium retention arrives to the clinic with the complaints of "heart skipping beats" and leg tremors. Which of the following should the nurse ask this client regarding these symptoms? 1. "Have you stopped taking your digoxin medication?" 2. "When was the last time you had a bowel movement?" 3. "Were you doing any unusual physical activity?" 4. "Are you using a salt substitute?"	Answer: 4 Rationale: The client has a history of sodium retention and might think that a salt substitute can be used. Advise clients who are taking a potassium supplement or potassium-sparing diuretic to avoid salt substitutes, which usually contain potassium. Although this client may be prescribed digoxin this is not the primary focus of this question. The client's bowel habits are not of concern at this time. The cardiac and musculoskeletal discomforts being reported are not consistent with physical exertion. Assessment Application Physiological Integrity
10.15 A 35-year-old female client comes into the clinic postoperative parathyroidectomy. Which of the following should the nurse tell this client? 1. Drink one glass of red wine per day. 2. Avoid the sun. 3. Milk and milk-based products will ensure an adequate calcium intake. 4. Red meat is the protein source of choice.	Answer: 3 Rationale: This client is at risk for developing hypocalcemia. This risk can be avoided if instructed to ingest milk and milk-based products, have adequate exposure to the sun, and avoid alcoholic beverages. The greatest dietary concern for this client is the adequacy of calcium intake. Protein monitoring is not indicated. Implementation Application Physiological Integrity

10.16 A client is admitted for treatment of hypercalcemia. The nurse realizes that this client's intravenous fluids will most likely be:
1. dextrose 5% and water.
2. dextrose 5% and $\frac{1}{4}$ normal saline.
3. dextrose 5% and $\frac{1}{2}$ normal saline.
4. normal saline.

Answer: 4
Rationale: Isotonic saline is used because sodium excretion is accompanied by calcium excretion through the kidneys. If isotonic saline is not used, the client is at risk for hyponatremia in addition to the hypercalcemia. The remaining solutions are hypotonic and do not have adequate sodium content.
Implementation
Analysis
Physiological Integrity

10.17 A 28-year-old male client is admitted with diabetic ketoacidosis. The nurse realizes that this client will have a need for which of the following electrolytes?
1. sodium
2. potassium
3. calcium
4. magnesium

Answer: 4
Rationale: One risk factor for hypomagnesemia is an endocrine disorder, including diabetic ketoacidosis. The client's levels of sodium, potassium, and calcium are not the primary needs of this client.
Diagnosis
Analysis
Physiological Integrity

10.18 An elderly client with peripheral neuropathy has been taking magnesium supplements. The nurse realizes that which of the following symptoms can indicate hypermagnesemia?
1. hypotension, warmth, and sweating
2. nausea and vomiting
3. hyper reflexia
4. excessive urination

Answer: 1
Rationale: Elevations in magnesium levels is accompanied by hypotension, warmth, and sweating. Lower levels are associated with nausea and vomiting, hypertension, and hyper reflexia. Urinary changes are not noted.
Assessment
Analysis
Physiological Integrity

10.19 A client is admitted with burns over 50% of his body. The nurse realizes that this client is at risk for which of the following electrolyte imbalances?
1. hypercalcemia
2. hypophosphatemia
3. hypernatremia
4. hypermagnesemia

Answer: 2
Rationale: Causes of hypophosphatemia include stress responses and extensive burns. Clients who experience burns are not at an increased risk for elevated levels of calcium, sodium, or magnesium.
Diagnosis
Analysis
Physiological Integrity

10.20 A client is diagnosed with hyperphosphatemia. The nurse realizes that this client might also have an imbalance of which of the following electrolytes?
1. calcium
2. sodium
3. potassium
4. chloride

Answer: 1
Rationale: Excessive serum phosphate levels cause few specific symptoms. The effects of high serum phosphate levels on nerves and muscles are more likely the result of hypocalcemia that develops secondary to an elevated serum phosphorus level. The phosphate in the serum combines with ionized calcium, and the ionized serum calcium level falls. There is no direct correlation between levels of phosphorus and that of sodium, potassium, or chloride.
Diagnosis
Analysis
Physiological Integrity

10.21 The nurse is reviewing a client's blood pH level. Which of the systems in the body regulate blood pH? (Select all that apply.)
1. renal
2. cardiac
3. buffers
4. respiratory

Answers: 1, 3, 4
Rationale: Three systems work together in the body to maintain the pH despite continuous acid production: buffers, the respiratory system, and the renal system. The cardiac system is responsible for circulating blood to the body.
Assessment
Analysis
Physiological Integrity

10.22 The nurse observes a client's respirations and notes that the rate is 30 per minute and the respirations are very deep. The metabolic disorder this client might be demonstrating is:
   1. hypernatremia.
   2. increasing carbon dioxide in the blood.
   3. hypertension.
   4. pain.
	Answer: 2
	Rationale: Acute increases in either carbon dioxide or hydrogen ions in the blood stimulate the respiratory center in the brain. As a result, both the rate and depth of respiration increase. The increased rate and depth of lung ventilation eliminates carbon dioxide from the body, and carbonic acid levels fall, which brings the pH to a more normal range. Hypernatremia is associated with profuse sweating and diarrhea. The respiratory rate in a client exhibiting hypertension is not altered. Pain may be manifested in rapid, shallow respirations.
	Diagnosis
	Analysis
	Physiological Integrity

10.23 The blood gases of a client with an acid–base disorder show a blood pH outside of normal limits. The nurse realizes that this client is:
   1. fully compensated.
   2. demonstrating anaerobic metabolism.
   3. partially compensated.
   4. in need of intravenous fluids.
	Answer: 3
	Rationale: If the pH is restored to within normal limits, the disorder is said to be fully compensated. When these changes are reflected in arterial blood gas (ABG) values but the pH remains outside normal limits, the disorder is said to be partially compensated. Anaerobic metabolism results when the body's cells become hypoxic. Although the client may be in need of intravenous fluids, this is not the most correct or definitive answer.
	Diagnosis
	Analysis
	Physiological Integrity

10.24 A client's blood gases show a pH greater of 7.53 and bicarbonate level of 36 mEq/L. The nurse realizes that the acid–base disorder this client is demonstrating is:
   1. respiratory acidosis.
   2. metabolic acidosis.
   3. respiratory alkalosis.
   4. metabolic alkalosis.
	Answer: 4
	Rationale: Arterial blood gases (ABGs) show a pH greater than 7.45 and bicarbonate level greater than 26 mEq/L when the client is in metabolic alkalosis. Respiratory and metabolic acidosis are both consistent with pH less than 7.35. Respiratory alkalosis is associated with a pH greater than 7.45 and a $Paco_2$ of less than 35 mm Hg. It is caused by respiratory related conditions.
	Diagnosis
	Application
	Physiological Integrity

10.25 An elderly postoperative client is demonstrating lethargy, confusion, and a respiratory rate of 8 per minute. The nurse sees that the last dose of pain medication administered via a patient controlled anesthesia (PCA) pump was within 30 minutes. Which of the following acid–base disorders might this client be experiencing?
   1. respiratory acidosis
   2. metabolic acidosis
   3. respiratory alkalosis
   4. metabolic alkalosis
	Answer: 1
	Rationale: Acute respiratory acidosis occurs due to a sudden failure of ventilation. Overdoses of narcotic or sedative medications can lead to this condition. The client condition being described is respiratory not metabolic in nature.
	Diagnosis
	Analysis
	Physiological Integrity

11.1 A client is brought into the emergency department with multiple stab wounds. The nurse realizes that these wounds can be classified as being:
1. unintentional.
2. intentional.
3. accidental.
4. related to disease process.

Answer: 2
Rationale: Most gunshot and stab wounds are examples of intentional injuries. Unintentional injuries result from actions which are not deliberate. Accidents result from unplanned events. Stab wounds are not related to the presence of a disease process.
Diagnosis
Application
Physiological Integrity

11.2 The nurse suspects that a client is a victim of abuse. Which of the following would provide this indication to the nurse?
1. spontaneously moving all four extremities
2. evidence of adequate hydration.
3. injuries that do not correlate with the client's story of the injury
4. caring attitude between client and spouse

Answer: 3
Rationale: There are clues to identifying violence related injuries. Some of these clues include injuries that do not correlate with the client's explanation of the injury. Spontaneously moving all extremities, adequate hydration, and the demonstration of a caring attitude are normal behaviors and not typically associated with abuse.
Diagnosis
Application
Physiological Integrity

11.3 The nurse is admitting a trauma client. What factors assist in determining the classification of trauma clients? (Select all that apply.)
1. height of fall
2. location of injury
3. mechanism of injury
4. vehicle speed

Answer: 1, 2, 3, 4
Rationale: Trauma clients are classified as Class 1, 2, or 3 based on factors that include mechanism of injury, vehicle speed, height of falls, and location of penetrating injuries. Class 3 trauma is the least severe.
Diagnosis
Application
Physiological Integrity

11.4 A trauma client has an airway obstruction and needs to be intubated. Which of the following acronyms can the nurse use to guide the assessment of the difficulty with intubating this client?
1. APIE
2. SMART
3. LEMON LAW
4. CAGE

Answer: 3
Rationale: The Lemon Law is an acronym for Look externally, Evaluate the 3-3-2 rule, Mallampati Classification, Obstruction, and Neck mobility. APIE, SMART, and CAGE are not acronyms associated with intubation.
Assessment
Application
Physiological Integrity

11.5 A trauma victim is presenting with a deviated trachea, jugular vein distention, and cyanosis. The nurse realizes that this client is most likely demonstrating:
1. cervical spine injury.
2. blunt trauma to the chest.
3. acceleration-deceleration injury.
4. tension pneumothorax.

Answer: 4
Rationale: Signs and symptoms of a tension pneumothorax include severe respiratory distress, hypotension, jugular vein distension, tracheal deviation toward the uninjured side, and cyanosis. The client with a cervical spine injury may present with alterations in sensation and movement. Blunt trauma to the chest would manifest with bleeding or bruising of the chest area. An acceleration-deceleration injury results when a moving object strikes a stationary body part.
Diagnosis
Analysis
Physiological Integrity

11.6 A client is admitted with trauma to the integumentary system. Which of the following are types of skin trauma? (Select all that apply.)
1. cutaneous
2. abrasion
3. laceration
4. contusion

Answer: 2, 3, 4
Rationale: Four specific injuries to the integument are contusions, abrasions, puncture wounds, and lacerations. Cutaneous is a term used to refer to the integument. It is not associated with trauma to the skin.
Assessment
Application
Physiological Integrity

11.7 A trauma client is being assessed with the Champion Revised Scoring System. What are the elements of this scoring system? (Select all that apply.) 　1. diastolic blood pressure 　2. heart rate 　3. Glasgow coma scale 　4. systolic blood pressure 　5. respiratory rate	Answer: 3, 4, 5 Rationale: The Champion Revised Scoring System analyzes three elements: the Glasgow Coma Scale, systolic blood pressure, and respiratory rate. The client then receives a total score. The highest score is 12. Although the diastolic blood pressure and heart rate are a part of the client's assessment, they are not included in the Champion Revised Scoring System. Implementation Application Physiological Integrity
11.8 A trauma client is in hypovolemic shock. The nurse should be prepared to administer which of the following types of blood products to this client? 　1. whole blood 　2. packed RBCs 　3. platelets 　4. plasma	Answer: 1 Rationale: Whole blood replaces blood volume and oxygen-carrying capacity in hemorrhage or shock. Packed RBCs do not replace the same level of volume as whole blood. Platelets are used for clotting and do not replace the volume or oxygen-carrying capabilities of whole blood. Plasma does not provide the oxygen-carrying capacity of whole blood. Planning Application Physiological Integrity
11.9 A trauma client needs whole blood transfusions and has a blood type of AB+. The nurse realizes that this client will need to receive which type of blood? 　1. O+ only 　2. AB+ only 　3. AB− only 　4. any type	Answer: 4 Rationale: A client with blood type AB+ can receive blood from any blood type. Diagnosis Application Physiological Integrity
11.10 A client is receiving a blood transfusion. Which of the following should the nurse do to ensure safe blood administration? 　1. Inject an intravenous diuretic through the blood tubing line. 　2. Return the empty bag and tubing to the blood bank after the infusion is completed. 　3. Administer the blood over eight hours. 　4. Stay with the client for the entire transfusion.	Answer: 2 Rationale: Empty blood bags and tubing should be returned to the blood bank after the transfusion has ended. Nothing should be administered through the blood tubing line. The blood should be administered within two hours. The client needs to be observed for the first 15 minutes and then as needed for the duration of the transfusion. Most sources recommend infusing blood over the course of four hours. Implementation Application Physiological Integrity
11.11 A client is going to be evaluated for brain death. Which of the following diagnostic tests will need to be done to make this evaluation? 　1. EEG 　2. EKG 　3. serum carbon dioxide level 　4. chest x-ray	Answer: 1 Rationale: Confirmation tests for brain death include an electroencephalogram and cerebral blood flow study. The EKG is used to monitor the heart. The serum carbon dioxide level may be used to assess blood gases. The chest x-ray is used to evaluate the lungs. Planning Analysis Physiological Integrity
11.12 The nurse is determining a client's cardiac output. Which of the following equations can the nurse use to make this assessment? 　1. heart rate × respiratory rate 　2. systolic blood pressure × heart rate 　3. stroke volume × heart rate 　4. mean arterial pressure × heart rate	Answer: 3 Rationale: Cardiac output is determined by multiplying the stroke volume (SV) by the heart rate (HR): $CO = SV \times HR$. Heart rate, respiratory rate, blood pressure, and arterial pressure are assessments used in critical care but are not included in the calculation of cardiac output. Assessment Application Physiological Integrity

11.13 A trauma client has multiple injuries and has lost approximately 25% of circulating blood volume. The nurse realizes that this client is in which stage of shock?
1. stage I
2. stage II
3. stage III
4. stage IV

Answer: 1
Rationale: In this phase of shock, circulating blood volume is reduced by 25% to 35%; however, with the body's compensatory mechanisms, blood pressure and tissue perfusion to vital organs is maintained, which prevents cell damage. During stage II shock, the client has experienced a fluid loss of 35% to 50%. Perfusion to vital organs is not sufficient. In stage III shock, the tissue anoxia becomes so generalized that treatment cannot reverse the damage. There is no stage IV shock.
Evaluation
Application
Physiological Integrity

11.14 A trauma client in stage II shock is demonstrating signs of pulmonary edema. The nurse realizes that this client is demonstrating:
1. heart failure.
2. ARDS.
3. SARs.
4. respiratory acidosis.

Answer: 2
Rationale: A complication of decreased perfusion of the lungs is acute respiratory distress syndrome (ARDS), or "shock lung." The exact mechanism that produces ARDS is unknown, but some contributing factors have been identified. The pulmonary capillaries become increasingly permeable to proteins and water, which results in noncardiogenic pulmonary edema. Surfactant production (which controls surface tension within alveoli) is impaired, and the alveoli collapse or fill with fluid. Heart failure is not manifested by pulmonary edema in stage II shock. SARs is an infection. Respiratory acidosis is manifested by alterations in blood gases not pulmonary edema.
Diagnosis
Analysis
Physiological Integrity

11.15 A client is diagnosed as being in the warm phase of septic shock. The nurse will expect to see which of the following signs and symptoms in this client?
1. hypotension
2. tachycardia
3. urine output less than 30 cc per hour
4. alert and anxious

Answer: 4
Rationale: In the warm phase of septic shock, a client will demonstrate normal blood pressure or a slight increase in blood pressure, increased pulse, rapid and deep respirations, warm flushed skin, alert, oriented, anxious, normal urine output, elevated body temperature, chills, weakness, nausea, vomiting, diarrhea, and decreased CVP. During the cold phase of septic shock, hypovolemia and oliguria result.
Assessment
Application
Physiological Integrity

11.16 A client is prescribed an infusion of nitroprusside sodium (Nipride). Which of the following should the nurse do to ensure a safe infusion of this medication?
1. Mix with dextrose 5% and $\frac{1}{2}$ normal saline.
2. Inject furosemide (Lasix) 20 mg into the transfusion bag.
3. Time the drops to infuse at the rate of 20 drops per minute.
4. Protect the infusion bag from light by keeping the wrapping provided from the pharmacy on the bag.

Answer: 4
Rationale: Nitroprusside sodium (Nipride) is a vasodilator and should be protected from light. This medication should be mixed with D5W only, be infused with a pump, and should not be mixed with any other medications in the infusion bag. The rate of medication administration is not standardized but determined by the physician based upon the client's condition.
Implementation
Application
Physiological Integrity

11.17 A client in shock is prescribed a vasoconstrictor. Which of the following would the nurse most likely be administering to this client?
1. dopamine (Dopastat)
2. dobutamine (Dobutrex)
3. isoproterenol (Isuprel)
4. metaraminol (Aramine)

Answer: 4
Rationale: Vasoconstricting drugs used to treat shock include norepinephrine (Levophed) and metaraminol (Aramine). Dopamine (Dopastat), Dobutamine (Dobutrex), and Isoproterenol (Isuprel) are vasoconstrictors but they can only be administered after fluid volume is restored.
Planning
Application
Physiological Integrity

12.1 A client who has never experienced a reaction to a bee sting comes into the emergency department with intense edema and redness at the site of the sting. The nurse realizes that this client is demonstrating:

1. mobilization of lymphocytic memory T cells.
2. activation of granulocytes.
3. creation of neutrophils.
4. circulation of eosinophils.

Answer: 1

Rationale: T lymphocytes mature into active T_{Helper}, cytotoxic T cells, or memory T cells. Memory cells stay inactive, sometimes for years, but activate immediately with subsequent exposure to the same antigen. They then proliferate rapidly, and produce an intense immune response. Memory cells are responsible for providing acquired immunity. Granulocytes protect against harmful microorganisms during a period of acute inflammation. Neutrophils are responsible for phagocytosis and chemotaxis. Eosinophils are also responsible for phagocytosis and provide protection against parasites.

Diagnosis

Analysis

Health Promotion and Maintenance

12.2 A client asks the nurse, "What's going to happen to me now that my spleen is gone?" What is an appropriate nursing response?

1. "You will have to avoid getting colds and flu."
2. "Your stomach will resume its function."
3. "Your liver and bone marrow will resume its function."
4. "It was not really necessary for you to have a spleen."

Answer: 3

Rationale: The spleen is not essential for life. If it is removed because of disease or trauma, the liver and the bone marrow assume its functions. The client will still be able to survive getting colds and the flu. The stomach function is not related to the spleen. Option 4, although not incorrect, does not adequately answer the client's question.

Implementation

Application

Health Promotion and Maintenance

12.3 The nurse is caring for a client with a localized inflammatory response. Which of the following are stages within the inflammatory response? (Select all that apply.)

1. basilar
2. cellular
3. vascular
4. tissue Repair

Answer: 2, 3, 4

Rationale: There are three stages in the inflammatory response: (1) a vascular response characterized by vasodilation and increased permeability of blood vessels, (2) a cellular response and phagocytosis, and (3) tissue repair. Basilar is not a phase of the inflammatory response.

Diagnosis

Application

Health Promotion and Maintenance

12.4 A client who is demonstrating an inflammatory response is prescribed a nonsteroidal anti-inflammatory drug (NSAID). The nurse realizes that this medication will:

1. Increase the production of histamine.
2. Increase the flow of serosanguineous drainage.
3. Reduce the production of serotonin.
4. Reduce prostaglandin synthesis.

Answer: 4

Rationale: Aspirin and other nonsteroidal anti-inflammatory drugs (NSAIDs) as well as the glucocorticoids, inhibit prostaglandin synthesis, and thereby reduce fever, pain, and inflammation. Histamine production is increased by the use of an NSAID drug. The flow of serosanguineous drainage is not involved in the actions associated with nonsteroidal anti-inflammatory medications. Serotonin is contained in the granules of basophils and is not impacted by NSAID usage.

Implementation

Analysis

Health Promotion and Maintenance

12.5 A client with a compromised immune system is admitted to the hospital with an infection. Which of the following will most likely be done to help this client?

1. Discharge the client early to recover from the infection at home.
2. Place the client in a semi-private room only.

Answer: 3

Rationale: Clients with suppressed or impaired immune function are more susceptible to disease and require protection from exposure to environmental elements. Isolation techniques should be employed to prevent the spread of disease and to protect immune suppressed clients. No information was given that would determine the need for a specific type of isolation.

Planning

Application

Physiological Integrity

---

3. Utilize isolation techniques to protect the client from further infection. 4. Place the client in respiratory isolation.	
12.6 One school district is not requiring vaccinations for children who are starting school. The nurse realizes that this action could cause: 1. healthier children. 2. a reduction in the number of colds and flu in the school. 3. a decrease in school costs. 4. an epidemic of an illness that could have been avoided with a vaccination.	Answer: 4 Rationale: For many diseases, the potential consequences of a single disease episode on the individual and society make prevention desirable, especially for highly-contagious diseases that are capable of causing epidemics. In these instances, immunization or vaccination is used to provide artificially-acquired immunity. The purpose of vaccination is to establish adequate levels of antibody or memory cells to provide effective immunity. Healthier children are not the product of reduced usage of immunizations. Immunizations will not impact the number of colds and flu outbreaks in a school system. High rates of illness may increase school costs. Evaluation Analysis Health Promotion and Maintenance
12.7 A client is having skin testing done to assess for allergies. The nurse realizes that evidence of an exposure to an antigen would be: 1. itching at the site. 2. an area of approximately 1 mm of induration and erythema. 3. only evident after five days. 4. an area of greater than 10 mm of induration and erythema.	Answer: 4 Rationale: Skin testing can assess cell-mediated immunity. A known antigen is injected intradermally. The site is then observed for induration and erythema, which typically peaks at 24 to 48 hours. An induration of at least 10 mm in diameter is a positive reaction that indicates previous exposure and sensitization to the antigen. Itching is not a sign of exposure to an antigen. Evaluation Application Health Promotion and Maintenance
12.8 An elderly client with a history of lung disease had a pneumococcal vaccination 10 years ago. Which of the following should be done for this client? 1. Draw a blood culture. 2. Remind the client that he needs a booster in five more years. 3. Remind the client that he does not need a flu vaccination. 4. Suggest that the client have a pneumococcal booster during this visit.	Answer: 4 Rationale: Pneumococcal vaccine is generally recommended for the same populations as influenza vaccine. A single dose of this vaccine confers lifetime immunity, although repeating immunization every six years may be considered for high-risk clients. A blood culture is used to diagnose the presence of an infection. The flu vaccine and the pneumococcal vaccine are not the same. Diagnosis Application Health Promotion and Maintenance
12.9 A client who received a vaccination two weeks prior returns to the clinic with a wound at the inoculation site. The nurse realizes that this client is: 1. experiencing a severe local reaction to the inoculation. 2. allergic to the inoculation. 3. scratching the inoculation site. 4. demonstrating signs of the disease that the inoculation was intended to prevent.	Answer: 1 Rationale: Moderate to severe local reactions may occur following administration of an immunization. Occasionally local ulcerations occur; when they do, warm, wet packs, or sterile wet-to-dry dressings may be prescribed. There is inadequate information to determine if the client has an allergy to the vaccine or scratching. It is unlikely the client has developed the disease which the inoculation was intended to prevent. Evaluation Analysis Health Promotion and Maintenance
12.10 A client asks the nurse how long it will be before a leg wound heals. The nurse realizes that healing occurs in three phases, which are: (Select all that apply.) 1. inflammation. 2. deconstruction.	Answer: 1, 3, 4 Rationale: Inflammation is the first phase of the healing process. The second phase of the healing process, known as *reconstruction*, may overlap the inflammatory phase. The ideal result of the healing process is *resolution*, which is the restoration of the original structure and function of the damaged tissue. Deconstruction means to breakdown. Implementation

3. reconstruction. 4. resolution. 5. dissolution.	Application Physiological Integrity

12.11 The nurse is assessing a client's arm for inflammation. What are cardinal signs of a localized inflammatory process? (Select all that apply.)
  1. purulent drainage
  2. pain
  3. hyperemia
  4. erythema
	Answer: 2, 3, 4
	Rationale: The cardinal signs of inflammation are erythema/redness, local heat caused by the increased blood flow to the injured area (hyperemia), swelling due to accumulated fluid at the site, pain from tissue swelling and chemical irritation of nerve endings, and loss of function caused by the swelling and pain. Purulent drainage typically accompanies an infection.
	Planning
	Application
	Physiological Integrity

12.12 A client who is recovering from an infectious process has a poor appetite. Which of the following nutrients is of utmost importance for this client to ingest to support the healing process?
  1. water
  2. protein
  3. carbohydrates
  4. fats
	Answer: 2
	Rationale: Adequate protein is necessary for tissue healing and the production of antibodies and white blood cells (WBCs). Lack of adequate protein increases the risk of infection. Water provides hydration. Hydration is needed for the body but is not the key nutrient for the promotion of healing. Carbohydrates are needed for energy. Fats are a source of warmth and excess are stored for later use.
	Planning
	Analysis
	Physiological Integrity

12.13 A client wants to know why he developed an infection after being cut on the leg with a piece of wood, but his friend who was also cut did not. Which of the following can the nurse explain to this client?
  1. "Maybe the wood that cut the friend wasn't dirty and infected."
  2. "You must have an autoimmune disorder."
  3. "The organism found you more susceptible to the creation of an infection."
  4. "Your friend will get an infection too. It will just occur later."
	Answer: 3
	Rationale: In order for a microorganism to cause infection, it must have disease-causing potential (virulence), be transmitted from its reservoir, and gain entry into a susceptible host. There is no evidence to indicate that the friend will develop an infection. The wood might not have been infected. An autoimmune disorder will not cause an infection in this situation.
	Evaluation
	Application
	Physiological Integrity

12.14 A client is resisting the use of incentive spirometry postoperatively. Which of the following can be provided as an explanation to the client for the use of this device?
  1. "It will help prevent the development of pneumonia."
  2. "It gives you something to do while recovering."
  3. "It will prevent you from getting a cold."
  4. "The doctor ordered it."
	Answer: 1
	Rationale: Hospital-acquired pneumonia is the second most common nosocomial infection, and has the highest morbidity and mortality. Explaining the correct rationale for the use of the device will produce a better chance of compliance in a client. The use of the incentive spirometry is not intended as a diversion tool. The incentive spirometry will not reduce the risk of getting a cold. Although the physician may have ordered the treatment, this response does not meet the client's need for information.
	Implementation
	Application
	Physiological Integrity

12.15 A client with methicillin-resistant *Staphylococcus aureas* (MRSA) is no longer responding to the medication vancomycin (Vancocin). The nurse realizes that this client is most likely demonstrating:
  1. a super infection.
  2. VISA.
  3. VRE.
  4. PRSP.
	Answer: 2
	Rationale: Vancomycin (Vancocin) has been the only uniformly effective drug for MRSA; however, in 1997, a new form of *S. aureus* emerged with intermediate resistance to vancomycin, which is known as vancomycin intermediate-resistant *Staphylococcus aureus* (VISA). There are no indications the client has a super infection, VRE (Vancomycin resistant enterococci), or PRSP (Penicillin resistant Streptococcus pneumoniae).
	Diagnosis
	Analysis
	Physiological Integrity

12.16 A client who was diagnosed with an infection is prescribed a macrolide antibiotic. Which of the following should the nurse instruct the client about taking this medication?

1. Take the medication on a full stomach.
2. Take the medication with a glass of milk.
3. Take the medication on an empty stomach.
4. Take the medication with a full glass of juice.

Answer: 3
Rationale: The most commonly prescribed macrolide is erythromycin (E-mycin), which should be taken on an empty stomach and without acidic juice. A full glass of water is suggested instead of milk or another beverage.
Implementation
Application
Physiological Integrity

12.17 The nurse is caring for a client in droplet precautions. Which of the following should the nurse wear when providing care to this client?

1. head covering and gown
2. shoe covering and gown
3. gloves only
4. mask and eye protection or face shield

Answer: 4
Rationale: To provide care to a client in droplet precautions, the nurse should wear a mask and eye protection or a face shield when entering the room. Head, shoe covers, and gowns will not protect the areas vulnerable to droplets. Gloves are not adequate protection to droplet secretions.
Planning
Application
Physiological Integrity

CHAPTER 13

13.1 During the physical assessment of a client, the nurse wants to include the client's immunity function. Which of the following techniques would provide the nurse with the best information?

1. ascultation of the heart
2. percussion of the lungs
3. palpation of the abdomen
4. inspection of the skin

Answer: 4
Rationale: Because of this diversity of organs and function, assessment of the immune system is often integrated throughout the history and physical examination. Assessing the skin for color, temperature, and moisture will provide clues as to the status of the client's immunological functioning. Data obtained from auscultation of the heart, percussion of the lungs, and palpation of the abdomen are important components of the client assessment. They will not provide information directly related to the immune status.
Assessment
Analysis
Health Promotion and Maintenance

13.2 A differential diagnosis for a client is food allergies. The nurse escorts the client into an examination room and begins to ask questions about what the client has most recently eaten. Which of the following has the nurse observed about this client?

1. anorexia
2. urticaria
3. obesity
4. cachexia

Answer: 2
Rationale: Urticaria, or hives, is the most common systemic response to food allergies. Anorexia refers to the loss of appetite and an inability to take in nutrition. Obesity reflects a state in which more calories are ingested than are exerted. Cachexia refers to a condition in which the client has inadequate nutritional intake.
Assessment
Application
Health Promotion and Maintenance

13.3 A client tells the nurse, "I've never had this before" and exposes an area of redness, itching, and skin thickness on his left hand. The nurse realizes that this client is demonstrating which of the following?

1. a type I allergic response
2. a type II allergic response
3. a type III allergic response
4. a type IV allergic response

Answer: 4
Rationale: Contact dermatitis is a classic example of a type IV reaction. Intense redness, itching, and thickening affect the skin in the area exposed to the antigen. Fragile vesicles are often present as well. Many antigens can provoke this response; poison ivy is a prime perpetrator. A Type I allergic response is typical of allergic asthma, allergic rhinitis, or anaphylactic shock. It is triggered when an allergen interacts with IgE bound to mast cells and basophils. Type II allergic responses are the result of an exogenous antigen such as a foreign tissue or cell. Type III responses include serum sickness in response to some drugs.
Diagnosis
Analysis
Health Promotion and Maintenance

13.4 The client is diagnosed with a type IV hypersensitivity response. The nurse realizes that this client will most likely need treatment with: 1. antihistamines. 2. cardiac output medications. 3. renal dialysis. 4. endotracheal intubation.	Answer: 1 Rationale: With a hypersensitivity response, supportive care is important to relieve discomfort. This often involves the administration of selected antihistamine or anti-inflammatory medications. Cardiac output medications may be indicated for type I hypersensitivity reactions. Type II hypersensitivity reactions may require management of renal failure. The establishment and maintenance of an airway priority actions for a type I hypersensitivity reaction. Planning Application Physiological Integrity
13.5 A client is found to be allergic to several allergens from the epicutaneous testing. Which of the following should be done next to help this client? 1. Undergo intradermal testing of the allergens. 2. Undergo patch testing. 3. Determine treatment. 4. Keep a food diary.	Answer: 3 Rationale: Epicutaneous (patch) testing involves the placement of a diluted allergenic extract on the skin. The skin is then pricked or punctured through the drop. After a reaction, the physician will begin to determine treatment for the client. Substances that cause a reaction to the prick test should not be tested intradermally. The epicutaneous testing is not a means of assessing food allergies. Food allergies are reviewed using a food diary. Planning Application Physiological Integrity
13.6 A client is demonstrating signs of anaphylactic shock. Which of the following should the nurse do first to assist this client? 1. Administer subcutaneous epinephrine. 2. Maintain an airway. 3. Provide calm reassurance. 4. Place on a cardiac monitor.	Answer: 2 Rationale: Establishing and maintaining a patent airway is of primary importance if a client demonstrates anaphylactic shock. While the remaining options may be completed after an anaphylactic shock, they are not the first actions to be completed. After an airway is established, epinephrine may be administered and a cardiac monitor connected. The provision of reassurance can take place after the other interventions have been performed. Implementation Application Physiological Integrity
13.7 A client tells the nurse, "I had this arthritis pain under control but then I learned I might lose my job." Which of the following should the nurse say in response to this client? 1. "Well, we better do everything to help you before you lose your health benefits." 2. "I'm sure you'll find another job." 3. "Stress can cause an exacerbation of the arthritis." 4. "Have you considered going on disability?"	Answer: 3 Rationale: The onset of an autoimmune disorder is frequently associated with an abnormal stressor, either physical or psychological. Autoimmune disorders are frequently progressive relapsing-remission disorders characterized by periods of exacerbation and remission. The nurse should not compound the client's anxiety by making statements which appear to assume the client will lose his job as in options 1 and 2. Arthritis is a condition which is associated with periods of remission and exacerbation. The client should be encouraged to remain as active as possible and avoid giving up. Implementation Analysis Physiological Integrity
13.8 A client with an autoimmune disorder tells the nurse, "My family keeps telling me that I don't look sick." The nurse should utilize which of the following nursing diagnoses to help this client? 1. *Interrupted Family Processes* 2. *Ineffective Protection* 3. *Ineffective Coping* 4. *Activity Intolerance*	Answer: 1 Rationale: This client states that his or her family does not recognize a disease process based upon the client's physical appearance. The best nursing diagnosis for this client would be *Interrupted Family Processes*. The client's appearance of health indicates they are adequately protected. The question does not contain data which supports a lack of coping or activity tolerance by the client. Diagnosis Application Psychosocial Integrity
13.9 A client is recovering from a skin graft where the thumb of his right hand is sutured to the skin on his abdomen. The nurse realizes this client has which of the following types of grafts?	Answer: 3 Rationale: An autograft, a transplant of the client's own tissue, is the most successful type of tissue transplant. Skin grafts are the most common examples of autografts. An allograph, also known as an allogeneic graft, is a graft of tissue

1. allograft 2. isograft 3. autograft 4. xenograft	obtained from the body of another animal of the same species but with a genotype that differs from the recipient, which is also called a homograft or homologous graft. A xenograft is a heterologous graft comprised of tissue from an animal to a human. Diagnosis Analysis Physiological Integrity

13.10 Before a bone marrow transplant, a client is prescribed ganciclovir (Cytovene). Which of the following should be included in the instructions to the client about this medication?
  1. It will prevent the development of herpes pneumonia.
  2. It will decrease the onset of bacterial infections.
  3. It will maintain cardiac output.
  4. It will prevent the development of cytomegaloviral pneumonia.
	Answer: 4
	Rationale: Prior to transplantation, several antibiotic and antiviral drugs may be prescribed. Ganciclovir (Cytovene) prevents the development of cytomegalovirus (CMV) pneumonia in bone marrow transplant recipients. The actions of ganciclovir do not include the prevention of herpes pneumonia, bacterial infections, or alterations in cardiac output.
	Planning
	Application
	Physiological Integrity

13.11 A client is prescribed a monoclonal antibody after an allograft on his left thigh. Which of the following should be done for this client?
  1. Instruct the client that side effects will occur after at least six doses of the medication.
  2. Encourage the client to have a chest x-ray one week after the first dose.
  3. Premedicate with hydrocortisone.
  4. Closely observe the client for four hours following the original dose.
	Answer: 3
	Rationale: Due to the high incidence of adverse effects, the first two doses of OKT3 are administered by a physician and the client is closely observed for two hours following each dose. Adverse reactions are possible after any of the treatments. A chest x-ray should be done before the first dose to ensure there is no pulmonary congestion. Nursing care includes premedicating with hydrocortisone to reduce potential adverse effects.
	Implementation
	Application
	Physiological Integrity

13.12 A client who received a kidney transplant six months prior is demonstrating an alteration in his blood-urea-nitrogen level. The nurse realizes that this client is demonstrating:
  1. a functional decline as an early indicator of rejection.
  2. a functional decline as an early indicator of acceptance.
  3. an expected response.
  4. an allergic response.
	Answer: 2
	Rationale: Laboratory studies should be conducted. A decline in abnormal renal function studies may serve as an early indicator of acceptance. The reduction in function is associated with rejection. The client's progress is individualized and not necessarily "expected." The manifestations are not consistent with an allergic response.
	Diagnosis
	Analysis
	Physiological Integrity

13.13 An HIV positive client comes into the clinic complaining of increasing pain in his feet and legs. The nurse realizes that this client is demonstrating:
  1. a reaction to the medication.
  2. an opportunistic infection.
  3. a secondary cancer.
  4. a nervous system manifestation of the disease.
	Answer: 4
	Rationale: Peripheral nervous system manifestations are also common in HIV-infected clients. Sensory neuropathies with manifestations of numbness, tingling, and pain in the lower extremities affect about 30% of clients with AIDS. The manifestations noted are not consistent with a medication reaction, opportunistic infection, or secondary cancer.
	Diagnosis
	Analysis
	Physiological Integrity

13.14 A young HIV female client tells the nurse she does not want to see the gynecologist because, "I'm going to die anyway." Which of the following should the nurse say in response to this client?	Answer: 1 Rationale: Forty percent of women with HIV infection have cervical dysplasia. Cervical cancer develops frequently and tends to be aggressive. Women with concurrent HIV infection and cervical cancer usually die of the cervical cancer, not AIDS. Because of this, it is recommended that women with HIV infection

1. "Having a PAP smear will help detect the onset of cervical cancer." 2. "Why do you think that you are going to die?" 3. "The gynecologist will help diagnose any Hodgkin's disease." 4. "But you still should be on birth control."	have Papanicolaou (Pap) smears every six months. While the nurse should investigate the feelings of the client, the emphasis is on preventative treatments. The gynecologist does not focus on the diagnosis of Hodgkin's disease. Safe sex practices and the use of contraceptives are within the scope of the gynecologist; however, this is not the primary focus of the interaction. Implementation Application Health Promotion and Maintenance
13.15 An HIV positive client is not adhering to the prescribed medication therapy. Which of the following actions by the nurse will best improve client compliance and long-term treatment of the disease process? 1. Confront the client about the noncompliant behavior. 2. Talk with the client about not adhering to the medication schedule. 3. Suggest that the client take the medication at bedtime to prevent nausea. 4. Refer the client to a social worker so that lower-cost medications can be obtained.	Answer: 2 Rationale: Provider-client relationships seem to have the most influence on adherence behavior. The nurse should talk with the client about not adhering to the medication schedule. Confronting the client would lead to alienation. There is nothing in the question to suggest that nausea is a side effect of the medication. There is no reason to assume that the noncompliance is due to a financial reason. Planning Analysis Health Promotion and Maintenance
13.16 An adolescent client asks the nurse about sexual practices and the onset of HIV. Which of the following should the nurse instruct this client? 1. Always use a condom. 2. Be sure to be tested for HIV every six months. 3. There is no such thing as safe sex. 4. The only safe sex is no sex.	Answer: 4 Rationale: All sexually-active individuals need to know how HIV is spread. Following are the only totally safe sex practices: no sex, long-term mutually monogamous sexual relations between two uninfected people, and mutual masturbation without direct contact. Implementation Application Health Promotion and Maintenance
13.17 An HIV-positive client is being treated for thrush. Client teaching by the nurse should include which of the following side effects? 1. "Hepatitis can develop as a side effect." 2. "Nausea, vomiting, and diarrhea are common side effects." 3. "There are few side effects associated with the medication to treat thrush." 4. "Skin discoloration is a common side effect."	Answer: 3 Rationale: Candidiasis or oral thrush is treated with either clotrimazole (Canesten) troches or nystatin (Mycostatin) suspension. There are few toxic responses noted with either medication. Hepatitis is a communicable disease and not transmitted via medication therapy. Planning Application Physiological Integrity
13.18 The nurse is preparing to instruct a class of young adults about ways to achieve safe sex. What should be included in the nurse's presentation? (Select all that apply.) 1. Avoid spermicidal agents. 2. Be HIV tested if entering into a new monogamous relationship and have the test repeated in six months.	Answer: 2, 3, 4 Rationale: Guidelines for safer sex include: practice mutual monogamy, limit the number of sexual partners, and do not engage in unprotected sex. When entering into a new monogamous relationship, both partners should undergo HIV testing initially and if both are negative, practice abstinence or safe sex for six months, followed by retesting; if results still indicate that both partners are negative, sexual activity can probably be considered safe. Latex condoms should be used for oral, vaginal, or anal intercourse; avoid natural or animal skin condoms, which allow passage of HIV. For vaginal or anal sex, lubricate the condom with the

3. Avoid sexual activity until both partners found HIV negative for two tests.
4. Only use water-based lubricants with condoms.

spermicidal agent nonoxynol-9 for additional protection; do not use an oil-based lubricant such as petroleum jelly, which can result in condom damage; water-based lubricants are acceptable.
Planning
Application
Health Promotion and Maintenance

CHAPTER 14

14.1 A client who is newly diagnosed with cancer says to the nurse, "I don't want to spend my final days on earth in a hospital bed." The best response by the nurse is:
1. "Why do you feel so negative about being in the hospital?"
2. "Please tell me more about how you are feeling right now."
3. "If I were you I would go home and enjoy the life you have left."
4. "I know how you feel. It must be hard to know that you are dying."

Answer: 2
Rationale: The nurse is in the unique position to provide physical as well as psychosocial support to the client diagnosed with cancer. This nurse needs to learn more about the client's feelings and not discount or add to the client's feelings of pending hospitalization.
Implementation
Analysis
Psychosocial Integrity

14.2 A client thinks she has cancer because her last Pap smear identified cervical dysplasia. The best response by the nurse is:
1. "This means the cells of your cervix have lost their useful function."
2. "This means the cells are abnormal because of irritation."
3. "This means the cells are normal."
4. "This confirms that the cells are cancerous."

Answer: 2
Rationale: Dysplastic cells show abnormal variation in size, shape, and appearance and a disturbance in their usual arrangement. Examples of dysplasia include changes in the cervix in response to continued irritation, such as from the human papillomavirus (HPV).
Implementation
Application
Psychosocial Integrity

14.3 A female client tells the nurse, "I want to stop taking birth control. I heard it causes cancer." Which of the following responses can the nurse make to this client?
1. "You heard correctly. They do cause cancer."
2. "This is entirely wrong and I wouldn't stop taking them."
3. "Some birth control pills with estrogen can increase the risk for breast cancer but they also decrease the risk for ovarian cancer."
4. "Aspirin is more dangerous than a birth control pill."

Answer: 3
Rationale: Estrogen-containing contraceptive pills have been implicated in breast cancer, but they also have been shown to decrease the risk of ovarian cancer. Investigators have not reached a final conclusion about the cancer risk posed by contraceptives.
Implementation
Application
Health Promotion and Maintenance

14.4 A 65-year-old male client is diagnosed with lymphoma while being treated for bladder cancer. The nurse realizes that this client is demonstrating:
1. metastasis.
2. a weakened immune system.
3. identification of the primary cancer.
4. two unrelated cancers.

Answer: 2
Rationale: Chemotherapy can weaken an immune system. When this occurs, the client is predisposed to the development of additional disease processes. There is not enough information to assume this second diagnosis of cancer is metastasis or a primary cancer.
Diagnosis
Analysis
Health Promotion and Maintenance

14.5 A client who is being treated for cancer says, "I thought the pain that I had before I was diagnosed with cancer was bad. This is horrible." The nurse's best response is:
1. "Pain is the main indication of cancer."
2. "The treatment for the cancer must not be working."
3. "Pain is a frame of mind."
4. "The pain might be worse because of the cancer treatment."

Answer: 4
Rationale: Chronic pain may be related to treatment or may indicate progression of the disease. Identifying the pain as treatment-related rather than tumor-related is extremely important because it has a definite effect on the client's psychological outlook. There are other signs of cancer other than pain. In some instances, pain is a late manifestation. There is not adequate data to indicate the treatment is ineffective. Pain is whatever the client perceives it to be. The "frame of mind" does not determine pain.
Evaluation
Application
Psychosocial Integrity

14.6 A client asks the nurse, "What does it matter what grade the tumor I had in my stomach?" The best response by the nurse is:
1. "It is a method of explaining the extent of the tumor to your insurance provider."
2. "It is a way to name the tumor."
3. "It explains if the tumor has spread."
4. "It explains how aggressive the tumor is."

Answer: 4
Rationale: There is an elaborate identification system for tumor classification. Staging is a way to describe if a tumor has spread within or beyond the tissue of origin. Although the insurance company may indicate a desire to know the type and grade of tumor, this is not the primary purpose for the system. Naming the tumor is the classification. Grading describes the aggressiveness of the tumor.
Implementation
Application
Physiological Integrity

14.7 A 30-year-old client has been informed of an abnormal mammogram and is to return to the radiology department for additional testing. The nurse realizes that this client will most likely need to have a:
1. chest x-ray.
2. computed tomography (CT) scan.
3. ultrasound.
4. nuclear scan.

Answer: 3
Rationale: Ultrasound imaging is useful for detecting masses in the denser breast tissue of young women. X-rays are most beneficial as an initial screening tool. X-rays lack the definition to distinguish between benign and malignant masses. Computed tomography is most beneficial when screening for renal and gastrointestinal cancers. Nuclear scans are not used for clients at this stage.
Planning
Application
Health Promotion and Maintenance

14.8 A client with abdominal cancer is asking why the physician wants to perform surgery. An appropriate response for the nurse to make to this client is:
1. "That's a good question."
2. "The physician must think this will help get rid of the cancer."
3. "Maybe the physician wants to confirm that you don't have cancer."
4. "Surgical resection is used for diagnosis and staging of 90% of all cancers."

Answer: 4
Rationale: Surgery is an important approach to cancer care. Surgical resection is used for diagnosis and staging of more than 90% of all cancers and for primary treatment of more than 60% of cancers. The goals of surgery have also expanded to include prophylaxis, diagnosis, treatment, reconstruction, and palliation. The remaining options are too vague, false, or include terminology that the client may not understand.
Implementation
Application
Health Promotion and Maintenance

14.9 A client is receiving bleomycin (Blenoxane) as part of his chemotherapy cancer treatment. Which of the following should the nurse do prior to his treatment?
1. Assess for diarrhea.
2. Evaluate the degree of hair loss since the last treatment.
3. Evaluate for motor weakness.
4. Measure vital signs and cardiovascular status.

Answer: 4
Rationale: The main toxic effect of antitumor antibiotics is damage to the cardiac muscle. Diarrhea, hair loss, and motor weakness are not related to the use of the antitumor antibiotics.
Implementation
Analysis
Physiological Integrity

14.10 A client with uterine cancer is prescribed a treatment in which radioactive material will be inserted and maintained within her vagina. Which of the following types of treatment does this describe?
1. brachytherapy
2. teletherapy
3. chemotherapy
4. extracavitary radiation

Answer: 1
Rationale: In brachytherapy, the radioactive material is placed directly into or adjacent to the tumor. This is a technique that delivers a high dose to the tumor and a lower dose to the normal tissues. Teletherapy involves the delivery of radiation from a source placed a distance from the client. Chemotherapy is the use of medications to kill cancerous cells. Intracavitary radiation is also known as brachytherapy. Extracavitary radiation is a nonexistent term.
Planning
Analysis
Physiological Integrity

14.11 A client is prescribed external radiation as part of his cancer treatment. Which of the following should be included in this client's instructions? (Select all that apply.)
1. Wash the skin with soap and water.
2. Do not wash off the treatment marks.
3. Use an electric razor to shave the treatment area.
4. Avoid applying heat or cold to the area.

Answer: 2, 3, 4
Rationale: Client teaching should include washing the skin with plain water, no soap; and do not apply deodorant, lotions, medications, perfume, or powder to the site. Take care not to wash off the treatment marks. Do not rub, scratch, or scrub treated skin areas. If necessary, use only an electric razor to shave the treated area. Apply neither heat nor cold (e.g., heating pad or ice pack) to the treatment site.
Planning
Application
Health Promotion and Maintenance

14.12 A client with cancer is diagnosed with pain associated with the cancer treatment. The nurse realizes that this client is most likely experiencing:
1. pain within a hollow visceral organ.
2. incisional pain.
3. metastatic bone pain.
4. no pain.

Answer: 2
Rationale: There are three categories or pain syndromes in clients with cancer: pain associated with direct tumor involvement, pain associated with treatment, and pain from a cause not related to either the cancer or therapy. The one choice that is associated with cancer treatment is incision pain.
Assessment
Analysis
Physiological Integrity

14.13 The nurse is planning a community health program for senior citizens about cancer detection. Which of the following acronyms would be helpful for the nurse to use in this educational session?
1. ACTION
2. ABC
3. CAREFUL
4. CAUTION

Answer: 4
Rationale: The American Cancer Society promotes early detection through public education using the CAUTION model: C= change in bowel or bladder habits, A= a sore that does not heal, U =unusual bleeding or discharge, T=thickening lump in breast or elsewhere, I=indigestion or difficulty swallowing, O=obvious change in wart or mole, and N=nagging cough or hoarseness.
Planning
Application
Health Promotion and Maintenance

14.14 The nurse is preparing to change the postoperative dressing of a client with a mastectomy. During the dressing change the client looks away. Which of the following should the nurse do to assist this client?
1. Hand the client a mirror so that she can look at the incision while the dressing is being changed.
2. Support the client; however, do not avoid discussing the incision.
3. Suggest that the client identify a family member who will have to do the dressing since the client refuses to learn.

Answer: 2
Rationale: The nurse should allow denial but not participate in the denial. The nurse should assist the client to cope with the changes in her appearance. It may be too soon for the client to assume responsibility for the dressing changes. The nurse should gradually allow the client to assume full responsibility.
Implementation
Application
Psychosocial Integrity

4. Recommend that the client receive home care upon discharge because the client will not be able to provide self dressing changes.	

14.15 The family of a client with terminal metastatic cancer asks the nurse for guidelines regarding when to call for help when the client is discharged to home. Which of the following would indicate this client needs medical intervention? (Select all that apply.)

1. rectal temperature greater than 101.5 F
2. difficulty breathing
3. onset of bleeding
4. resting comfortably, and reading
5. extreme hunger
6. improvement in ankle edema

Answer: 2, 3, 5
Rationale: The nurse should instruct the client and family to call the physician or nurse for help with any of the following signs or symptoms: an oral temperature greater than 101.5°F (38.6°C); severe headache; significant increase in pain at usual site, especially if the pain is not relieved by the medication regimen; severe pain at a new site; difficulty breathing; new bleeding from any site, such as rectal or vaginal bleeding; confusion, irritability, or restlessness; withdrawal; greatly decreased activity level; frequent crying; verbalizations of deep sadness or a desire to end life; changes in body functioning, such as the inability to void or severe diarrhea or constipation; changes in eating patterns, such as refusal to eat, extreme hunger, or a significant increase in nausea and vomiting; and appearance of edema in the extremities or significant increase in edema already present.
Implementation
Application
Physiological Integrity

14.16 A client who was treated for bladder cancer 15 years ago tells the nurse, "I live each day like it is my last yet plan for the future." The nurse realizes that this client is demonstrating which phase of cancer survival?

1. diagnosis and treatment
2. extended survival
3. watchful waiting
4. permanent survival

Answer: 4
Rationale: Permanent survival is said to begin when the survival period has gone on long enough that the risk of recurrence is small. The first stage in the "three seasons of cancer survival" is diagnosis and treatment. During this phase diagnosis takes place but the emphasis is on treatment. Extended survival begins at the end of treatment. Watchful waiting refers to the period when time must pass to determine the success of treatment.
Evaluation
Analysis
Psychosocial Integrity

14.17 A client is informed that the tumor removed from his abdomen had well-defined borders, was encapsulated, and totally removed. The nurse realizes that this client has just learned the tumor was most likely:

1. malignant.
2. metastatic.
3. benign.
4. one that would not respond to chemotherapy.

Answer: 3
Rationale: Characteristics of a benign neoplasm include well-defined borders, displaces other surrounding tissues, is slow-growing, encapsulated, easily removed, and does not recur. Malignant neoplasm grows aggressively, is not cohesive, and is irregular in shape. Metastatic growths infiltrate to other areas. If the tumor is benign, chemotherapy would not be necessary.
Diagnosis
Analysis
Physiological Integrity

CHAPTER 15

15.1 A client who is scheduled for abdominal surgery is concerned about an unsightly scar. During the preoperative teaching session, the nurse should explain that:

1. a scar will be unavoidable.
2. the surgeon will most likely not be concerned about scar formation.
3. plastic surgery can remove the scar at a later date.
4. it will depend upon the location and angle of the incision.

Answer: 4
Rationale: Surgical incisions that are parallel to the lines of cleavage within the dermis will heal more easily and with less scarring that those created across cleavage lines. Some degree of scarring will most likely take place. Although the surgeon will take into consideration the client's postoperative appearance, the surgical procedure will mandate the degree of scarring left. Plastic surgery is not an option for all clients.
Implementation
Application
Psychosocial Integrity

15.2 An adolescent client has extensive acne over his face and upper neck. The nurse realizes that this condition is caused by:
1. inflamed sebaceous glands.
2. blocked endocrine glands.
3. blocked exocrine glands.
4. inflamed ceruminous glands.

Answer: 1
Rationale: Blocked sebaceous glands cause a pimple or comedomes to appear on the surface of the skin. Acne is an inflammation of the sebaceous glands.
Diagnosis
Application
Physiological Integrity

15.3 The nurse assesses a client's skin color as "pasty white." When documenting findings, the nurse should use which of the following to describe this client's skin color?
1. erythema
2. pallor
3. cyanosis
4. jaundice

Answer: 2
Rationale: Pallor, or paleness of the skin, may occur with shock, fear, anger, anemia, or hypoxia. Erythema refers to redness. The presence of cyanosis indicates a bluish discoloration. Jaundice is a yellowish tone that is caused by an excess of bilirubin.
Diagnosis
Comprehension
Physiological Integrity

15.4 A client with thick wavy hair comes into the clinic. The nurse realizes that this client's hair is indicative of:
1. poor nutrition.
2. hormone deficiency.
3. adequate nutrition.
4. vitamin deficiency.

Answer: 3
Rationale: Many factors, including nutrition and hormones, influence hair growth. The client discussed does not have any outward appearance of deficiencies or malnourishment.
Diagnosis
Application
Physiological Integrity

15.5 A client is waiting to have a skin biopsy and asks, "What is going to happen when this is done?" Which of the following would be an appropriate response for the nurse to make?
1. "Didn't your doctor tell you?"
2. "Maybe you shouldn't have it done."
3. "I'm not sure."
4. "Let me check to see exactly what you are having done and then we can talk more about what you can expect."

Answer: 4
Rationale: Regardless of the type of diagnostic test, the nurse is responsible for explaining the procedure and any special preparation needed and for supporting the client. To answer the client's inquiry with a question is not therapeutic. The nurse should not discourage the client from obtaining treatments ordered.
Implementation
Application
Physiological Integrity

15.6 The nurse is conducting a focused interview about a client's integumentary status. Which of the following client characteristics would cause the nurse to focus on risk factors for skin cancer?
1. blond hair and blue eyes
2. female, age 35
3. home in Portland, Maine
4. is a child daycare worker

Answer: 1
Rationale: Risk factors for skin cancer include male gender, age over 50, family history of skin cancer, extended exposure to sunlight, tendency to sunburn, light-colored hair or eyes, residence in high altitudes or near the equator, and exposure to radiation, x-rays, or petroleum products.
Planning
Analysis
Physiological Integrity

15.7 The nurse is preparing to assess a client's integumentary status. Which of the following techniques should the nurse use to conduct this assessment?
1. inspection
2. inspection and percussion
3. inspection and palpation
4. percussion and palpation

Answer: 3
Rationale: Physical assessment of the skin, hair, and nails is conducted by inspection and palpation. Percussion employs tapping to assess structures beneath the skin's surface.
Planning
Application
Physiological Integrity

15.8 During the assessment of a client's integumentary status, the nurse notes: "vitiligo present bilateral hands." This documentation means that: 1. the client has nodules with ulcerations. 2. the client has dark, asymmetrical colored patches. 3. the client has grouped vesicles. 4. the client has an abnormal loss of melanin in patches.	Answer: 4 Rationale: Vitiligo is an abnormal loss of melanin in patches, and typically occurs over the face, hands, or groin. Diagnosis Application Physiological Integrity
15.9 After the completion of an integumentary status assessment, the nurse documents: "+1 edema right lower leg." This documentation means: 1. slight pitting, no obvious distortion. 2. deep pitting, no obvious distortion. 3. pitting is obvious, extremities are swollen. 4. pitting remains with obvious distortion.	Answer: 1 Rationale: Edema or accumulation of fluid in the body's tissues is recorded as +1, +2, +3, or +4. The designation +1 means that the client has slight pitting in the right lower leg with no obvious distortion. Diagnosis Analysis Physiological Integrity
15.10 The nurse is assessing the integumentary status of a 79-year-old female. Which of the following findings are considered common in older adults? (Select all that apply.) 1. keratoses 2. skin tags 3. urticaria 4. photoaging	Answer: 1, 2, 4 Rationale: Common skin lesions in older adults include skin tags, keratoses, lentigines, angiomas, telangiectases, venous lakes, and photoaging. Urticaria (hives) is an integumentary disorder that is not normal. Assessment Application Health Promotion and Maintenance
15.11 The nurse is planning to assess an African American's integumentary status. Which of the following findings would indicate the presence of cyanosis in this client? 1. yellow hue in the eyes 2. bluish-tinged nail beds 3. cherry-red lips 4. orange-green cast to the skin	Answer: 2 Rationale: Cyanosis is more readily assessed in the nail beds, oral mucous membranes, and conjunctivae. A yellowish hue refers to the presence of jaundice. Cherry red lips are associated with carbon monoxide poisoning. Orange-green cast to the skin is not associated with any specific disorder. Diagnosis Application Physiological Integrity
15.12 The nurse is planning to document the appearance of herpetic lesions found over a client's nose and mouth region. Which of the following terms would the nurse most likely use to describe this finding? 1. scaly 2. pustular 3. pruritic 4. ulcerated	Answer: 4 Rationale: The term "ulcerated" is most likely used to describe pressure ulcers, skin cancer, and herpes simplex. Scaly lesions are characteristic of eczema. Pustular lesions are associated with acne. Pruritic refers to itching. Diagnosis Application Physiological Integrity
15.13 During the assessment of an elderly client's integumentary status, the nurse notes small areas of hyperpigmentation on the client's hands. The nurse realizes that this finding is due to:	Answer: 1 Rationale: The nurse is describing "liver spots" or small areas of hyperpigmentation over the client's hands. This is due to hyperplasia of melanocytes, especially in sun-exposed areas of the client's epidermis. Alterations in vitamin D production, reduced blood perfusion, and changes in adipose tissue are not associated with excessive pigmentation.

1. hyperplasia of melanocytes in sun-exposed areas. 2. reduced vitamin D production. 3. decreased blood perfusion of the dermis. 4. redistribution of adipose tissue.	Diagnosis Application Physiological Integrity
15.14 A client is seen in the clinic after having a biopsy done which sampled a small section of dermis and subcutaneous fat. The nurse realizes that this client has had: 1. an incisional skin biopsy. 2. a punch skin biopsy. 3. an excisional skin biopsy. 4. a shave skin biopsy.	Answer: 2 Rationale: A punch skin biopsy is done to differentiate benign lesions from skin cancers. An instrument is used to remove a small section of dermis and subcutaneous fat. The punch biopsy provides a full thickness specimen for analysis. The incisional biopsy involves the removal of a portion of a tumor or lesion. The excisional biopsy is the removal of an entire lesion or tumor. The shave biopsy is the scraping of a layer of cells for analysis. Diagnosis Analysis Physiological Integrity
15.15 A client is scheduled for a test to diagnose the presence of a herpes infection. The nurse realizes that the client is most likely going to have: 1. a patch test. 2. a Tzanck test. 3. a potassium chloride test. 4. a Wood's light examination.	Answer: 2 Rationale: The Tzanck test is used to diagnose herpes infections but does not differentiate herpes simplex from herpes zoster. Patch testing is used to assess allergens. The Wood's light test is used to assess for tinea infections. Diagnosis Application Physiological Integrity

CHAPTER 16

16.1 A client with a history of pruritis says, "The itching seems to improve when I take my allergy medicine." The nurse realizes that this is most likely because: 1. the client is distracted from the itching because of the allergies. 2. the client's pruritis is improving. 3. the allergy medication is reducing histamine release. 4. the client is taking other medication of which the nurse is not aware.	Answer: 3 Rationale: The irritant that causes the itching releases histamine. Antihistamines may relieve pruritis for some clients. The allergies are the cause of the itching so option 1 is not realistic. Pruritis is improving as a result of the histamine release caused by the medication. There is no indication the client is taking other medications. Evaluation Analysis Physiological Integrity
16.2 A 47-year-old female client with a history of sun exposure is concerned that she has a disease because, "There are broken blood vessels on my cheeks." The nurse realizes that this client is describing: 1. nevus flammeus. 2. telangiectases. 3. venus lakes. 4. skin tags.	Answer: 2 Rationale: Telangiectases are single dilated capillaries or terminal arteries that appear often on the cheeks and nose. These lesions are most common in older adults and result from photoaged skin. The lesions appear as broken veins. Nevus flammeus is a congenital vascular condition involving the capillaries. Venus lakes do not exist. Skin tags are soft papules on a pedicle. Diagnosis Analysis Physiological Integrity
16.3 A client is receiving his first ultraviolet light therapy treatment for psoriasis. Which of the following should be included in this client's teaching? 1. The treatment will be the same length every time. 2. There is no anticipated damage to the eyes or mucous membranes.	Answer: 3 Rationale: Clients with generalized psoriasis or with psoriasis over 30% of the body will most likely be treated with phototherapy. To avoid damage to the eyes they will need to be shielded during the treatment and the client can expect areas of erythema approximately eight hours after the treatment. The treatment is measured in seconds with a gradual increase in exposure times. Implementation

3. The skin will appear reddened in approximately eight hours after the treatment. 4. This is the treatment of choice for clients with psoriasis on 10% of the body.	Application Physiological Integrity
16.4 A female client comes into the clinic with eyelid redness and edema. Which of the following would be appropriate for the nurse to include in the assessment of this client? 　1. Ask if the client has recently been in a public swimming pool. 　2. Ask the client if she shaves her legs. 　3. Ask the client if she has recently changed her facial soap. 　4. Ask the client if she has been thoroughly removing all of her eye makeup.	Answer: 4 Rationale: This client is experiencing folliculitis, a bacterial infection of the hair follicle on the eyelid. This condition is found more frequently on the scalp and extremities. When found on the eyelids, it is called a stye. It is caused by a bacterial infection of the hair follicle, most commonly caused by *Staphylococcus aureus*. The client's complaints are in the orbital area. An infection caused by the swimming pool would encompass the entire body. Shaving would involve the legs. The complaints are not generalized on the face but localized in the eye area, so the facial soap is not the culprit. Assessment Application Physiological Integrity
16.5 A female client comes into the clinic concerned that while on a recent vacation she noticed several small patches of skin that "just won't tan." The nurse realizes that this client might be experiencing: 　1. tinea capitis. 　2. tinea corporis. 　3. tinea versicolor. 　4. tinea cruris.	Answer: 3 Rationale: Tinea versicolor is a fungal infection of the upper chest, back, and sometimes the arms. The lesions are yellow, pink, or brown sheets of scaling skin. The patches do not have pigment and do not tan when exposed to ultraviolet light. Tinea capitis refers to a fungal infection of the head and scalp. Tinea corporis is a fungal infection that covers most of the body. The lesions are round and scaling. Tinea cruris refers to a fungal infection of the groin region. Diagnosis Analysis Physiological Integrity
16.6 The mother of a 12-year-old child states that she is concerned about her daughter's hair. She reports that her daughter frequently scratches her scalp and the hair "is clumpy and smells really bad." Which of the following should the nurse do to assist this mother? 　1. Suggest that the daughter be checked for head lice. 　2. Suggest that the daughter have a blood glucose level drawn. 　3. Suggest that the daughter wash her hair. 　4. Suggest that the daughter have a haircut.	Answer: 1 Rationale: Pediculosis capitis is an infestation with head lice. It is more common in female children Manifestations of head lice include pruritis, scratching, and erythema of the scalp. If untreated, the hair appears matted and crusted with a foul-smelling substance. There are no indications from the information provided that the child has diabetes. Although hygiene may be an issue, the greatest indicator points toward the presence of head lice. There is no need to encourage a haircut at this time. Implementation Application Physiological Integrity
16.7 A 68-year-old male client comes into the clinic with a "strange painful rash" located on the left side of his upper chest. The nurse realizes that this client might be experiencing: 　1. herpes simplex. 　2. herpes zoster. 　3. verruca plana. 　4. condylomata acuminata.	Answer: 2 Rationale: This client is most likely experiencing herpes zoster. Vesicles appear on the skin and usually appear unilaterally on the face, trunk, or thorax. The client often experiences severe pain for up to 48 hours before and during eruption of the lesions. The pain may continue for weeks to months. Herpes simplex is usually located on the face, mouth, or genital regions. The clinical manifestations that this client reports are inconsistent with verruca or condylomata. Diagnosis Application Physiological Integrity

16.8 A female client comes into the clinic with an itchy reddened area on both hands. Which of the following assessment techniques should the nurse include in the client's assessment? 1. Ask the client to remove her shoes and stockings. 2. Listen to the client's lungs. 3. Assess the client's hand grasp strength. 4. Ask the client if she has changed soap or perfume.	Answer: 4 Rationale: This client's description fits that of contact dermatitis. This is caused by a hypersensitivity response or chemical irritation. The major sources known to cause contact dermatitis are dyes, perfumes, poison plants, chemicals, or metals. A focused assessment is indicated. There are no reports of the rash on her legs or feet. Respiratory complications are not present. It is not necessary to assess this client's musculoskeletal strength. Assessment Application Physiological Integrity
16.9 A 57-year-old female client complains of "strange pimples" over her buttocks region. The nurse realizes that this client might be experiencing: 1. contact dermatitis. 2. acne vulgaris. 3. acne conglobata. 4. acne rosacea.	Answer: 3 Rationale: Acne conglobata is a chronic type of acne of unknown cause that begins in middle adulthood. It causes serious skin lesions consisting of comedones, papules, pustules, nodules, cysts, and scars. This acne occurs primarily on the back, buttocks, and chest. Diagnosis Application Physiological Integrity
16.10 The nurse is preparing a teaching plan for a group of community teenagers about acne. Which of the following should be included in this teaching plan? (Select all that apply.) 1. Avoid eating greasy foods. 2. Sun exposure is permitted when protected with sunscreen, but avoid sunburn. 3. Wash the affected skin area at least six times per day. 4. Use a cotton ball saturated in rubbing alcohol after washing the skin. 5. Keep hair clean with frequent shampoos. 6. Squeeze pimples when they occur.	Answer: 2, 5 Rationale: The teaching plan for the client with acne should include: wash the skin with a mild soap and water at least twice a day; shampoo the hair often enough to prevent oiliness; eat a regular, well-balanced diet; foods do not cause or increase acne; expose the skin to sunlight, but avoid sunburn; get regular exercise and sleep; try to avoid putting your hands on your face; and do not squeeze a pimple. Planning Application Health Promotion and Maintenance
16.11 A 52-year-old male client of English descent is diagnosed with basal cell cancer on the face and forehead. Which of the following should the nurse include when teaching this client about his diagnosis? 1. This is a virulent form of skin cancer. 2. This type of skin cancer tends to reoccur. 3. This type of skin cancer should be left alone. 4. This type of skin cancer is rare.	Answer: 2 Rationale: Basal cell cancer tends to reoccur. Tumors larger than 2 cm have a high rate of return. Basal cell cancer is the most common but least aggressive type of skin cancer. No cancer should be left alone. Malignant melanoma is the most virulent form of skin cancer. Implementation Application Physiological Integrity
16.12 A client with skin cancer is recovering from a surgical procedure in which the layers of the lesion were shaved off. The nurse realizes that this client most likely has had: 1. complete surgical excision of the lesion.	Answer: 2 Rationale: In Mohs surgery, thin layers of the tumor are horizontally shaved off. A frozen section of the tissue is stained at each level to determine tumor margins. A surgical excision is the total removal of the lesion not just layers. Curettage is the shaving of abnormal tissue within 1 to 2 mm of the margin. Electrodesiccation refers to the use of a low-voltage transmission to the base of the tumor.

2. Mohs surgery.	Evaluation
3. curettage.	Analysis
4. electrodesiccation.	Physiological Integrity

16.13 A 35-year-old female client is diagnosed with advanced malignant melanoma. The nurse realizes that this client:

1. has an uncertain prognosis.
2. has a poor prognosis due to her age.
3. will be completely cured with surgery.
4. will need chemotherapy and radiation.

Answer: 1
Rationale: The prognosis for survival for people diagnosed with malignant melanoma is determined by tumor thickness, ulceration, metastasis, site, age, and gender. Younger clients and women have a somewhat better chance of survival. There is no evidence that the client will be completely cured with surgery or will need chemotherapy and radiation.
Diagnosis
Analysis
Physiological Integrity

16.14 The nurse instructs a client with melanoma to "eat foods rich in protein and calories." This intervention is most likely associated with which of the following nursing diagnosis?

1. *Impaired Skin Integrity*
2. *Hopelessness*
3. *Anxiety*
4. *Fluid Volume Deficit*

Answer: 1
Rationale: When planning care for a client with *Impaired Skin Integrity,* interventions should include monitoring for infection, wound care, careful hand washing, and adequate caloric and protein intake for wound healing. Psychological alterations such as hopelessness and anxiety cannot be managed by a diet rich in protein and calories. Fluid volume is not directly impacted by a diet high in protein and calories.
Implementation
Analysis
Physiological Integrity

16.15 A client confined to bed has slid to the bottom of the bed. Which of the following should the nurse do to adjust this client's body position?

1. Pull the client up in bed.
2. Slide the client up in bed.
3. Lift the client up in bed.
4. Do nothing.

Answer: 3
Rationale: Clients in hospital beds are subject to shearing forces when the head of the bed is elevated and the torso slides down toward the foot of the bed. Pulling the client up in bed subjects the client to shearing forces. For this reason, always lift clients up in bed with the assistance of support staff as indicated.
Planning
Application
Physiological Integrity

16.16 A client in a wheelchair has a history of sacral pressure ulcer formation. Which of the following instructions should be included in the client's teaching?

1. Shift the weight every 15 minutes to one hour.
2. Sit on a donut.
3. Stay in one position as long as possible.
4. Have a family pull the client up in the wheelchair.

Answer: 1
Rationale: Sitting uninterrupted in a wheelchair should be avoided. The client should be repositioned every hour. If the client can move, teach them to shift their weight every 15 minutes. Avoid the use of donut devices because they cause a reduction in blood perfusion and contribute to pressure ulcer formation. Pulling the client up in the chair may result in skin shear.
Planning
Application
Physiological Integrity

16.17 A 40-year-old male client says, "I wish I could have all of these tattoos removed." Which of the following solutions could the nurse suggest to this client?

1. chemical peeling
2. skin graft
3. dermabrasion
4. a blepharoplasty

Answer: 3
Rationale: Dermabrasion is a method of removing facial scars, severe acne, and pigment from unwanted tattoos. The area is sprayed with a chemical to cause light freezing and is then abraded with sandpaper or a revolving wire brush to remove the epidermis and a portion of the dermis. Chemical peeling involves a process that smoothes the skin by removing the surface layers. Skin grafting involves removing skin from another body area and will cause scarring; it is not an acceptable management tool for this client's problem. Blepharoplasty is a cosmetic surgical procedure on the eyes. This cannot be used to remove the tattoos.
Implementation
Application
Health Promotion and Maintenance

16.18 A 55-year-old client who is recovering from a face lift says, "I think this was a waste of time and money. I look horrible!" Which of the following would be an appropriate nursing response?

1. "It takes a while for the skin to heal."
2. "You could use makeup."
3. "I would complain to the doctor."
4. "What did you expect?"

Answer: 1

Rationale: This client needs to be reminded that there will be bruising and swelling that might take several weeks to disappear. It might also take a year for healing to complete and the final results to appear. The client's reports are normal when faced with an alteration in appearance. The use of makeup is not needed and is premature. Filing a complaint with the doctor is not indicated. The client's emotional state warrants an empathetic response; asking the client what they expected is not a therapeutic response.

Implementation

Application

Psychosocial Integrity

16.19 A client with a history of basal cell skin cancer asks the nurse what to do to avoid having the cancer recur. Which of the following would be appropriate for the nurse to instruct this client?

1. Avoid the sun at all costs.
2. Sun exposure between the hours of 10:00 A.M. and 3:00 P.M. is best.
3. Always use a sunscreen of SPF 15 or higher.
4. Sunscreen is not needed on cloudy days.

Answer: 3

Rationale: The client should be instructed on the use of a sunscreen of SPF 15 or higher. It is unrealistic to instruct a client to always avoid the sun. The hours of 10:00 to 3:00 P.M. are the worst for sun exposure. Sunscreen is needed even on cloudy days.

Implementation

Application

Health Promotion and Maintenance

CHAPTER 17

17.1 A client comes into the clinic to be seen for a burn that appears moist with blisters. The nurse realizes that this client most likely has experienced a:

1. first-degree burn.
2. superficial second-degree burn.
3. deep second-degree burn.
4. third-degree burn.

Answer: 2

Rationale: Partial thickness, or second-degree, burns can either be superficial or deep. This client's burn, which appears moist with blisters, is consistent with a superficial second-degree burn. A first-degree burn would involve only the surface layer of skin. Redness would be expected. Deep second-degree and third-degree burns would be deeper and involve more damage to the dermis, epidermis, and underlying tissue.

Diagnosis

Analysis

Physiological Integrity

17.2 A female client comes into the clinic complaining of nausea and vomiting after spending the weekend at a seaside resort. Which of the following should be the most important assessment for the nurse?

1. normal rest and sleep pattern
2. typical meal pattern
3. if the client had to change time zones when traveling to the resort
4. if the client has been sunburned

Answer: 4

Rationale: Sunburns result from exposure to ultraviolet light. Because the skin remains intact, the manifestations in most cases are mild and are limited to pain, nausea, vomiting, skin redness, chills, and headache. The client has not reported concerns which will support issues with sleep pattern, diet, and travel.

Assessment

Application

Physiological Integrity

17.3 The family of a client with third-degree burns wants to know why the "scabs are being cut off" of the client's leg. What is the most appropriate response by the nurse to this family?

1. "I'll ask the doctor to come and talk with you about the treatment plan."
2. "The client asked for the scabs to be removed."

Answer: 4

Rationale: The client's family is describing eschar, which is the hard crust of burned necrotic tissue. Eschar needs to be removed to promote wound healing.

Implementation

Application

Physiological Integrity

---

3. "The scabs are removed to check for blood flow to the burned area."
4. "The scabs are really old burned tissue and need to be removed to promote healing."

17.4 A client with third-degree burns is prescribed gastrointestinal medication. The primary action of this drug is:
1. to prevent the onset of a Curling's ulcer.
2. to treat a preexisting duodenal ulcer.
3. for the antiemetic properties.
4. to ensure adequate peristalsis.

Answer: 1
Rationale: Dysfunction of the gastrointestinal system is directly related to the size of the burn wound. This can lead to a cessation of intestinal motility, which causes gastric distention, nausea, vomiting, and hematemesis. Stress ulcers or Curling's ulcers are acute ulcerations of the stomach or duodenum that form following the burn injury. There is no evidence to support the presence of a preexisting duodenal ulcer. Although peristalsis is desired, it is not the primary area of gastrointestinal concern. There is no data presented to indicate the presence of nausea or vomiting.
Evaluation
Analysis
Physiological Integrity

17.5 A client comes into the physician's office after sustaining chemical burns to the left side of his face and right wrist. The nurse realizes that this client needs to be treated:
1. in the outpatient ambulatory clinic.
2. in the emergency room.
3. in a burn center.
4. in the doctor's office and then at home.

Answer: 3
Rationale: Adult clients who should be treated at burn centers include those with burns that involve the hands, feet, face, eyes, ears, or perineum. Clients having small or noninvasive burns may be managed at an outpatient clinic are mild in nature. The emergency room is a location for evaluation of a burn. The physician's office like the ambulatory clinic can manage mild burns.
Diagnosis
Analysis
Health Promotion and Maintenance

17.6 A client is coming into the emergency department with third-degree burns over 25% of his body. The nurse should prepare which of the following solutions for intravenous infusion for this client?
1. 5% dextrose in water
2. 5% dextrose in 0.45 normal saline
3. warmed lactated Ringer's
4. 5% dextrose in normal saline

Answer: 3
Rationale: Warmed Ringer's lactate solution is the intravenous fluid most widely used during the first 24 hours after a burn injury because it most closely approximates the body's extracellular fluid composition.
Planning
Application
Physiological Integrity

17.7 The nurse notes that a client with third-degree burns is demonstrating a reduction in his serum potassium level. The nurse realizes that this finding is consistent with:
1. the resolution of burn shock.
2. the onset of burn shock.
3. the onset of renal failure.
4. the onset of liver failure.

Answer: 1
Rationale: Potassium levels are initially elevated during burn shock but will decrease after burn shock resolves as fluid shifts back to intracellular and intravascular compartments.
Evaluation
Analysis
Physiological Integrity

17.8 A client who is being treated with topical mafenide acetate for third-degree burns is demonstrating facial and neck edema. The nurse realizes that this client most likely:
1. is reacting positively to the medication.
2. needs an increase in dosage of the medication.

Answer: 3
Rationale: Approximately 3% to 5% of clients develop a hypersensitivity to mafenide, which can manifest as facial edema. The manifestation of facial and neck edema is considered an adverse reaction. There is inadequate information presented to assess response to the medication.
Diagnosis
Analysis
Physiological Integrity

---

3. is developing a hypersensitivity to the medication. 4. is not responding to the medication.	
17.9 Following surgical debridement, a client with third-degree burns does not bleed. The nurse realizes that this client: 1. will no longer need this procedure. 2. will need to be premedicated prior to the next procedure. 3. should have an escharotomy instead. 4. will need to have the procedure repeated.	Answer: 4 Rationale: Surgical debridement is the process of excising the burn wound by removing thin slices of the wound to the level of viable tissue. If bleeding does not occur after the procedure, it will be repeated. It is an assumption that clients having debridement will all require premedication. An escharotomy involves removal of the hardened crust covering the burned area. Evaluation Analysis Physiological Integrity
17.10 The nurse is providing care to a client with a third-degree burn on his left thigh and left forearm. During wound care, the nurse applies Elase to the burned areas. Which of the following types of wound debridement is this nurse using? 1. mechanical 2. enzymatic 3. surgical 4. topical	Answer: 2 Rationale: Enzymatic debridement involves the use of a topical agent to dissolve and remove necrotic tissue. An enzyme such as Elase is applied in a thin layer directly to the wound and covered with one layer of fine mesh gauze. A topical antimicrobial agent is then applied and covered with a bulky wet dressing. Mechanical debridement may be performed by applying and removing gauze dressings, hydrotherapy, irrigation, or using scissors and tweezers. Surgical debridement is the process of excising the wound to the fascia or removing thin slices of the burn to the level of viable tissue. Topical treatments are key in the care of a burn but do not involve debridement. Implementation Application Physiological Integrity
17.11 A client is being seen in the emergency department after sustaining a burn to his arms and legs. List all of the information the nurse should collect during the first interview with this client.	Answer: Time of injury; cause of injury; first aid treatment; past medical history; age; medications; body weight; and allergies. Rationale: In most cases, the client is awake and oriented and able to relate the information during the emergent phase of care. Because changes in sensorium will become evident within the first few hours following a major burn injury, the nurse obtains as much information as is possible immediately on the client's arrival. Assessment Application Physiological Integrity
17.12 A client with third-degree burns is being treated with high-volume intravenous fluids and has a urine output of 40 cc per hour. The nurse realizes that this urine output: 1. is normal for this client. 2. provides evidence that the client is dehydrated. 3. provides evidence that the client is over-hydrated. 4. is indicative of pending renal failure.	Answer: 1 Rationale: Intake and output measurements indicate the adequacy of fluid resuscitation, and should range from 30 to 50 mL per hour in an adult. Evaluation Analysis Physiological Integrity
17.13 A client with third-degree burns to his right arm is scheduled for passive range of motion to the extremity every two hours. Which of the following should the nurse do prior to this exercise session? 1. Empty the client's indwelling catheter collection bag.	Answer: 4 Rationale: The nurse should anticipate this client's needs for analgesia and administer pain medication to promote the client's comfort during the exercise session. Arm exercise is not related to the amount of urine in the catheter bag. Linen changes do not impact range of motion activities. The burn's dressing is changed according to the physician's orders or as needed.

2. Change the client's bed linens. 3. Change the dressing on the burn. 4. Medicate for pain.	Planning Application Physiological Integrity
17.14 A client with third-degree burns to her face just learned that she will have extensive scarring once the burn heals. Which of the following nursing diagnoses would be applicable to this client at this time? 1. *Potential for Infection* 2. *Powerlessness* 3. *Fluid Volume Deficit* 4. *Risk for Ineffective Airway Clearance*	Answer: 2 Rationale: This client can begin to experience powerlessness in that she has no control over the outcome of healing or scar formation to her face. The nurse should allow the client to express feelings in efforts to help the client cope with the news of potential scarring. The client with a third-degree burn is at risk for infection, however, this question is focused on the impact of her facial scarring. There is inadequate information to determine the client's risk for fluid volume deficits or ineffective airway clearance. Further, this is not the focus of the question. Diagnosis Analysis Psychosocial Integrity
17.15 An obese client is brought into the emergency department after being burned in an explosion. Name the burn assessment method that would provide the best information about the total body surface area injured by the burn.	Answer: Lund and Browder burn assessment chart Rationale: Although useful in emergency care situations, the rule of nines is not accurate for estimating total body surface area (TBSA) for adults who are short, obese, or very thin. The Lund and Browder burn assessment chart is a method of estimating TBSA affected by a burn injury that is more accurate than the "rule of nines" because it accounts for changes in body surface area across the lifespan. Assessment Application Physiological Integrity
17.16 A client with a burn tells the nurse, "I thought burns were supposed to hurt. I have no pain." The nurse realizes that this client most likely has: 1. a superficial burn. 2. a superficial partial-thickness burn. 3. a deep partial-thickness burn. 4. a full-thickness burn.	Answer: 4 Rationale: Pain sensations with full-thickness burns are absent. Diagnosis Analysis Physiological Integrity

CHAPTER 18

18.1 A client asks the nurse, "Why is the doctor concerned about my pituitary gland?" The nurse realizes that this gland regulates: 1. renal function. 2. eight hormone related functions. 3. bone density. 4. arterial blood flow.	Answer: 2 Rationale: The pituitary gland is often called the "master gland" because its hormones regulate many body functions. The anterior pituitary secretes at least six major hormones. The posterior pituitary stores and releases antidiuretic hormone and oxytocin. The pituitary influences renal function, bone density, and arterial blood flow via the hormones that it releases. Planning Analysis Physiological Integrity
18.2 A male client tells the nurse that his wife is having difficulty conceiving. Which of the following hormones should be evaluated in the client regarding his wife's issue? 1. growth hormone 2. prolactin 3. thyroid-stimulating hormone 4. follicle-stimulating hormone	Answer: 4 Rationale: In men, follicle stimulating hormone is involved in the development and maturation of sperm. Growth hormone, prolactin, and thyroid-stimulating hormone do not have a direct influence on male fertility. Diagnosis Analysis Health Promotion and Maintenance
18.3 A client is admitted with dehydration and excessive urination. The nurse realizes that the client might	Answer: 1 Rationale: Antidiuretic hormone, or ADH, decreases urine production by causing the renal tubules to reabsorb water from the urine and return it to the circulating

be experiencing an alteration in which of the following hormones?
1. ADH
2. FSH
3. ACTH
4. TSH

blood. This client is demonstrating excessive urination which might indicate an alteration in this hormone. FSH (follicle-stimulating hormone) functions in ovum and sperm formation. ACTH (adrenocorticotropic hormone) stimulates the adrenal function. TSH (thyroid-stimulating hormone) stimulates thyroid function. Alteration in these hormones does not have as direct of a relationship to the client's symptoms as ADH does.
Diagnosis
Analysis
Physiological Integrity

18.4 A client is scheduled for a thyroidectomy. Which of the following should the nurse include when teaching this client about recovery after the procedure?
1. Exercise will be restricted for up to six months after the surgery.
2. A low- or no-sodium diet will be prescribed.
3. Physical therapy sessions will need to be continued.
4. There might be hormone replacement medications needed since the parathyroid glands will most likely also be removed.

Answer: 4
Rationale: The parathyroid glands are embedded on the posterior surface of the lobes of the thyroid gland. They secrete parathyroid hormone in response to dropping levels of calcium in the blood. These glands also participate with phosphorous regulation. This client will most likely need medication or supplements since these glands will be missing after the surgery. Lengthy exercise restriction or physical therapy is not generally indicated following thyroidectomy. A sodium-restricted diet would not ordinarily be necessary.
Planning
Analysis
Health Promotion and Maintenance

18.5 A female client comes into the clinic to be seen for fatigue and a cold that "won't go away" that began when she got a new job and her mother moved in with her family. The nurse realizes that this client might be experiencing:
1. an increase in epinephrine secretion.
2. an increase in glucocorticoid secretion.
3. a drop in mineralocorticoid secretion.
4. a reduction in norepinephrine secretion.

Answer: 2
Rationale: The glucocorticoids include cortisol and cortisone. These hormones affect carbohydrate metabolism and are released in times of stress. An excess of glucocorticoids in the body depresses the inflammatory response and inhibits the effectiveness of the immune system. Alteration in epinephrine, norepinephrine, or mineralocorticoids would have an influence on cardiovascular function and fluid and electrolyte balance, but would not influence immune response as much as an increase in glucocorticoid secretion.
Diagnosis
Analysis
Physiological Integrity

18.6 A client who is prescribed to have a hemoglobin A1c level drawn asks the nurse about the purpose of the test. Which of the following would be an appropriate response for the nurse to make to this client?
1. "It's a blood test to check for menopausal symptoms."
2. "It's a blood test to check for kidney functioning."
3. "It's to check for thyroid functions."
4. "It's to check for pancreas functioning."

Answer: 4
Rationale: The diagnostic tests of the pancreas are primarily to identify, confirm, and monitor glucose levels in clients with diabetes mellitus. The hemoglobin A1c is one of these tests. Hemoglobin A1c does not measure kidney or thyroid function, nor does it evaluate menopausal symptoms.
Planning
Application
Physiological Integrity

18.7 The nurse is planning to conduct a physical assessment for a client's endocrine functioning. Which of the following will the nurse be able to assess on this client?

Answer: 3
Rationale: The only endocrine organ that can be palpated is the thyroid gland. The anatomical location of the pancreas, adrenal glands, and the parathyroid glands prohibits direct examination by palpation or percussion.

1. palpation of the pancreas 2. percussion of the adrenal glands 3. palpation of the thyroid gland 4. palpation of the parathyroid glands	Planning Application Health Promotion and Maintenance
18.8 During an assessment the nurse notes that the client's eyes are extremely wide open and bulging. The nurse realizes that this finding is consistent with: 1. diabetes mellitus. 2. hyperthyroidism. 3. hypofunction of the adrenal glands. 4. hypofunction of the anterior pituitary gland.	Answer: 2 Rationale: Exophthalmos or protruding eyes may be seen in hyperthyroidism. This is not a finding that is associated with diabetes mellitus, hypofunction of the adrenal glands, or hypofunction of the pituitary gland. Diagnosis Analysis Physiological Integrity
18.9 The nurse realizes an alteration in growth hormone can lead to changes in an individual's physical stature. The condition that can occur with abnormally high levels of growth hormone in adults is: 1. dwarfism. 2. acromegaly. 3. hirsutism. 4. gynecomastia.	Answer: 2 Rationale: Extremely large bones may indicate acromegaly which is caused by excessive growth hormone. Extremely short stature may indicate dwarfism, which is caused by insufficient growth hormone. Hirsutism, or abnormal hair growth, is associated with adrenal hormone access. Gynecomastia, or development of breast tissue in men, is frequently associated with androgen therapy. Diagnosis Application Health Promotion and Maintenance
18.10 A client comes into the clinic demonstrating symptoms of hypocalcemic tetany. Which of the following assessments did the nurse conduct to determine the client's condition? 1. Place a tuning fork over one of the client's fingers. 2. Measure the client's blood pressure. 3. Tap a finger in front of the client's ear at the angle of the jaw. 4. Measure capillary blood.	Answer: 3 Rationale: The nurse most likely assessed the client for Chvostek's sign by tapping a finger in front of the client's ear at the angle of the jaw. Decreased calcium levels will cause the client's lateral facial muscles to contract. This demonstrates tetany. Placing a tuning fork over the client's finger evaluates the client's ability to perceive vibrations, but does not evaluate the muscle response of tetany. Blood pressure measurement may give the nurse valuable information about the client's fluid and electrolyte status, but does not evaluate tetany. A capillary blood level for serum calcium would give a measurement, but does not assess for the clinical symptoms of tetany. Diagnosis Analysis Physiological Integrity
18.11 An elderly client who is seen in the clinic has a palpable thyroid gland. The nurse realizes that this finding indicates: 1. nothing. This can be normal in the elderly client. 2. the onset of hypertension. 3. the onset of diabetes mellitus. 4. an explanation for a reduced urine output.	Answer: 1 Rationale: Elderly clients' thyroid glands could be more fibrotic and nodular as a normal finding. Without other assessments or supporting data, a palpable thyroid gland does not explain the onset of hypertension, diabetes mellitus, or reduction in urine output. Diagnosis Application Health Promotion and Maintenance
18.12 A client learns that the results of his water deprivation test showed no changes in urine osmolality. The nurse realizes that this finding is consistent with: 1. diabetes insipidus. 2. diabetes mellitus. 3. syndrome of inappropriate antidiuretic hormone. 4. nothing. No pathology is present.	Answer: 4 Rationale: In clients without pathology, there is no change in urine and plasma osmolality. Diabetes insipidus and syndrome of inappropriate antidiuretic hormone would result in changes in urine osmolality. Water deprivation testing is not used to detect diabetes. Diagnosis Application Health Promotion and Maintenance

18.13 A client being treated with medication for a seizure disorder is scheduled for a serum T3 and T4 level. The nurse realizes that this client's results might be:
1. falsely elevated.
2. falsely reduced.
3. normal.
4. indicative of pending parathyroid hormone disease.

Answer: 2
Rationale: The value of T3 and T4 blood levels might be decreased by certain medications including phenytoin (Dilantin), which is a medication commonly prescribed for seizure disorders. Measurement of T3 and T4 levels are not indicative of parathyroid disease.
Assessment
Analysis
Physiological Integrity

18.14 A middle-aged female client is found to have a decrease in her cortisol level. The nurse realizes that this finding is consistent with:
1. hyperthyroidism.
2. Cushing's syndrome.
3. Addison's disease.
4. nothing.

Answer: 3
Rationale: A cortisol level is a serum test done to measure the amount of total cortisol in the serum and evaluate adrenal cortex function. Decreased levels are consistent with Addison's disease and hypothyroidism. Cushing's syndrome would reveal an elevated cortisol level.
Diagnosis
Application
Physiological Integrity

18.15 After the most recent physician's office visit and blood work, the client learns that the oral glucose tolerance test scheduled for the next week is not needed. The client says to the nurse, "This is good news if I don't need additional testing." The nurse realizes that the cancellation of this test could indicate:
1. consistently high fasting blood glucose levels.
2. no evidence of type 1 diabetes mellitus.
3. normal renal functioning.
4. normal liver functioning.

Answer: 1
Rationale: An oral glucose tolerance test is done to diagnose diabetes mellitus if prior fasting blood sugar levels are inconsistent. However, the test will not be done if the client's fasting blood sugars are consistently high or greater than 200 mg/dl. Cancellation of the test does not indicate absence of evidence of type 1 diabetes, or normal liver or renal function.
Evaluation
Analysis
Physiological Integrity

CHAPTER 19

19.1 During the assessment of a client with a hyperthyroidism, the nurse notes smooth, fine hair and warm, dry skin. These findings are indicative of:
1. nothing. These are normal findings in hyperthyroidism.
2. misdiagnosis.
3. the client has another underlying disease.
4. inconsistency with the diagnosis of hyperthyroidism.

Answer: 1
Rationale: The client with hyperthyroidism can present with smooth and warm skin and the hair may become fine. There is inadequate information provided to assume the client has been misdiagnosed or has another underlying disease.
Assessment
Analysis
Physiological Integrity

19.2 A postoperative parathyroidectomy client has a temperature of 103°F with a rising systolic blood pressure. What should the nurse do for this client?
1. Nothing. These are normal postoperative findings.
2. Apply a cooling blanket.
3. Apply ice to the groin.
4. Administer aspirin as prescribed.

Answer: 2
Rationale: These findings are indicative of a pending thyroid storm. Treatment includes cooling the client without inducing shivering and not providing aspirin, which would increase free levels of thyroid hormone. The client must be cooled without inducing shivering. Ice could likely cause shivering. The surgical site is the throat not the groin.
Implementation
Application
Physiological Integrity

19.3 A client with hyperthyroidism tells the nurse, "The medicine isn't working because I'm not feeling any better." Which of the following would be an appropriate response for the nurse to make to this client?
1. "Be sure to tell the doctor about how you are feeling."
2. "You are right. Maybe the medication isn't working."
3. "It can take several weeks for the medication to begin working."
4. "It sounds like you need another medication to add to the one you are already taking."

Answer: 3
Rationale: Antithyroid medications inhibit thyroid hormone production but have no effect on already-produced and circulating thyroid hormone. It can take several weeks before the client experiences the effects.
Diagnosis
Analysis
Physiological Integrity

19.4 The nurse is preparing a client for a thyroidectomy. Which of the following instructions should the nurse include during this preparation?
1. Review scar expectations and how the use of plastic surgery is often helpful.
2. Remind the client to avoid iodine and salt.
3. Explain how the bed will need to be flat after surgery.
4. Instruct about how to support the neck with the hands.

Answer: 4
Rationale: The only correct option is instructing about how to support the neck with both hands after the surgery. Typically the scar will fade to a small line, so plastic surgery is not needed. Iodine is given preoperatively and the bed is usually in a semi-Fowler's position.
Planning
Application
Physiological Integrity

19.5 A postoperative thyroidectomy client wants to know when her "eyes will go back to being normal." The nursing diagnosis most appropriate for this client's concern would be:
1. *Disturbed Body Image.*
2. *Disturbed Sensory Perception: Visual.*
3. *Coping.*
4. *Powerlessness.*

Answer: 1
Rationale: This client is experiencing a disturbed body image. The nurse should establish a trusting relationship; encourage the client to verbalize feelings about self and to ask questions about the illness and treatment. Establishing trust facilitates open sharing of feelings and perceptions. The client's eye problems are not related to visual disorders. There is no supportive information provided to make assumptions about the client's coping skills or feelings of powerlessness.
Diagnosis
Analysis
Psychosocial Integrity: Coping and Adaptation

19.6 A client with myxedema tells the nurse, "I watch what I eat but my cholesterol continues to go up." An appropriate response for the nurse to make to this client would be:
1. "Maybe you don't realize how much fat is in the foods that you eat."
2. "It's a normal part of aging."
3. "What are you eating at bedtime?"
4. "The thyroid gland malfunction can affect your cholesterol level."

Answer: 4
Rationale: Deficient amounts of thyroid hormone can cause abnormalities in lipid metabolism, with elevated serum cholesterol and triglyceride levels. As a result, the client is at increased risk for atherosclerosis and cardiac disorders. The role of the nurse during this interaction is to provide education and support. Option 1 makes assumptions about the client's dietary intake. Comments about aging and eating at bedtime are not therapeutic.
Implementation
Application
Physiological Integrity

19.7 The family of an elderly client with hypothyroidism says, "I try to keep her clean but she has all of these open areas on her legs and arms." Which of the following would be appropriate for the nurse to instruct this family?
1. "Make sure she has a daily bath."
2. "Use firm consistent strokes when bathing."

Answer: 3
Rationale: The client with hypothyroidism has dry skin and edema which increase the risk of skin breakdown. Hot water, rough massage, and alcohol-based products increase skin dryness. The client should only bathe when necessary, with warm—not hot—water. Gentle motions should be used. Alcohol-free oils and lotions should be used.
Implementation
Application
Physiological Integrity

3. "Use warm water." 4. "Follow the bath with a rubbing alcohol massage."	
19.8 The nurse is assessing a female client with hyperparathyroidism. Which of the following assessment findings would be consistent with this diagnosis? 1. muscle atrophy 2. diarrhea 3. weight gain 4. hypotension	Answer: 1 Rationale: Hyperparathyroidism affects the musculoskeletal, renal, cardiovascular, gastrointestinal, and metabolic systems. Muscle atrophy is seen as a musculoskeletal effect. This client could also demonstrate constipation, weight loss, and hypertension. Assessment Analysis Physiological Integrity
19.9 The nurse is providing care to a client with hypoparathyroidism. Which of the following assessment findings would be consistent with this diagnosis? (Select all that apply.) 1. facial grimacing 2. smooth, soft skin 3. abdominal cramps 4. increased dental caries 5. hair loss 6. arrhythmias	Answer: 1, 3, 5, 6 Rationale: Hypoparathyroidism affects the musculoskeletal, integumentary, gastrointestinal, cardiovascular, and central nervous systems. Assessment findings would include facial grimacing (musculoskeletal), abdominal cramps (gastrointestinal), hair loss (integumentary), and arrhythmias (cardiovascular). Smooth, soft skin and increased dental caries are not common findings in the client with hypoparathyroidism. Assessment Analysis Physiological Integrity
19.10 A client says to the nurse, "I didn't realize this steroid medicine would make me lose weight in my legs." The nurse realizes that this client is demonstrating signs of: 1. poor wound healing. 2. muscle wasting. 3. risk for compression fractures. 4. increased susceptibility to infections.	Answer: 2 Rationale: Long-term use of steroids can place a client at risk for developing Cushing's syndrome. One characteristic of this syndrome is muscle weakness and wasting, particularly in the extremities. Poor wound healing, risk for compression fractures, and increased susceptibility to infections are all common in clients who are being treated with steroids. However, these problems would not manifest in limb weight loss as described. Evaluation Analysis Physiological Integrity
19.11 The nurse is providing care to a client who is postoperative from a bilateral adrenalectomy. Which of the following interventions would be helpful to assess for the onset of adrenal insufficiency? 1. Change dressing using clean technique. 2. Question the order for cortisol administration. 3. Place on fluid restriction. 4. Monitor strict intake and output.	Answer: 4 Rationale: Removal of an adrenal gland, especially a bilateral adrenalectomy, results in adrenal insufficiency. Addisonian crisis and hypovolemic shock may occur. Cortisol is often given on the day of surgery and in the postoperative period to replace inadequate hormone levels. Intravenous fluids are also administered. The nurse should monitor intake and output. While care should be taken during dressing changes to avoid infection, this will not prevent adrenal insufficiency. Planning Application Physiological Integrity
19.12 A client with Cushing's syndrome tells the nurse, "I seem to catch a cold every couple of weeks." Which of the following nursing interventions would be appropriate for this client? 1. Encourage daily weights. 2. Plan for frequent rest periods. 3. Assess for protein and vitamin intake. 4. Review coping strategies.	Answer: 3 Rationale: The client with Cushing's syndrome is at risk for infection due to the overproduction of glucocorticoids. The nurse should teach the importance of increasing intake of protein and vitamins C and A, which are all needed to support and repair body tissues. Rest periods and daily weights are recommended in the care of a client with Cushing's, but neither will directly address the problem of frequent infections as much as the diet change. There is no indication of a need to review or change coping strategies. Planning Application Physiological Integrity

19.13 A client tells the nurse, "I am rarely outside in the sun and I'm getting such a tan!" Which of the following should the nurse assess in this client?

1. Ask if the client is still taking the prescribed steroid for her Addison's disease.
2. Ask the client what time of day they are outdoors.
3. Palpate the client's thyroid gland.
4. Auscultate the client's lung sounds.

Answer: 1
Rationale: Addison's disease (failure of the adrenal glands to produce hormones) could develop if a client abruptly stops taking steroids for a chronic health condition. One symptom of this disease process is hyperpigmentation. In Caucasian clients, the skin looks deeply tanned in both exposed and unexposed areas. Auscultation of lung sounds and palpation of the thyroid gland would not help in determining the cause of this skin change. The client has already reported limited time being spent outdoors. This is not the best answer selection.
Assessment
Application
Physiological Integrity

19.14 A client comes into the emergency department with Addisonian crisis. Which of the following should the nurse be prepared to administer to assist this client?

1. warm blankets
2. intravenous fluids
3. thyroid replacement hormone
4. blood transfusion

Answer: 2
Rationale: The client with Addisonian crisis (hyposecretion of adrenal hormones) may have a high fever, weakness, abdominal pain, severe hypotension, circulatory collapse, shock, and coma. Treatment of the crisis is rapid intravenous replacement of fluids and glucocorticoids. Fluid balance is usually restored in four to six hours. The client experiencing an Addisonian crisis may have a high fever so warm blankets would not promote comfort or therapeutic action. There is no thyroid hormone insufficiency. There are no indications the client is in need of a blood transfusion.
Planning
Application
Physiological Integrity

19.15 A 35-year-old female client on oral contraceptives is prescribed steroid therapy. Which of the following should be included when teaching the client about this medication?

1. weigh daily
2. nothing
3. avoid salt
4. consider adding another form of contraception

Answer: 4
Rationale: Corticosteroids may impair the effectiveness of oral contraceptives. Avoiding excess salt and monitoring weight daily may assist the client in limiting the adverse effects of the steroids that some experience; however, the need to ensure adequate methods of contraception takes priority. The nurse must fulfill their role as an educator. As an "educator," taking action is paramount.
Implementation
Application
Health Promotion and Maintenance

CHAPTER 20

20.1 A client says, "I'm glad I only have diabetes. Many of my friends have heart problems." Which of the following would be an appropriate response for the nurse to make to this client?

1. "You are lucky."
2. "I bet your friends have diabetes too."
3. "I agree."
4. "Diabetes can affect your heart if it is not controlled."

Answer: 4
Rationale: Diabetes is the sixth leading cause of death by disease in the United States, primarily because of the widespread cardiovascular effects that result in atherosclerosis, coronary artery disease, and stroke. People with diabetes are two to four times more likely to have heart disease, and two to six times more likely to have a stroke than people who do not have diabetes.
Implementation
Application
Health Promotion and Maintenance

20.2 A client tells the nurse, "I eat all the time but I'm losing weight and I can't stop going to the bathroom!" The nurse realizes that this client is describing:

1. neuropathy.
2. polyphagia and polyuria.
3. polyphagia and polydipsia.
4. retinopathy and polyphagia.

Answer: 2
Rationale: The client with diabetes can develop a triad of symptoms: polyuria (frequent urination), polyphagia (hunger, excessive eating), and polydipsia (excessive thirst). This client described polyphagia and polyuria. Neuropathy would be manifested by pain or numbness in the feet. Retinopathy would result in visual changes.
Assessment
Application
Physiological Integrity

20.3 An elderly client with type 2 diabetes says, "I don't want to be on the needle for the rest of my life." Which of the following would be an appropriate response for the nurse to make to this client?

1. "I'll teach you how to give yourself insulin."
2. "The needle barely hurts."
3. "You need it for now. There's a chance you won't need it after you get well."
4. "You can always refuse to take it."

Answer: 3

Rationale: Elderly clients who are recovering from surgery or a serious illness often require insulin for type 2 diabetes to maintain blood glucose levels. Offering education as in option 1 does not meet the client's voiced concerns. Dismissal of the needle's discomfort does not address the nature of the client's concerns. Refusal of potentially life saving treatments is not in the best interest of the client.
Implementation
Application
Psychosocial Integrity

20.4 A client is scheduled for an oral glucose tolerance test. Which of the following medications should the client be instructed to stop for three days before the test?

1. multiple vitamin
2. blood pressure medication
3. heart-regulating medication
4. warfarin (Coumadin)

Answer: 1

Rationale: There are a variety of medications that could interfere with the results of an oral glucose tolerance test. These medications include steroids, oral contraceptives, synthetic estrogen, phenytoin (Dilantin), Vitamin C, aspirin, thiazide diuretics, and nicotinic acid. Since the type of blood pressure medication or heart-regulating medication is not provided, the most logical choice for the client to avoid for three days prior to the test would be the multiple vitamin because it could contain vitamin C.
Implementation
Analysis
Physiological Integrity

20.5 A client with type 2 diabetes says, "I was feeling really shaky yesterday so I drank a few ounces of orange juice and felt better." Which of the following should the nurse instruct this client?

1. "If this happens again, check your blood glucose level with your monitor."
2. Nothing. This is an appropriate intervention for the client to make.
3. "Call the doctor if this happens again."
4. "Go to the emergency room if this happens again."

Answer: 1

Rationale: Self-monitoring of blood glucose allows the person with diabetes to monitor and achieve metabolic control and decrease the danger of hypoglycemia. Self-monitoring is useful when the person has symptoms of hypoglycemia. Medical intervention would not be necessary if self-treatment is successful.
Implementation
Application
Health Promotion and Maintenance: Prevention and/or Early Detection of Health Problems

---

20.6 A client with diabetes is being started on an insulin pump. At home, this client takes 36 units of NPH and 18 units of regular insulin. The nurse should calculate the daily basal dose for this client at:

1. 54 units.
2. 49 units.
3. 25 units.
4. 1 unit.

Answer: 3

Rationale: The correct daily basal dose is 25 units. To calculate the basal dose for a client on an insulin infusion, total the number of units of insulin the client currently takes at home. Multiply this figure by 90%. To find the daily basal dose, multiply by 50%. The hourly dose is calculated by dividing this figure by 24.
Implementation
Application
Physiological Integrity

20.7 The nurse is instructing a client with type 1 diabetes about care during sick days. Which of the following should be included in these instructions?

1. Monitor blood glucose level every eight hours.
2. Administer insulin dose as prescribed.

Answer: 2

Rationale: General guidelines for care for a person with diabetes during sick days include taking insulin as prescribed; monitoring blood glucose and/or urine ketones at least every two to four hours; drink plenty of water or calorie-free fluids; rest as much as possible; and contact the physician with fever, vomiting, shortness of breath, abdominal pain, dehydration, chest pain, diarrhea, vision changes, or persistently high blood glucose levels/ketones in the urine.

3. Administer one-half of the prescribed insulin dose. 4. Limit rest to only eight hours per day.	Planning Application Physiological Integrity
20.8 The nurse is preparing to mix 20 units of NPH insulin with 8 units of regular insulin into one syringe for injection. Select the order of the steps the nurse should follow as listed below: 1. Wipe tops of both vials with alcohol. 2. Inject 8 units of air into the regular insulin vial. 3. Inject 20 units of air into the NPH insulin vial. 4. Withdraw 20 units of NPH insulin into the syringe. 5. Withdraw 8 units of regular insulin into the syringe.	Answer: 1, 3, 2, 5, 4 Rationale: The correct order for mixing two insulins begins with cleansing the vials with alcohol. Then air should be injected into the long-acting insulin. Air is then injected into the short acting insulin, which is placed into the syringe first. The procedure ends with placing the long-acting insulin into the syringe. Implementation Application Physiological Integrity
20.9 A client who is prescribed repaglinide (Prandin) for type 2 diabetes tells the nurse about episodes of hypoglycemia when taking the medication. Which of the following would be appropriate for the nurse to assess in this client? 1. Ask the client if he is also taking a calcium channel blocker. 2. Ask the client if he is still taking the prescribed furosemide (Lasix). 3. Ask the client if he is waiting two hours to eat as recommended. 4. Ask the client if he is taking any over-the-counter pain relievers such as ibuprofen (Motrin).	Answer: 4 Rationale: Calcium channel blockers and thiazide diuretics could cause hyperglycemia with this medication. Having the client wait two hours to eat with this medication would cause hypoglycemia and is incorrect. Nonsteroidal anti-inflammatory agents such as ibuprofen (Motrin) would intensify the action of this medication and could encourage hypoglycemia. Assessment Application Physiological Integrity
20.10 A client with diabetes says, "I am watching everything that I eat and only buy sugar-free sodas but I still can't lose any weight!" Which of the following could the nurse say to this client? 1. "Sugar-free doesn't mean no calories." 2. "Are you sure you are only buying sugar-free items?" 3. "Everyone cheats every now and then." 4. "How much water are you drinking everyday?"	Answer: 1 Rationale: Nutritive sweeteners are often included in foods labeled as "sugar-free." The caloric content of these substances is similar to that of table sugar but cause less elevation in blood glucose. The nurse should instruct the client regarding the caloric content of these sweeteners. It is counterproductive for the nurse to question the client in a manner which attacks their credibility. Making assumptions the client is cheating is inappropriate. Hydration is important but is not the best answer selection. Assessment Application Health Promotion and Maintenance
20.11 A client with type 2 diabetes wants to lose 20 lbs and asks the nurse to help plan her meal pattern. Which of the following would be appropriate for this client to aid with weight loss and blood glucose level maintenance? 1. Eat the largest meal of the day for breakfast and two small meals for lunch and dinner. 2. Plan for three equal-sized meals with one or two snacks.	Answer: 2 Rationale: There are no specific guidelines for a type 2 diet but it is recommended that the client consume three meals of equal size, evenly spaced at four to five hours apart with one or two snacks. Any of the other suggestions would not encourage a normal blood glucose level or weight loss. Planning Application Health Promotion and Maintenance

3. Plan for a small breakfast, moderate-sized lunch, and large dinner with a bedtime snack. 4. Plan for a small breakfast and dinner with a large lunch and a bedtime snack.	

20.12 A postoperative client with type 2 diabetes says, "I was under better control before the operation. Now I'm on insulin." Which of the following could the nurse say to this client?
  1. "It happens."
  2. "Didn't your doctor tell you that you would be on insulin now?"
  3. "Giving injections is easy."
  4. "It's just until you are able to take your other medication and start to recover from the surgery."
	Answer: 4
	Rationale: Oral hypoglycemic agents may be withheld for one to two days before the surgery and regular insulin is often administered to the client with type 2 diabetes during the perioperative period.
	Implementation
	Application
	Physiological Integrity

20.13 A client with type 1 diabetes comes into the emergency department with deep respirations, lethargy, and extreme thirst. The nurse realizes that this client is demonstrating:
  1. insulin overdose.
  2. the onset of the flu.
  3. possible diabetic ketoacidosis (DKA).
  4. hypoglycemia.
	Answer: 3
	Rationale: The symptoms of diabetic ketoacidosis (DKA) include thirst, malaise, lethargy, fruity breath odor, and Kussmaul's respirations. Clients who are experiencing insulin overdose or hypoglycemia would likely exhibit symptoms such as perspiration, cool moist skin, mental status changes, and cardiac symptoms. Although blood sugar disturbances can be caused by viral illnesses such as the flu, the nurse should consider DKA first.
	Diagnosis
	Analysis
	Physiological Integrity

20.14 A client with type 2 diabetes is admitted to the intensive care unit with a blood glucose level of 850. Which of the following should be done while providing care to this client?
  1. Restrict fluids.
  2. Permit activity as tolerated.
  3. Monitor blood pressure every eight hours.
  4. Discontinue insulin infusion when blood glucose level decreases to 250 mg/dl.
	Answer: 4
	Rationale: Treatment for this client is focused on correcting fluid and electrolyte imbalances, provide insulin to lower blood glucose level, and support the client during this life-threatening metabolic condition. The client should be on an insulin infusion until the blood glucose level drops to approximately 250 mg/dl. Bed rest with adequate fluid intake is indicated. Vital sign monitoring should be frequent, at least every four hours.
	Implementation
	Application
	Physiological Integrity

20.15 A client with type 2 diabetes asks, "What can I do to prevent heart problems?" Which of the following can the client do to avoid this long-term complication?
  1. Stop smoking.
  2. Avoid high-sugar-content fruits.
  3. Limit exercise to two times per week.
  4. Restrict fluids.
	Answer: 1
	Rationale: Risk factors that contribute to the development of macrovascular disease of diabetes are hypertension, hyperlipidemia, cigarette smoking, and obesity. It is best if the client would stop smoking. A balanced diet including fruit and daily exercise are recommended to maintain overall health. Fluids need not be restricted in a plan to prevent heart disease.
	Planning
	Application
	Health Promotion and Maintenance

20.16 A client with diabetes says, "I think I have a back problem. My feet are getting numb." The nurse realizes that this client could be describing:	Answer: 2 Rationale: The person with polyneuropathy commonly has distal paresthesias that are described as numbness or tingling. Mononeuropathy involves a single nerve or nerve group and can occur in any body system. Visceral neuropathy

1. mononeuropathy. 2. polyneuropathy. 3. visceral neuropathy. 4. gastroparesis.	affects specific organs, usually abdominal organs. Gastroparesis is a delay in gastric emptying that is often caused by hypoglycemia. Diagnosis Analysis Physiological Integrity
20.17 The nurse determines that a client has evidence of peripheral vascular disease associated with diabetes. Which of the following findings did the nurse most likely assess? 1. even hair distribution on legs 2. feet warm and dry bilaterally 3. dusky skin tone 4. skin between toes intact	Answer: 3 Rationale: Evidence of peripheral vascular disease includes hair loss on legs and feet; shiny, thin skin; feet that are cool to the touch; feet and ankles that are a darker color than leg; dependent rubor; thick toenails; changes in pulses; nocturnal pain; pain at rest; intermittent claudication; and patchy areas of gangrene on feet and toes. Diagnosis Analysis Physiological Integrity
20.18 A client with diabetes says, "I want to check my feet everyday but I can't lift my legs because of arthritis in my knees." Which of the following techniques could the nurse instruct this client? 1. "Check the inside of socks when changing for any bleeding." 2. "Only wear soft shoes and slippers." 3. "Don't worry about it unless pain in the feet is present." 4. "Prop a mirror against the wall and lift the foot, checking for any skin breakdown."	Answer: 4 Rationale: The client with diabetes is at risk of reduced circulation, infection, and ulcerations of the legs and feet. The diabetic client must frequently assess their lower extremities. Suggest the use of a hand mirror to check the bottom of the feet and the heels if the client is unable to lift their feet/legs off of the floor. The presence of blood will not alert the client to all potential leg problems. Wearing of soft shoes and slippers may increase the client's risk for foot injury. The sensation of pain may be hindered or reduced in the diabetic client. Implementation Application Health Promotion and Maintenance
20.19 During a visit, the home care nurse finds a safety hazard in the home of a client with diabetes. Which of the following did the nurse assess in this client's home? 1. throw rugs in the kitchen and bathroom 2. night lights 3. grab bars next to the commode 4. shower chair	Answer: 1 Rationale: The presence of hazardous environmental factors increases the risk of falls or other accidents. Throw rugs in the kitchen and bathroom are a source for potential falls or trips. These are a safety hazard for this client. Night lights, grab bars, and shower chairs are considered to be devices that increase client safety. Evaluation Analysis Safe, Effective Care Environment
20.20 A client with diabetes tells the nurse, "I plan to lose 30 lbs. in two months." The nurse realizes that this client: 1. has set a goal that is achievable. 2. is highly motivated. 3. needs bariatric surgery. 4. is not being realistic with the goal.	Answer: 4 Rationale: The nurse needs to teach constructive problem-solving techniques with the client. Problem-focused behaviors include setting attainable and realistic goals. The client is setting a goal that is most likely not attainable given the timeframe. Although the client may appear motivated, the primary concern in this question is likely inability of this goal to be achieved. There is no information provided to assess the need for bariatric surgery. Evaluation Analysis Health Promotion and Maintenance

21.1 A client is seen coughing immediately after swallowing a bit of food. The nurse realizes that this client might have an impairment of:
1. the tongue.
2. the hard palate.
3. the soft palate.
4. the esophagus.

Answer: 3
Rationale: The soft palate is primarily muscle that contracts when swallowing food. The hard palate is primarily bone. Neither the tongue nor the esophagus are issues associated with this client's coughing when swallowing food.
Diagnosis
Analysis
Physiological Integrity

21.2 A client states, "My mouth is always dry!" The nurse realizes that this client might experience an inability to break down carbohydrates because:
1. the saliva includes an enzyme needed for carbohydrate breakdown.
2. the saliva includes a vitamin that is needed for carbohydrate breakdown.
3. the saliva includes a mineral that is needed for carbohydrate breakdown.
4. the saliva includes a hormone that is needed for carbohydrate breakdown.

Answer: 1
Rationale: Saliva provides enzymes, such as amylase, that begin the chemical breakdown of starches while food is still in the mouth.
Diagnosis
Analysis
Health Promotion and Maintenance

21.3 A client learns that he has an "incompetent pyloric sphincter." The nurse realizes that this client could experience:
1. difficulty swallowing.
2. reduced saliva production.
3. pain with digestion of fats.
4. inconsistent gastric emptying.

Answer: 4
Rationale: The pyloric sphincter controls emptying of the stomach into the duodenal portion of the small intestine. The difficulty being demonstrated by the client is taking place in the gastrointestinal system after the food has been swallowed or requires saliva. There is not information included in the question concerning the client experiencing pain.
Assessment
Analysis
Health Promotion and Maintenance

21.4 A client is diagnosed with a vitamin B$_{12}$ deficiency. The nurse realizes that this client has an impairment of his stomach's:
1. mucous cells.
2. zymogenic cells.
3. parietal cells.
4. enteroendocrine cells.

Answer: 3
Rationale: Parietal cells secrete hydrochloric acid and intrinsic factor. Intrinsic factor is necessary for the absorption of vitamin B$_{12}$ in the small intestines. Mucous cells produce mucous which clings to the lining of the stomach providing protection from gastric juice. Zymogenic cells produce pepsinogen. Enteroendocrine cells produce hormonelike substances which diffuse into the blood.
Planning
Analysis
Physiological Integrity

21.5 A client says, "I drink fluids throughout the day but I seem to be always hungry!" The nurse realizes that this client's gastric emptying is:
1. delayed.
2. sluggish.
3. impaired.
4. normal.

Answer: 4
Rationale: Gastric emptying depends on the volume, chemical composition, and osmotic pressure of the gastric contents. The stomach empties large volumes of liquid content more rapidly, while gastric emptying is slowed by solids and fats. The absence of feelings of fullness rule out delayed or sluggish emptying by the stomach. There is inadequate information to assess additional problems such as impaired gastric emptying.
Diagnosis
Analysis
Health Promotion and Maintenance

21.6 A client tells the nurse about the "new vitamin pill" she started taking because it won't "break down until it

Answer: 4
Rationale: Almost all food products and water as well as vitamins and most electrolytes are absorbed in the small intestines. The client is taking a vitamin

---

reaches the large intestines." The nurse realizes that the benefits of this vitamin are:
   1. excellent.
   2. better than most.
   3. average.
   4. useless.
	that won't metabolize until it reaches the large intestine, which means it will not be used by the body.
	Evaluation
	Analysis
	Health Promotion and Maintenance

21.7 A client states, "What's the purpose of a gallbladder anyway? I hear about people getting their gallbladder removed all of the time!" Which of the following would be beneficial for the nurse to instruct the client about this organ?
   1. There is no known function.
   2. It stores bile until it is needed for digestion of fats.
   3. It houses crystals that the body cannot digest.
   4. It stores food until needed by the body.
	Answer: 2
	Rationale: The gallbladder stores bile until it is needed by the body for digestion.
	Implementation
	Application
	Health Promotion and Maintenance

21.8 The nurse learns that a client has severely restricted her protein intake because she "didn't want to gain any weight." The nurse realizes that this client is at risk for developing:
   1. carbohydrate malfunctioning.
   2. incomplete anabolic processes.
   3. extreme weight gain.
   4. ketoacidosis.
	Answer: 2
	Rationale: In the process of anabolism, simpler molecules combine to build more complex structures, as seen with the bonding of amino acids to form proteins. The action of carbohydrates is not directly related to protein intake. The loss of protein intake will not promote excessive weight gain. Ketoacidosis requires protein intake.
	Diagnosis
	Analysis
	Health Promotion and Maintenance

21.9 During the calculation of a client's caloric intake, the nurse learns that the client ingests 175 grams of carbohydrates per day. This volume of carbohydrate translates into how many calories?
   1. 175
   2. 350
   3. 700
   4. 1575
	Answer: 3
	Rationale: One gram of carbohydrates equals four calories. This client is ingesting 700 calories from carbohydrates per day.
	Implementation
	Application
	Health Promotion and Maintenance

21.10 A client says, "I'm on a diet where I can eat meat and cheese as much as I want!" The nurse realizes that this client is at risk for:
   1. increase in adipose tissue.
   2. vitamin E deficiency.
   3. sustained biologic functioning.
   4. skin lesions.
	Answer: 1
	Rationale: When a person consumes more than the body requires of fats, the excess is stored as adipose tissue, which increases the risk of obesity and heart disease.
	Diagnosis
	Analysis
	Health Promotion and Maintenance

21.11 The nurse learns that a client is taking excessive amounts of vitamins A and E. Which of the following is the client at risk for developing?
   1. an autoimmune disorder
   2. diarrhea
   3. polyuria
   4. vitamin toxicity
	Answer: 4
	Rationale: Vitamins A and E are fat-soluble vitamins in that they are stored in the fat cells of the body. Excessive amounts of the fat-soluble vitamins can lead to toxicity. The onset of an autoimmune disorder is not a result of vitamin toxicity. The excess vitamins will not be excreted from the body through diarrhea or polyuria.
	Assessment
	Analysis
	Health Promotion and Maintenance

21.12 A client with diabetes tells the nurse that she eats a sweet potato each day because it "naturally lowers blood	Answer: 3 Rationale: Vitamin B_6, or pyridoxine, is found in meat, poultry, fish, potatoes, tomatoes, sweet potatoes, and spinach. Vitamin B_1 is found in lean meats, liver

sugar levels." In addition to this information, which vitamin is this client ingesting on a daily basis?

1. vitamin B_1
2. vitamin B_2
3. vitamin B_6
4. vitamin B_{12}

and eggs. Vitamin B_2 is prevalent in liver, egg white, whole grains, and meat. Vitamin B_{12} is contained in liver, meat, poultry, and dairy foods (excluding butter).
Assessment
Analysis
Health Promotion and Maintenance

21.13 The nurse is preparing to assess a client's abdomen. Which assessment technique should this nurse use last?

1. inspection
2. percussion
3. palpation
4. auscultation

Answer: 3
Rationale: When assessing the abdomen, use palpation last because pressure on the abdominal wall and contents may interfere with bowel sounds and cause pain. Inspection is the first assessment tool used followed by auscultation, and then palpation.
Planning
Application
Physiological Integrity

21.14 During the auscultation of a client's abdomen, the nurse observes a high-pitched, tinkling, rushing sound that is followed with several seconds of growling. The correct way to document this finding is:

1. "borborygmus present."
2. "cheilosis present."
3. "bruit present."
4. "normal bowel sounds."

Answer: 1
Rationale: Normal bowel sounds occur every 5 to 15 seconds. Borborygmus is a hyperactive, high-pitched, tinkling, rushing, or growing bowel sound. Cheilosis refers to the lesions found at the corners of the mouth. Bruit is the blowing sound heard in response to the restriction of blood flow through vessels. Normal bowel sounds are clicking or gurgling and occur every 5 to 15 seconds.
Assessment
Application
Health Promotion and Maintenance

21.15 An older client tells the nurse that he is noticing that he wants more "salt and spices" on his foods. The nurse realizes that this client is experiencing:

1. a sodium deficiency.
2. a vitamin deficiency.
3. an age-related change in taste.
4. changing food preferences.

Answer: 3
Rationale: An age-related change is commonly seen in elderly clients. Taste is less acute because the tongue atrophies. There is a corresponding tendency to excessively season food when this occurs. Vitamin and mineral deficiencies are not associated with a reduction in taste sensation. There is no information presented which will support the client has had a change in food preferences.
Assessment
Analysis
Health Promotion and Maintenance

21.16 A client asks, "How much calcium should I be taking each day?" An appropriate response for the nurse to make is:

1. 8 mg.
2. 15 mg.
3. 150 mg.
4. 1000 mg.

Answer: 4
Rationale: The recommended amount of calcium is 1000 mg per day for adults. This amount changes to 1200 mg for post-menopausal women.
Implementation
Application
Health Promotion and Maintenance

21.17 A client with type 2 diabetes says, "I've never heard about the liver having anything to do with my blood sugar." Which of the following could the nurse instruct this client?

1. The liver releases stored glucose in times of low blood sugar levels.
2. The liver has nothing to do with blood glucose control.
3. The liver synthesizes vitamins.
4. The liver controls blood pressure.

Answer: 1
Rationale: The liver releases glucose during times of hypoglycemia and takes up glucose during times of hyperglycemia and stores it as glycogen or converts it to fat.
Implementation
Application
Health Promotion and Maintenance

22.1 A female client has a body mass index (BMI) of 27. Which of the following would be an appropriate documentation by the nurse?
1. normal weight
2. overweight
3. obese
4. metabolic syndrome

Answer: 2
Rationale: A body mass index (BMI) of 25 to 29.9 kg/m² is classified as overweight; obesity is a BMI of 30 kg/m² or greater.
Diagnosis
Application
Health Promotion and Maintenance

22.2 A female client has a waist-to-hip ratio of 0.5. The nurse realizes that this client is at risk for developing:
1. hypertension.
2. heart disease.
3. hyperlipidemia.
4. This client is not at risk.

Answer: 4
Rationale: The risk for hyperinsulinemia, abnormal lipids, and heart disease is lower in people with lower body obesity than in those with upper body obesity. This result does not indicate an abnormal ratio.
Evaluation
Analysis
Health Promotion and Maintenance

22.3 The nurse hears a mother say to her child, "If you behave, we'll stop and get you an ice cream cone when we're done here." The nurse realizes that this mother:
1. is using food as a reward.
2. is frustrated with the child's behavior.
3. is anxious.
4. is hungry.

Answer: 1
Rationale: Sociocultural influences that contribute to obesity include overeating at family meals, rewarding behavior with food, religious and family gatherings that promote food intake, and sedentary lifestyles.
Diagnosis
Analysis
Health Promotion and Maintenance

22.4 During a physical assessment, the nurse suspects that the client might be experiencing metabolic syndrome. Which of the following assessment findings would provide evidence for this nurse's assumption?
1. difficulty ambulating
2. low waist-to-hip ratio
3. blood pressure 150/96
4. heart rate 72 and regular

Answer: 3
Rationale: Individuals with metabolic syndrome are found to have three or more of the following: increased waist circumference, hypertension, elevated blood triglycerides and fasting blood glucose, and low HDL cholesterol. A low-waist-to hip ratio is preferred and the heart rate is within normal limits.
Assessment
Application
Health Promotion and Maintenance

22.5 The nurse is reviewing the lipid panel of a client with a BMI of 31. Which of the following would be expected in this client?
1. elevated HDL
2. normal TH level
3. low LDL
4. low HDL

Answer: 4
Rationale: High-density lipoprotein (HDL) levels are reduced in obese clients, whereas low-density lipoprotein (LDL) levels are elevated. This BMI value indicates obesity. There is no relationship between the BMI and the TH.
Diagnosis
Application
Health Promotion and Maintenance

22.6 A client with a BMI of 29 says, "I cut out all my sweet snacks last week and I still can't lose any weight." Which of the following would be appropriate for the nurse to do or say in response?
1. Refer the client to a dietician.
2. Document that "client states no longer eating sweet snacks."
3. "You didn't gain the weight overnight."
4. "Let's calculate how many calories you are not eating each day."

Answer: 4
Rationale: A pound of body fat is equivalent to 3500 kcal. To lose one pound, therefore, a person must reduce daily caloric intake by 250 kcal for 14 days or increase activity enough to burn the equivalent kcal. A physician's order is required for a dietary referral. Documenting the client's comments is not the priority. Discussing the time it took for the client to gain the weight will not promote a therapeutic environment.
Implementation
Application
Health Promotion and Maintenance

22.7 A male client who lives alone has a BMI of 34. Which of the following strategies could the nurse suggest to help this client reduce overeating?
1. Eat out more often to control portion size.
2. Read a book while eating to distract him.
3. Prepare a meal and eat it in the dining room.
4. Cook once a week and store the leftovers to reduce the need to cook again.

Answer: 3
Rationale: There are a variety of strategies to assist a client with a weight problem. Eating out in restaurants should be reduced. Reading or watching television should not be encouraged. Cooking so much that there are leftovers is also not a good strategy. The nurse should suggest that the client prepare the meal in one room and then eat it in another to restrict eating in the kitchen.
Implementation
Application
Health Promotion and Maintenance

22.8 An overweight client tells the nurse, "Every Monday at work we have bagels. I can't stop myself! Sometimes I eat two!" The nurse realizes that this client is describing:
1. appetite stimulation by external cues.
2. extreme hunger.
3. carbohydrate addiction.
4. metabolic syndrome.

Answer: 1
Rationale: Most overweight people are stimulated to eat by external cues, such as the proximity to food and the time of day. In contrast, hunger and satiety are the cues that regulate eating in adults of normal weight. The client's reports involve eating with no mention of hunger. There is no information provided to support the presence of any addiction or metabolic disorder.
Diagnosis
Application
Health Promotion and Maintenance

22.9 A female client learns that she has regained 15 lbs. that she had lost the previous year. Which of the following could the nurse suggest to this client?
1. A new diet in which the weight could be lost again in two weeks.
2. Maybe her body wants to have the extra 15 lbs.
3. Remind her that she is still not obese.
4. Return to the diet, exercise, and behavior change techniques that worked before.

Answer: 4
Rationale: The potential risks associated with regaining weight make maintenance a critical issue. Clients are encouraged to continue exercise, self-monitoring, and treatment support. Long-term weight loss and maintenance mean a lifelong commitment to significant lifestyle changes, including food and eating habits, activity and exercise routines, and behavior modification.
Implementation
Application
Health Promotion and Maintenance

22.10 A 45-year-old male client says, "I'm gaining weight but I'm not eating any differently than I did years ago." The nurse realizes that this client is:
1. probably not being truthful.
2. justifying his weight gain.
3. demonstrating a change in metabolism with aging.
4. looking for the nurse to approve the weight gain.

Answer: 3
Rationale: Adults commonly gain about 20 pounds between early and middle adulthood. Encourage clients to reduce the amount of calories consumed because energy needs change.
Diagnosis
Application
Health Promotion and Maintenance

22.11 An overweight female client states, "I'm trying to stick to my diet and exercise plan but my husband tells me that I'm fine the way I am." An appropriate nursing diagnosis for this client would be:
1. *Imbalanced Nutrition: More than Body Requirements.*
2. *Ineffective Therapeutic Regimen Management.*
3. *Activity Intolerance.*
4. *Chronic Low Self-Esteem.*

Answer: 2
Rationale: Family and social support is critical to successful adherence to the therapeutic regimen. There is no information provided to support the client's lack of adherence to the dietary plan. There is no information provided to support activity intolerance or the lack of self-esteem.
Diagnosis
Application
Psychosocial Integrity

22.12 An elderly client who uses a walker tells the nurse, "I'm so alone now that my family is gone." The nurse realizes that this client might be at risk for developing:
  1. obesity.
  2. malnutrition.
  3. psychosis.
  4. immobility.
	Answer: 2
	Rationale: Older clients are at increased risk for malnutrition. Functional limitations can impair the ability to shop and cook. Psychosocial issues also contribute to the problem. Loss of appetite is a problem that is commonly seen with depression. Social isolation and loneliness contribute to the problem. There is no information provided to support selections of obesity, psychosis, or immobility.
	Diagnosis
	Analysis
	Psychosocial Integrity

22.13 A client is being assessed for malnutrition. The nurse realizes laboratory test findings that indicate malnutrition include: (Select all that apply.)
  1. elevated serum albumin.
  2. elevated red blood cell count.
  3. low serum sodium.
  4. low serum potassium.
  5. low white blood cell count.
	Answer: 4 and 5
	Rationale: The standard measurements to assess for malnutrition include height, weight, calculation of body mass index (BMI), and skinfold measurements. A BMI of less than 18 to 20 kg/m² may indicate malnutrition. The following laboratory results may also be seen in severe malnutrition: reduced serum albumin; reduced total lymphocyte count; and low potassium levels.
	Diagnosis
	Analysis
	Health Promotion and Maintenance

22.14 A malnourished client is demonstrating ongoing diarrhea that occurs after every meal. The nurse realizes that this client could be experiencing:
  1. pending cardiovascular overload.
  2. malabsorption.
  3. carbohydrate intolerance.
  4. a food allergy.
	Answer: 2
	Rationale: Abnormalities in gastrointestinal function can lead to malabsorption and diarrhea with refeeding. The diarrhea occurs after each meal, not with foods that may cause an allergy or only with carbohydrates. This is not related to cardiovascular problems.
	Evaluation
	Analysis
	Physiological Integrity

22.15 A client is prescribed a hypertonic solution with vitamins and minerals to be administered through a peripheral intravenous access line. The nurse realizes that this client is prescribed:
  1. total parenteral nutrition.
  2. enteral nutrition.
  3. short-term total parenteral nutrition.
  4. partial parenteral nutrition.
	Answer: 4
	Rationale: Partial parenteral nutrition may be given through a peripheral vein. Total parenteral nutrition should be administered through a central vein. Enteral nutrition is delivered directly into the gastrointestinal system. A peripherally-inserted central catheter (PICC) line may be used for short-term TPN.
	Diagnosis
	Analysis
	Physiological Integrity

22.16 The mother of a 12-year-old female child states, "My daughter saw an older child who was extremely overweight. Ever since that time my daughter won't eat." The nurse realizes that the child might be experiencing:
  1. an irrational fear of gaining weight.
  2. defiance.
  3. normal preadolescent behavior.
  4. a power struggle with the parent.
	Answer: 1
	Rationale: Anorexia nervosa typically begins during adolescence. Clients with anorexia nervosa have a distorted body image and irrational fear of gaining weight. Defiant behaviors involve rebellion. The child is not demonstrating that type of behavior. It is not normal for a preadolescent female to discontinue eating. The child is not demonstrating behaviors consistent with a power struggle.
	Diagnosis
	Analysis
	Psychosocial Integrity

22.17 A 33-year-old female client states, "I eat anything I want and just have a laxative for dessert!" The nurse realizes that this client is exhibiting:	Answer: 2 Rationale: In bulimia and after binge eating, the client may induce vomiting or take excessive quantities of laxatives or diuretics. Anorexic behaviors involve avoidance of eating. Laxative use is not a healthful means to control body weight. There is no discussion of the client's perceived body image.

1. anorexia.
     2. bulimia.
     3. an effective way to ensure a
         normal weight.
     4. distorted body image.
	Diagnosis
	 Analysis
	 Health Promotion and Maintenance

22.18 A 19-year-old female client is being assessed for bulimia. The mother asks what diagnostic tests can be done to determine the presence of bulimia. What is the nurse's best response?
     1. "You should ask the doctor about this."
     2. "She will need a psychiatric evaluation to determine the diagnosis."
     3. "There is no specific test that can determine bulimia."
     4. "Bulimia is rarely diagnosed correctly."
	Answer: 3
	 Rationale: There is no specific diagnostic test for bulimia. A psychiatric evaluation may be indicated after a diagnosis is made. The information being sought by the client's mother can be provided by the nurse. It is not necessary to refer her to the physician. Bulimia can be diagnosed by a competent physician when adequate information is present.
	 Implementation
	 Application
	 Health Promotion and Maintenance

22.19 A client is admitted for treatment of malnutrition. Which of the following assessment findings would suggest to the nurse the client is experiencing a vitamin C deficiency?
     1. smooth tongue
     2. bleeding gums
     3. muscle cramps
     4. ataxia
	Answer: 2
	 Rationale: Physical assessment information to suggest a vitamin C deficiency includes swollen bleeding gums, delayed wound healing, weakness, depression, and easy bruising. A smooth tongue is consistent with an iron deficiency. Thiamine deficiencies include the presence of muscle cramps and ataxia.
	 Diagnosis
	 Analysis
	 Physiological Integrity

CHAPTER 23

23.1 The nurse learns that an elderly client with ill-fitting dentures has been using an over-the-counter preparation for a gum sore over the last month. Which of the following should the nurse instruct this client?
     1. Continue to use the preparation.
     2. Stop wearing the dentures.
     3. Change the preparation.
     4. Make an appointment to see the physician.
	Answer: 4
	 Rationale: The nurse should instruct the client to seek medical attention for any oral lesion that does not heal within one week. Because the current over-the-counter (OTC) remedy is not effective, the client should see the physician before using a different OTC preparation. Not wearing the dentures can lead to nutritional problems and social isolation.
	 Implementation
	 Application
	 Health Promotion and Maintenance

23.2 A client with a long history of chewing tobacco says, "I've been chewing for years. I'm not going to get cancer." Which of the following would be an appropriate nursing response?
     1. "Use of smokeless tobacco has been linked to oral cancer."
     2. "You are probably one of the lucky ones."
     3. "I guess you're right."
     4. "It's not my body."
	Answer: 1
	 Rationale: Reducing or eliminating tobacco use (smoking and smokeless tobacco) can significantly reduce the incidence of oral cancer. Emphasize the relationship between smokeless tobacco and oral cancer.
	 Implementation
	 Application
	 Health Promotion and Maintenance

23.3 A client who is in need of a radical neck dissection for cancer continues to delay the surgery. Which of the following nursing diagnoses would best describe the reason for this client's delay?	Answer: 4 Rationale: Radical surgery of the head or neck seriously affects body image. An altered speech pattern and any disfigurement affect the ability to feel attractive or effective in work or social roles. Clients may defer lifesaving surgery to postpone disfiguring interventions or therapies. Impaired verbal communication,

1. *Impaired Verbal Communication* 2. *Imbalanced Nutrition: Less than Body Requirements* 3. *Risk for Ineffective Airway Clearance* 4. *Disturbed Body Image*	imbalanced nutrition, and risk for ineffective airway clearance are all potential postoperative diagnoses for this client but they do not address the reason for delay of the surgery. Diagnosis Analysis Psychosocial Integrity
23.4 The nurse is preparing to instruct a client who is newly-diagnosed with gastroesophageal reflux disease (GERD) about dietary considerations. Which of the following should the nurse include in these instructions? (Select all that apply.) 1. "Be sure to eat at least one citrus fruit per day." 2. "Alcohol should be limited to two drinks per day." 3. "Meals should be small and more frequent." 4. "Avoid peppermint." 5. "Avoid eating up to three hours before bedtime."	Answer: 3, 4, 5 Rationale: Acidic foods such as tomato products, citrus fruits, spicy foods, and coffee should be eliminated from the diet. Fatty foods, chocolate, peppermint, and alcohol relax the lower esophageal sphincter or delay gastric emptying, so they should be avoided. The client should be advised to maintain ideal body weight, eat smaller meals, refrain from eating for three hours before bedtime, and stay upright for two hours after meals. Elevating the head of the bed on 6- to 8-inch blocks often is beneficial. Stopping smoking is a necessary lifestyle change. Avoiding tight clothing and avoiding bending may help to relieve symptoms. Planning Application Health Promotion and Maintenance
23.5 The nurse is preparing the morning medications for a client with gastroesophageal reflux disease (GERD). Which of the following nursing interventions would be appropriate for this client's medications? 1. Hold the antacids for at least two hours after oral medications are taken. 2. Provide all prescribed medications at 10:00 A.M. 3. Provide the antacids first and then follow with the oral medications. 4. Provide the antacids only at the hour of sleep.	Answer: 1 Rationale: Antacids interfere with the absorption of many drugs given orally and should be separated by at least two hours. Planning Application Physiological Integrity
23.6 The nurse is assessing a client with gastrointestinal dysfunction who says, "I was having chest pain so bad last week I thought I was having a heart attack!" The nurse suspects that the client was experiencing: 1. diverticulitis. 2. hiatal hernia. 3. constipation. 4. bowel obstruction.	Answer: 2 Rationale: Manifestations of hiatal hernia include reflux, heartburn, substernal chest pain, occult bleeding, a feeling of fullness, dysphagia, belching, and indigestion. Diverticulitis, constipation, and bowel obstruction would generally not have substernal burning or pain symptoms. Diagnosis Analysis Physiological Integrity
23.7 A client who is experiencing difficulty swallowing is diagnosed with esophageal cancer after having a barium swallow. The nurse realizes that the diagnostic test must have displayed: 1. a narrow esophageal lumen. 2. a tumor. 3. metastasis. 4. blood.	Answer: 1 Rationale: Diagnostic tests for esophageal cancer include barium swallow, esophagoscopy, chest x-ray, computed tomography (CT) scan, magnetic resonance imaging (MRI), and serum blood tests. With a barium swallow, esophageal cancer is seen as a narrowing of the lumen or an irregular mucosal pattern. Other testing would be needed to detect an actual tumor, metastasis, and any bleeding. Evaluation Analysis Physiological Integrity

23.8 A client with nausea says, "I'm tired of taking this medication. All it does is make me nauseated." Which of the following could the nurse instruct this client? 1. Encourage the client to stop taking the medication. 2. Nothing. 3. Suggest eating a dry cracker to help with the nausea. 4. Suggest that the client take the medication with a heavy meal.	Answer: 3 Rationale: In most cases, nausea and vomiting are self-limiting and require no treatment. Dry food such as soda crackers may reduce nausea and promote comfort. Discontinuing the medication will also stop the desired action for which the medication has been prescribed. Taking no action does not meet the needs of the client. Taking medication with a heavy meal may increase the nausea being experienced. Implementation Application Physiological Integrity
23.9 A client with chronic gastritis says, "I've stopped taking the medication because I feel so much better now that I drink ginger tea." The nurse realizes that this client: 1. is using a complementary therapy for the symptoms. 2. cannot afford the medication. 3. needs to see the doctor immediately. 4. is in denial of the disease.	Answer: 1 Rationale: Complementary therapies such as herbal remedies or aromatherapy may be appropriate to recommend for clients with gastritis. Recommendations may include ginger in the form of powder, capsules, or made into a tea taken before or after meals. This action on the part of the client does not indicate denial or financial ability to continue the medication; however, the physician should be made aware of the fact that the client is not taking the prescribed medication. Evaluation Analysis Health Promotion and Maintenance
23.10 A client tells the nurse, "I get these tremendous stomach pains in the middle of the night and they disappear after I eat something. No wonder I can't lose any weight!" The nurse suspects that this client is experiencing: 1. gastroesophageal reflux disease (GERD). 2. acute gastritis. 3. chronic gastritis. 4. peptic ulcer disease.	Answer: 4 Rationale: Pain is the classic symptom of peptic ulcer disease. The pain is typically described as gnawing, burning, aching, or hunger-like and is experienced in the epigastric region, and sometimes radiates to the back. The pain occurs when the stomach is empty (two to three hours after meals and in the middle of the night) and is relieved by eating with a classic "pain-food-relief" pattern. This classic pattern is not typical of gastroesophageal reflux disease (GERD), acute gastritis, or chronic gastritis. Diagnosis Analysis Physiological Integrity
23.11 The nurse learns that a client who is being treated for peptic ulcer disease is still "having problems." Which of the following should the nurse instruct this client? 1. Make sure the client is eating a bland diet. 2. Avoid eating breakfast. 3. Have the largest meal of the day at lunchtime. 4. smoking cessation techniques	Answer: 4 Rationale: Smoking should be discouraged, because it slows the rate of healing and increases the frequency of relapses. Diet therapy for peptic ulcer disease includes having the client eat several small meals per day and avoid foods that produce symptoms, rather prescribing a particular diet such as a bland diet. Implementation Application Physiological Integrity
23.12 A client with peptic ulcer disease says, "I feel so much better now that I've stopped eating." The nurse realizes that this client is at risk for: 1. *Sleep Pattern Disturbance.* 2. *Imbalanced Nutrition: Less than Body Requirements.* 3. *Pain.* 4. *Fluid Volume Overload.*	Answer: 2 Rationale: In an attempt to avoid discomfort, the client with peptic ulcer disease (PUD) may gradually reduce food intake, and sometimes jeopardize nutritional status. Anorexia and early satiety are additional problems associated with PUD. The client is not at increased risk for pain, sleep pattern disturbance, or fluid volume overload due to this action. Diagnosis Analysis Physiological Integrity
23.13 A client who is recovering from surgery for stomach cancer a month ago continues to experience dumping	Answer: 1 Rationale: Dumping syndrome is typically self-limiting, and lasts 6 to 12 months after surgery; however, a small percentage of people continue to experience

syndrome. Which of the following should the nurse instruct this client?

1. "It's usually self-limiting and will resolve within 6 to 12 months."
2. "It will be a problem for the rest of your life."
3. "There's no treatment."
4. "Only eat a clear liquid diet."

long-term symptoms. A clear liquid diet is not recommended as a treatment for postoperative dumping syndrome. A small percentage of postoperative clients may continue to have dumping syndrome. Treatment options for dumping syndrome include dietary modifications.
Implementation
Application
Physiological Integrity

23.14 A client who had stomach cancer surgery two years ago comes into the clinic fearful that the "cancer is back because I'm so tired all of the time." The nurse realizes that this client is likely experiencing:

1. a return of the stomach cancer.
2. metastasis.
3. ineffective coping.
4. vitamin deficiency.

Answer: 4
Rationale: The cells of the stomach produce intrinsic factor, which are required for the absorption of vitamin B_{12}. Vitamin B_{12} deficiency leads to pernicious anemia. Because of hepatic stores of vitamin B_{12}, symptoms of anemia may not be seen for one to two years after surgery. There are no clinical manifestations presented to support the reoccurrence or metastasis of the cancer. The client is seeking clarification of their condition not demonstrating an inability to cope.
Assessment
Analysis
Health Promotion and Maintenance

23.15 A client who is in the post-gastric surgery stage for cancer is denying that he has cancer. The nurse should:

1. remind the client of the diagnosis.
2. ask a clinical psychologist to talk with the client.
3. do not argue with the client, but continue to provide emotional support as needed.
4. explain how many people with cancer live long, productive lives.

Answer: 3
Rationale: The nursing diagnosis *Anticipatory Grieving* is appropriate for this client. The nurse should not negate denial because denial is a coping mechanism that protects the client from hopelessness. There is no real need to remind the client of the diagnosis. The client is acting in a manner with can often be anticipated. At this point, there is no need for the clinical psychologist to intervene. Making a referral to the clinical psychologist is beyond the duties of the nurse. The client is not emotionally prepared to discuss cancer survival at this time.
Implementation
Application
Psychosocial Integrity

CHAPTER 24

24.1 During a physical assessment, the nurse learns that a client has pain in the right shoulder and scapula most evenings after eating dinner. Which of the following should the nurse ask to further assess these findings?

1. "Have you been told you have high blood pressure?"
2. "Have you been restricting your diet?"
3. "How much water do you drink each day?"
4. "Have you changed your exercise program?"

Answer: 2
Rationale: The symptoms being reported are associated with cholelithiasis. Additional manifestations include age, family history of gallstones, race or ethnicity, obesity, hyperlipidemia, rapid weight loss, female gender, use of oral contraceptives, pregnancy, fasting, prolonged parenteral nutrition, cirrhosis, ileal disease or resection, sickle cell anemia, and glucose intolerance.
A client who exhibits the symptoms described may alter their diet to increase comfort. Blood pressure, water intake, and exercise would likely not influence these symptoms.
Assessment
Application
Physiological Integrity

24.2 A client is scheduled for extracorporeal shock wave lithotripsy for gallstones. Which of the following should be included in the care of this client after the procedure?

1. Admit to the hospital until the stones have been passed.
2. Nothing.
3. Instruct about the potential for nausea, vomiting, and hematuria postprocedure.

Answer: 3
Rationale: Nursing care after the procedure includes monitoring for biliary colic that may result from the gallbladder contracting to remove stone fragments, nausea, and transient hematuria. Hospitalization and frequent vital sign monitoring are not indicated. Doing nothing is not appropriate.
Implementation
Application
Physiological Integrity

---

4. Monitor vital signs for eight hours postprocedure.	

24.3 A client who is admitted to the hospital with an acutely inflamed gallbladder says, "I suddenly feel better. The pain was really bad but then it completely stopped." The nurse should:
  1. contact the physician immediately.
  2. suggest that the client prepare to be discharged.
  3. see when the client last received pain medication.
  4. do nothing.
	Answer: 1
	Rationale: Rupture of an acutely inflamed gallbladder may be heralded by abrupt but transient pain relief as contents are released from the distended gallbladder into the abdomen. Promptly report this change to the physician.
	Diagnosis
	Analysis
	Physiological Integrity

24.4 A client comes into the clinic complaining of "gaining weight only in the stomach." The nurse realizes that this client is exhibiting signs of:
  1. splenomegaly.
  2. portal hypertension.
  3. esophageal varices.
  4. hepatic encephalopathy.
	Answer: 2
	Rationale: Portal hypertension has several effects when prolonged. The client is demonstrating signs of ascites, which is the accumulation of fluid in the peritoneal cavity. Splenomegaly, esophageal varices, and hepatic encephalopathy may be associated with portal hypertension, but are not the cause of ascites.
	Diagnosis
	Analysis
	Physiological Integrity

24.5 A client with hepatitis is complaining of "itchy skin" and "odd colored bowel movements." The nurse realizes that this client is in which phase of acute hepatitis?
  1. preicteric
  2. icteric
  3. posticteric
  4. prodromal
	Answer: 2
	Rationale: The icteric phase of acute hepatitis is characterized by jaundice, pruritis, clay-colored stools, brown urine, and an improvement in appetite. Preicteric and prodromal phase are the same and begin with the onset of signs of infection and last for about one week. The posticteric phase marks the beginning of regeneration of hepatic cells. This phase lasts for several months.
	Diagnosis
	Analysis
	Physiological Integrity

24.6 While providing care to a client with hepatitis B, the nurse is exposed to this client's blood. What should the nurse do?
  1. Nothing.
  2. Prepare to be treated with interferon.
  3. Report the exposure and prepare to receive hepatitis B immune globulin (HBIG).
  4. Report the exposure and prepare to receive immune globulin (IG).
	Answer: 3
	Rationale: Hepatitis B postexposure prophylaxis is indicated for people exposed to the hepatitis B virus. Hepatitis B immune globulin (HBIG) is given to provide for short-term immunity. Candidates for postexposure prophylaxis include those with known or suspected percutaneous or permucosal contact with blood infected with the hepatitis B virus.
	Planning
	Application
	Health Promotion and Maintenance

24.7 A client with hepatic cirrhosis begins to bleed. Which of the following should the nurse anticipate being included in the physician's orders?
  1. Administer nadolol (Corgard).
  2. Administer folic acid.
  3. Administer vitamin K.
  4. Administer packed red blood cells (PRBCs).
	Answer: 4
	Rationale: When bleeding is acute, packed red blood cells, fresh frozen plasma, or platelets may be administered to restore blood components and promote hemostasis. Corgard is a beta-blocker used to treat angina. Folic acid is a supplement used to treat and prevent anemia. Vitamin K does aid in the clotting process, but is not the priority treatment in an acute situation.
	Planning
	Application
	Physiological Integrity

24.8 A client who is prescribed lactulose is complaining of "diarrhea with cramps" throughout most of the	Answer: 2 Rationale: Lactulose pulls water into the bowel lumen, which increases the number of daily stools. The dose should be adjusted to achieve two to three soft stools per day.

day. The nurse realizes that this client is demonstrating:

1. intolerance of the medication and it should be discontinued.
2. the need to adjust the dose of the medication.
3. an expected outcome from taking the medication.
4. an allergy to the medication.

Evaluation
Analysis
Physiological Integrity

24.9 The family and friends of a liver transplant client is concerned because they have not been permitted to see the client after the surgery. The nurse realizes that this means:

1. nothing. This is a common restriction.
2. the client's condition is not stable.
3. the client is prone to developing an infection and is in isolation.
4. the client's condition is critical.

Answer: 1
Rationale: Restrictions on the number of visitors and the time they may spend with the client are common in transplant clients to protect the client from infection. There is inadequate information to assess for postoperative complications. While the client has an increased risk for the development of infection, they are not in isolation. There is no indication the client is in critical condition.
Evaluation
Analysis
Physiological Integrity

24.10 The nurse is preparing to instruct a client with pruritis caused by jaundice about the care of the skin. Which of the following should be included in these instructions? (Select all that apply.)

1. Bathe with hot water.
2. Apply lotion to keep the skin moist.
3. Use soap when bathing.
4. Alcohol-based products work the best.
5. Scratching is permitted.
6. Take another antihistamine if the itching continues.

Answer: 2
Rationale: Nursing care for the client with jaundice and pruritis focuses on measures to prevent dry skin. Those measures include using warm (not hot) water when bathing, applying an emollient or lubricant as needed to keep skin moist, avoid soap or preparations with alcohol, and do not rub the skin. Dry skin contributes to pruritus. Antihistamines should be administered cautiously.
Planning
Application
Physiological Integrity

24.11 A client who is being evaluated for liver trauma that was sustained in a motor vehicle accident is found to have a negative peritoneal lavage. The nurse realizes that this client is demonstrating:

1. severe liver lacerations.
2. clotting factor malfunction.
3. no bleeding from the liver.
4. hematoma formation.

Answer: 3
Rationale: Diagnostic peritoneal lavage is often used along with computed tomography (CT) scan to diagnose liver trauma. If blood is immediately detected, the client is taken directly to surgery for abdominal exploration. If frank bleeding is not apparent, a liter of isotonic fluid is instilled into the abdomen, then drained and sent for laboratory analysis.
Diagnosis
Analysis
Physiological Integrity

24.12 A client tells the nurse that his bowel movements are "weird" in that they look "soapy" and "smell really bad." The nurse realizes that this client might be experiencing:

1. an obstructed gallbladder.
2. turner's sign.
3. cullen's sign.
4. steatorrhea.

Answer: 4
Rationale: Steatorrhea is fatty, frothy, foul-smelling stools caused by a decrease in pancreatic enzyme secretion. Gallbladder obstruction manifestations are consistent with pain not stool changes. Cullen's sign is a bluish-grey discoloration in the periumbilical area. Turner's sign is grey-blue discoloration at the flank area. Both may be seen in clients with pancreatic disease.
Assessment
Analysis
Physiological Integrity

24.13 A client with acute pancreatitis is being discharged. Which of the following should the nurse include when providing discharge instructions to this client? 1. Avoid all alcohol. 2. Resume a regular diet. 3. Limit smoking. 4. A fever is common.	Answer: 1 Rationale: Alcohol can cause stones to form, blocking pancreatic ducts and the outflow of pancreatic juice. Continued alcohol intake is likely to cause further inflammation and destruction of the pancreas. Avoid alcohol entirely. Diet modifications and smoking cessation are necessary in the client with pancreatitis. Fever should be reported. Planning Application Health Promotion and Maintenance
24.14 A client with acute pancreatitis is uncomfortable in bed. Which of the following positions might improve this client's comfort level? 1. Lay flat in bed. 2. Elevate the head 45 degrees. 3. Lay on the stomach. 4. Assist to a standing position and ambulate.	Answer: 2 Rationale: Assist to a comfortable position, such as a side-lying position with knees flexed and head elevated 45 degrees. The client may experience an increase in discomfort if lying flat on their back or abdomen. Standing may intensify discomfort. Implementation Application Physiological Integrity
24.15 The family of a client with acute pancreatitis arrives to the care area with a large bag of personal items and food. What should the nurse instruct this family about the care of the client? 1. Only bring foods the client requests. 2. Bring high-calorie foods to support the client's caloric needs. 3. Bring fresh fruits. 4. Avoid bringing food to the client.	Answer: 4 Rationale: Remind family and visitors to avoid bringing food into the client's room. The sight or smell of food may stimulate secretory activity of the pancreas through the cephalic phase of digestion. Implementation Application Physiological Integrity

CHAPTER 25

25.1 The nurse is assessing a client with a pancreatic disorder. The nurse realizes the client might be experiencing digestive problems that affect which section of the intestines? 1. duodenum 2. jejunum 3. ileum 4. appendix	Answer: 1 Rationale: Both pancreatic enzymes and bile from the liver enter the small intestine at the duodenum. Assessment Application Health Promotion and Maintenance
25.2 A client says, "I drink so much water every day you'd think I would have diarrhea, not constipation!" An appropriate response for the nurse to make to this client is: 1. "You're obviously not drinking enough water!" 2. "Are you sure you're drinking as much as you think you are?" 3. "You are dehydrated." 4. "Your body only absorbs about 1 liter of the water."	Answer: 4 Rationale: Although up to 10 liters of food, liquids, and secretions enter the gastrointestinal tract each day, most is digested and absorbed in the small intestine; less than 1 liter reaches the large intestine. This does not indicate dehydration. The other responses are not examples of therapeutic communication. Implementation Application Health Promotion and Maintenance
25.3 A client has been diagnosed with internal hemorrhoids. The nurse realizes that these hemorrhoids are most likely located:	Answer: 4 Rationale: The anorectal junction separates the rectum from the anal canal and may be the site of internal hemorrhoids.

1. at the cecum. 2. at the hepatic flexure. 3. at the splenic flexure. 4. at the anorectal junction.	Diagnosis Analysis Physiological Integrity
25.4 The nurse is instructing a client about how to increase intra-abdominal pressure in order to facilitate a bowel movement. In this example, the nurse is instructing the client about: 1. peristalsis. 2. Valsalva's maneuver. 3. Crede procedure. 4. splinting.	Answer: 2 Rationale: Closing the glottis and contracting the diaphragm and abdominal muscles to increase intra-abdominal pressure, or Valsalva's maneuver, facilitates expulsion of feces. Peristalsis is associated with bowel elimination, not the expulsion of feces. The Crede procedure is associated with urinary elimination. Splinting is done post-operatively or to decrease pain sensation. Implementation Application Physiological Integrity
25.5 A client comes into the outpatient clinic for testing because of chronic constipation. The nurse realizes that this client might have evidence of: 1. internal hemorrhoids. 2. diarrhea. 3. external hemorrhoids. 4. appendicitis.	Answer: 3 Rationale: Frequent bouts of constipation may lead to external hemorrhoids at the area of the external hemorrhoidal plexus. Internal hemorrhoids are less likely to be associated with constipation. The client has reported constipation not diarrhea. Appendicitis is an emergent condition. It is not associated with chronic constipation. Planning Analysis Physiological Integrity
25.6 A client is scheduled for a test to visualize the entire colon. The nurse should provide preprocedure instructions for: 1. a flexible sigmoidoscopy. 2. a colonoscopy. 3. an endoscopic retrograde cholangiopancreatogram. 4. an MRI of the abdomen.	Answer: 2 Rationale: Direct visualization of the entire large intestine colonoscopy is accomplished by using a flexible tube. A flexible sigmoidoscopy is the visualization of the anus, rectum, and sigmoid colon. An endoscopic retrograde cholangiopancreatogram is not used to visualize the colon. An MRI will not provide direct visualization. Planning Application Health Promotion and Maintenance
25.7 The nurse is beginning the interview of an older client with a bowel disorder. Which of the following might be an appropriate question to begin this interview? 1. "I see here that you have a problem with constipation." 2. "Many people your age become bowel-fixated." 3. "Do you have any other health-related problems?" 4. "Older people always worry about their bowels."	Answer: 3 Rationale: Clients may feel embarrassed to talk about bowel elimination patterns. To promote effective rapport, ask about less personal information first. The other responses are not therapeutic. Planning Application Health Promotion and Maintenance
25.8 The nurse is assessing a client with diarrhea. Which of the following would be appropriate for the nurse to ask during the focused assessment? 1. "Tell me about your work responsibilities." 2. "Have you been feeling blue or sad recently?" 3. "Are you still taking the medication for depression?" 4. "Are you still taking the prescribed sleeping medication?"	Answer: 1 Rationale: Assess the client's lifestyle for any patterns of psychologic stress and/or depression, which may alter bowel elimination. Depression may be associated with constipation, whereas diarrhea may occur in situations of high stress and anxiety. Assessment Application Psychosocial Integrity

25.9 The nurse is preparing to assess a client's abdomen. Place in order the steps the nurse should follow when performing this assessment.
  1. Percussion
  2. Inspection
  3. Auscultation
  4. Palpation
	Answer: 2,3,1,4
	Rationale: The techniques of inspection, auscultation, percussion, and palpation are used. Palpation is the last method used in assessing the abdomen because pressure on the abdominal wall and contents may interfere with bowel sounds and cause pain, thereby ending the examination.
	Planning
	Application
	Health Promotion and Maintenance

25.10 During the auscultation of a client's abdomen the client states, "Something must be wrong—you've been listening down there forever!" The nurse should respond with:
  1. "I am having trouble listening with this stethoscope."
  2. "I'm not sure what I'm listening to."
  3. "Now I have to start counting all over again."
  4. "I need to listen over all the major areas of your stomach."
	Answer: 4
	Rationale: Normal bowel sounds (gurgling or clicking) occur every 5 to 15 seconds. Listen for at least 5 minutes in each of the four quadrants to confirm the absence of bowel sounds.
	Assessment
	Application
	Psychosocial Integrity

25.11 During the assessment of a client's perianal area the nurse notes "donut-shaped red tissue." This finding is indicative of:
  1. anal fissures.
  2. prolapsed rectum.
  3. internal hemorrhoids.
  4. external hemorrhoids.
	Answer: 2
	Rationale: Doughnut-shaped red tissue at the anal area may appear with a prolapsed rectum. Fissures are painful longitudinal breaks in the skin. A red mass is associated with internal hemorrhoids. Internal hemorrhoids cannot be viewed with an external inspection of the perianal area.
	Diagnosis
	Application
	Physiological Integrity

25.12 After testing a client's stool sample for occult blood the nurse notes the finding as being "trace." Which of the following should the nurse say to this client?
  1. Nothing.
  2. "The results are inconclusive and the doctor will talk with you more about any next steps."
  3. "You have cancer and need to be checked."
  4. "Everyone has some blood in their stool."
	Answer: 2
	Rationale: Normal stool has no blood. The nurse should not diagnose the client's condition based on this finding. The best response would be for the nurse to suggest the client talk with the physician about the finding.
	Implementation
	Application
	Physiological Integrity

25.13 A client has recently lost her mother to colon cancer. Which of the following should the nurse suggest to this client?
  1. "You should make sure you get checked monthly."
  2. "Have you talked with a psychologist about your loss?"
  3. "Is your father still alive?"
  4. "Have you considered being checked for the same condition?"
	Answer: 4
	Rationale: Colon cancer is one of the most common inherited cancer syndromes. Monthly checking would be too frequent. There is no indication the client has abnormal or unresolved psychological concerns related to the loss of her mother. The father's current status is not the primary concern for this client's preventative health plan.
	Implementation
	Application
	Health Promotion and Maintenance

25.14 An elderly client says, "I drink milk and take calcium. I don't know why the osteoporosis is getting worse." An appropriate response for the nurse to say to this client is:	Answer: 3 Rationale: A common age-related change with the small intestines is the decreased ability to absorb calcium and vitamin D. The client's reports indicate ingestion of both milk and a calcium supplement. The nurse needs to look at

1. "Maybe you need to drink more milk." 2. "There's nothing that can be done to stop it." 3. "Older people sometimes have difficulty absorbing calcium and vitamin D." 4. "You may need hip replacement surgery in the future."	causes beyond nutrition. Advising the client there are no treatment options is incorrect. There is no indication the client will require joint replacement surgery. Implementation Application Health Promotion and Maintenance
25.15 A client is scheduled for an abdominal ultrasound. Which of the following should the nurse provide as preprocedure instructions? 1. "No special instructions are needed." 2. "Do not eat anything 2 hours before the test." 3. "Take clear liquids only after midnight." 4. "Be sure to stop eating or drinking for at least 8 hours before the test."	Answer: 4 Rationale: For an abdominal ultrasound, tell client not to eat or drink for 8-12 hours prior to the examination. This will allow easier visualization of all structures. A full bladder or stomach can block the view. Implementation Application Health Promotion and Maintenance

CHAPTER 26

26.1 A client tells the nurse about "diarrhea when eating ice cream." The nurse realizes that this client might be experiencing: 1. disease of the colon. 2. inflammation of the small intestines. 3. cholera. 4. lactose intolerance.	Answer: 4 Rationale: When the lactose in milk is not broken down and absorbed, the lactose molecules exert an osmotic draw, which causes diarrhea. Diagnosis Analysis Physiological Integrity
26.2 The nurse is providing care to a client admitted with acute diarrhea. Which of the following interventions would assist in this client's care? 1. Provide a normal diet as tolerated. 2. Hold all medications until the diarrhea stops. 3. Provide clear liquids, in small amounts. 4. Encourage normal activities of daily living in the hospital room.	Answer: 3 Rationale: This client should have limited food intake, reintroducing solid foods slowly. Therefore, clear liquids are the best approach. The nurse should provide antidiarrheal medication as prescribed. Because of the potential for orthostatic hypotension, this client should be instructed to move slowly and not engage in normal activities of daily living until the blood pressure is assessed. Planning Application Physiological Integrity
26.3 The nurse is caring for a client with a fecal impaction. Which of the following types of enemas will best assist this client? 1. normal saline 2. oil retention 3. tap water 4. soap suds	Answer: 2 Rationale: Oil retention enemas instill mineral or vegetable oil into the bowel to soften the fecal mass. The instilled oil is retained overnight or for several hours before evacuation. The normal saline enema is used to soften the fecal mass and promote defecation in the least irritating manner. Tap water enemas soften the bowel and irritate the bowel to promote defecation. Soap suds provide an increased means to irritate the bowel to promote a bowel movement. Planning Application Physiological Integrity

26.4 A client with irritable bowel syndrome asks the nurse, "Why did the doctor order something for depression?" How should the nurse respond? 1. "Didn't the doctor tell you that you are depressed?" 2. "Bowel disorders cause depression." 3. "You should probably ask the doctor." 4. "These medications help with the symptoms associated with your bowel problem."	Answer: 4 Rationale: Antidepressant drugs, including tricyclics and selective serotonin reuptake inhibitors (SSRIs), may help relieve abdominal pain associated with IBS. Implementation Application Physiological Integrity
26.5 The nurse is implementing a bowel retraining program for a client. Which of the following should be included in this client's plan of care? 1. Assess the client to determine the best time of day to use the commode for defecation. 2. Keep the bedpan near the client at all times. 3. Instruct the client to not attempt to use the bathroom unattended. 4. Stay with the client while defecating.	Answer: 1 Rationale: Placing the client in a normal position to defecate at a consistent time of day stimulates the defecation reflex and helps reestablish a pattern of stool evacuation. Ideally, the bowel retraining program should focus on use of the commode or toilet. Providing the client with assistance to the bathroom is a safety measure and does not influence the success of the bowel retraining program. Remaining with the client may reduce comfort level and interfere with defecation. Planning Application Physiological Integrity
26.6 A client comes into the emergency department with suspected appendicitis. Which of the following should the nurse do for this client? 1. Provide a hot water bottle to place over the abdomen. 2. Provide with clear water to drink. 3. Inspect the abdomen and assess bowel sounds. 4. Provide with antacids and a bisacodyl (Dulcolax) suppository.	Answer: 3 Rationale: Keep the client with suspected appendicitis NPO, and do not administer laxatives or enemas, which may cause perforation of the appendix. No heat should be applied to the abdomen; this may increase circulation to the appendix and also cause perforation. Implementation Application Physiological Integrity
26.7 The nurse can detect no bowel sounds on a client recovering from bowel surgery. This finding should be noted as: 1. borborygmy. 2. possible paralytic ileus. 3. hyperactive bowel sounds. 4. atonic bowel.	Answer: 2 Rationale: Paralytic ileus, or ileus, is defined as an impaired propulsion or forward movement of bowel contents. The client will not have bowel sounds upon auscultation. Borborygmy are loud, hyperactive bowel sounds. Hyperactive bowel sounds are an increase in sound and frequency. Atonic is a term used to refer to the loss of muscular tone. Diagnosis Analysis Physiological Integrity
26.8 A client is diagnosed with gastroenteritis. The nurse should assess which of the following serum laboratory values first? 1. sodium 2. bicarbonate 3. calcium 4. potassium	Answer: 4 Rationale: Electrolyte and acid–base imbalances may result from gastroenteritis. Extensive vomiting can lead to metabolic alkalosis due to the loss of hydrochloric acid from the stomach. When diarrhea predominates, metabolic acidosis is more likely. Potassium is lost in either case, which leads to hypokalemia. Assessment Application Health Promotion and Maintenance
26.9 Only three children out of a group of 12 developed signs of enteritis. Which of the following could be an	Answer: 1 Rationale: The process of grinding hamburger allows *E. coli* to be mixed throughout the meat. The signs presented are consistent with *E. coli* exposure.

indication of the source of the children's health problem?

1. The three children ate hamburgers.
2. Nine children ate hotdogs.
3. Most of the children drank canned soda.
4. All of the children ate ice cream.

Hotdogs, canned soda, and ice cream are not associated with the bacteria.
Diagnosis
Application
Health Promotion and Maintenance

26.10 A 28-year-old female client is diagnosed with inflammatory disease of the small bowel. The nurse realizes that this client most likely is experiencing:

1. ulcerative colitis.
2. chronic diarrhea.
3. gastroenteritis.
4. Crohn's disease.

Answer: 4
Rationale: In Crohn's disease, a patchy pattern of involvement is seen, which affects primarily the small intestine. Ulcerative colitis affects the large intestine. Chronic diarrhea is not supported by the information provided. Gastroenteritis results from ingesting contaminated foods or beverages.
Diagnosis
Application
Physiological Integrity

26.11 A client with Crohn's disease is recovering from a bowel resection. The nurse realizes that this client will:

1. never have another recurrence of the disease.
2. possibly have a recurrence in another portion of the bowel.
3. develop ulcerative colitis.
4. experience intestinal strictures.

Answer: 2
Rationale: The disease process tends to recur in other areas following removal of affected bowel segments. The processes involving Crohn's disease and ulcerative colitis are different. There is no increased risk for the development of intestinal strictures.
Evaluation
Analysis
Physiological Integrity

26.12 A client with Crohn's disease is demonstrating *Imbalanced Nutrition: Less than Body Requirements.* Which of the following should be included in this client's plan of care?

1. a low-calorie, high-milk diet
2. a low-calorie, low-residue diet
3. the DASH diet
4. a high-calorie, low-fat diet

Answer: 4
Rationale: Provide a diet with high-kilocalorie, high-protein, and low-fat diet and restrict milk and milk products if lactose intolerance is present. The Crohn's client needs an elevation in calories related to the nutrients lost as a result of diarrhea. This will eliminate options 1 and 2. There is no DASH diet.
Planning
Application
Health Promotion and Maintenance

26.13 A client is suspected as having sprue. Which of the following should the nurse instruct this client about his diet?

1. Avoid all milk products.
2. A vegetarian diet is the best treatment for this condition.
3. Gluten products must be eliminated from the diet.
4. All whey products must be eliminated from the diet.

Answer: 3
Rationale: The client with celiac sprue is placed on a gluten-free diet. This treatment is generally successful, as long as the client avoids gluten totally.
Implementation
Application
Health Promotion and Maintenance

26.14 A client who is newly diagnosed with short bowel syndrome, asks "Now what do I need to do? I'm so tired of being sick." The nurse should respond with:

1. "It's going to be difficult in the beginning."
2. "Sometimes minor diet changes will alleviate the problem."
3. "I think more surgery is in your future."
4. "It will be a life-long challenge for you."

Answer: 2
Rationale: Management of short bowel syndrome focuses on alleviating symptoms. Clients often simply require frequent, small, high-kilocalorie, high-protein feedings. Advising the client there will initially be difficulty promotes negativity and may not be correct information. Surgery is not utilized to manage short bowel syndrome. The client is seeking information related to the management of the condition. Advising the client it will be a life-long challenge does not address their verbalized concerns.
Implementation
Application
Health Promotion and Maintenance

26.15 A client with cancer of the rectum is scheduled for surgery and the placement of a permanent ostomy. Which of the following types of ostomies will this client most likely have performed during the surgery? 1. duodenal 2. double-barrel 3. sigmoid 4. transverse loop	Answer: 3 Rationale: A sigmoid colostomy is the most common permanent colostomy performed, particularly for cancer of the rectum. It is usually created during an abdominoperineal resection. The duodenal, double-barrel, and transverse loop colonoscopy are not in the correct area to manage cancer in this location. Planning Analysis Physiological Integrity
26.16 A client is being seen for a "sudden lump" in his groin after lifting a heavy box to a shelf. The nurse realizes that this client might be experiencing: 1. an indirect inguinal hernia. 2. a direct inguinal hernia. 3. a femoral hernia. 4. an incisional hernia.	Answer: 1 Rationale: Although indirect inguinal hernias are congenital defects, they often are not evident until adulthood, when increased intra-abdominal pressure and dilation of the inguinal ring allow abdominal contents to enter the channel. Direct inguinal hernias are acquired defects that result from weakness of the posterior inguinal wall. Direct inguinal hernias usually affect older adults. Femoral hernias are also acquired defects in which a peritoneal sac protrudes through the femoral ring. Inadequate information is provided to support the presence of an incisional hernia. Diagnosis Analysis Physiological Integrity
26.17 A client learns that a small bowel obstruction was caused by an appendectomy he had 5 years ago. The nurse realizes that this obstruction was most likely caused by: 1. an untreated infection of the appendix. 2. adhesions. 3. undiagnosed femoral hernia. 4. umbilical hernia.	Answer: 2 Rationale: In adults, adhesions develop following abdominal surgery or inflammatory processes. Adhesions usually produce a simple obstruction or single blockage in one portion of the intestine. An untreated infection would have resulted in peritonitis. There is inadequate information provided to support femoral or umbilical hernias. Diagnosis Analysis Physiological Integrity
26.18 The nurse is providing medications to a client with diverticular disease. Which of the following medications should the nurse question for this client? 1. docusate (Colace) 2. metronidazole (Flagyl) 3. trimethoprim-sulfamethoxazole (Bactrim) 4. bisacodyl (Dulcolax) suppository	Answer: 4 Rationale: Although a stool softener such as docusate (Colace) may be prescribed, it is important to note that laxatives can further increase intraluminal pressure in the colon and should be avoided for the client with diverticular disease. Systemic broad-spectrum antibiotics effective against usual bowel flora are prescribed to treat acute diverticulitis. Oral antibiotics such as metronidazole (Flagyl) and ciprofloxacin (Cipro) or trimethoprim-sulfamethoxazole (Septra, Bactrim) may be prescribed if manifestations are mild. Implementation Analysis Safe, Effective Care Environment
26.19 An unlicensed assistive staff member says to the nurse, "I need for you to assess a client. He has something coming out of his rectum." The nurse realizes that the assistant most likely observed: 1. internal hemorrhoids. 2. colostomy. 3. prolapsed hemorrhoids. 4. femoral hernia.	Answer: 3 Rationale: Prolapsed hemorrhoids will be visible from the rectum and anal area. Internal hemorrhoids are not visible by an external examination as they are inside. The colostomy and femoral hernia are not located in the rectal area. Evaluation Application Safe, Effective Care Environment
26.20 The nurse is providing discharge instructions to a client who is recovering from anal-rectal surgery. Which of the following should be included in these instructions? (Select all that apply.)	Answer: 2, 3 Rationale: Teach the importance of maintaining a high-fiber diet and liberal fluid intake to increase stool bulk and softness and thereby decrease discomfort with defecation. Stress the importance of responding to the urge to defecate to prevent constipation. Teach the client to keep the perianal region clean and dry. If a dressing is in place, instruct to avoid soiling it with urine or feces during

1. Do not remove the dressing.
2. Change the dressing if it becomes soiled with urine or feces.
3. Use the sitz bath.
4. Use the antibiotic until all drainage stops.
5. Avoid bowel movements.

elimination. Following removal of the dressing, teach to clean the area gently with soap and water following a bowel movement. Discuss the use of sitz baths for cleaning and comfort. Suggest taking an analgesic if necessary prior to defecation, but caution that some analgesics may promote constipation. Teach signs and symptoms of infection or other possible complications to report to the physician. If an antibiotic has been prescribed, provide written and verbal instructions about its use, its desired effects, and possible adverse effects and their management.
Implementation
Application
Health Promotion and Maintenance

CHAPTER 27

27.1 During the assessment of a client with multiple injuries, the nurse notices a large hematoma located at the left costovertebral angle. Which additional body system should this nurse assess?
1. gastrointestinal
2. renal
3. spinal
4. respiratory

Answer: 2
Rationale: The two kidneys are located outside the peritoneal cavity and on either side of the vertebral column at the levels of T12 through L3, which is also termed the costovertebral angle. Although multiple systems may be injured, the location of the hematoma described would not cause initial concern about a gastrointestinal, spinal, or respiratory injury.
Planning
Analysis
Physiological Integrity

27.2 A client is admitted with an infection of the ureters. The nurse realizes that this infection could include which of the following structures of the kidney?
1. cortex
2. medulla
3. pelvis
4. adrenal glands

Answer: 3
Rationale: The renal pelvis is continuous with the ureters. The cortex and medulla are deeper within the renal tissue and not an extension of the ureters as is the case of the renal pelvis. The adrenal glands are located just above the kidneys, but are not considered a part of the urinary system.
Assessment
Analysis
Physiological Integrity

27.3 The nurse is studying the process of net filtration pressure within the kidney. Which of the following forces create net filtration pressure?
1. glomerular filtration rate
2. permeability of the filtration membrane
3. tubular reabsorption
4. hydrostatic and osmotic pressure

Answer: 4
Rationale: Net filtration pressure is responsible for the formation of filtrate and is determined by two forces: hydrostatic pressure (the push) and osmotic pressure (the pull). Glomerular filtration rate is a measure (mL/min) of filtration across the glomerular membrane into Bowman's capsule. This is influenced by membrane permeability, as well as blood pressure and blood flow. Tubular reabsorption is the process by which water and electrolytes are returned to the blood.
Assessment
Analysis
Physiological Integrity

27.4 A client is experiencing a sudden decrease in systemic blood pressure. Which of the following will occur within the kidney to help control this blood pressure drop?
1. Juxtaglomerular cells will release renin.
2. Glomerular filtration rate (GFR) will increase.
3. Renal vessels will dilate.
4. Hydrostatic pressure will increase.

Answer: 1
Rationale: A drop in systemic blood pressure often triggers the juxtaglomerular cells to release renin. Renin acts on angiotensinogen to release angiotensin I, which is in turn converted to angiotensin II. Angiotensin II activates vascular smooth muscle throughout the body, which causes systemic blood pressure to rise. Thus, the renin-angiotensin mechanism is a factor in renal autoregulation, even though its main purpose is the control of systemic blood pressure. Increased glomerular filtration rate (GFR), dilation of renal vessels, and increased hydrostatic pressure will all cause a further drop in blood pressure.
Evaluation
Analysis
Physiological Integrity

27.5 A client with renal failure is demonstrating signs of an altered blood pH. Which of the following kidney functions aids in the maintenance of normal blood pH?
1. glomerular filtration rate (GFR)
2. hydrostatic pressure

Answer: 3
Rationale: Tubular secretion is important for disposing of substances not already in the filtrate. This process eliminates undesirable substances that have been reabsorbed by passive processes and rids the body of excessive potassium ions. It is also a vital force in the regulation of blood pH. Glomerular filtration rate (GFR), hydrostatic pressure, and tubular reabsorption contribute to urine formation and maintenance of fluid and electrolyte balance, but not necessarily to pH balance.

3. tubular secretion 4. tubular reabsorption	Evaluation Analysis Physiological Integrity

27.6 A client is voiding large amounts of highly diluted urine. The nurse realizes the dilution or concentration of urine is determined by which of the following?
    1. presence of urea
    2. quantity of chloride
    3. patency of the ureters
    4. action of antidiuretic hormone
	Answer: 4
	Rationale: The dilution or concentration of urine is largely determined by the action of antidiuretic hormone. This hormone causes the pores of the collecting tubules to enlarge, so that increased amounts of water move into the interstitial space. The end result is that water is reabsorbed and urine is more highly concentrated. When not secreted, the filtrate passes through the system without further water reabsorption, so that the urine is more dilute. Presence of urea, quantity of chloride, or the patency of the ureters would not cause large amounts of dilute urine, but rather more concentrated urine.
	Evaluation
	Analysis
	Physiological Integrity

27.7 The nurse is collecting a sample of a client's urine for composite analysis. Which of the following is the largest component of urine, by weight?
    1. urea
    2. water
    3. sodium
    4. chloride
	Answer: 1
	Rationale: The largest component of urine by weight is urea. Urine is composed, by volume, of about 95% water and 5% solutes. Sodium and chloride make up a smaller percentage of the solute composition of urine.
	Implementation
	Analysis
	Physiological Integrity

27.8 A client experienced a temporary reduction of oxygen. The nurse realizes that this drop in oxygen level will have which impact on the client's renal functioning?
    1. nothing
    2. stimulate the absorption of calcium and phosphate
    3. stimulate bone marrow to produce more red blood cells
    4. produce large amounts of dilute urine
	Answer: 3
	Rationale: Erythropoietin stimulates the bone marrow to produce red blood cells in response to tissue hypoxia. The stimulus for the production of erythropoietin by the kidneys is decreased oxygen delivery to kidney cells. This short-term reduction of oxygen would not cause absorption of calcium and phosphate, which exist normally in a reciprocal concentrations; or the production of large amounts of dilute urine, which may be caused by inadequate antidiuretic hormone (ADH).
	Diagnosis
	Analysis
	Physiological Integrity

27.9 A client is participating in rehabilitation for bladder retraining. Which of the following bladder layers houses the detrusor muscle?
    1. epithelial mucosa
    2. muscle layer
    3. connective tissue mucosa
    4. fibrous layer
	Answer: 2
	Rationale: The muscle layer, called the detrusor muscle, consists of fibers arranged in inner and outer longitudinal layers and in a middle circular layer. The epithelial mucosa, connective tissue mucosa, and fibrous layer do not contain muscle.
	Implementation
	Analysis
	Physiological Integrity

27.10 After stating the need to "go to the bathroom," a client voids 450 cc of urine. The nurse realizes that this client's urine output is considered:
    1. too low.
    2. concentrated.
    3. too high.
    4. normal.
	Answer: 4
	Rationale: The size of the bladder varies in the amount of urine it contains. In healthy adults, the bladder holds about 300 to 500 mL of urine. This client's amount of 450 cc is within the "normal" range. No indicators of color were given to be able to determine if the urine was concentrated.
	Evaluation
	Analysis
	Physiological Integrity

27.11 The nurse is preparing to catheterize a client after the client has just independently voided. The purpose of this catheterization is to:
    1. serve as a urine output baseline.
    2. support the diagnosis of kidney stones.
	Answer: 3
	Rationale: A post-voiding residual urine test is done to evaluate the bladder's ability to empty urine. A urine output baseline would best be measured by a 24-hour collection. Kidney stones are diagnosed by clinical picture along with x-ray, CAT scan, or actual passage of stones. Renal function is best evaluated by a combination of urine and serum studies.

3. evaluate the ability of the bladder to empty urine. 4. evaluate renal function.	Implementation Application Physiological Integrity

27.12 A client is admitted with possible renal calculi. The nurse realizes that the diagnostic test this client might need to help with this health problem is:
    1. intravenous pyelogram.
    2. 24-hour urine.
    3. routine urinalysis.
    4. kidney biopsy.
	Answer: 1
	Rationale: Radiologic examinations include an intravenous pyelogram, a retrograde pyelogram, and a renal arteriogram or angiogram. These examinations are useful in visualizing (via x-ray film) the urinary tract to identify abnormal size, shape, and function of the kidneys, the kidney pelvis, and ureters; and to detect renal calculi, tumors, or cysts. Routine urinalysis and 24-hour urine studies provide information about the volume and content of the urine, but are not diagnostic of calculi. Kidney biopsy provides a microscopic view of the kidney tissue and would not be diagnostic of calculi.
	Planning
	Application
	Physiological Integrity

27.13 During the assessment of a client's urinary system, the nurse learns that the client has painful urination. This finding should be documented as:
    1. dysuria.
    2. hematuria.
    3. oliguria.
    4. polyuria.
	Answer: 1
	Rationale: Painful urination is termed dysuria. Hematuria is the presence of blood in the urine. Oliguria is the term used to describe a urine output less than 400 mL within 24 hours. Polyuria is used to describe high-volume urine output.
	Diagnosis
	Application
	Physiological Integrity

27.14 While auscultating a client's renal arteries, the nurse hears a "whooshing." This finding might be indicative of:
    1. venous stenosis.
    2. acute renal failure.
    3. chronic renal failure.
    4. renal artery stenosis.
	Answer: 4
	Rationale: Auscultate the renal arteries by placing the bell of the stethoscope lightly in the areas of the renal arteries, which are located in the left and right upper abdominal quadrants. Systolic bruits or "whooshing" sounds may indicate renal artery stenosis. Renal failure (acute or chronic) may result from renal artery stenosis, but has multiple other causes and is diagnosed by blood and urine studies, physical exam and potentially renal biopsy. Auscultation of venous blood flow is not possible with a stethoscope.
	Diagnosis
	Application
	Physiological Integrity

27.15 During the assessment of a client's renal system, the nurse is unable to palpate the kidneys. This finding is indicative of:
    1. inflammation.
    2. chronic renal disease.
    3. nothing.
    4. polycystic kidney disease.
	Answer: 3
	Rationale: The kidneys are normally not palpable. The kidneys may or may not be palpable in clients with inflammation, chronic renal disease, and polycystic kidney disease.
	Assessment
	Application
	Physiological Integrity

27.16 The nurse is able to percuss a dull tone over a client's bladder. This finding is suggestive of:
    1. normal.
    2. colon cancer.
    3. pregnancy.
    4. urinary retention.
	Answer: 4
	Rationale: A dull percussion tone over the bladder of a client who has just urinated may indicate urinary retention. Colon cancer and pregnancy would not produce bladder dullness and are best diagnosed by other means such as HCG level (pregnancy) and colonoscopy (colon cancer). A dull tone heard over a bladder in a person who has just voided would not be normal. It would be expected that the bladder would be empty just after voiding.
	Assessment
	Application
	Physiological Integrity

27.17 A 65-year-old female comes into the clinic to be seen for urinary incontinence. The nurse realizes that this symptom can indicate: 1. nothing. This is common with aging.	Answer: 2 Rationale: Urinary incontinence is not a normal sign of aging and therefore should be evaluated further for this client. Incontinence is not indicative of reduced renal blood flow. Multiple causes could contribute to urinary incontinence (including medications), but further evaluation is needed.

2. something else is going on and the client needs to be evaluated. 3. decreased renal blood flow. 4. medications are causing the incontinence.	Planning Analysis Physiological Integrity
27.18 A client is unable to provide a urine specimen for culture. Which of the following can be done to obtain this sterile specimen? 1. Suggest the client wait a few minutes and try again. 2. Give the client a glass of warm water. 3. Instruct the client to obtain the specimen the next morning. 4. Prepare to catheterize the client for the specimen.	Answer: 4 Rationale: If a client is unable to void for a urine culture specimen, it may be necessary to obtain the specimen with a urinary catheterization. Although increasing liquids and waiting may help the client to produce urine, because this is a sterile specimen, catheterization is a good option. Planning Application Physiological Integrity
27.19 Upon a routine urinalysis, a client is found to have +3 ketones in the urine. Which of the following should be done following this finding? 1. Nothing. This is normal. 2. Suggest that the client be tested for diabetes. 3. Schedule a renal ultrasound. 4. Schedule a renal MRI.	Answer: 2 Rationale: +1 to +3 ketones in the urine is suggestive of ketoacidosis, starvation, or a high-protein diet. Renal ultrasound or a renal MRI are useful in detecting structural problems within the kidney; they would not be useful in this case. The presence of +1 to +3 ketones is not normal. Diagnosis Analysis Physiological Integrity
27.20 While conducting the functional health pattern assessment, the nurse would like to assess the client's nutritional-metabolic status in relation to the renal system. Which of the following questions would provide the most information about this status? 1. "Do you ever have swelling in your ankles?" 2. "How many times a day do you urinate?" 3. "Describe your usual energy level." 4. "Do you have any pain or burning when you urinate?"	Answer: 1 Rationale: Questions to assess a client's nutritional-metabolic status within the renal functional health pattern assessment include questions about how much coffee, tea, or alcohol does the client drink in a 24-hour period; has the client ever limited their fluid intake? Ask the client if they limit the amount of salt they eat. Ask the client whether they have swelling in their ankles; if so, what do they do to address the swelling? Urination frequency, energy level, and pain or burning on urination are important assessment points, but do not directly relate to nutritional-metabolic status in relation to renal function. Ask the client to explain each of their answers in order to obtain the most thorough information. Assessment Application Physiological Integrity
27.21 An elderly female client is demonstrating signs of bladder dysfunction. Which of the following are characteristics of age-related bladder changes? (Select all that apply.) 1. decreased blood flow 2. urinary retention more common 3. increase in nocturia 4. increased risk of hyponatremia 5. large amounts of residual urine present after voiding	Answer: 2, 3, 5 Rationale: Age-related bladder changes include urinary retention, frequency, urgency, nocturia, larger amounts of residual urine present after voiding, and some stress incontinence (especially in women who have had several children). Decreased blood flow is not a common cause of age–related bladder changes. Evaluation Analysis Health Promotion and Maintenance
27.22 A client is scheduled for a renal angiogram. Of the following, select the interventions that would be most	Answer: 1, 3, 5 Rationale: Interventions to prepare a client for a renal angiogram include assessing for allergy to iodine, seafood, or other contrast dye from other x-ray

appropriate to prepare this client for the diagnostic test. (Select all that apply.)

1. Keep NPO for 8 to 12 hours before the test.
2. Place on a clear liquid diet.
3. Hold any anticoagulant therapy.
4. Monitor urine output.
5. Provide bowel cleansing preparations.

procedures, provide a laxative or cleansing enema usually the night before, and the client should be NPO for 8–12 hours prior to the test. Anticoagulants should be discontinued.

Implementation
Application
Physiological Integrity

CHAPTER 28

28.1 A married female client has a history of repeated urinary tract infections (UTIs). Which of the following should the nurse include while assessing this client?

1. employment status
2. height and weight
3. activity status
4. preferred method of birth control

Answer: 4
Rationale: Risk factors for urinary tract infections (UTIs) include sexual intercourse, use of diaphragm and spermicidal compounds for birth control, and pregnancy. Employment status, height and weight, and activity status do not have a direct relationship to repeated UTI.

Assessment
Application
Physiological Integrity

28.2 Which one of the following methods of bladder emptying would be preferred for an elderly client who is prone to developing urinary tract infections (UTIs)?

1. intermittent catheterization
2. indwelling urinary catheterization
3. Crede maneuver
4. timed intervals for taking client to bathroom to void

Answer: 1
Rationale: Intermittent catheterization carries a lower risk of infection than an indwelling catheter, and is preferred for clients who are unable to empty their bladder by voiding. The Crede maneuver is a technique used to assist clients with spinal cord injury to empty the bladder. Timed intervals to take the client to void would not be effective if they are not able to empty their bladder by voluntary voiding. The urine would remain in the bladder and be a site for infection to develop.

Planning
Application
Physiological Integrity

28.3 A client is diagnosed with chronic pyelonephritis. The nurse realizes that this client is prone to developing:

1. cystitis.
2. chronic renal failure.
3. acute renal failure.
4. renal calculi.

Answer: 2
Rationale: Chronic pyelonephritis involves chronic inflammation and scarring of the tubules and interstitial tissues of the kidney. It is a common cause of chronic renal failure. Cystitis may cause acute pyelonephritis and acute renal failure. Renal calculi are generally caused by dietary intake and not by chronic pyelonephritis.

Diagnosis
Analysis
Physiological Integrity

28.4 A client with an indwelling urinary catheter is demonstrating signs of asymptomatic bacteriuria. Which of the following would be the best course of action for this client?

1. Begin oral antibiotic therapy for three days.
2. Begin intravenous antibiotic therapy.
3. Remove the catheter and begin antibiotic therapy.
4. Remove the catheter and monitor for continued signs of bacteriuria.

Answer: 3
Rationale: Antibiotics and urinary anti-infectives are not generally recommended to treat asymptomatic bacteriuria in catheterized clients. The preferred treatment for catheter-associated urinary tract infection (UTI) is to remove the indwelling catheter, then administer a 10 to 14 day course of antibiotic therapy to eliminate the infection. Removing the catheter without the initiation of antibiotic therapy would not solve the problem. The infection could worsen.

Planning
Analysis
Physiological Integrity

28.5 A client asks the nurse for ways to prevent recurrent urinary tract infections. Which of the following is an appropriate nursing response?

Answer: 1
Rationale: An appropriate response to this client is to avoid douching. Instruct women to cleanse the perineal area from front to back after voiding and defecating. Teach women to void before and after sexual intercourse to flush out bacteria introduced into the urethra and bladder. Teach measures to maintain the

1. "Avoid douching." 2. "Use feminine hygiene sprays." 3. "Wear clean nylon underpants." 4. "Clean the perineal area from back to front."	integrity of perineal tissues: avoid bubble baths, feminine hygiene sprays, and vaginal douches; wear cotton briefs and avoid synthetic materials such as nylon; if postmenopausal, use hormone replacement therapy or estrogen cream. Implementation Application Health Promotion and Maintenance
28.6 A male client comes into the emergency department with symptoms of renal colic. The nurse realizes that this client most likely has a calculi that is obstructing the: 1. renal pelvis. 2. bladder. 3. ureter. 4. urethra.	Answer: 3 Rationale: Renal colic, which is acute, severe flank pain on the affected side, develops when a stone obstructs the ureter and causes ureteral spasm. Calculi in the bladder, renal pelvis, or urethra would not cause flank pain or colic. Diagnosis Analysis Physiological Integrity
28.7 A male client has a history of calcium calculi. Which of the following medications can be prescribed to help this client? 1. penicillin (Pentids) 2. furosemide (Lasix) 3. allopurinol (Alloprim) 4. NSAIDs	Answer: 2 Rationale: A thiazide diuretic, which is frequently prescribed for calcium calculi, acts to reduce urinary calcium excretion and is very effective in preventing further stones. Furosemide (Lasix) is a thiazide diuretic. Penicillin (Pentids) is an antimicrobial. Allopurinol (Alloprim) is used to reduce serum levels of uric acid. NSAIDs (nonsteroidal anti-inflammatory drugs) are used to reduce pain and fever. Neither penicillin, allopurinol, nor NSAIDs would influence the formation of calcium stones. Planning Analysis Health Promotion and Maintenance
28.8 A male client is admitted for removal of a bladder papilloma. Which of the following should the nurse assess in this client? 1. history of cigarette smoking 2. pedal pulses 3. daily fluid intake 4. appetite level	Answer: 1 Rationale: Carcinogenic breakdown products of certain chemicals and from cigarette smoke are excreted in the urine and stored in the bladder, which possibly causes a local influence on abnormal cell development. Cigarette smoking is the primary risk factor for bladder cancer. The risk in smokers is twice that of non-smokers. Daily fluid intake, pedal pulses, and appetite are all important assessments but these findings would not indicate an increased risk for bladder papilloma. Assessment Application Physiological Integrity
28.9 A client is discharged after photocoagulation for a bladder papilloma. Which of the following should be included in this client's discharge instructions? 1. Make an appointment for follow-up in three years. 2. Make an appointment for follow-up in one year. 3. Make an appointment for follow-up in three months. 4. Make an appointment for follow-up if symptoms return.	Answer: 3 Rationale: Following cystoscopic tumor resection, clients are followed at three-month intervals for tumor recurrence. A follow-up appointment would be needed to evaluate and concerns or issues. Follow-up needs to be timely and one or three years would be too long. The client would be encouraged to make a follow-up appointment at any time if the symptoms occur, no matter what the timeframe. Recurrences may develop anywhere in the urinary tract, including the renal pelvis, ureter, or urethra. Implementation Application Health Promotion and Maintenance
28.10 A client had a renal stent removed. Which of the following should be included in the care of this client? 1. Encourage ambulation. 2. Ensure an adequate protein intake. 3. Monitor blood pressure. 4. Monitor urine output.	Answer: 4 Rationale: Monitor urine output closely for the first 24 hours after stents or ureteral catheters are removed. Edema or stricture of ureters may impede output and lead to hydronephrosis and kidney damage. Ambulation, adequate protein intake, and blood pressure monitoring are all important in the care of this client; however, ensuring that urine output is adequate following stent removal is the highest priority. Implementation Application Physiological Integrity

28.11 A male client with a urinary stoma says, "I looked at it while you were out of the room. It's not so bad." The nurse realizes that this client is demonstrating: 1. anger. 2. denial. 3. grief. 4. coping.	Answer: 4 Rationale: The client may initially use defensive coping mechanisms such as denial, minimization, and dissociation from the immediate situation to reduce anxiety and maintain psychological integrity. Adaptive mechanisms include learning as much as possible about the surgery and its effects, practicing procedures, setting realistic goals, and rehearsing various alternative outcomes. Accepting the stoma as part of the self is vital to adapting to the changed body image and is indicated by a willingness to provide self-care. Grief and anger may also be expressed by the client with a new stoma, but the client's statement demonstrates a coping behavior. Evaluation Analysis Psychosocial Integrity
28.12 A middle-aged male client comes into the clinic for "frequency" and "small amounts of urine at a time." The nurse realizes that this client might be experiencing symptoms of: 1. cystitis. 2. benign prostatic hypertrophy (BPH). 3. renal calculi. 4. bladder cancer.	Answer: 2 Rationale: Benign prostatic hypertrophy (BPH) is a common cause of urinary retention; difficulty initiating and maintaining urine flow is often the presenting complaint in men with BPH. Cystitis symptoms may include frequency but would be coupled with burning, pain during urination, and hematuria. Renal calculi would likely cause flank pain. Bladder cancer symptoms would include hematuria. Assessment Analysis Physiological Integrity
28.13 A female client is admitted with an overdistended bladder. Which of the following diagnostic tests can be done to confirm the diagnosis of urine retention? 1. bladder scan 2. renal scan 3. intravenous pyelography (IVP) 4. MRI	Answer: 1 Rationale: Urinary retention is confirmed using a bladder scan or by inserting a urinary catheter (if possible) and measuring the urine output. Renal scan, intravenous pyelography (IVP), and MRI will provide information about the structure of the kidney and vascular flow in the renal system, but are not the tests of choice in determining urine retention. Planning Application Physiological Integrity
28.14 While being catheterized for urinary retention, the client becomes diaphoretic and pale. Which of the following can be done to help this client? 1. Nothing. This is a normal response. 2. Provide the client with fluids. 3. Clamp the catheter after draining 500 cc of urine. 4. Pull the urinary catheter.	Answer: 3 Rationale: Some clients may experience a vasovagal response and become pale, sweaty, and hypotensive if the bladder is rapidly drained. The vasovagal response is not to be an expected response in each client during catheterization. The nurse should be aware that it is a possible response in some clients and be able to recognize and respond to it. Draining urine in 500 mL increments and clamping the catheter for 5 to 10 minutes between increments may prevent this response. Pulling the catheter or replacing fluids will not address the symptoms. Implementation Application Physiological Integrity
28.15 An elderly client with diabetes is diagnosed with a flaccid bladder. Which of the following should be included in the care of this client? 1. ways to maintain an alkaline urine 2. instruction about the use of anticholinergic medications 3. remind to restrict fluids 4. begin instructing about the Credé method for bladder emptying	Answer: 4 Rationale: The Credé method (applying pressure to the suprapubic region with the fingers of one or both hands), manual pressure on the abdomen, and the Valsalva maneuver (bearing down while holding one's breath) promote bladder emptying for the client with a spastic or flaccid bladder. Altering the pH of the urine, use of anticholinergics, or restricting fluids would not assist the client to adapt to the neurogenic issue that is causing flaccid bladder. Planning Application Physiological Integrity

28.16 A female client is admitted with multiple medical problems and incontinence, regardless of the position or situation. The type of incontinence that this client is most likely experiencing is:
1. urge.
2. stress.
3. total.
4. overflow.

Answer: 3
Rationale: Total incontinence is loss of all voluntary control over urination, and urine loss occurs without stimulus and in all positions. Urge incontinence occurs when the client must void immediately when the urge is perceived. Stress incontinence is the result of coughing or laughing. Overflow incontinence results when the bladder is filled beyond capacity.
Assessment
Analysis
Physiological Integrity

28.17 An 80-year-old female client says to the nurse, "I can't hold my water very well so I don't leave the house much." Which of the following is an appropriate nursing response?
1. "I understand."
2. "This is not something you have to live with. Talk with your doctor about this problem."
3. "I guess it's hard getting older."
4. "Do you get enjoyment out of watching television?"

Answer: 2
Rationale: Although urinary incontinence rarely causes serious physical effects, it frequently has significant psychosocial effects, and can lead to lowered self-esteem, social isolation, and even institutionalization. Inform all clients that urinary incontinence is not a normal consequence of aging and that treatments are available. The nurse must give a response that addresses the problem while being empathetic. Asking the client about their television viewing has no relevance on the issue that has been expressed by the client.
Implementation
Application
Psychosocial Integrity

28.18 A male client needs to increase the acidity of his urine. Which foods should this client increase in his diet?
1. cranberries, grapes, and tomatoes
2. sardines and herring
3. green vegetables and oranges
4. beans, chocolate, and dairy products

Answer: 1
Rationale: Acidifying foods include cheese, cranberries, eggs, grapes, meat and poultry, plums and prunes, tomatoes, and whole grains. Sardines, herrings, oranges, green vegetables, beans, chocolate, and dairy products tend to have an alkaline influence on the urine.
Implementation
Application
Health Promotion and Maintenance

28.19 A client who is recovering from spinal surgery had "an accident" while attempting to reach the bathroom to void. The type of incontinence this client most likely experienced is:
1. urge.
2. stress.
3. functional.
4. total.

Answer: 3
Rationale: Functional incontinence results from physical, environmental, or psychosocial causes. Impaired mobility is one such cause. Urge incontinence occurs when the client must void immediately when the urge is perceived. Stress incontinence is the result of coughing or laughing. Total incontinence is loss of all voluntary control over urination, and urine loss occurs without stimulus and in all positions.
Diagnosis
Analysis
Physiological Integrity

28.20 A client is scheduled for a lithotripsy for renal calculi. The purpose of a bowel preparation prior to this procedure is to:
1. ensure that there is no evidence of constipation prior to the procedure.
2. increase comfort.
3. reduce postoperative pain.
4. ensure maximum visualization of the kidney and the stones.

Answer: 4
Rationale: Fecal material in the bowel may impede fluoroscopic visualization of the kidney and stone. Bowel preparation would not contribute to patient comfort or reducing postoperative pain. Constipation prior to the procedure has no bearing on the procedure if bowel preparation is completed.
Planning
Application
Physiological Integrity

28.21 A client is participating in bladder retraining activities. Of the following, select the toileting activities that can reduce episodes of incontinence. (Select all that apply.)

1. intermittent straight catheterization
2. scheduled toileting
3. habit training
4. external catheter placement at bedtime
5. use of adult incontinence protection devices

Answer: 2, 3

Rationale: Behavioral techniques such as scheduled toileting, habit training, and bladder training are used to reduce the frequency of incontinence. Scheduled toileting is toileting at regular intervals (e.g., every 2 to 4 hours). Habit training is toileting the client on a schedule that corresponds with the normal pattern. Intermittent straight catheterization is not a toileting activity. Use of adult incontinence protection devices does not reduce periods of incontinence.

Implementation
Application
Physiological Integrity

28.22 A client is being instructed on how to perform Kegel exercises. Which of the following should be included in these instructions? (Select all that apply.)

1. These should be performed at least once per day.
2. These should be performed for at least several months.
3. While voiding, stop the flow of urine and hold for a few seconds.
4. Tighten the muscles around the anus to resist defecation.
5. Take a deep breath and hold while performing the exercises.

Answer: 3, 4

Rationale: Kegel exercises should begin by identifying the pelvic muscles with these techniques: stop the flow of urine during voiding and hold for a few seconds, tighten the muscles at the vaginal entrance around a gloved finger or tampon, or tighten the muscles around the anus as though resisting defecation. The client should perform theses exercises by tightening pelvic muscles, holding for 10 seconds, and relaxing for 10 to 15 seconds. The client should keep abdominal muscles and breathing relaxed while performing exercises. The exercises should be performed twice per day and work up to four times a day. Encourage exercising at a specific time each day or in conjunction with another daily activity. It is important to establish a routine because these exercises should be continued for life. Assistive devices, such as vaginal cones and biofeedback, may be useful for clients who have difficulty identifying appropriate muscle groups.

Implementation
Application
Health Promotion and Maintenance

CHAPTER 29

29.1 An elderly client is admitted to the hospital with cardiac complications associated with diabetes. Which of the following concerns should the nurse have regarding this client's medications?

1. What are the costs of the client's medications?
2. Is the client is taking the prescribed dosage?
3. Is the client receiving too much medication because of renal function?
4. What vitamin supplements is this client taking?

Answer: 3

Rationale: Decreased glomerular filtration rate (GFR) in the older adult also reduces the clearance of drugs excreted through the kidneys. This reduced clearance prolongs the half-life of drugs and may necessitate lower drug doses and longer dosing intervals. Common medications affected by decreased GFR include cardiac medications and anti-diabetic agents. Assessing the client's compliance with the prescribed dose is important in any circumstance but is not specific to this scenario. Use of vitamin supplements also requires assessment, but is not specific to the situation described. The cost of the medications might be an issue if it was suspected that the client was not taking their medications. The scenario given indicates that there is a possible complication related to medications that are being taken by the client.

Planning
Analysis
Physiological Integrity

29.2 A client is diagnosed with hypertension caused by polycystic kidney disease. Which of the following might be helpful to control this client's blood pressure?

1. kidney transplant
2. renal dialysis
3. peritoneal dialysis
4. ACE inhibitors

Answer: 4

Rationale: Hypertension associated with polycystic disease is generally controlled using angiotensin-converting enzyme (ACE) inhibitors or other antihypertensive agents. Renal transplant or dialysis is indicated when kidney function cannot control the wastes from metabolic processes.

Planning
Analysis
Physiological Integrity

29.3 Three weeks after being treated for strep throat, a client comes into the clinic with signs of acute glomerulonephritis. Which of the following symptoms will the nurse most likely find upon assessment of this client?
1. periorbital edema
2. hunger
3. polyuria
4. polyphagia

Answer: 1
Rationale: Acute proliferative glomerulonephritis is characterized by an abrupt onset of hematuria, proteinuria, salt and water retention, and evidence of azotemia that occurs 10 to 14 days after the initial infection. The urine often appears brown or cola-colored. Salt and water retention increase extracellular fluid volume, which leads to hypertension and edema. The edema is primarily noted in the face, particularly around the eyes or periorbital edema. Dependent edema, which affects the hands and upper extremities in particular, may also be noted. Other manifestations may include fatigue, anorexia, nausea and vomiting, and headache. Hunger (polyphagia) and polyuria are symptomatic of diabetes mellitus.
Assessment
Application
Physiological Integrity

29.4 The nurse is planning the care of a client with chronic glomerulonephritis. The goal of treatment for this client should include:
1. achieving maximum independence.
2. maintaining renal functioning.
3. returning to work as soon as possible.
4. lifestyle changes.

Answer: 2
Rationale: Management of all types of glomerulonephritis—acute and chronic, primary and secondary—focuses on identifying the underlying disease process and preserving kidney function. In most glomerular disorders, there is no specific treatment to achieve a cure. Treatment goals are to maintain renal function, prevent complications, and support the healing process. Although maintenance of independence, returning to work, and lifestyle adaptation may be included in the plan of care, they are not priorities.
Planning
Application
Physiological Integrity

29.5 Which of the following interventions would be appropriate for a client with *Excess Fluid Volume* related to chronic glomerulonephritis?
1. Document energy level.
2. Schedule activities to conserve energy.
3. Weigh daily on the same scale.
4. Assess for signs of infection.

Answer: 3
Rationale: Weigh daily using a consistent technique (i.e., time of day, scale, and clothing). Accurate daily weights are the best indicator of approximate fluid balance. Energy level and signs of infection do not address the issue of fluid volume excess.
Planning
Application
Physiological Integrity

29.6 A client with chronic kidney disease is diagnosed with hypertension. The nurse realizes that this client's blood pressure needs to be controlled because:
1. blood pressure control can slow the decline of kidney function.
2. it is the easiest diagnosis to treat.
3. there are medications available to treat this disorder.
4. everyone should have low-normal blood pressure.

Answer: 1
Rationale: Management of hypertension to maintain the blood pressure within normal limits is vital to prevent kidney damage. When hypertension is secondary to kidney disease, adequate blood pressure control can slow the decline of renal function. Hypertension is not always easily diagnosed. The goal of having this client's blood pressure under control is directly related to their chronic kidney disease. The idea of everyone having low-normal blood pressure does not apply to this client because of the new diagnosis and history of chronic kidney disease.
Diagnosis
Analysis
Physiological Integrity

29.7 A client who is diagnosed with renal cancer states, "I only lost a few pounds! I had no other symptoms!" The nurse realizes that the only consistent symptom of renal cancer is:
1. nausea.
2. vomiting.
3. hematuria.
4. flank pain.

Answer: 3
Rationale: Renal tumors are often silent and have few manifestations. The classic triad of symptoms, which is gross hematuria, flank pain, and a palpable abdominal mass, is seen in only about 10% of people with renal cell carcinoma. Hematuria, often microscopic, is the most consistent symptom. Systemic manifestations include fever without infection, fatigue, and weight loss. Nausea and vomiting are not frequent symptoms of renal cancer.
Diagnosis
Analysis
Physiological Integrity

29.8 Which of the following should be included when providing instructions to a client who is post-nephrectomy for kidney cancer?
1. ways to limit fluids
2. early recognition of a urinary tract infection (UTI)
3. organ donor information
4. promote high-impact sports and activities

Answer: 2
Rationale: If renal cancer was detected at an early stage and cure is anticipated, teaching should focus on protecting the remaining kidney, including: measures to prevent infection, renal calculi, hydronephrosis, and trauma; maintain a fluid intake of 2000 to 2500 mL per day, and increase the amount during hot weather or strenuous exercise; urinate when the urge is perceived, and before and after sexual intercourse; properly clean the perineal area; manifestations of urinary tract infection (UTI), and the importance of early and appropriate evaluation and intervention; manifestations of prostatic hypertrophy; avoid contact sports such as football or hockey; and measures to prevent motor vehicle accidents and falls, which could damage the kidney.
Planning
Application
Physiological Integrity

29.9 An elderly client is scheduled for a CT scan with and without contrast dye. Which of the following should be done prior to this CT scan?
1. Keep the client NPO.
2. Monitor renal functioning.
3. Assess for level of responsiveness.
4. Assess vital signs.

Answer: 2
Rationale: Common nephrotoxins associated with acute tubular necrosis include the aminoglycoside antibiotics and radiologic contrast media. Many other drugs, heavy metals such as mercury and gold, and some common chemicals such as ethylene glycol (antifreeze) are also potentially toxic to the renal tubule. The risk for acute tubular necrosis is higher when nephrotoxic drugs are given to older clients or clients with preexisting renal insufficiency, and when used in combination with other nephrotoxins. Dehydration increases the risk by increasing the toxin concentration in nephrons. Monitoring responsiveness and vital signs are important assessments, but do not address the specific risks of this examination. The specific location of the body for the CT scan is not indicated, therefore, it is not known if the client would need to be kept NPO prior to the test.
Planning
Analysis
Physiological Integrity

29.10 A client with acute renal failure (ARF) is prescribed furosemide (Lasix). The nurse realizes that this medication will be helpful to the client because:
1. it will reduce edema.
2. it is the gentlest diuretic to use.
3. it will keep sodium in the body.
4. it will preserve protein.

Answer: 1
Rationale: If restoration of renal blood flow does not improve urinary output, a potent loop diuretic such as furosemide (Lasix) or an osmotic diuretic such as mannitol (Osmitrol) may be given with intravenous fluids. The purpose is twofold. First, if nephrotoxins are present, the combination of fluids and potent diuretics may, in effect, "wash out" the nephrons and reduce toxin concentration. Second, establishing urine output may prevent oliguria, and reduce the degree of azotemia and fluid and electrolyte imbalances. Furosemide also may be used to manage salt and water retention associated with acute renal failure (ARF). This type of diuretic helps to eliminate sodium. It does not preserve protein. Medications are not typically described by their "gentleness." Each client's response to a medication can be unique.
Evaluation
Analysis
Physiological Integrity

29.11 A client is scheduled to have an arteriovenous (AV) fistula created for renal dialysis. Which of the following interventions are appropriate for this client? (Select all that apply.)
1. Ensure the use of the dominant hand and arm for placement.
2. Always use the nondominant hand and arm for blood pressure readings.
3. The fistula can be used immediately after its creation.

Answer: 2 and 4
Rationale: The nondominant arm is preferable for fistula placement. A functional arteriovenous (AV) fistula has a palpable pulse and a bruit on auscultation. The arm in which the fistula is placed should not be used for blood pressure reading or for venipuncture and that arm should be marked as not available for these purposes. It takes about a month for the fistula to mature.
Planning
Application
Physiological Integrity

---

4. A functioning fistula has a palpable pulse and bruit. 5. Venipunctures should be performed on the arm with the fistula.	
29.12 A client who is recovering from acute renal failure is being discharged. Which of the following should the nurse include in this client's instructions? 1. Avoid alcohol consumption. 2. Use over-the-counter medications as needed. 3. Resume a normal diet. 4. Instruct to weigh self at least once a week.	Answer: 1 Rationale: Because alcohol can increase the nephrotoxicity of some materials, discourage alcohol ingestion. Additional client teaching needs for home care include avoiding exposure to nephrotoxins, particularly those in over-the-counter products, preventing infection and other major stressors that can slow healing, monitoring weight, blood pressure, and pulse, manifestations of relapse, continuing dietary restrictions, and knowing when to contact the physician. Implementation Application Physiological Integrity
29.13 A client is admitted with signs of chronic renal failure. Which of the following is indicative of metabolic acidosis? 1. low urine output 2. muscle cramps 3. diarrhea 4. Kussmaul's respirations	Answer: 4 Rationale: As renal failure advances, hydrogen-ion excretion and buffer production are impaired, which leads to metabolic acidosis. Respiratory rate and depth increase, as with Kussmaul's respirations, to compensate for metabolic acidosis. Low urine output, muscle cramps, and diarrhea are often associated with chronic renal failure, but the clearest indication of metabolic acidosis is Kussmaul's respirations. Diagnosis Analysis Physiological Integrity
29.14 A client with diabetes and heart disease is diagnosed with chronic renal failure. The nurse realizes that this client should NOT be prescribed which of the following classifications of medications? 1. beta-blockers 2. calcium channel blockers 3. oral antihyperglycemic agents 4. analgesics	Answer: 3 Rationale: Drugs such as meperidine (Demerol), metformin (Glucophage), and other oral antihyperglycemic agents eliminated by the kidney are avoided entirely. Beta-blockers, calcium channel blockers, and analgesics may be used with dosage adjustment. Implementation Application Physiological Integrity
29.15 A client with chronic renal failure is trying to decide between hemodialysis and peritoneal dialysis. Which of the following are advantages of peritoneal dialysis for this client? (Select all that apply.) 1. minimal vascular complications 2. liberal intake of fluids 3. better metabolite elimination 4. lower risk of infection 5. better self-management	Answer: 1, 2, 5 Rationale: Peritoneal dialysis has several advantages over hemodialysis. Heparinization and vascular complications associated with an arteriovenous (AV) fistula are avoided. The clearance of metabolic wastes is slower but more continuous. More liberal intake of fluids and nutrients is often allowed for the client on continuous ambulatory peritoneal dialysis (CAPD). While glucose absorbed from dialysate can increase blood glucose levels in the diabetic, regular insulin can be added to the infusion to manage hyperglycemia. The client on peritoneal dialysis is better able to self-manage the treatment regimen, which reduces feelings of helplessness. The major disadvantages of peritoneal dialysis include less effective metabolite elimination and risk of infection (peritonitis). Peritoneal dialysis may not be effective for overweight clients with no residual kidney function. Serum triglyceride levels increase with peritoneal dialysis. Finally, the presence of an indwelling peritoneal catheter may cause a body image disturbance. Implementation Application Physiological Integrity
29.16 A client who received a kidney transplant 7 years ago is seen for increasing blood pressure and	Answer: 3 Rationale: Chronic rejection may develop months to years following the transplant. The presenting manifestations of chronic rejection—progressive

proteinuria. The nurse realizes that this client is demonstrating signs of:
1. renal artery stenosis.
2. acute kidney rejection.
3. chronic kidney rejection.
4. pyelonephritis.

azotemia, proteinuria, and hypertension—are those of progressive renal failure. Acute rejection most commonly occurs in the weeks that immediately follow transplant. Renal artery stenosis manifests with a bruit over the surgical anastomosis site. Pyelonephritis manifests with abdominal discomfort and low-grade fever.
Diagnosis
Analysis
Physiological Integrity

29.17 Which of the following interventions would be appropriate for a client in renal failure with the diagnosis of *Imbalanced Nutrition: Less than Body Requirements?*
1. Schedule meals for three times each day.
2. Provide mouth care before meals.
3. Provide antiemetics after meals.
4. Weigh once per week.

Answer: 2
Rationale: Interventions for this nursing diagnosis should include monitoring food and nutrient intake as well as episodes of vomiting; weighing daily before breakfast; administering antiemetic agents 30 to 60 minutes before eating; assisting with mouth care prior to meals and at bedtime; serving small meals and provide between-meal snacks; arranging for a dietary consultation; monitoring nutritional status by tracking weight, laboratory values such as serum albumin and BUN, and anthropometric measurements; and administering parenteral nutrition as prescribed.
Planning
Application
Physiological Integrity

29.18 Which of the following should be assessed in an elderly client with age-related renal dysfunction?
1. activity status
2. recreational activities
3. evidence of medication or drug toxicity
4. daily meal pattern

Answer: 3
Rationale: With age-related changes in kidney functioning, there is a decrease in glomerular filtration rate (GFR). This can lead to a decrease in the clearance of drugs, primarily through the kidneys. The nurse should assess this client for drug toxicity. Recreational activities, activity status, and meal patterns may all be influenced by declining renal function; however, the clearance of medications is the priority assessment.
Assessment
Application
Physiological Integrity

29.19 A client is diagnosed with postrenal acute renal failure. The nurse realizes that this type of renal failure can be caused by:
1. enlarged prostate.
2. hypovolemia.
3. sepsis.
4. drug toxicity.

Answer: 1
Rationale: Causes for post renal acute renal failure include calculi, cancer, external compression, prostatic enlargement, strictures, and blood clots. Hypovolemia, sepsis, and drug toxicity would be considered prerenal causes.
Assessment
Analysis
Physiological Integrity

29.20 A client is diagnosed with 45% of normal glomerular filtration. The nurse realizes that this client is experiencing:
1. acute renal failure.
2. renal insufficiency.
3. chronic renal failure.
4. end-stage renal disease.

Answer: 2
Rationale: Renal insufficiency is where the glomerular filtration rate is 20% to 50% of normal. Acute renal failure, chronic renal failure, and end-stage renal disease are not defined by this criteria alone.
Diagnosis
Analysis
Physiological Integrity

CHAPTER 30

30.1 When assessing the adult heart, the nurse expects to hear the following normal heart sounds:
1. S1 then S2.
2. S2 then S3.
3. S3 then S4.
4. S2 then S1.

Answer: 1
Rationale: The normal sequence of heart sounds is S1, then S2. S3 and S4 are considered abnormal heart sounds in adults.
Assessment
Application
Physiological Integrity

30.2 The S1 heart sound corresponds to which of the following physiological events? 　1.　closure of the semilunar valves 　2.　ejection of blood from the atria 　3.　closure of the AV valves 　4.　the onset of relaxation	Answer: 3 Rationale: S1 corresponds to the closure of the AV valves. Closure of the semilunar valves corresponds to S2. Valves produce heart sounds, not ejection of blood or relaxation of the muscle. Assessment Application Physiological Integrity
30.3 The nurse listens to adult heart sounds and expects to hear _____ beats per minute when a normal sinus rhythm is present. 　1.　30-60 　2.　60-90 　3.　100-130 　4.　130-160	Answer: 2 Rationale: The normal range expected for a normal sinus rhythm is 60-100 beats per minute. While rate is only one determinant of how the ECG rhythm is named, it is important to be able to select a heart rate in the normal range. A rate of 30-60 is bradycardia, while a rate greater than 100 is considered tachycardia. Assessment Application Physiological Integrity
30.4 The client is admitted to the hospital for evaluation and diagnosis of cardiovascular pathology. The client is scheduled for an ejection fraction study. Correct facts that will guide client teaching include: (Select all that apply.) 　1.　an ejection fraction (EF) study will measure the percentage of total blood in the ventricle ejected from the heart with each beat. 　2.　an ejection fraction (EF) provides information about how effectively the heart is pumping. 　3.　the normal ejection fraction is 95-100%. 　4.　stroke volume times heart rate equals cardiac output.	Answer: 1, 2, 4 Rationale: Correct facts that will guide teaching include: an ejection fraction (EF) study will measure the percentage of total blood in the ventricle ejected from the heart with each beat; an EF provides information about how effectively the heart is pumping; and stroke volume times heart rate equals cardiac output. Normal ejection fraction is 50-70%. Implementation Synthesis Health Promotion and Maintenance
30.5 When the nurse assesses an apical heart rate and hears _____, it is called tachycardia. 　1.　less than 60 beats per minute 　2.　60-90 beats per minute 　3.　greater than 100 beats per minute 　4.　90 beats per minute	Answer: 3 Rationale: The normal heart rate range is 60-100 beats per minute. A heart rate that is greater than 100 beats per minute is called tachycardia. A heart rate that is less than 60 beats per minute is called bradycardia. A heart rate that is between 60-90 beats per minute would be considered within the normal range. Analysis Application Physiological Integrity
30.6 When the nurse assesses apical heart rate and hears _____, it is called bradycardia. 　1.　less than 60 beats per minute 　2.　60-90 beats per minute 　3.　greater than 100 beats per minute 　4.　greater than 150 beats per minute	Answer: 1 Rationale: The normal heart rate range is 60-100 beats per minute. A heart rate that is less than 60 beats per minute is called bradycardia. A heart rate that is greater than 100 beats per minute is called tachycardia. Analysis Application Physiological Integrity
30.7 At which location will S1 be heard the loudest? 　1.　left sternal border at the fifth intercostal space	Answer: 2 Rationale: S1 is the sound produced by the atrioventricular (AV) valves closing. The apex of the heart is located lower on the left chest wall than the base of the heart. The loudest sounds can be heard over the apex of the heart. The sound is

2. left midclavicular line at the fifth intercostal space 3. right sternal border at the third intercostal space 4. right midclavicular line at the fifth intercostal space	audible at the left sternal boarder, but would not be as loud. This sound would not normally be audible on the right midclavicular line at the fifth intercostal space, not at the right sternal border. Assessment Application Physiological Integrity
30.8 At what location will S2 be heard the loudest? 1. left sternal border at the fifth intercostal space 2. left midclavicular line at the fifth intercostal space 3. right midclavicular line at the third intercostal space 4. right sternal border at the second intercostal space	Answer: 4 Rationale: S2 is the sound produced by the closure of the aortic and pulmonic valves, and is best heard at the base of the heart, which is at the second intercostal space at the right sternal border. S1 is best heard at the left fifth intercostal space. The right midclavicular line at the third intercostal space is not optimal for auscultating heart sounds. The base of the heart is actually located higher on the chest wall than the apex. Assessment Application Physiological Integrity
30.9 In the client with hypovolemic shock, the nurse realizes that the heart sounds will change in the which of the following ways? 1. diminished S1 and S2 2. accentuated S2 and diminished S1 3. diminished S2 and accentuated S1 4. no change in S1 or S2	Answer: 3 Rationale: Diminished S2 occurs due to a fall in blood pressure and accentuated S1 occurs because of the tachycardia. The three earliest signs of hypovolemic shock are tachycardia, delayed capillary refill, and restlessness. Analysis Synthesis Physiological Integrity
30.10 When listening to heart sounds, the nurse expects to hear S1 and S2. The presence of an additional sound immediately following S2 is called _____, which can result from _____. 1. S4, increased resistance to ventricular filling 2. S3, ventricular volume overload 3. S4, inflammation of the pericardial sac 4. S3, a stenotic mitral valve	Answer: 2 Rationale: S3 is an abnormal (pathologic) heart sound heard immediately following S2 in adults. It is often called a ventricular gallop and results from conditions such as congestive heart failure (CHF), mitral valve regurgitation, or tricuspid valve regurgitation. S4 immediately precedes S1 and can result from conditions such as anemia or a change in ventricular compliance. Analysis Synthesis Physiological Integrity
30.11 The nurse is caring for a client admitted with a grade III heart murmur heard during midsystole. The nurse realizes that the following cardiac conditions could result in this assessment finding: (Select all that apply.) 1. atrioventricular (AV) valve disease 2. mitral valve prolapse 3. aortic stenosis 4. cardiomyopathy	Answer: 3 and 4 Rationale: Midsystolic murmurs are associated with semilunar valve and hypertrophic cardiomyopathies. A grade III murmur can be heard clearly and can be categorized as systolic (between S1 and S2), diastolic (between S2 and S1), pansystolic (all of systole), or continuous (heard throughout systole and all or part of diastole). Murmurs associated with atrioventricular (AV) valve disease or mitral valve prolapse would more often be heard during early or mid-diastole. Analysis Synthesis Physiological Integrity
30.12 The client's ECG shows the following characteristics: PR interval .08, QRS .08, and isoelectric ST segment. The nurse realizes that these characteristics indicate:	Answer: 3 Rationale: Application of the normal ECG measurements helps the nurse interpret an ECG and identify if normal conduction is present. Rhythms will be named based on measurements taken from the ECG. ECG waveforms reflect the direction of electrical flow in relation to a positive electrode. Current flowing

1. normal conduction from the SA node to the ventricles, normal conduction through the ventricles, and normal ST segment.
2. faster than normal conduction from the SA node to the ventricles, faster than normal conduction through the ventricles, and normal ST segment.
3. faster than normal conduction from the SA node to the ventricles, normal conduction through the ventricles, and normal ST segment.
4. normal conduction from the SA node to the ventricles, normal conduction through the ventricles, and abnormal ST segment.

toward the positive electrode produces an upward (positive) waveform; current flowing away from the positive electrode produces a downward (negative) waveform. Current flowing perpendicular to the positive pole produces a biphasic (both positive and negative) waveform. Absence of electrical activity is represented by a straight line called the isoelectric line. The PR interval is normally 0.12 to 0.20 second (up to 0.24 second is considered normal in clients over age 65). PR intervals greater than 0.20 second indicate a delay in conduction from the SA node to the ventricles. The normal duration of a QRS complex is from 0.06 to 0.10 second. QRS complexes greater than 0.10 second indicate delays in transmitting the impulse through the ventricular conduction system. The ST segment, the period from the end of the QRS complex to the beginning of the T wave, should be isoelectric. An abnormal ST segment is displaced (elevated or depressed) from the isoelectric line.
Analysis
Application
Physiological Integrity

30.13 The client is having a treadmill test. Which of the following is an important teaching point?
1. A patient gown and slippers should be worn for the test.
2. Smoking is permitted up until the time of the test.
3. There are no restrictions prior to the test in the foods eaten as long as small meals are planned the day of the test.
4. Comfortable clothing and shoes should be worn for the test.

Answer: 4
Rationale: Client teaching is based on understanding how the test will be conducted. Comfortable and safe clothing is essential for this test. Slippers may not be safe, secure shoes for walking during this test as speed is increased. The patient may be more comfortable in exercise clothing instead of a patient gown. Smoking is discouraged prior to the testing. The diet may be restrictive regarding the amount and types of foods allowed in order to prevent nausea and oxygen deprivation to the cardiac muscle.
Implementation
Application
Physiological Integrity

30.14 The client is being evaluated for left atrium thrombus due to a dysrhythmia (altered heart rhythm). Which of the following common cardiac tests will be ordered to assess for thrombus? (Select all that apply.)
1. pericardiocentesis
2. cardiac catheterization
3. computed tomography (CT)
4. transesophageal echocardiography (TEE)

Answer: 4
Rationale: Transesophageal echocardiography (TEE) allows visualization of: adjacent cardiac and extracardiac structures, left atrium for thrombus, dissection of the aorta, endocarditis, left ventricle function, and repairs being made during cardiac surgery. Pericardiocentesis is a procedure to remove fluid from the pericardial sac. Cardiac catheterization is used to identify coronary artery disease (CAD) or valve disease, measure pulmonary artery or heart chamber pressures, obtain a biopsy, evaluate artificial valves, or to angioplasty or stent an area in the coronary arteries. A computed tomography (CT) scan can show calcium deposits in coronary arteries. For this client, the TEE test can assess for left atrial thrombi and is an expected test.
Analysis
Synthesis
Physiological Integrity

30.15 Place the following statements regarding cardiac catheterization in the correct order.
1. Inject contrast.
2. Heart activity is filmed.
3. Thread catheter to heart chamber.
4. Catheter insertion in the leg.
5. Peripheral IV insertion.

Answer: 5,4,3,1,2
Rationale: A peripheral IV is started before the procedure so that IV access is available for emergency drugs that may be needed. The catheter is then inserted in the leg, then threaded to the heart chamber. The contrast is then injected, and the heart activity is filmed.
Implementation
Synthesis
Physiological Integrity

30.16 Pericardiocentesis would be utilized in which of the following client situations?
  1. chest pain
  2. slow heart rhythm
  3. cardiac tamponade
  4. suspected damage to a heart valve

Answer: 3
Rationale: In the case of cardiac tamponade, this procedure would be considered an emergency procedure. The procedure would be used to remove fluid from the pericardial sac, which is preventing the heart from effectively pumping blood. This procedure would not be recommended in clients with chest pain, slow heart rhythm, or with suspected damage to a heart valve.
Analysis
Application
Physiological Integrity

30.17 An older adult is being evaluated for age-related cardiac changes. Common age-related changes include which of the following? (Select all that apply.)
  1. decreased cardiac output
  2. increased cardiac output
  3. increased blood pressure
  4. decreased stroke volume

Answer: 1, 3
Rationale: Decreased cardiac output occurs with aging under physiologic stress due to decreased myocardial efficiency and contractility. In the aging heart, stroke volume may increase (not decrease) in order to compensate for tachycardia and can lead to increased blood pressure.
Assessment
Application
Physiological Integrity

30.18 The client is being interviewed by the nurse. Which functional health pattern is related to asking the client if they have had tests to check the function of their heart?
  1. cognitive-perceptual
  2. health perception-health management
  3. nutritional-metabolic
  4. activity-exercise

Answer: 2
Rationale: Functional health patterns can be used to guide interview questions. The category of health perception-health management assists the nurse to gather information about past heart problems, treatments for problems, previous diagnoses, previous tests and findings, and medications the client has been prescribed. The cognitive-perceptual pattern refers to the client's ability to understand and process information. The nutritional-metabolic pattern assesses intake patterns. The activity-exercise pattern refers to the client's level of physical activity.
Assessment
Application
Physiological Integrity

30.19 An important nutritional-metabolic interview question to ask clients who are being evaluated for heart conditions is:
  1. "Have you had a recent weight gain or loss?"
  2. "Is there any change in your usual bowel elimination?"
  3. "Has there been a change in your usual daily activities?"
  4. "Have you experienced chest pain in the last week?"

Answer: 1
Rationale: Weight gain can be linked to abnormal retention of fluids, which can affect heart function. Weight loss can be linked to level of nutrition or dehydration. The nutritional-metabolic functional health pattern guides questions that are related to weight gain or loss. Questions regarding elimination, daily activity, and chest pain are all important questions to ask but are categorized under other functional health patterns.
Assessment
Synthesis
Physiological Integrity

30.20 A common lab test related to heart assessment is a lipid profile. Which of the following statements is true regarding this test?
  1. A normal triglyceride level is 40–190 mg/dl.
  2. LDL is measured and should be over 130 mg/dl.
  3. Cholesterol must be checked, and fasting and normal values are 140–200 mg/dl.
  4. HDL is not part of this test.

Answer: 1
Rationale: A normal triglyceride level is 40–190 mg/dl. LDL should be under 130 mg/dl (not over). HDL is measured with a lipid profile and should be 37–70 mg/dl for men or 40–88 mg/dl for women. Cholesterol, when measured alone, does not need to be done after fasting. The normal cholesterol range is 140–200 mg/dl. In order to measure triglycerides and lipoproteins (HDL and LDL), the client must be fasting for 12 hours.
Analysis
Application
Physiological Integrity

31.1 The following clients come to the clinic for a physical exam. Which client has signs and symptoms of hypertension that require further assessment?
1. a 55-year-old African American male with a blood pressure of 120/100
2. a 30-year-old Hispanic female with a blood pressure of 118/70
3. a 60-year-old African American female with a blood pressure of 118/60
4. a 48-year-old Caucasian male with a blood pressure of 124/80

Answer: 1
Rationale: African Americans have a higher prevalence of hypertension. Hypertension affects about one-third of Americans over 50. Consistent blood pressure readings greater than 140 mmHg systolic or 90 mmHg diastolic define hypertension. The other clients had systolic and diastolic blood pressure readings that are considered below the hypertension levels.
Planning
Synthesis
Physiological Integrity

31.2 Cardiovascular heart disease (CHD) is a large problem in the United States. Clients with which of the following may require closer evaluation for CHD? (Select all that apply.)
1. diabetes
2. hyperlipidemia
3. hypotension
4. positive family history

Answer: 1, 2, 4
Rationale: Diabetes and hyperlipidemia are both disease conditions that contribute to coronary heart disease (CHD). Positive family history in some cases is considered a nonmodifiable risk factor for CHD. Hypotension is not associated with development of CHD.
Assessment
Application
Physiological Integrity

31.3 A nurse is conducting teaching about risk factor management for cardiovascular heart disease at a senior center. The most important information for the nurse to include is to:
1. stop smoking.
2. eat in moderation.
3. exercise when able.
4. reduce saturated fats in the diet.

Answer: 1
Rationale: Cigarette smoking is the leading independent risk factor for coronary heart disease. The answers related to diet are not specific enough. Exercise needs to be regular.
Implementation
Synthesis
Health Promotion and Health Maintenance

31.4 The client asks the nurse about metabolic syndrome. The most accurate answer for the nurse to provide is:
1. "This syndrome is not a concern for females unless they smoke."
2. "This syndrome is caused by obesity, physical inactivity, and genetic factors."
3. "This syndrome can be avoided by taking daily vitamins and drinking 64 fluid ounces of water a day."
4. "This syndrome affects only older adults beyond the age of 65."

Answer: 2
Rationale: Metabolic syndrome is caused by obesity, physical inactivity, and genetic factors. The syndrome is not directly related to smoking and age. Daily vitamin and fluid consumption have not been found to alter the syndrome.
Implementation
Application
Health Promotion and Health Maintenance:

31.5 Drugs used to treat hyperlipidemia:
1. act by increasing the LDL levels and decreasing the HDL levels.
2. include lovastatin (Mevacor), which acts by lowering LDL levels.
3. do not include angiotensin-converting enzyme inhibitors.
4. include bile acid sequestrants as first-line drugs to lower cholesterol levels.

Answer: 2
Rationale: The statin drugs specifically lower LDL. Hyperlipidemia drugs are meant to lower LDL and raise HDL, not the opposite. Angiotensin-converting enzyme (ACE) inhibitors are appropriate to add to drug treatment for high-risk clients. Bile acid sequestrant drugs are not the first-line drugs but may be added to statins when combination treatment is needed.
Evaluation
Application
Physiological Integrity

31.6 A client on the Pritikin Diet is eating foods high in complex carbohydrates and fiber, low in cholesterol, and low in fat. The program also includes: 1. exercising three times a week for 30 minutes and eating high-protein red meats. 2. supervised exercise twice a week and a daily multivitamin. 3. aerobic exercise daily for 30 minutes and only organic foods. 4. walking 45 minutes daily and vitamin supplements including vitamins C, E, and folate.	Answer: 4 Rationale: The Pritikin Diet program incorporates walking each day for 45 minutes and taking a vitamin that includes supplements of C, E, and folate. This diet is not limited to organic foods only. Assessment Application Health Promotion and Health Maintenance
31.7 A client who is taking atorvastatin (Lipitor) should be monitored for: 1. blood glucose and uric acid levels. 2. constipation and sudden back pain. 3. serum cholesterol and liver enzymes. 4. renal function.	Answer: 3 Rationale: The nurse should be observing lab work for the current cholesterol level and to ensure that liver enzymes remain normal. Blood glucose, uric acid level, renal function, constipation, and sudden back pain are generally not associated with the use of this drug. Analysis Application Physiological Integrity
31.8 The nurse is assessing a client who presents with chest pain. The client has been previously diagnosed with chest pain and now reports an increase in the frequency and duration of the chest pain. Appropriate nursing care for this type of chest pain includes: 1. bed rest with bathroom privileges. 2. aspirin 325 mg a day per physician order. 3. Pepto Bismol 30 cc prn. 4. atropine (Atropair) 0.4 mg IVP.	Answer: 2 Rationale: Aspirin is considered helpful due to the antiplatelet effects. Bed rest with bathroom privileges would not necessarily be indicated in this situation. Pepto Bismol is used to treat heartburn or upset stomach. Atropine (Atropair) is used to dry secretions and stimulate cardiac function, not for chest pain. Planning Application Physiological Integrity
31.9 A 52-year-old obese male client who is admitted with elevated triglycerides and a history of smoking two packs of cigarettes a day for 20 years: 1. is not at risk for coronary artery disease. 2. is at risk for coronary artery disease. 3. possesses all nonmodifiable risk factors for coronary artery disease that cannot be overcome. 4. possesses all modifiable risk factors for coronary artery disease that can be overcome.	Answer: 2 Rationale: Age is a nonmodifiable risk factor and obesity, elevated triglycerides, and smoking are modifiable risk factors. Together the risk factors place the client at higher risk to develop coronary artery disease. Analysis Synthesis Physiological Integrity
31.10 The nurse is caring for an adult client who is admitted with chest pain that began four hours ago. Which of the following tests will be most specific in identifying acute heart damage?	Answer: 3 Rationale: Troponin is primarily located in cardiac muscle and can indicate myocardial infarction or unstable angina. Troponin elevates at 2 to 4 hours after a myocardial infarction. CPK and CK-MB will elevate with myocardial damage, but will take longer to rise and are not as specific as troponin. Cholesterol level is not helpful in diagnosis of myocardial damage.

1. CPK 2. CK-MB 3. troponin 4. cholesterol	Analysis Application Physiological Integrity

31.11 When a client's ECG shows frequent premature ventricular contractions (PVCs), the nurse expects that the physician will create an order for: (Select all that apply.)
    1. oxygen.
    2. beta-blockers.
    3. antidysrhythmic agents.
    4. isoproterenol (Isuprel).
	Answer: 1, 2, 3
	Rationale: Physician orders for oxygen, beta-blockers, and antidysrhythmic agents are all expected for a client whose ECG shows frequent premature ventricular contractions (PVCs). Isoproterenol (Isuprel) is not needed at this time since the client's blood pressure is not mentioned, just the abnormal heart rhythm.
	Planning
	Application
	Physiological Integrity

31.12 The nurse realizes that the client in the critical care unit with ventricular tachycardia will require which of the following? (Select all that apply.)
    1. immediate assessment and probable emergency intervention by the nurse
    2. close observation for one hour prior to calling the physician
    3. defibrillation to convert the rhythm in the awake client
    4. cardioversion, if sustained and symptomatic
	Answer: 1, 4
	Rationale: The nurse should immediately assess the client to see how the potentially life-threatening rhythm is being tolerated. The nurse should be prepared to cardiovert the client in ventricular tachycardia with a pulse according to standing orders. The nurse in critical care needs to be aware of standing orders for each client prior to an emergent event and needs to have the necessary emergency equipment nearby. Observation prior to calling a physician is not an appropriate action when a potentially life-threatening rhythm is identified. Defibrillation is only conducted in ventricular tachycardia when the client is pulseless; otherwise, time is taken to synchronize for cardioversion.
	Implementation
	Synthesis
	Physiological Integrity

31.13 The priority of care for a client with a junctional escape rhythm is:
    1. eliminate caffeine from the diet.
    2. assess the client for symptoms associated with the rhythm.
    3. prepare for a pacemaker insertion.
    4. contact the physician immediately for emergency orders.
	Answer: 2
	Rationale: Junctional escape rhythms may be monitored if the client is not symptomatic. It is most important to assess the client to see how they are affected by the rhythm. Then, calling the physician to report the rhythm may be appropriate. Eliminating caffeine or preparing for a pacemaker insertion are not appropriate actions for this client with a junctional escape rhythm. No indication of symptoms relating to the rhythm were given.
	Analysis and Planning
	Synthesis
	Physiological Integrity

31.14 The nurse is caring for a client who develops atrial fibrillation with a heart rate above 100 beats per minute. Place the following nursing actions in sequence from the highest priority to the lowest priority.
    1. Check the patency of an intermittent IV.
    2. Assess the client for comfort level and vital signs.
    3. Call the physician to report the dysrhythmia.
    4. Check the client's chart for lab results from today's tests.
	Answer: 2, 1, 4, 3
	Rationale: Assess the client first. Check the patency of the IV in case it is needed for anticipated medication orders. Check for lab results prior to calling the physician because the nurse will be asked the results of lab tests today before orders are given.
	Implementation
	Synthesis
	Physiological Integrity

31.15 Sinus bradycardia (rate 56) is identified in a sleeping client on telemetry. The nurse realizes that the priority is to: 1. call the physician and report the dysrhythmia.	Answer: 3 Rationale: The priority is to awaken the patient to determine how the heart rate is affected with activity. Normally the heart rate should increase when the client is awakened. The client should also be evaluated to determine how the dysrhythmia is affecting heart function. Many clients who are asymptomatic while in sinus bradycardia heart rhythm will be observed and not have any

2. check the medication administration record to see if a drug is ordered prn that will help slow the heart rate. 3. awaken the client and see how the heart rate responds. 4. call for an immediate 12-lead EKG.	further intervention. Common reasons for sinus bradycardia that should be considered by the nurse include: athletic conditioning, a conduction disorder, or sleep. Notifying the physician without assessing a patient response would not be appropriate. Ordering an EKG would require a physician's order first. Planning Application Physiological Integrity
31.16 A client is in sinus tachycardia. The nurse realizes that the needed interventions are to: (Select all that apply.) 1. observe the client for effects on cardiac function. 2. administer two tablets of acetaminophen (Tylenol) per physician order if an elevated temperature is present. 3. administer normal saline 0.9% IV at the ordered rate of 200 ml per hour if hypovolemia is suspected as the cause. 4. administer atropine (Atropair) IV push to halt the tachycardia.	Answer: 1, 2, 3 Rationale: Appropriate nursing interventions for a client who is in sinus tachycardia is observe the client for effects on cardiac function; administer two tablets of acetaminophen (Tylenol) per physician order if elevated temperature is present; and administer normal saline 0.9% IV at the ordered rate of 200 ml per hour if hypovolemia is suspected as the cause. Care is focused on determining how the client tolerates the elevated heart rate and treating underlying causes. Two common underlying causes are fever and hypovolemia. Atropine (Atropair) is indicated in the treatment of a heart rate that is too slow (not too fast) and administration would worsen tachycardia. Implementation Synthesis Physiological Integrity
31.17 The nurse notes an ECG rhythm with a rate of 80, a regular rhythm, a 1:1 relationship of P:QRS, a PR interval of 0.16, and a QRS complex measurement of 0.8. The nurse realizes that this rhythm is evidence of: 1. sinus tachycardia. 2. sinus bradycardia. 3. normal sinus rhythm. 4. ventricular rhythm.	Answer: 3 Rationale: The criteria listed all meet the normal ranges and therefore the rhythm as described is a normal sinus rhythm. Sinus tachycardia would have a rate of greater than 100 and sinus bradycardia would have a rate of less than 60. The parameters do not reflect a ventricular rhythm. Analysis Synthesis Physiological Integrity
31.18 The client has a pacemaker that creates a pacer spike before each QRS on the ECG when the intrinsic heart rate falls below 70. The nurse realizes that this is: 1. normal, because the demand pacemaker is responding to the heart rate drop at the preset level. 2. abnormal, because the demand pacemaker is not effectively pacing both the atria and ventricle. 3. abnormal, because the asynchronous pacemaker is not functioning as designed. 4. normal, because the asynchronous pacemaker is responding to the heart rate change as designed.	Answer: 1 Rationale: A demand pacemaker is set to begin firing at an intrinsic heart rate that is determined to be the lowest acceptable rate. The pacemaker is preset by the physician. An asynchronous pacemaker delivers a pacing stimulus at a set rate and does not respond to the client's intrinsic heart rate. The pacer spike shows up before the QRS interval on an ECG strip. Analysis Synthesis Physiological Integrity
31.19 The term *pacemaker noncapture* requires the nurse to do the following: (Select all that apply.)	Answer: 2, 3, 4 Rationale: Administering nitroglycerin would not be indicated for a pacemaker malfunction. Administration of nitroglycerin is used to treat chest pain according

1. Administer nitroglycerin sublingual stat times one dose from standing orders.
2. Contact the physician and describe what is documented on the ECG strip.
3. Assess the client to determine their response to the pacemaker noncapture.
4. Document the event by printing an ECG strip and making it part of the client's record.

to physician orders. Actions that the nurse should take when noncapture exists include: contact the physician and describe what is documented on the ECG strip; assess the client to determine their response to the pacemaker noncapture; and document the event by printing an ECG strip and making it part of the client's record. Pacemaker noncapture can indicate the pacemaker output is set too low, a pacemaker lead is broken, the pacemaker battery is low, or a high-pacing threshold exists.
Implementation
Synthesis
Physiological Integrity

31.20 The client has a pacemaker with one pacing spike seen on the ECG before every QRS complex. There is no change in the pacemaker rhythm over time, with rest or with activity. The nurse realizes that this means that the type of pacemaker is:
1. demand pacing.
2. dual-chamber pacing.
3. atrial single-chamber pacing.
4. asynchronous pacing.

Answer: 4
Rationale: Considerations when determining the type of pacemaker include the pacing spike frequency noted on the ECG, the location within each complex, and whether it is fixed or intermittent. An asynchronous pacemaker produces the description provided. A demand pacemaker spike varies with the heart rate. A dual-chamber pacer normally produces two pacing spikes; one before the P wave and one before the QRS. An atrial pacer would produce a spike, normally with a P wave that follows it prior to the QRS.
Analysis
Synthesis
Physiological Integrity

CHAPTER 32

32.1 The nurse is assessing a client with chronic heart failure. What type of abnormal sounds would the nurse most likely auscultate?
1. expiratory wheezes
2. friction rub
3. harsh vesicular
4. crackles

Answer: 4
Rationale: Fluid accumulates in the alveolar spaces with left-sided heart failure. This fluid causes the crackle sound at the end of inspiration. Expiratory wheezes, friction rub, and harsh vesicular sounds are not associated with chronic heart failure.
Assessment
Synthesis
Physiological Integrity

32.2 When caring for a chronic heart failure client with left-sided failure, the nurse would most likely hear which of the following statements from the physician after a cardiac catheterization?
1. "Pressures in the left ventricle and atrium are increased."
2. "Pressures in the left ventricle and atrium are decreased."
3. "Pressures in the right ventricle and atrium match the left ventricle pressures."
4. "Pressures in the right ventricle are reflective of how both sides of the heart are functioning."

Answer: 1
Rationale: As the heart loses its ability to eject blood effectively from the left ventricle upon contraction, blood is retained in the left ventricle after systole and the chamber pressure rises due to the additional fluid. This client is in left-sided heart failure, so pressure is higher in the left side of the heart, not the right side.
Analysis
Application
Physiological Integrity

32.3 Two signs that are indicative of heart failure are:
1. S1, S2 and flat neck veins.
2. S3 and distended neck veins.
3. S2 is heard the loudest and followed by S1.
4. S5 and flat neck veins.

Answer: 2
Rationale: The abnormal S3 sound is reflective of the heart's attempts to fill an already distended ventricle. Neck veins distend because of the increased venous pressure. S1 and S2 are normal heart sounds. Flat neck veins are considered a normal finding.
Analysis
Application
Physiological Integrity

32.4 When obtaining the health history of a client who is being assessed for possible congestive heart failure, it is significant when the client says:
1. "I break out into a cold sweat when I eat a large meal."
2. "I am sleepy after I eat lunch each day."
3. "I have to prop myself up on three pillows to sleep at night. I cannot breathe otherwise."
4. "I feel better with my legs down when I sit up in my favorite chair."

Answer: 3
Rationale: Needing to prop oneself up with pillows at night in order to breathe describes orthopnea, which is consistent with congestive heart failure (CHF). Congestive heart failure produces a volume excess, congestion in the lungs, and dyspnea when trying to lie down. Diaphoresis and sleepiness after meals and comfort when legs are dependent are all notable findings, but are not related to a diagnosis of CHF.
Assessment
Synthesis
Physiological Integrity

32.5 A client is admitted with acute heart failure. The nurse realizes that acute heart failure is associated with an abrupt onset of:
(Select all that apply.)
1. cardiomyopathy.
2. heart valve disease.
3. coronary heart disease (CHD).
4. myocardial infarction (MI).

Answer: 4
Rationale: Clients often present for care with signs of acute heart failure when they have had a myocardial infarction (MI). Cardiomyopathy, valve disease, and coronary heart disease (CHD) are all associated with chronic heart failure.
Assessment
Application
Physiological Integrity

32.6 Blood tests are ordered for a client who is diagnosed with possible congestive heart failure (CHF). The most specific test to most accurately indicate CHF is:
1. liver function.
2. urinalysis and blood urea nitrogen (BUN).
3. atrial natriuretic factor (ANF).
4. serum electrolytes.

Answer: 3
Rationale: While liver function, urinalysis, blood urea nitrogen (BUN), and serum electrolytes are appropriate tests for this diagnosis, atrial natriuretic factor (ANF) provides the strongest indicator because it measures the hormones released by the heart muscle in response to changes in blood volume.
Analysis
Synthesis
Physiological Integrity

32.7 The nurse is caring for a client who now has invasive hemodynamic monitoring. The highest priority of care for this client is:
1. prevent infection at the catheter site by changing the dressing as ordered.
2. set alarm limits and turn monitor alarms on.
3. explain to family members why the monitoring is in use.
4. coil IV tubing on the bed.

Answer: 2
Rationale: Alarms are safety devices that warn of a disconnected line or hemodynamic instability. Alarms should always be investigated by the nursing staff. To keep clients safe, only suspend alarms when drawing blood or changing tubing and never turn alarms off. Prevention of infection by managing the dressing is important, but is not the priority of care. Keeping the family involved by explaining the use of the alarms is important, but is not the priority of care. Coiling the IV tubing around the bed is contraindicated.
Implementation
Synthesis
Safe, Effective Care Environment

32.8 The client in critical care has an invasive hemodynamic pressure monitoring line. The appropriate landmark to use when calibrating and leveling hemodynamic monitoring equipment is:
1. the second intercostal space, right sternal border.
2. the right atrial position at the fourth intercostal space, midaxillary line.
3. the left ventricular position at the third intercostal space, midclavicular line.

Answer: 2
Rationale: Calibration and leveling should be done every shift to ensure that accurate pressures are recorded. The right atrial position should be marked on the chest wall so that all caregivers use a consistent reference point for calibrating and leveling. The pressure monitoring is done within the right atrium, not the left atrium or outside of the heart.
Planning
Application
Safe, Effective Care Environment

4. the second intercostal space, left sternal border.	
32.9 The nurse is caring for an ICU client whose fluid volume status needs to be closely watched. The most likely type of monitoring that will be used is: 1. arterial pressure monitoring. 2. pulmonary artery pressure monitoring. 3. central venous pressure monitoring. 4. intra-aortic balloon pump monitoring.	Answer: 3 Rationale: Central venous pressure (CVP) monitoring can be accomplished with a central IV line and an IV pump or a monitoring system. It would be the least complicated method to monitor fluid status. If the client is acutely ill with a cardiac condition, then CVP can be obtained from a pulmonary artery pressure monitoring system as well. Arterial pressure monitoring would not be indicative of only venous pressure. An intra-aortic balloon pump would not be used for pressure monitoring. Implementation Synthesis Physiological Integrity
32.10 A pulmonary artery (PA) catheter is used in critical care clients who: 1. cannot tolerate hemodynamic monitoring. 2. require a peripheral intravenous catheter for medication administration. 3. would benefit from having the right ventricle pressures measured every shift. 4. require evaluation of left ventricular pressures through pulmonary artery wedge pressure readings.	Answer: 4 Rationale: Pulmonary artery (PA) catheters can be used to evaluate pulmonary artery pressures, left ventricular pressures, measure cardiac output, and manipulate fluid volume status in acutely ill clients. PA catheters are a form of hemodynamic monitoring. The PA catheter does not measure right ventricular pressures and would not be used to administer medications. It is a central arterial catheter, not a peripheral line. Implementation Application Physiological Integrity
32.11 The nurse is teaching a client who has started taking digoxin (Lanoxin) for left-sided heart failure. The highest priority information to teach is: 1. how to manage nausea that can be associated with taking digoxin. 2. foods that should be eaten while taking digoxin. 3. check the pulse each day before taking the medication and do not take the medication if the pulse is under 60 beats per minute without talking to the physician. 4. check the pulse each day and write down the beats per minute on a notepad.	Answer: 3 Rationale: All four answers provide important teaching information, but the highest priority for teaching is for the client to know that it may not be safe to take the drug when the pulse rate is under 60 bpm and to contact the physician. Implementation Synthesis Physiological Integrity
32.12 Typical medications taken by heart failure clients include: (Select all that apply.) 1. promethazine (Phenergan). 2. furosemide (Lasix). 3. digoxin (Lanoxin). 4. enalapril (Vasotec).	Answer: 2, 3, 4 Rationale: Furosemide (Lasix), digoxin (Lanoxin), and enalapril (Vasotec) are all medications that are frequently prescribed for heart failure clients. Furosemide (Lasix) is a diuretic. Digoxin (Lanoxin) is a cardiac glycoside. Enalapril (Vasotec) is an ACE inhibitor. Promethazine (Phenergan) is not specific to care of heart failure clients (it is used as an antiemetic, antihistamine, or a sedative). Implementation Application Physiological Integrity
32.13 The elderly client has just returned home from the hospital after treatment for chronic heart failure. The client experiences a pulse rate increase from 80 beats per minute to 102 beats	Answer: 4 Rationale: The pulse rate increase indicates that activity is not being tolerated. Rest should help bring the heart rate back to the pre-exercise level. Recommending that the client do household tasks in the morning, to ignore the pulse rate and become more active, and to rest for 30 minutes between laundry

per minute when walking between the kitchen and the utility room to do laundry. Which of the following are appropriate nursing actions for the home health nurse?

1. Encourage the client to accomplish tasks like laundry early in the morning before fatigue is an issue.
2. Recommend that the client ignore the pulse rate and become more active in order to build stamina.
3. Encourage the client to rest for 30 minutes between each load of laundry completed.
4. Encourage the client to keep a chair near the washer/dryer unit and sit to rest when the client feels their pulse rate increase.

loads are not practical strategies for an elderly client with compromised heart function. All home activities should be performed at a comfortable pace for the client.
Implementation
Application
Physiological Integrity

32.14 The nurse recognizes which of the following as a sign of decreased cardiac output and tissue perfusion in a client with heart failure?

1. decreased mental alertness.
2. increased urine output
3. abdominal distention
4. strong peripheral pulses

Answer: 1
Rationale: A change in mentation is a common sign of decreased cardiac output and tissue perfusion. Urine output would decrease, not increase. Pulses would weaken, not be strong. Abdominal distention is unrelated.
Evaluation
Application
Physiological Integrity

32.15 The nurse is assessing a client who arrives at the hospital with dyspnea, orthopnea, cyanosis, clammy skin, a productive cough with pink, frothy sputum, and crackles. The nurse realizes that the client is likely suffering from which of the following conditions?

1. chronic heart failure
2. pulmonary edema
3. endocarditis
4. angina

Answer: 2
Rationale: The signs and symptoms are indicative of pulmonary edema. Not all clients have frothy, pink sputum. The presence of this symptom differentiates this from chronic heart failure. Endocarditis would manifest with pain and potentially fever. Angina is chest pain. Pulmonary edema is considered a medical emergency.
Analysis
Application
Physiological Integrity

32.16 The most important first action the nurse should initiate on a client who arrives to the hospital in pulmonary edema is:

1. initiate a peripheral intravenous catheter.
2. seek an order to medicate for discomfort.
3. monitor the blood glucose level.
4. administer oxygen and attach a pulse oximeter.

Answer: 4
Rationale: When dealing with this medical emergency, take steps to improve the oxygenation and airway first. Then move on to the rest of the ABCs. Initiating an IV would follow starting the administration of oxygen. However, often more than one caregiver is present and these two actions can be done simultaneously. The nurse would not likely be medicating the client until the ABCs have been addressed. The blood glucose level is not related to pulmonary edema.
Implementation
Synthesis
Physiological Integrity

32.17 Which of the following is important to keep in mind when caring for clients with possible endocarditis?

1. Endocarditis can be treated by open heart surgery to clean the heart valves.
2. Endocarditis is unrelated to fever so medicate clients with ordered antipyretic and observe.

Answer: 3
Rationale: Endocarditis can be prevented in clients at risk by administering antibiotics prior to procedures. Endocarditis carries serious risks for damage to heart valves. Fever may be present in endocarditis. Open heart surgery is not an appropriate treatment for this condition.
Planning
Application
Physiological Integrity

---

3. Endocarditis can be prevented in clients at risk by administering antibiotics prior to procedures.
4. Endocarditis does not pose a high risk for damage to affected heart valves.

32.18 Clinical signs and symptoms of pericarditis include: (Select all that apply.) 1. pericardial friction rub. 2. abdominal discomfort and nausea. 3. chest pain. 4. bradycardia.	Answer: 1, 3 Rationale: Pericardial friction rub and chest pain are hallmark signs of pericarditis, in addition to fever. Abdominal discomfort, nausea, and bradycardia are not associated with pericarditis. Assessment Application Physiological Integrity
32.19 Cardiac tamponade is treated with: 1. antidysrhythmic drugs and oxygen. 2. oxygen and rest. 3. pericardiocentesis. 4. chest x-ray and antibiotics.	Answer: 3 Rationale: When cardiac tamponade occurs, it is considered a medical emergency and pericardiocentesis is performed to remove the fluid or blood that has collected around the heart and is preventing the heart from pumping effectively. Oxygen, rest, antibiotics, and antidysrhythmic medications may be indicated after the pericardiocentesis is performed. Planning Application Physiological Integrity
32.20 What is the initial indication of valve disease? 1. A murmur is heard during physical exam. 2. It is discovered by accident on a chest x-ray. 3. It is discovered only through cardiac catheterization. 4. An echocardiography study is done to preventatively check the valves.	Answer: 1 Rationale: A murmur that is detected during physical exam prompts other tests to evaluate valve function. A chest x-ray would not be a diagnostic test that would indicate a cardiac valve problem. Cardiac catheterization is not the only method of determining a valve problem. Echocardiography studies are not routinely done as a preventative measure to check valves. Assessment Application Physiological Integrity

CHAPTER 33

33.1 A client is admitted with a disorder that is affecting his bone marrow. The nurse realizes that this disorder will negatively impact which body system? 1. gastrointestinal 2. hematologic 3. musculoskeletal 4. nervous	Answer: 2 Rationale: All blood cells originate from cells in the bone marrow that are called stem cells or hemocytoblasts. The direct negative affects of a bone marrow disorder would be on the hematological system of the body, not the gastrointestinal, musculoskeletal, or nervous systems. Assessment Analysis Physiological Integrity
33.2 A client needs a blood transfusion. The nurse realizes that the function of the blood includes: (Select all that apply.) 1. digestion of protein. 2. oxygenation of body tissues. 3. transmit impulses. 4. aids in joint mobility. 5. regulate fluid and electrolyte balance.	Answer: 2, 5 Rationale: The functions of blood include transporting oxygen, nutrients, hormones, and metabolic wastes; protecting against invasion of pathogens; maintaining blood coagulation; and regulating fluids, electrolytes, acids, bases, and body temperature. Digesting proteins, transmitting impulses, and aiding in joint mobility are not functions of blood cells and would not require a blood transfusion. Diagnosis Analysis Physiological Integrity
33.3 A client is diagnosed with an abnormally low red blood cell (RBC) count. The nurse realizes that this disorder is:	Answer: 3 Rationale: Anemia, the most common red blood cell (RBC) disorder, is an abnormally low RBC count or reduced hemoglobin content. Polycythemia is an abnormally high RBC count. Leukemia is a form of cancer. Bacteremia is an infection that spreads to the bloodstream.

1. polycythemia. 2. leukemia. 3. anemia. 4. bacteremia.	Diagnosis Analysis Physiological Integrity

33.4 The nurse sees that a client's hemoglobin level is low. The purpose of hemoglobin is to:
    1. remove toxic wastes.
    2. bind with urea.
    3. filter sodium.
    4. transport oxygen.
	Answer: 4
	 Rationale: Hemoglobin is the oxygen-carrying protein within red blood cells (RBCs). It consists of the heme molecule and globin, a protein molecule. Removing toxic wastes, binding with urea, and filtering sodium are not done by hemoglobin.
	 Diagnosis
	 Analysis
	 Physiological Integrity

33.5 A client with a low red blood cell count is receiving a blood transfusion. The nurse realizes that the body needs which length of time to create more red blood cells?
    1. 2 weeks
    2. 10 days
    3. 3 to 5 days
    4. 48 hours
	Answer: 3
	 Rationale: The complete sequence from stem cell to red blood cell (RBC) takes 3 to 5 days.
	 Diagnosis
	 Analysis
	 Physiological Integrity

33.6 A client has a low red blood cell count. The nurse realizes that the client's body will produce more red blood cells (RBCs) in response to:
    1. hypoxia.
    2. calcium.
    3. eating.
    4. activity.
	Answer: 1
	 Rationale: The stimulus for red blood cell (RBC) production is tissue hypoxia. Calcium levels, eating, and activity levels will not stimulate RBC production.
	 Diagnosis
	 Analysis
	 Physiological Integrity

33.7 A client is experiencing a disorder in which large amounts of red blood cells (RBCs) are being destroyed. An outcome of this disorder can be demonstrated as:
    1. dysphagia.
    2. jaundice.
    3. nausea.
    4. anxiety.
	Answer: 2
	 Rationale: During disease processes that cause increased hemolysis or impaired liver function, bilirubin accumulates in the serum, which causes a yellowish appearance of the skin and sclera or jaundice. Dysphagia is difficulty swallowing and would not be a result of blood cells being destroyed. Nausea and anxiety are not typical outcomes of this type of disorder.
	 Diagnosis
	 Analysis
	 Physiological Integrity

33.8 During the analysis of a client's complete blood count, the nurse deter-mines that the client's white blood cell (WBC) count is elevated. This is also considered:
    1. lymphoma.
    2. leukopenia.
    3. polycythemia.
    4. leukocytosis.
	Answer: 4
	 Rationale: Leukocytosis is a higher-than-normal white blood cell (WBC) count. Leukopenia is a reduction of the number of leukocytes in the blood of 5000 or less. Polycythemia is an increase in the total red cell mass of the blood. Lymphoma is cancer of the lymph system.
	 Diagnosis
	 Analysis
	 Physiological Integrity

33.9 A client has an inflammation of his gastrointestinal tract. When interpreting the labwork for this client, the nurse expects an increase in which of the following types of white blood cells (WBCs)? Select all that apply.
    1. lymphocytes
    2. basophils
    3. eosinophils
    4. neutrophils
	Answer: 2, 4
	 Rationale: Basophils, which comprise less than 1% of the white blood cell (WBC) count, contain histamine, heparin, and other inflammatory mediators. Basophils increase in number during allergic and inflammatory reactions. Neutrophils are active phagocytes, the first cells to arrive at a site of injury. Their numbers increase during inflammation. Immature forms of neutrophils (bands) are released during inflammation or infections, and are referred to as having a shift to the left (so named because immature cell frequencies appear on the left side of the graph) on a differential blood count. Eosinophils comprise 1% to 3% of circulating WBCs, but are found in large numbers in the mucosa of the intestines and lungs. Their numbers increase during allergic reactions and parasitic

infestations. Basophils, which comprise less than 1% of the WBC count, contain histamine, heparin, and other inflammatory mediators. Basophils increase in numbers during allergic and inflammatory reactions. Lymphocytes comprise 20% to 30% of the WBC count. Lymphocytes mature in lymphoid tissue into B cells and T cells. B cells are involved in the humoral immune response and antibody formation, whereas T cells take part in the cell-mediated immunity process.
Assessment
Analysis
Physiological Integrity

33.10 A client who is diagnosed with a blood disorder has a platelet value of >400,000/ml. The nurse interprets this to mean that this client is exhibiting: 1. thrombocytosis. 2. anemia. 3. leukemia. 4. thrombocytopenia.	Answer: 1 Rationale: An excess of platelets is thrombocytosis. Thrombocytopenia is a decrease in the number of platelets in circulating blood; it can result from decreased or defective platelet production or from accelerated platelet destruction. Anemia is related to low hemoglobin, low levels of iron or oxygen in the blood, or blood loss. Leukemia is a diagnosis given in which the white blood cells are low. Diagnosis Analysis Physiological Integrity
33.11 A client is diagnosed with a disorder in which deoxygenated blood is having difficulty returning to the heart and lungs for reoxygenation. In which part of the peripheral vascular system is the origin of this client's disorder? 1. arteries 2. arterioles 3. capillaries 4. venules	Answer: 4 Rationale: In the capillary beds, oxygen and nutrients are exchanged for metabolic wastes, and deoxygenated blood begins its journey back to the heart through venules, the smallest vessels of the venous network. Arteries and arterioles are vessels within the arterial network, not the venous network. Diagnosis Analysis Physiological Integrity
33.12 A client with some blood loss is maintaining a blood pressure of 100/60 mmHg. The nurse interprets this to mean that the client's blood pressure is being maintained through the help of: 1. arterioles. 2. venules. 3. capillaries. 4. veins.	Answer: 1 Rationale: The smaller arterioles are less elastic than arteries but contain more smooth muscle, which promotes their constriction (narrowing) and dilation (widening). In fact, arterioles exert the major control over arterial blood pressure. With blood loss, the arterioles would constrict as a compensation mechanism to increase blood pressure. This would not happen at the capillary level and is possible in the arterial system, not the venous system. Diagnosis Analysis Physiological Integrity
33.13 A client is diagnosed with an alteration in peripheral vascular resistance. The nurse realizes that this resistance is determined by: (Select all that apply.) 1. blood flow. 2. blood viscosity. 3. vessel length. 4. blood pressure. 5. vessel diameter.	Answer: 2, 3, 5 Rationale: Peripheral vascular resistance is determined by blood viscosity, vessel length, and vessel diameter. Blood flow and blood pressure, in addition to peripheral vascular resistance, all affect arterial circulation. Diagnosis Analysis Physiological Integrity
33.14 A client's blood pressure is 128/98 mmHg. The nurse interprets this to mean that the diastolic blood pressure reading represents: 1. pressure at the peak of ventricular contraction. 2. pressure at the peak of atrial contraction. 3. pressure at the closure of the mitral valve. 4. pressure at the peak of ventricular relaxation.	Answer: 4 Rationale: The lowest pressure exerted during ventricular relaxation (diastole) is the diastolic blood pressure. The highest pressure exerted against the arterial walls at the peak of ventricular contraction (systole) is called the systolic blood pressure. Blood pressure is a measurement of ventricular relaxation and constriction, not of atrial relaxation or constriction. It is not directly reflective of valves opening and closing. Diagnosis Analysis Physiological Integrity

33.15 A client is demonstrating a sign of blood pressure stabilization accompanied by a decreased urine output. The nurse explains that the body mechanism responsible for this blood pressure stabilization is:
1. response to chemoreceptors in the aortic arch.
2. renal conservation of sodium and water.
3. change in body temperature.
4. intake of dietary fat and protein.

Answer: 2
Rationale: Blood pressure is influenced by many factors. The kidneys help maintain blood pressure by excreting or conserving sodium and water. When blood pressure decreases, the kidneys initiate the renin-angiotensin mechanism. This stimulates vasoconstriction, which results in the release of the hormone aldosterone from the adrenal cortex, and increases sodium ion reabsorption and water retention. In addition, pituitary release of antidiuretic hormone (ADH) promotes renal reabsorption of water. The net result is an increase in blood volume and a consequent increase in cardiac output and blood pressure. With the changes described, the kidneys are compensating and causing the changes. The changes are not reflective of intervention influenced by the chemoreceptors in the aortic arch, body temperature changes, or dietary intake.
Diagnosis
Analysis
Physiological Integrity

33.16 A client is admitted with an enlarged lymph node. The nurse explains to the client that the purpose of the lymph system is to:
1. filter blood.
2. break down old red blood cells.
3. synthesize lymphocytes.
4. remove infectious organisms.

Answer: 4
Rationale: Lymph nodes are small aggregates of specialized cells that assist the body's immune system by removing foreign material, infectious organisms, and tumor cells from lymph. Filtering blood, breaking down or synthesizing cells are not functions of the lymph system.
Diagnosis
Application
Physiological Integrity

33.17 The nurse is preparing to assess a client's hematologic, peripheral vascular, and lymphatic systems. Which of the following assessment techniques is not typically utilized for this assessment?
1. inspection
2. palpation
3. percussion
4. auscultation

Answer: 3
Rationale: Percussion is not typically used to assess the hematologic, peripheral vascular, and lymphatic systems. The techniques used to assess these systems includes inspection of the skin for such changes as edema, ulcerations, or alterations in color and temperature; auscultation of blood pressure; and palpation of the major pulse points of the body and lymph nodes.
Assessment
Application
Health Promotion and Maintenance

33.18 During the assessment, a client's pedal pulses are increased. The nurse should document this finding as:
1. +1.
2. +2.
3. +3.
4. +4.

Answer: 3
Rationale: The correct documentation for this finding is +3. Pulses should be described as increased, normal, diminished, or absent. Scales that range from 0 to 4+ are sometimes used as follows: 0 = absent; 1+ = diminished; 2+ = normal; 3+ = increased; and 4+ = bounding.
Diagnosis
Application
Health Promotion and Maintenance

33.19 During the assessment of a client's lower extremities, the nurse notes slight pitting. This assessment finding should be documented as:
1. 1+.
2. 2+.
3. 3+.
4. 4+.

Answer: 2
Rationale: The correct documentation of this finding is 2+. Edema can be graded on a scale of from 1+ to 4+: 1+ = no visible change in the leg or slight pitting; 2+ = no marked change in the shape of the leg or pitting slightly deeper; 3+ = leg visibly swollen and deep pitting; and 4+ = leg very swollen and pitting very deep.
Diagnosis
Application
Health Promotion and Maintenance

33.20 A client is admitted to the hospital with an inflammatory disorder. The nurse expects that the physician will order which of the following diagnostic tests?
1. red blood cell count
2. hemoglobin
3. sedimentation rate
4. platelet count

Answer: 3
Rationale: The erythrocyte sedimentation rate test is done as a measure of general inflammation within the body, which is increased in many illnesses. Changes with hemoglobin, platelet, or red blood cell levels are not indicative of inflammation.
Diagnosis
Analysis
Physiological Integrity

34.1 Upon analysis, a client's red blood cells (RBCs) appear microcytic and hypochromic. The nurse interprets this information to mean that this client is demonstrating signs of:
1. iron deficiency anemia.
2. acute blood loss anemia.
3. chronic blood loss anemia.
4. vitamin B_{12} deficiency anemia.

Answer: 3
Rationale: Chronic blood loss depletes iron stores as red blood cell (RBC) production attempts to maintain the RBC supply. The resulting RBCs are microcytic (small) and hypochromic (pale). Iron deficiency anemia results in a fewer number of RBCs being produced. The RBCs that are produced are microcytic, hyperchromic, and malformed. With Vitamin B_{12} deficiency anemia, the RBCs that are produced are macrocytic (large) and misshapen (oval rather than concave). Acute blood loss anemia would result in low level of RBCs in circulation.
Diagnosis
Analysis
Physiological Integrity

34.2 A client with chronic gastritis is experiencing "tingling" in his hands. The nurse realizes that this client might be demonstrating signs of:
1. iron deficiency anemia.
2. acute blood loss anemia.
3. folic acid deficiency anemia.
4. vitamin B_{12} deficiency anemia.

Answer: 4
Rationale: Manifestations of vitamin B_{12} deficiency anemia develop gradually as bodily stores of the vitamin are depleted. Pallor or slight jaundice and weakness develop. Because vitamin B_{12} is important for neurologic function, paresthesias in the extremities and problems with proprioception develop. These manifestations may progress to difficulty maintaining balance due to spinal cord damage. Tingling hands are directly related to Vitamin B_{12}, not iron, folic acid or acute blood loss.
Diagnosis
Analysis
Physiological Integrity

34.3 The nurse is providing information to a client who is prone to developing sickle cell crises. Which of the following should the nurse include in these instructions?
1. Do not get overheated.
2. Ensure an adequate fluid intake.
3. Plan for a moderate to large amount of exercise every day.
4. Seek out air conditioning or other ways to keep cool during hot, humid days.

Answer: 2
Rationale: The client should ensure an adequate fluid intake. Conditions likely to trigger sickling include hypoxia, low environmental or body temperature, excessive exercise, anesthesia, dehydration, infections, or acidosis.
Planning
Application
Health Promotion and Maintenance

34.4 A client in sickle cell crisis is experiencing edema of the hands and feet. The nurse realizes that this edema is caused by:
1. fluid overload.
2. poor venous return.
3. small vessel infarction.
4. dehydration.

Answer: 3
Rationale: A vasoocclusive or thrombotic crisis occurs when sickling develops in the microcirculation. Obstruction of blood flow triggers vasospasm that halts all blood flow in the vessel. Lack of blood flow leads to tissue ischemia and infarction. Infarction of small vessels in the extremities causes painful swelling of the hands and feet; large joints also may be affected.
Diagnosis
Analysis
Physiological Integrity

34.5 A client is being treated for acquired hemolytic anemia. Which of the following assessment findings would suggest that the condition is severe?
1. misshaped limbs due to pathological fractures
2. enlarged spleen
3. jaundice
4. bradycardia

Answer: 1
Rationale: The manifestations of acquired hemolytic anemia depend on the extent of hemolysis and the body's ability to replace destroyed red blood cells (RBCs). When the condition is severe, bone marrow expands, and bones may be deformed or may develop pathologic fractures. An enlarged spleen and jaundice are not severe findings for this anemia, but may be present. Bradycardia is not related to this condition. Tachycardia would be anticipated with the continued anemia.
Diagnosis
Application
Physiological Integrity

34.6 A client with aplastic anemia is demonstrating signs of blood cell production. Which of the following should be done to support this client?

Answer: 3
Rationale: Treatment focuses on removing the causative agent, if known, and using blood transfusions. Transfusions may be discontinued as soon as the bone marrow resumes blood cell production. Complete recovery may take months.

1. Continue with blood transfusions as prescribed. 2. Report the finding. 3. Plan to discontinue blood transfusions. 4. Plan to administer fresh frozen plasma.	Bone marrow transplant may be the treatment of choice in some instances. Reporting the finding would be important, but not directly supporting to the client. Blood transfusions of any kind would not be indicated when there is indication that the bone marrow is resuming blood cell production. Evaluation Application Physiological Integrity
34.7 The nurse is providing dietary instructions to a vegetarian client with iron deficiency anemia. Which of the following should be included in these instructions? 1. Consider adding animal sources of iron and protein to the diet. 2. Ensure an adequate intake of vitamin C when consuming non-animal-based proteins. 3. Drink at least 12 glasses of water every day. 4. Avoid exercise at least 30 minutes after completing a meal or snack.	Answer: 2 Rationale: Heme iron makes up about one-half of the iron from animal sources. Nonheme iron includes the remaining iron from animal sources and all the iron from plants, legumes, and nuts. Heme iron promotes absorption of nonheme iron from other foods when both forms are consumed at the same time. Absorption of nonheme iron is also enhanced by vitamin C and inhibited by tea and coffee. Since the client is a vegetarian, suggesting animal sources of iron and protein would not be appropriate. Water consumption and physical activity would have no bearing on this issue. Implementation Application Health Promotion and Maintenance
34.8 A client is prescribed an oral iron preparation. Which of the following would be appropriate for the nurse to instruct this client about this medication? (Select all that apply.) 1. Take with orange juice. 2. Nausea is expected with this medication. 3. Take with an antacid. 4. Take 2 hours before a scheduled tetracycline dose. 5. Take with vitamin E replacements.	Answer: 1, 4 Rationale: Instructions regarding oral iron preparations should include: avoid the use of drugs that might interact with iron such as antacids, allopurinol (Alloprim), chloramphenicol (Chlorofair), tetracyclines, and vitamin E; administer iron preparations with orange juice to enhance absorption; if using an elixir, give it through a straw to prevent staining the teeth; monitor for manifestations of iron toxicity such as nausea, diarrhea, or constipation; and if the client is also taking tetracyclines, schedule the dose of iron 2 hours before tetracycline (iron reduces the absorption of tetracycline). Also, warn the client that his bowel movements may be black or tarry green. Implementation Application Physiological Integrity
34.9 The nurse is planning to instruct a client with secondary polycythemia about ways to prevent blood stasis. Which of the following should be included in these instructions? 1. Leg pain is normal. 2. Elevate feet and legs when sitting. 3. Restrict fluids. 4. Black stools are to be expected.	Answer: 2 Rationale: Discuss measures to prevent blood stasis: elevate legs and feet when sitting, use support stockings, and continue treatment measures. Teach the client and family the importance of maintaining adequate hydration, and increase fluid intake during hot weather and when exercising. Instruct the client to report manifestations of thrombosis such as leg or calf pain; chest pain; neurologic symptoms or bleeding manifested as black, tarry stools, and vomiting blood or coffee-ground emesis. Planning Application Physiological Integrity
34.10 A client diagnosed with leukemia says, "If I have too many white blood cells and white blood cells fight infections, why do I have to be careful not to be exposed to germs?" An appropriate response for the nurse to make is: 1. "Leukemia means you have the wrong kind of white blood cells." 2. "That's not what leukemia is." 3. "The white blood cells with leukemia aren't effective to fight infections." 4. "Your bone marrow can become infected."	Answer: 3 Rationale: Leukemic cells are not effective in the normal immune functions of white blood cells (WBCs), which increases the risk for infection. The cells are not "wrong," just not the right type at the right level to fight infection. The risk is not of bone marrow infection, but overall systemic infection. The client has a basic understanding of the diagnosis and just needs clarification. Implementation Application Physiological Integrity

34.11 A 17-year-old client with edematous lymph nodes and headaches is diagnosed with leukemia. The nurse suspects that this client most likely has:
  1. acute lymphocytic leukemia (ALL).
  2. chronic lymphocytic leukemia (CLL).
  3. acute myeloid leukemia (AML).
  4. chronic myeloid leukemia (CML).
	Answer: 1
	Rationale: Lymphocytic leukemias infiltrate the spleen, lymph nodes, CNS, and other tissues. Acute lymphoblastic leukemia is the most common type of leukemia in children.
	Diagnosis
	Analysis
	Physiological Integrity

34.12 A client who is undergoing treatment for leukemia is scheduled for a bone marrow transplant. The nurse determines that this client is in which phase of treatment for the disorder?
  1. induction
  2. maintenance
  3. rehabilitative
  4. postremission
	Answer: 4
	Rationale: Once remission has been achieved, postremission chemotherapy is continued to eradicate any additional leukemic cells, prevent relapse, and prolong survival. A single chemotherapeutic agent, combination therapy, or bone marrow transplant may be used for postremission treatment. The other phases of treatment do not include a bone marrow transplant.
	Planning
	Analysis
	Physiological Integrity

34.13 The nurse is preparing an analgesic for a client with leukemia. Which of the following routes is preferred for this client?
  1. intramuscular
  2. intravenous
  3. oral
  4. subcutaneous
	Answer: 3
	Rationale: A client with leukemia is prone to developing infections as well as possible blood coagulation abnormalities. Administration of an analgesic through a route that would penetrate the skin, could lead to bleeding or infection at the insertion site. The oral route is the route of choice for administering an analgesic to this client.
	Planning
	Application
	Physiological Integrity

34.14 A client is diagnosed with stage II A Hodgkin's lymphoma. The nurse interprets this information to mean that the extent of this disorder is limited to:
  1. a single lymph node with systemic symptoms.
  2. two or more lymph nodes on the same side without systemic symptoms.
  3. upper abdominal lymph nodes without systemic symptoms.
  4. an extranodal site involvement with systemic symptoms.
	Answer: 2
	Rationale: Stage II A means the disorder involves two or more lymph node regions on the same side of the diaphragm without systemic symptoms.
	Assessment
	Analysis
	Physiological Integrity

34.15 A college-aged client who is in the hospital for Hodgkin's disease treatment is visited by friends who bring a pizza and cola to the client's room. Which of the following can the nurse do to ensure the client's comfort?
  1. Ask the visitors to leave.
  2. Ask the visitors to eat the pizza in the lounge.
  3. Encourage the client to eat as much pizza as possible.
  4. Provide the client with an antiemetic and suggest something else for the client to eat with the visitors.
	Answer: 4
	Rationale: The effects of malignant lymphoma and its treatment with chemotherapy and/or radiation therapy can contribute to nausea and interfere with nutritional status. Nausea, a sensation of abdominal fullness, and fear of vomiting often limit food intake. Crackers and hard candy often relieve queasiness; whereas hot, spicy, sweet, or strong-smelling foods may increase nausea. Alternative nausea relief measures may be effective. Having the visitors eat in the lobby would be excluding the client. Allowing the client to eat as much as desired without addressing any current nausea would not be most helpful to the client.
	Implementation
	Application
	Physiological Integrity

34.16 A client with idiopathic thrombocytopenia purpura continues to experience symptoms of the disease after completing several courses of	Answer: 2 Rationale: A splenectomy is the treatment of choice if the client with idiopathic thrombocytopenia purpura relapses when glucocorticoids are discontinued. The spleen is the site of platelet destruction and antibody production. This surgery often

prednisone (Meticorten) therapy. The nurse anticipates that which of the following will most likely be indicated for this client?
1. life-long prednisone therapy
2. splenectomy
3. aspirin therapy
4. weekly platelet transfusions

cures the disorder, although relapse may occur years after splenectomy. Aspirin therapy would be contraindicated in this situation and would most likely result in bleeding. Platelet transfusions are ineffective with this disorder since the problem is that the platelets are being produced adequately, but destroyed. Life-long prednisone therapy is rarely prescribed and prednisone therapy was not effective for this client.
Planning
Analysis
Physiological Integrity

34.17 A client with hemophilia is admitted with acute bleeding. Until the cause of the bleeding is determined, the nurse should be prepared to do which of the following interventions?
1. Infuse packed red blood cells.
2. Infuse normal saline.
3. Infuse heparin.
4. Infuse fresh-frozen plasma.

Answer: 4
Rationale: Fresh-frozen plasma replaces all clotting factors except platelets. When the cause of bleeding is not yet determined, fresh-frozen plasma may be administered intravenously until a definitive diagnosis is made. Red packed cells and normal saline would increase volume, but not replace the clotting factors. Heparin would be contraindicated as it would promote further bleeding.
Planning
Application
Physiological Integrity

34.18 A client with disseminated intravascular coagulation is not responding to infusions of fresh frozen plasma and platelets. Which of the following interventions might be indicated for this client? Select all that apply.
1. Begin heparin injections.
2. Begin heparin infusion.
3. Begin normal saline infusion.
4. Prepare for a bone marrow biopsy.

Answer: 1, 2
Rationale: When bleeding is the major manifestation of disseminated intravascular coagulation (DIC), fresh frozen plasma and platelet concentrates are given to restore clotting factors and platelets. Heparin may be administered. Heparin interferes with the clotting cascade and may prevent further clotting factor consumption due to uncontrolled thrombosis. It is used when bleeding is not controlled by plasma and platelets, as well as when the client has manifestations of thrombotic problems such as acrocyanosis and possible gangrene. Long-term heparin therapy, by injection or continuous infusion with a portable pump, may be necessary for clients with chronic DIC. Normal saline would not help with the clotting. The diagnosis has already been determined and bone marrow aspiration would not be indicated, just a change in treatment.
Planning
Application
Physiological Integrity

34.19 A client who is undergoing chemotherapy for lymphoma says, "I thought I was ugly before this all started. Now I know for sure I'm disgusting to look at." Which of the following is this client most at risk for developing related to their comments?
1. changed body image perception
2. reduced sexual response
3. altered taste sensation
4. inability to cope with the diagnosis and treatment

Answer: 1
Rationale: Radiation and chemotherapy lead to changes in appearance and body function, further altering body image. Reactions to this diagnosis vary and may include refusal to look in a mirror, discuss the effects of the disease or treatment, unwillingness to participate in rehabilitation, inappropriate treatment decisions, increasing dependence on others or refusal to provide self-care, hostility, withdrawal, and signs of grieving.
Diagnosis
Analysis
Psychosocial Integrity

34.20 A client who is being treated for malignant lymphoma is experiencing pruritis. Which of the following interventions would be appropriate for this client? (Select all that apply.)
1. Bathe with cool water.
2. Vigorously rub the skin after bathing.
3. Apply lavender-scented body lotion.
4. Keep room temperature above normal.
5. Cleanse bedding and clothing in mild detergent with a second rinse cycle.

Answer: 1, 5
Rationale: The nurse should provide and teach measures to promote comfort and relieve itching. These measures include: use cool water and a mild soap to bathe; blot skin dry; apply plain cornstarch or nonperfumed lotion or powder to the skin unless contraindicated; use lightweight blankets and clothing; maintain adequate humidity and a cool room temperature; and wash bedding and clothes in mild detergent and use a second rinse cycle.
Implementation
Application
Physiological Integrity

35.1 The nurse measures a client's blood pressure as 144/88 mmHg. Which of the following interventions would be most appropriate for this client?

1. Provide stress-reduction techniques.
2. Inform the physician so anti-hypertensive medication can be prescribed.
3. Offer the client a glass of water.
4. Remeasure the blood pressure in a few minutes.

Answer: 4
Rationale: There is no evidence that this client has had previously high blood pressure readings. The nurse should remeasure the blood pressure in a few minutes in the event the reading was because of physical activity or anxiety. Hypertension is defined as systolic blood pressure of 140 mmHg or higher, or diastolic pressure of 90 mmHg or higher, based on the average of three or more readings taken on separate occasions. The client may not feel stressed or need anti-hypertensive medication. Offering a glass of water would have no effect on the blood pressure.
Implementation
Application
Health Promotion and Maintenance

35.2 A client with diabetes is beginning treatment for hypertension. The nurse shares with the client that the blood pressure reading goal is:

1. 140/90 mmHg.
2. 135/85 mmHg.
3. 130/80 mmHg.
4. 120/80 mmHg.

Answer: 3
Rationale: Hypertension management focuses on reducing the blood pressure to less than 140 mmHg systolic and 90 mmHg diastolic. The ultimate goal of hypertension management is to reduce cardiovascular and renal morbidity and mortality. The risk of cardiovascular complications decreases when the average blood pressure is less than 140/90; when the client also has diabetes or renal disease, the treatment goal is a blood pressure less than 130/80.
Planning
Analysis
Physiological Integrity

35.3 The nurse is instructing a client with hypertension about lifestyle modifications. Which of the following would be appropriate to include in the teaching for this client? (Select all that apply.)

1. Review the DASH diet.
2. Begin a walking program, and progress to 30 minutes 5 to 6 days each week.
3. Plan a weight lifting regimen.
4. Eliminate dairy products from the diet.
5. Restrict fluid intake.

Answer: 1, 2
Rationale: Lifestyle modifications are recommended for all clients whose blood pressure falls within the prehypertension range and everyone with intermittent or sustained hypertension. These modifications include weight loss, dietary changes, restricted alcohol use and cigarette smoking, increased physical activity, and stress reduction. Dietary approaches to managing hypertension focus on reducing sodium intake, maintaining adequate potassium and calcium intakes, and reducing total and saturated fat intake. The DASH diet has proven beneficial effects in lowering blood pressure. Regular exercise reduces blood pressure and contributes to weight loss, stress reduction, and feelings of overall well-being. Previously sedentary clients are encouraged to engage in aerobic exercise for 30 to 45 minutes per day most days of the week. Isometric exercise, such as weight training, may not be appropriate, as it can raise the systolic blood pressure.
Implementation
Application
Health Promotion and Maintenance

35.4 A client is being started on enalapril (Vasotec). The most common complaint from clients who routinely take this medication is:

1. increased thirst.
2. reduced urine output.
3. persistent cough.
4. sore throat.

Answer: 3
Rationale: Primary adverse affects for both ACE I and ARBs include persistent cough, first dose hypotension, and hyperkalemia.
Implementation
Application
Physiological Integrity

35.5 A client's blood pressure continues to be elevated despite being prescribed an ACE inhibitor for several weeks. Which of the following would be most appropriate for the nurse to do at this time?

1. Ask if the client is taking the prescribed medication.
2. Suggest to the physician that another medication be added.

Answer: 1
Rationale: Noncompliance, or failure to follow the identified treatment plan, is a continuing risk for any client with a chronic disease. Prescribed medications may have undesirable effects; whereas hypertension itself often has no symptoms or noticeable effects. The nurse should inquire about reasons for noncompliance with the recommended treatment plan by assessing for factors that can contribute to noncompliance, such as adverse drug effects. If it is determined that the client is not taking the prescribed medication, the other interventions would not be indicated at this time.

---

3. Schedule the client to have the blood pressure checked again in a week. 4. Realize the client is anxious because of the diagnosis.	Assessment Application Health Promotion and Maintenance
35.6 A client is undergoing diagnostic testing to determine the cause of hypertension. Which of the following would be included if a secondary cause for this disorder is suspected? 1. serum electrolytes 2. abdominal CT scan 3. MRI of the carotid arteries 4. intravenous pyelogram	Answer: 4 Rationale: Intravenous pyelogram, renal ultrasound, renal angiogram, and CT or MRI may be done when secondary hypertension is suspected. Planning Analysis Physiological Integrity
35.7 During the abdominal assessment of an elderly client, the nurse palpates a mass in the mid-abdomen. Which of the following should the nurse do next? 1. Percuss the mass. 2. Ask the client to cough. 3. Get the physician. 4. Auscultate the mass.	Answer: 4 Rationale: Further assessment is needed before the physician would be contacted, typically first by phone. Most abdominal aneurysms are asymptomatic, but a pulsating mass in the mid- and upper abdomen and a bruit (the sound auscultated over turbulent or restricted blood flow) over the mass are found on exam. If an aneurysm is suspected, asking the client to cough and percussing the mass would be inappropriate responses that could increase the pressure on the weakened site. Assessment Application Physiological Integrity
35.8 The nurse suspects a client who is recovering from an abdominal aortic aneurysm repair is experiencing graft leaking. Which of the following are indications of this event? (Select all that apply.) 1. urine output 45 cc/hr 2. complaint of groin pain 3. abdominal dressing dry and intact 4. respiratory rate 16 and regular 5. complaint of back discomfort	Answer: 2, 5 Rationale: The nurse should monitor for and report any of the following manifestations of graft leakage: ecchymoses of the scrotum, perineum, or penis; a new or expanding hematoma; increased abdominal girth; weak or absent peripheral pulses; tachycardia; hypotension; decreased motor function or sensation in the extremities; decreased hemoglobin and hematocrit; increased abdominal, pelvic, back, or groin pain; decreased urinary output (less than 30 mL/hour); decreased CVP, pulmonary artery pressure, or pulmonary artery wedge pressure. These manifestations may signal graft leakage and possible hemorrhage. Pain may be due to pressure from an expanding hematoma or bowel ischemia. The other findings listed are considered within normal limits. Diagnosis Application Physiological Integrity
35.9 The nurse suspects that a client is experiencing the effects of peripheral atherosclerosis. Which of the following did the nurse most likely assess in this client? 1. rubor with extremity elevation 2. normal hair distribution bilaterally over lower extremities 3. peripheral pulses present bilaterally 4. complaints of leg pain upon rest	Answer: 4 Rationale: Manifestations of peripheral atherosclerosis include intermittent claudication; pain at rest; paresthesias; diminished or absent peripheral pulses; pallor with extremity elevation; rubor with extremities in dependent position; thin, shiny, hairless skin; thickened toenails; and areas of skin discoloration or skin breakdown. Assessment Application Health Promotion and Maintenance
35.10 A client is having segmental pressure measurements conducted to help diagnose peripheral vascular disease. Which of the following would indicate the presence of this disorder? 1. thigh pressure higher than the arm 2. calf pressure higher than the arm	Answer: 3 Rationale: Noninvasive studies often are sufficient to diagnose peripheral vascular disease. Segmental pressure measurements use sphygmomanometer cuffs and a Doppler device to compare blood pressures between the upper and lower extremities and within different segments of the affected extremity. In peripheral vascular disease (PVD), the blood pressure may be lower in the legs than in the arms.

3. calf pressure lower than the arm 4. no difference between the arm or leg	Implementation Application Physiological Integrity

35.11 A client is demonstrating signs of ineffective peripheral tissue perfusion. Which of the following interventions would be appropriate for this client?
    1. Encourage client to reduce level of exercise.
    2. Discuss smoking cessation techniques.
    3. Keep extremities cool.
    4. Assist with pillow placement under knees.
	Answer: 2
	Rationale: Interventions for a client who is experiencing ineffective peripheral tissue perfusion include assessing peripheral pulses, pain, color, temperature, and capillary refill every 4 hours and as needed; positioning with extremities dependent; instructing to avoid smoking; discussing the benefits of regular exercise; using a foot cradle and lightweight blankets, socks, and slippers to keep extremities warm; avoiding electric heating pads or hot water bottles; encouraging frequent position changes; and instructing to avoid crossing legs or using a pillow under the knees.
	Implementation
	Application
	Physiological Integrity

35.12 A male client is diagnosed with thromboangiitis obliterans. Appropriate teaching for this client includes:
    1. medications are the only cure.
    2. surgical procedures can be performed to cure this disorder.
    3. management depends upon the client's willingness to stop smoking.
    4. nothing can help manage this disorder.
	Answer: 3
	Rationale: The prognosis for thromboangiitis obliterans depends significantly on the client's ability and willingness to stop smoking. With smoking cessation and good foot care, the prognosis for saving the extremities is good, even though no cure is available.
	Implementation
	Application
	Physiological Integrity

35.13 A client is being discharged on long-term oral anticoagulant therapy for arterial thrombus formation in the lower extremity. Which of the following should be included in this client's discharge instructions?
    1. Slight bleeding from the nose is expected.
    2. Contact the physician's office for follow-up laboratory studies.
    3. Pain in the limb is a sign of healing.
    4. Take two doses of the prescribed anticoagulant if a dose is missed one day.
	Answer: 2
	Rationale: When preparing the client and family for home or community-based care related to an acute arterial occlusion, discuss the following topics as necessary: incision care; manifestations of complications to be reported, including symptoms of infection or occlusion of the graft or artery; long-term anticoagulant therapy, including the reason, prescribed dose, follow-up laboratory testing and appointments, interactions with other drugs, and manifestations of excessive bleeding; any activity restrictions or dietary modifications; lifestyle modifications to slow atherosclerosis and control hypertension; and measures to promote peripheral circulation and maintain tissue integrity. Nasal bleeding is not expected. Pain in the limb could indicate another clot has formed. Anti-coagulant medications should never be "doubled" even in the case of a missed dose. The client would be encouraged to notify the physician if a dose is missed.
	Implementation
	Application
	Health Promotion and Maintenance

35.14 A client is demonstrating signs of thrombophlebitis. With this disorder, the nurse realizes that three mechanisms occur, which include: (Select all that apply.)
    1. pooling of blood in the vessel.
    2. blood hypercoagulation.
    3. sluggish blood flow.
    4. elevated systemic blood pressure.
    5. vessel damage.
	Answer: 2, 3, 5
	Rationale: Three pathologic factors, called Virchow's triad, are associated with thrombophlebitis: stasis of blood, vessel damage, and increased blood coagulability. Blood does not pool in the vessel, it is restricted. Systemic blood pressure elevation is not a mechanism of this problem.
	Diagnosis
	Analysis
	Physiological Integrity

35.15 A client is seen for increasing edema in his left lower extremity and pain in the limb with ambulation. Which of the following disorders do these symptoms suggest?
    1. arterial occlusion
    2. deep vein thrombosis
	Answer: 2
	Rationale: The manifestations of deep vein thrombosis (DVT) are primarily due to the inflammatory process that accompanies the thrombus. Calf pain is the most common symptom, and it may be described as tightness or a dull, aching pain in the affected extremity, particularly upon walking. Tenderness, swelling, warmth, and erythema may be noted along the course of involved veins. The affected extremity may be cyanotic and often is edematous. Rarely, a cord may be palpated

3. superficial vein thrombosis (SVT) 4. varicose veins	over the affected vein. A positive Homan's sign is an unreliable indicator of DVT. A DVT is not an arterial or a primary superficial vein problem. Varicose veins are tortuous veins with valve insufficiency. Diagnosis Analysis Physiological Integrity
35.16 A client with a deep vein thrombosis (DVT) is going to be weaned from intravenous heparin. The nurse anticipates that oral warfarin sodium should be prescribed: 1. the same day the heparin is discontinued. 2. the day before the heparin is discontinued. 3. 4 to 5 days before the heparin is discontinued. 4. the same day as the heparin is started.	Answer: 3 Rationale: Oral anticoagulation with warfarin may be initiated concurrently with heparin therapy. Overlapping heparin and warfarin therapy for 4 to 5 days is important because the full anticoagulant effect of warfarin is delayed, and it may actually promote clotting during the first few days of therapy. Planning Application Physiological Integrity
35.17 The nurse is planning care for a client who was diagnosed with deep vein thrombosis (DVT). Which of the following should be included in this plan of care? 1. activity as tolerated 2. Measure and apply graduated compression stockings. 3. Encourage the client to sit out of bed several hours every day. 4. Assist client with putting on tight-fitting pants.	Answer: 2 Rationale: The plan of care for a client with deep vein thrombosis (DVT) includes: possible bed rest, the duration of which is determined by the extent of leg edema; elevate legs 15 to 20 degrees, with the knees slightly flexed, above the level of the heart to promote venous return and discourage venous pooling; elastic antiembolism/compression stockings or pneumatic compression devices are also frequently ordered to stimulate the muscle-pumping mechanism that promotes the return of blood to the heart; when permitted, walking is encouraged; avoid prolonged standing or sitting; avoid leg crossing and tight-fitting garments or stockings that bind. Planning Application Physiological Integrity
35.18 A client who is being treated for a deep vein thrombosis (DVT) complains of chest pain and shortness of breath. Which of the following should the nurse do first? 1. Elevate the head of the bed and begin oxygen therapy. 2. Measure the client's blood pressure. 3. Assess the extremity with the thrombosis. 4. Assess the pulses on the extremity with the thrombosis.	Answer: 1 Rationale: Immediately report client complaints of chest pain and shortness of breath, anxiety, or a sense of impending doom. The manifestations of pulmonary embolism are similar to those of myocardial infarction. Prompt intervention to restore pulmonary blood flow can reduce the risk of significant adverse effects. Initiate oxygen therapy, elevate the head of the bed, and reassure the client who is experiencing manifestations of pulmonary embolism. Oxygen therapy and elevating the head of the bed promote ventilation and gas exchange in those alveoli that are well perfused, and help to maintain tissue oxygenation. The other interventions are not the priority and would delay the initiation of required interventions in this situation. Implementation Application Physiological Integrity
35.19 A 75-year-old female is diagnosed with chronic venous insufficiency. Which of the following instructions are appropriate for this client? 1. Keep legs in a dependent position as much as possible. 2. Avoid the use of knee-high hose or girdles. 3. Limit ambulation. 4. Dangle legs over the side of the bed several times per day.	Answer: 2 Rationale: Nursing care for the client with chronic venous insufficiency includes: elevate the legs while resting and during sleep; walk as much as possible, but avoid sitting or standing for long periods of time; when sitting, do not cross legs or allow pressure on the back of the knees, such as sitting on the side of the bed; do not wear anything that pinches legs, such as knee-high hose, garters, or girdles; wear elastic hose as prescribed; and keep the skin on the feet and legs clean, soft, and dry. Implementation Application Physiological Integrity

35.20 An elderly male client is prescribed elastic graduated compression stockings. The nurse should instruct this client to:
  1. wear the stockings continuously, except when showering.
  2. expect areas of skin breakdown under the stockings.
  3. wear the stockings primarily while sleeping.
  4. remove the stockings once per day and while sleeping.
	Answer: 4
	Rationale: The client who is prescribed elastic graduated compression stockings should be instructed to wear the elastic stockings during the majority of waking hours, and remove them once during the daytime and while sleeping. Skin breakdown is not anticipated with wearing the stockings and would need to be reported to the physician.
	Implementation
	Application
	Physiological Integrity

CHAPTER 36

36.1 The nurse observes a client breathing through an open mouth. Which of the following functions is being bypassed by mouth breathing?
  1. cooling the air
  2. neutralizing the air
  3. filtering the air
  4. separating the air
	Answer: 3
	Rationale: The nasal hairs filter the air as it enters the nares. The rest of the cavity is lined with mucous membranes that contain olfactory neurons and goblet cells that secrete thick mucus. The mucus not only traps dust and bacteria but also contains lysozyme, an enzyme that destroys bacteria as they enter the nose. As mucus and debris accumulate, mucosal ciliated cells move it toward the pharynx, where it is swallowed. The mucosa is highly vascular, warming air that moves across its surface. Cooling of the air would not be happening with nasal breathing. The air would not be neutralized or separated with nasal breathing, so it is not being bypassed with mouth breathing.
	Assessment
	Analysis
	Health Promotion and Maintenance

36.2 A client with a head cold is demonstrating a change in speech tone and volume. The nurse realizes that the sinus cavities are affected because:
  1. the client is sneezing.
  2. the client is coughing.
  3. the client is afebrile.
  4. the sinuses play a role in speech.
	Answer: 4
	Rationale: Sinuses lighten the skull, assist in speech, and produce mucus that drains into the nasal cavities to help trap debris. Sneezing and coughing are not specific to sinus infections only. The client would most likely be febrile (have a fever), not afebrile, with an infection.
	Assessment
	Analysis
	Health Promotion and Maintenance

36.3 A client is diagnosed with a middle ear infection. The nurse realizes that the portion of the client's airway that is affected is the:
  1. nasopharynx.
  2. oropharynx.
  3. laryngopharynx.
  4. nares.
	Answer: 1
	Rationale: The eustachian tubes also open into the nasopharynx, and connect it with the middle ear. This is the opening from the nasal passages to the back of the throat. The oropharynx is the mouth to throat location. Nares are the openings that enter the nose. The laryngopharynx is the area from the back of the throat to the deeper part of the throat.
	Diagnosis
	Analysis
	Health Promotion and Maintenance

36.4 During the assessment of a client, the nurse locates the approximate position of the larynx. This can be found by identifying:
  1. the clavicle.
  2. the Adam's apple.
  3. the first rib.
  4. the shoulder joint.
	Answer: 2
	Rationale: The larynx is framed by cartilages and connected by ligaments and membranes. The thyroid cartilage is formed by the fusion of two cartilages; the fusion point is visible as the Adam's apple. The clavicle, first rib, and shoulder joint are too far down and are not near the location of the larynx.
	Assessment
	Application
	Health Promotion and Maintenance

36.5 During an assessment, a client begins to cough. The nurse realizes that this means:
  1. the client has a cold.
  2. the client is nervous.
	Answer: 3
	Rationale: If anything other than air enters the larynx, a cough reflex expels the foreign substance before it can enter the lungs. This protective reflex does not work if the person is unconscious. It does not indicate the actuality that the client has a cold. Being nervous is not typically associated with coughing.

3. something other than air was entering the larynx.	Assessment Analysis Health Promotion and Maintenance
4. the client is not fully conscious.	

36.6 The nurse wants to assess the apex of a client's right lung. In which of the following locations should the nurse place the stethoscope to assess this client?
   1. intercostal space, sixth rib near the sternum
   2. intercostal space, fourth rib near the axillary line
   3. below the scapula
   4. near the right clavicle
	Answer: 4
	Rationale: The apex of each lung lies just below the clavicle; whereas the base of each lung rests on the diaphragm. The scapulae are located posterior to the lungs.
	Assessment
	Application
	Health Promotion and Maintenance

36.7 A client's blood oxygen saturation level is 99% on room air. The nurse realizes that the oxygenated blood is transported to the heart through which of the following structures?
   1. pulmonary arteries
   2. pulmonary veins
   3. bronchial arteries
   4. bronchial veins
	Answer: 2
	Rationale: The vascular system of the lungs consists of the pulmonary arteries, which deliver blood to the lungs for oxygenation; and the pulmonary veins, which deliver oxygenated blood to the heart. Bronchial arteries and veins are located within the lungs and are not directly involved with transporting oxygenated blood to the heart.
	Assessment
	Application
	Health Promotion and Maintenance

36.8 A client is demonstrating poor exhalation. The nurse realizes that this client is at risk for developing:
   1. pleurisy.
   2. pulmonary edema.
   3. increased carbon dioxide levels.
   4. reduced oxygen capacity of red blood cells.
	Answer: 3
	Rationale: During expiration, the carbon dioxide is expelled. If the client cannot exhale effectively, carbon dioxide can build up. Pleurisy is pain upon inspiration. Pulmonary edema may accumulate as a result of poor inhalation, not exhalation. Poor exhalation does not have an effect on the oxygen carrying capacity of red blood cells.
	Diagnosis
	Analysis
	Physiological Integrity

36.9 A client is diagnosed with a fracture of one floating rib. Which of the following ribs is most likely fractured?
   1. 1
   2. 5
   3. 9
   4. 12
	Answer: 4
	Rationale: The first seven ribs articulate with the body of the sternum. The eighth, ninth, and tenth ribs articulate with the cartilage immediately above the ribs. The eleventh and twelfth ribs are called floating ribs, because they are unattached.
	Assessment
	Application
	Physiological Integrity

36.10 During the assessment of a client's respiratory status, the nurse locates the manubrium and the body of the sternum, which is also called the:
   1. Adam's apple.
   2. angle of Louis.
   3. intercostal space.
   4. xiphoid process.
	Answer: 2
	Rationale: The junction between the manubrium and the body of the sternum is called the manubriosternal junction or the angle of Louis. Intercostal space refers to the space between the ribs. Xiphoid process is on the end tip of the sternum. The Adam's apple is located on the larynx.
	Assessment
	Application
	Health Promotion and Maintenance

36.11 During pulmonary function tests, a client is found to have approximately 500 mL of air that moves in and out of the lungs during normal quiet breathing. The nurse realizes that this finding is considered:
   1. tidal volume.
   2. expiratory reserve volume.
   3. residual volume.
   4. vital capacity.
	Answer: 1
	Rationale: Tidal volume (TV) is the amount of air (approximately 500 mL) that is moved in and out of the lungs with each normal, quiet breath. **Tidal volume (TV)** is the amount of air (approximately 500 mL) moved in and out of the lungs with each normal, quiet breath. Inspiratory reserve volume (IRV) is the amount of air (approximately 2100 to 3100 mL) that can be inhaled forcibly over the tidal volume. Expiratory reserve volume (ERV) is the approximately 1000 mL of air that can be forced out over the tidal volume. The residual volume is the volume of air (approximately 1100 mL) that remains in the lungs after a forced expiration. **Vital capacity (VC)** refers to the sum of TV+ IRV+ ERV and is approximately 4500 mL in the healthy client.

Evaluation
Analysis
Health Promotion and Maintenance

36.12 During the assessment of a client's respirations, the nurse observes the expiration phase as being almost twice as long as the inspiration phase. This finding is consistent with:
1. chronic lung disease.
2. heart failure.
3. respiratory distress.
4. normal respiration.

Answer: 4
Rationale: During normal respiration, a single inspiration lasts for about 1 to 1.5 seconds; whereas an expiration lasts for about 2 to 3 seconds.
Assessment
Application
Health Promotion and Maintenance

36.13 The nurse counts a client's respirations at 30 per minute. From this finding, the nurse is concerned that the client is:
1. developing pneumonia.
2. attempting to expel increased carbon dioxide in the blood.
3. going into respiratory arrest.
4. in pain.

Answer: 2
Rationale: When carbon dioxide concentration in the blood increases or the pH decreases, the respiratory rate increases. There is not enough data provided to indicate pneumonia. With respiratory arrest or pain, the respirations would typically be decreased.
Diagnosis
Analysis
Physiological Integrity

36.14 A client is diagnosed with a low iron count. The nurse realizes that this client might demonstrate signs of:
1. increased carbon dioxide in the blood.
2. nausea.
3. anxiety.
4. poor tissue oxygenation.

Answer: 4
Rationale: Oxygen is carried in the blood either bound to hemoglobin or dissolved in the plasma. Oxygen is not very soluble in water, so almost all oxygen that enters the blood from the respiratory system is carried to the cells of the body by hemoglobin. Each hemoglobin molecule is made of four polypeptide chains, and each chain is bound to an iron-containing heme group. The iron groups are the binding sites for oxygen; each hemoglobin molecule can bind with four molecules of oxygen.
Diagnosis
Analysis
Physiological Integrity

36.15 During the assessment of a client's nasal cavities, the nurse notes watery nasal discharge and pale turbinates. These findings are consistent with:
1. allergies.
2. infection.
3. cocaine use.
4. sinus infection.

Answer: 1
Rationale: Allergies may be indicated by watery nasal drainage, pale turbinates, and polyps on the turbinates. Drainage from allergies infection or a sinus infection would be colored and thicker. Perforation of the septum may occur with chronic cocaine abuse.
Diagnosis
Application
Health Promotion and Maintenance

36.16 During a nap, the nurse notes that a client's respirations periodically stop. This finding should be documented as:
1. tachypnea.
2. bradypnea.
3. apnea.
4. atelectasis.

Answer: 3
Rationale: Apnea is the cessation of breathing that lasts from a few seconds to a few minutes. Tachypnea is increased respiration, and bradypnea is slow respirations. Atelectasis describes an illness, which is not evident in this situation.
Assessment
Application
Physiological Integrity

36.17 During the palpation of a client's chest for expansion, the nurse notices a decrease in expansion of the right side. This finding is consistent with: (Select all that apply.)
1. emphysema.
2. pneumonia.
3. pleural effusion.
4. heart failure.
5. pneumothorax.

Answer: 2, 3, 5
Rationale: Thoracic expansion is decreased on the affected side in atelectasis, pneumonia, pneumothorax, and pleural effusion. Bilateral chest expansion is decreased in emphysema. Heart failure would not result in a change in chest expansion.
Diagnosis
Analysis
Health Promotion and Maintenance

36.18 The nurse percusses hyperresonance over a client's lungs. This finding is consistent with: 　1. pneumonia. 　2. atelectasis. 　3. chronic asthma. 　4. pleural effusion.	Answer: 3 Rationale: Hyperresonance is heard in clients with chronic asthma and pneumothorax. Pneumonia, atelectasis, and pleural effusion might result in hyporesonance. Diagnosis Application Health Promotion and Maintenance
36.19 The nurse is preparing to auscultate a client's lungs. Breath sounds that would be considered abnormal include: (Select all that apply.) 　1. crackles. 　2. vesicular. 　3. bronchovesicular. 　4. wheezes. 　5. bronchial.	Answer: 1, 4 Rationale: The three different types of normal breath sounds are vesicular, bronchovesicular, and bronchial. Normally, there are no crackles, wheezes, or friction rubs. Assessment Application Health Promotion and Maintenance
36.20 During the assessment of a client's voice sounds, the nurse hears increased and clear sounds over the client's right lower lobe. This finding is consistent with: 　1. emphysema. 　2. lobar pneumonia. 　3. asthma. 　4. pleural effusion.	Answer: 2 Rationale: Voice sounds are increased and clearer over lobar pneumonia. Voice sounds are decreased or absent over areas of atelectasis, asthma, pleural effusion, and pneumothorax. Assessment Application Health Promotion and Maintenance

CHAPTER 37

37.1 A client tells the nurse he has a "cold" every spring that lasts for a few weeks. The nurse suspects that the client is experiencing: 　1. acute viral rhinitis. 　2. allergic rhinitis. 　3. vasomotor rhinitis. 　4. atrophic rhinitis.	Answer: 2 Rationale: Rhinitis, inflammation of the nasal cavities, is the most common upper respiratory disorder. Rhinitis may be either acute or chronic. Acute viral rhinitis is the common cold. Allergic rhinitis, or hay fever, results from a sensitivity reaction to allergens such as plant pollens. It tends to occur seasonally. The etiology of vasomotor rhinitis is unknown. Although its manifestations are similar to those of allergic rhinitis, it is not linked to allergens. Atrophic rhinitis is characterized by changes in the mucous membrane of the nasal cavities. Diagnosis Analysis Health Promotion and Maintenance
37.2 A client says, "My nose is always congested and it just seems to get worse with the nasal spray I've been using." The nurse realizes that this client is describing: 　1. an incorrect use of the nasal spray. 　2. an acute sinus infection that needs to be treated with antibiotics. 　3. a side effect of the nasal spray. 　4. rebound nasal congestion.	Answer: 4 Rationale: Chronic use of nasal sprays may lead to rhinitis medicamentosa, a rebound phenomenon of drug-induced nasal irritation and inflammation. The nasal spray is being used correctly. The worsening nasal congestion is not considered a side effect. No other signs indicate that the client has a bacterial sinus infection. Diagnosis Analysis Health Promotion and Maintenance
37.3 A middle-age client is seen in the clinic for a continuing cough after recovering from the flu a "few weeks ago." The nurse realizes that this client might be demonstrating: 　1. viral pneumonia. 　2. sinus infection.	Answer: 4 Rationale: The respiratory epithelial necrosis caused by influenza increases the risk for secondary bacterial infections. Tracheobronchitis, which is inflammation of the trachea and bronchi, may develop. While tracheobronchitis is not a serious health risk, its manifestations may persist for up to 3 weeks. Cough is not common with otitis media. No other signs of sinus infection were described. The cough has continued, not changed, so tracheobronchitis is probable. No other signs or symptoms were listed for the visit.

3. otitis media.	Assessment
4. tracheobronchitis.	Analysis
	Physiological Integrity

37.4 A client who was diagnosed with the flu is demonstrating rapid, shallow respirations. Which of the following is this client most at risk for developing?
  1. atelectasis
  2. pneumonia
  3. dehydration
  4. increased tidal volume
	Answer: 1
	Rationale: Muscle aches, malaise, and elevated temperature may increase the respiratory rate and alter the depth of respirations, and decrease effective alveolar ventilation. Shallow respirations also increase the risk of atelectasis, which is lack of ventilation and decreased, not increased tidal volume in an area of lung. A client would be at risk for pneumonia if they had decreased mobility. Rapid respirations may contribute to water loss that occurs naturally with the process of breathing, but would not be large enough to induce dehydration.
	Diagnosis
	Analysis
	Physiological Integrity

37.5 A client tells the nurse, "After I leave here, I need to get to the dentist. My upper teeth are hurting and I don't know why." Which of the following should the nurse do?
  1. End the visit so the client can get to the dentist.
  2. Assess the client for a sinus infection.
  3. Reschedule the appointment at another time.
  4. Tell the client there is nothing wrong with his teeth.
	Answer: 2
	Rationale: Manifestations of sinusitis include pain and tenderness across the infected sinuses, plus headache, fever, and malaise. The pain usually increases when the client leans forward. When the maxillary sinuses are involved, pain and pressure are felt over the cheek. The pain may be referred to the upper teeth. The client has a medical need and is in a medical setting. It would not be appropriate to end or reschedule the appointment. Until an assessment is performed and a diagnosis is made or ruled out, it would be incorrect to tell the client that nothing is wrong.
	Assessment
	Application
	Physiological Integrity

37.6 During an assessment, the nurse learns that the only thing that helps a client with a daily morning headache is "taking a mentholated cough drop" before eating breakfast. The nurse realizes that this client is experiencing:
  1. acute rhinitis.
  2. allergic rhinitis.
  3. symptoms of sinusitis.
  4. after-effects from the flu.
	Answer: 3
	Rationale: Complementary therapies are often used to aid in the symptoms of sinusitis. Aromatherapy using herbs such as basil, marjoram, or eucalyptus in a vaporizer or on a handkerchief; herbal teas made from goldenseal, yarrow, or coltsfoot, hot or cold compresses or steam inhalation; using cough drops with menthol; and acupressure may be employed. Rhinitis is inflammation of the nasal passages. A mentholated cough drop would not relieve inflammation. It was not mentioned that the client had any history of having the flu.
	Assessment
	Analysis
	Physiological Integrity

37.7 The nurse suspects that a client is demonstrating signs of tonsillitis. Which of the following would be indications of this disorder? (Select all that apply.)
  1. hoarse voice
  2. thirst
  3. nuchal rigidity
  4. pain around the ears
  5. low grade fever
	Answer: 1, 4, 5
	Rationale: Manifestations of tonsillitis include sore throat, possible dysphagia and otalgia, tender, swollen anterior cervical lymph nodes, hoarse voice, red and swollen pharyngeal mucous membranes and/or tonsils, possible visible exudate on pharyngeal membranes and/or tonsils, fever, general malaise, arthralgia, and myalgia. The client with tonsillitis complains of a sore throat, difficulty swallowing, general malaise, fever, and otalgia (pain referred to the ear). Thirst and nuchal rigidity (pain when bending the neck) are not suggestive of tonsillitis.
	Assessment
	Application
	Physiological Integrity

37.8 A client with epiglottitis is allergic to penicillin. The nurse realizes that the antibiotic of choice for this client is:
  1. dexamethasone (Dexasone).
  2. ciprofloxacin (Cipro).
  3. ampicillin and sulbactam (Unasyn).
  4. ampicillin (Amcill).
	Answer: 2
	Rationale: If the client is allergic to penicillin, a combination of clindamycin (Cleocin) and either trimethoprim-sulfamethoxazole (TMP-SMZ) or ciprofloxacin (Cipro) may be used. Dexamethasone (Dexasone) is a systemic corticosteroid. Ampicillin (Amcill) contains penicillin.
	Planning
	Analysis
	Physiological Integrity

37.9 A middle-age adult client who is diagnosed with pertussis is complaining of right-sided thoracic pain. The nurse realizes that this client should be assessed for: (Select all that apply.) 　1. pleural effusion. 　2. pneumothorax. 　3. pulmonary emboli. 　4. rib fractures.	Answer: 2, 4 Rationale: Complications of pertussis in adolescents and adults may occur as a result of increased intrathoracic pressure during prolonged coughing spells. These may include pneumothorax, weight loss, inguinal hernia, rib fracture, and cough syncope. Pleural effusion is a collection of fluid in the lungs. Pulmonary emboli is a clot in a lung. These are not a result of pertussis. Assessment Application Physiological Integrity
37.10 A young adult male client is seen in the emergency department after sustaining injuries from a motorcycle accident. During the assessment, the client's nose begins to bleed. Which of the following should the nurse include in the assessment of this client? 　1. use of cocaine or other substance abuse 　2. normal dietary intake pattern 　3. normal activity status 　4. employment status	Answer: 1 Rationale: Epistaxis, or nosebleed, may be precipitated by a number of factors. Trauma (picking the nose or blunt trauma) can cause epistaxis, as can drying of nasal mucous membranes, infection, substance abuse (e.g., cocaine), arteriosclerosis, or hypertension. Normal dietary intake and activity status would not directly impact a nose bleed and are not priority assessment areas for this situation and setting. The client's employment status would not typically relate to a motorcycle accident and then nasal bleeding. Assessment Application Physiological Integrity
37.11 A client is receiving anterior nasal packing for a nose bleed. Which of the following should be included in the instructions for this client? 　1. Remove the packing in the morning. 　2. The packing will stay in place for at least 5 days. 　3. The packing will be in place for at least 24 hours and up to 3 days. 　4. The packing will be needed for at least one week.	Answer: 3 Rationale: Anterior nasal packs are usually left in place for 24 to 72 hours. If epistaxis is caused by a bleeding disorder, the packing may be left in place for 4 to 5 days while the disorder is treated. Implementation Application Physiological Integrity
37.12 While engaging in a high school sports activity, an adolescent sustains an injury to the nose. Which of the following indicates that the client has a nasal fracture? 　1. shortness of breath 　2. diaphoresis 　3. drop in blood pressures 　4. periorbital ecchymosis	Answer: 4 Rationale: Manifestations of a fractured nose include epistaxis, deformity or displacement to one side, crepitus, periorbital edema and ecchymosis (bruising), and nasal bridge instability. Shortness of breath, diaphoresis, and a decrease in blood pressure are not typical anticipated responses to clients who experience a nasal fracture. Assessment Application Physiological Integrity
37.13 A client with multiple facial and nasal injuries needs a nasogastric tube placed. Which of the following is the appropriate method to place this tube? 　1. Place the tube through the client's mouth. 　2. Place the tube through the client's unobstructed nare. 　3. Place the tube through the obstructed nare. 　4. Place the tube after the edema in the nares subsides.	Answer: 2 Rationale: The nasogastric tube is inserted through the unobstructed nare to avoid mucosal trauma; however, a large gastric tube may interfere with nasal breathing, and necessitate close monitoring. A tube would not be able to be placed through an obstructed nare. The nasal edema may persist for a long period of time, so waiting would not be appropriate. A tube placed through the client's mouth would be an orogastric tube. Planning Application Physiological Integrity

37.14 While eating a meal in the hospital, a client begins to demonstrate difficulty breathing and signs of choking. The nurse realizes that the client is experiencing: 1. laryngeal obstruction. 2. pulmonary emboli. 3. epiglottitis. 4. an acute myocardial infarction.	Answer: 1 Rationale: The most common cause of laryngeal obstruction in adults is ingested meat that lodges in the airway. Risk factors for food aspiration include ingesting large boluses of food and chewing them insufficiently, consuming excess alcohol, and wearing dentures. A foreign body in the larynx causes pain, laryngospasm, dyspnea, and inspiratory stridor. The most common manifestations of laryngeal obstruction are coughing, choking, gagging, obvious difficulty breathing with use of accessory muscles, and inspiratory stridor. Diagnosis Application Physiological Integrity
37.15 The nurse observes a client's respirations during sleep and notes the absence of respirations that lasts from 15 to 45 seconds. This finding is consistent with: 1. laryngeal spasm. 2. sleep apnea. 3. respiratory acidosis. 4. renal failure.	Answer: 2 Rationale: Manifestations of obstructive sleep apnea include: loud, cyclic snoring; periods of apnea that lasts 15 to 120 seconds during sleep; gasping or choking during sleep; restlessness and thrashing during sleep; daytime fatigue and sleepiness; morning headache; personality changes, depression; intellectual impairment; impotence; and hypertension. Diagnosis Application Physiological Integrity
37.16 A female client is seen for "increased hoarseness" and a change in "voice quality." What is an appropriate assessment question for the nurse to ask this client? 1. "What medications are you currently taking?" 2. "Have you recently experienced a cold?" 3. "Have you recently visited another country?" 4. "What is your occupation?"	Answer: 4 Rationale: Hoarseness and a breathy voice quality are manifestations of benign vocal cord tumors. In adults, vocal cord nodules are often referred to as "singer's nodules"; cheerleaders and public speakers may also develop them. Voice abuse also contributes to the development of vocal cord polyps, as does cigarette smoking and chronic irritation from industrial pollutants. Assessment questions usually start with the causes that would be easiest to eliminate. The client with a cold would exhibit additional signs and symptoms. The list of medications and recent travel history would have a rare relevance to this client's specific complaints. Planning Application Health Promotion and Maintenance
37.17 A client who is scheduled for a partial laryngectomy asks if he will still be able to talk after the surgery. An appropriate nursing response to this client is: 1. "No." 2. "You will have to ask your physician." 3. "Yes, but it might sound a little different." 4. "You will, but with an electronic device."	Answer: 3 Rationale: In a partial laryngectomy, 50% or more of the larynx is removed. The voice generally is well-preserved, although it may be changed by the surgery. Implementation Application Physiological Integrity
37.18 The nurse is providing care to a client with a new tracheostomy. Which of the following is appropriate to include in this client's care? (Select all that apply.) 1. Remove the dressing with sterile gloves. 2. Suction the client prior to care using sterile technique. 3. Clean the inner cannula with sterile normal saline. 4. Remove crusted secretions with hydrogen peroxide and flush with normal saline. 5. Apply new dressing in a V shape.	Answer: 2, 4, 5 Rationale: The steps in tracheostomy care include: suction the client prior to care using sterile technique; wear a clean glove to remove the dressing; wear sterile gloves to clean and place a new dressing; use hydrogen peroxide to remove crusted secretions but flush with normal saline afterward to prevent skin irritation; remove the inner cannula and clean with hydrogen peroxide; rinse the inner cannula with normal saline; place a new commercially-prepared dressing or use gauze refolded into a V shape. Implementation Application Physiological Integrity

37.19 While recovering at home from a total laryngectomy, a client notices an increase in left shoulder weakness. This symptom is consistent with: 1. normal recovery. 2. damage to the spinal accessory nerve. 3. side effect of neck radiation therapy. 4. medication complication.	Answer: 2 Rationale: Manifestations of potential complications of laryngectomy that should be reported to the physician include loss of hearing or facial expression due to auditory or facial nerve injury, or shoulder drop due to damage to the spinal accessory nerve. Evaluation Analysis Physiological Integrity
37.20 A client with laryngeal cancer is found to have carcinoma in situ. The nurse realizes that the staging of this cancer is: 1. stage 0. 2. stage I. 3. stage II. 4. stage III.	Answer: 1 Rationale: In stage 0, the laryngeal tumor is found to be carcinoma in situ without any lymph node involvement. Assessment Analysis Physiological Integrity

CHAPTER 38

38.1 A client states, "I've been sick for days and all the doctor does is take a chest x-ray, hand me prescriptions, and tell me I have bronchitis." The nurse realizes that this client's treatment: 1. is appropriate for the diagnosis. 2. should include more diagnostic tests. 3. is inadequate for the diagnosis of bronchitis. 4. should include hospitalization.	Answer: 1 Rationale: The diagnosis of acute bronchitis typically is based on the history and clinical presentation. A chest x-ray may be ordered to rule out pneumonia, because the presenting manifestations can be similar. Other diagnostic testing and hospitalization are rarely indicated. Treatment is symptomatic and includes rest, increased fluid intake, and the use of aspirin or acetaminophen to relieve fever and malaise. Many physicians prescribe a broad-spectrum antibiotic such as erythromycin or penicillin, because approximately 50% of acute bronchitis is bacterial in origin. An expectorant cough medication is recommended for use during the day and a cough suppressant for night to facilitate rest. Evaluation Analysis Physiological Integrity
38.2 A client who is diagnosed with primary atypical pneumonia tells the nurse that he "doesn't feel too sick." The nurse's best response is: 1. "Give it a few days and you will." 2. "You're lucky." 3. "You must be recovering from the illness." 4. "This type of pneumonia is usually mild in its effects."	Answer: 4 Rationale: Pneumonia that is caused by mycoplasma pneumoniae is generally classified as primary atypical pneumonia, because its presentation and course significantly differ from other bacterial pneumonias. Young adults are the primary affected population. Primary atypical pneumonia is highly contagious with manifestations similar to those of viral pneumonia; systemic manifestations of fever, headache, myalgias, and arthralgias often predominate. Because of the typically mild nature and predominant systemic manifestations, mycoplasmal and viral pneumonia are often referred to as "walking pneumonias." Predicting that the client should expect to feel bad soon or is "lucky" are not appropriate responses. Since the illness is typically mild, the client may not feel very sick while in the acute phase, not just during recovery. Implementation Application Physiological Integrity
38.3 A client who was admitted with symptoms of hypoxia, is changed from a face mask to a nasal cannula for oxygen delivery. The nurse realizes that this client's condition is: 1. deteriorating. 2. improving. 3. stabilizing. 4. compounded with another health issue.	Answer: 2 Rationale: Low-flow oxygen delivery systems include the nasal cannula, simple face mask, partial rebreathing mask, and nonrebreathing mask. A nasal cannula can deliver 24% to 45% oxygen concentrations with flow rates of 2 to 6 L/min. The nasal cannula is comfortable and does not interfere with eating or talking. A simple face mask delivers 40% to 60% oxygen concentrations with flow rates of 5 to 8 L/min. This client's condition is most likely improving. Implementation Analysis Physiological Integrity

38.4 A client who is being treated at home for pneumonia is demonstrating signs of increased confusion. The nurse interprets this information to mean that this client:

1. is experiencing a side effect of the prescribed medication.
2. is improving.
3. could be experiencing a worsening of the pneumonia.
4. should increase fluid intake.

Answer: 3

Rationale: Clients with pneumonia usually are treated in the community, unless their respiratory status is significantly compromised such as an altered mental status. There is no evidence to support that this client is experiencing a side effect of medication or dehydration. This client needs to be seen by a physician.

Diagnosis

Analysis

Physiological Integrity

38.5 A client who is in the hospital is diagnosed with sudden acute respiratory syndrome (SARS). The best nursing intervention for this client is to implement:

1. standard precautions.
2. standard precautions and droplet precautions.
3. standard precautions and contact precautions.
4. standard, contact, and airborne precautions.

Answer: 4

Rationale: Because healthcare workers are at risk for developing sudden acute respiratory syndrome (SARS) after caring for infected clients, infection control precautions should be immediately instituted when SARS is suspected. Standard precautions should be implemented in addition to contact and airborne precautions.

Implementation

Application

Health Promotion and Maintenance

38.6 A client with a lung abscess is being discharged from the hospital. Appropriate discharge instructions for this client should include:

1. complete the entire prescription of antibiotics.
2. expect symptoms to become worse.
3. return to routine activities of daily living.
4. lung abscesses rarely cause other problems once treatment is started.

Answer: 1

Rationale: Client and family teaching focuses on the importance of completing the prescribed antibiotic therapy. Most lung abscesses are successfully treated with antibiotics; however, treatment may last up to 1 month or more. Emphasize the importance of completing the entire course of therapy to eliminate the infecting organisms. Teach about the medication, including its name, dose, and desired and adverse effects. Stress the need to contact the physician if symptoms do not improve or if they become worse. Infection from lung abscess can spread not only to lung and pleural tissue but systemically, and cause sepsis.

Implementation

Application

Physiological Integrity

38.7 A client who is on isoniazid (INH) for pulmonary tuberculosis tells the nurse he doesn't like taking the medication because it makes his "fingers burn." The nurse concludes that the client is experiencing:

1. a common side effect of isoniazid (INH) that will go away after completing the medication.
2. a common side effect of isoniazid (INH) that can be treated with pyridoxine.
3. a long-term complication of isoniazid (INH) that has no treatment.
4. a common complication of isoniazid (INH) that can be treated with vitamin B_{12} injections.

Answer: 2

Rationale: Peripheral neuropathy—numbness, tingling, or a burning sensation of the extremities—may occur with isoniazid (INH). Pyridoxine or vitamin B_6 often is prescribed to prevent this adverse effect.

Evaluation

Analysis

Physiological Integrity

38.8 A client who had a Mantoux test for tuberculosis two days ago has a 2 mm area of erythema at the site of the test. The nurse concludes that this client's response: 1. is negative. 2. is positive for tuberculosis. 3. should be followed up with a tine test. 4. is unable to determine the presence of tuberculosis.	Answer: 1 Rationale: Intradermal PPD or Mantoux test is read within 48 to 72 hours, the peak reaction period, and recorded as the diameter of induration (raised area, not erythema) in millimeters. The area on the client is erythematous, not an induration. No followup is needed as this client's response is by definition a negative one. Assessment Application Health Promotion and Maintenance
38.9 A client tells the nurse he had the bacilli Calmette-Guerin (BCG) vaccination as a child because his mother had tuberculosis. This client will be screened for tuberculosis by: 1. conducting a tine test. 2. conducting a Mantoux test. 3. conducting both the tine and Mantoux tests. 4. conducting a chest x-ray.	Answer: 4 Rationale: After vaccination with BCG, a positive reaction to tuberculin testing is common. Periodic chest x-rays may be required for screening purposes. Planning Analysis Health Promotion and Maintenance
38.10 A client who is taking rifampin (Rifadin) as part of his treatment for tuberculosis wants to make an appointment for a urologist because his urine is "bright orange." The nurse realizes that this client is experiencing: 1. a secondary urinary tract infection. 2. a common side effect of rifampin (Rifadin) therapy. 3. the onset of a kidney stone. 4. early renal failure.	Answer: 2 Rationale: Rifampin (Rifadin) causes body fluids, including sweat, urine, saliva, and tears, to turn red-orange. This is not harmful. Evaluation Analysis Physiological Integrity
38.11 The nurse is providing care to a client with pulmonary tuberculosis. Which of the following should the nurse do to ensure personal protection while caring for this client? 1. wear a gown and eye goggles 2. wear a gown and surgical mask 3. wear a gown and HEPA mask 4. wear a gown and sterile gloves	Answer: 3 Rationale: Nursing staff should use personal protective devices to reduce the risk of transmission during client care. The Occupational Safety and Health Administration (OSHA) requires use of a HEPA-filtered respirator for protection against occupational exposure to tuberculosis. Surgical masks are ineffective to filter droplet nuclei, which necessitates the use of protective devices capable of filtering bacteria and particles smaller than 1 micron. Planning Application Health Promotion and Maintenance
38.12 A client is diagnosed with histoplasmosis. Which of the following elements of this client's history would help explain the reason for the disease? 1. lives in a city with chemical plants 2. drives a vehicle that uses diesel fuel 3. is an electrical engineer 4. works part-time for his grandparents' fresh poultry business	Answer: 4 Rationale: Histoplasmosis, an infectious disease caused by Histoplasma capsulatum, is the most common fungal lung infection in the United States. The organism is found in the soil and is linked to exposure to bird droppings and bats. Infection occurs when the spores are inhaled and reach the alveoli. Assessment Application Health Promotion and Maintenance

38.13 A client with lung cancer is demonstrating signs of complete tumor response after two courses of chemotherapy. The nurse concludes that this response is:
  1. good for a long-term survival from the disease.
  2. an indication that radiation therapy is needed.
  3. an indication that surgery can be performed.
  4. a contraindication for further chemotherapy.
	Answer: 1
	Rationale: Fifty percent of clients with tumors at early stages achieve complete tumor remission with combination chemotherapy. When a complete tumor response is achieved in the first few cycles of chemotherapy, the chances for long-term survival are much greater.
	Evaluation
	Analysis
	Physiological Integrity

38.14 A client who is receiving radiation therapy for lung cancer complains of ongoing fatigue. Appropriate teaching for this client includes that:
  1. this is a complication of radiation therapy and will continue for years.
  2. there is nothing that can help the fatigue.
  3. frequent rest periods and good nutrition can help with the fatigue.
  4. restricting caloric intake often helps with the fatigue.
	Answer: 3
	Rationale: Adequate rest and nutrition are important to alleviate the symptoms of radiation fatigue, which is common in clients who are receiving radiation therapy for lung cancer. The fatigue is generally temporary. The fatigue effects due to radiation do not last for years, only during treatment. Restricting calories would only contribute to continued fatigue.
	Implementation
	Application
	Physiological Integrity

38.15 A client is diagnosed with pleurisy. The nurse instructs the client to alleviate the associated chest pain by:
  1. only taking the prescribed analgesic when the pain is severe.
  2. teaching the client how to splint the affected area when coughing.
  3. advising the client to maintain bed rest.
  4. warning the client to expect a fever to develop.
	Answer: 2
	Rationale: Nursing care for the client with pleuritis is directed toward promoting comfort, including administration of NSAIDs and analgesics. Positioning and splinting the chest while coughing also are helpful. Teach the client and family that pleuritis is generally self-limited and of short duration. Discuss symptoms to report to the physician: increased fever, productive cough, difficulty breathing, or shortness of breath. Provide information about prescription and nonprescription NSAIDs and analgesics, including the drug ordered, how to use it, and its desired and possible adverse effects.
	Planning
	Application
	Physiological Integrity

38.16 A 20-year-old client who is asking questions about smoking cessation tells the nurse about an upcoming class on scuba diving. The nurse identifies that this client might be at risk for developing:
  1. pleural effusion.
  2. pleurisy.
  3. pneumothorax.
  4. hemothorax.
	Answer: 3
	Rationale: Primary pneumothorax affects previously healthy people, usually tall, slender men between ages 16 and 24. The cause of primary pneumothorax is unknown. Risk factors include smoking and familial factors. Air-filled blebs tend to form in the apices of the lungs. This is considered to be a benign condition, although recurrences are common. Certain activities also increase the risk of spontaneous pneumothorax, such as high altitude flying and rapid decompression during scuba diving.
	Diagnosis
	Analysis
	Health Promotion and Maintenance

38.17 The nurse observes air bubbles in a client's chest tube water seal chamber. The nurse interprets this finding as:
  1. normal.
  2. an emergency.
	Answer: 1
	Rationale: Periodic air bubbles in the water-seal chamber are normal and indicate that trapped air is being removed from the chest. This is not an emergency situation, or one that indicates a worsening condition. The nurse would need a physician's order to remove a chest tube. The client still needs the chest tube in place.

3. an indication that the pneumothorax is worsening. 4. an indication to remove the chest tube.	Evaluation Analysis Physiological Integrity
38.18 During the assessment of a client's respiratory status, the nurse notes paradoxical lung movements. This finding is consistent with: 1. flail chest. 2. pleurisy. 3. pneumothorax. 4. pneumonia.	Answer: 1 Rationale: Physiologic function of the chest wall is impaired as the flail segment is sucked inward during inhalation and moves outward with exhalation. This is known as paradoxic movement. Diagnosis Application Physiological Integrity
38.19 The nurse is providing care to a client with a differential diagnosis of carbon monoxide poisoning. Which of the following would be consistent with this diagnosis? (Select all that apply.) 1. cherry red mucous membranes 2. circumoral pallor 3. diarrhea 4. nausea 5. dizziness	Answer: 1, 4, 5 Rationale: The manifestations of carbon monoxide poisoning depend on the level of carboxyhemoglobin saturation. When hemoglobin is 10% to 20% saturated with carbon monoxide, symptoms include headache, dizziness, dyspnea, and nausea. A characteristic "cherry-red" color of the skin and mucous membranes may be seen. With increasing levels, confusion, visual disturbances, irritability, hallucinations, hypotension, seizures, and coma develop. Permanent neurologic deficit can occur in survivors of severe acute carbon monoxide poisoning. Assessment Analysis Physiological Integrity
38.20 A client is diagnosed with a tension pneumothorax. Which of the following would be consistent with this diagnosis? (Select all that apply.) 1. hypertension 2. distended neck veins 3. bradycardia 4. absent breath sounds on the affected side 5. tracheal deviation toward unaffected side	Answer: 2, 4, 5 Rationale: Manifestations of a tension pneumothorax include hypotension, shock, distended neck veins, severe dyspnea, tachypnea, tachycardia, decreased respiratory excursion, absent breath sounds on affected side, and tracheal deviation toward unaffected side. Assessment Application Physiological Integrity

CHAPTER 39

39.1 A client with asthma tells the nurse the asthma is exacerbated by fresh fruit. The nurse realizes that the classification of this trigger is: 1. exposure to an allergen. 2. emotional stress. 3. pharmacologic. 4. psychosocial.	Answer: 3 Rationale: Common pharmacologic triggers include aspirin and other NSAIDs, sulfites (which are used as preservatives in wine, beer, fresh fruits, and salad), and beta-blockers. Assessment Analysis Health Promotion and Maintenance
39.2 A client is being instructed on the use of a metered-dose inhaler for asthma. How long should the client wait before providing a second puff of the medication? 1. 3 to 5 seconds 2. 10 seconds 3. 20 to 30 seconds 4. no need to wait between puffs	Answer: 3 Rationale: The client should be instructed to wait 20 to 30 seconds before repeating the procedure for a second puff. Implementation Application Physiological Integrity
39.3 A client is prescribed a medication to reduce the need for inhaled corticosteroids while controlling asthma symptoms. The	Answer: 4 Rationale: Leukotriene modifiers interfere with the inflammatory process in the airways, and improve airflow, decrease symptoms, and reduce the need for short-acting bronchodilators. They are used for maintenance therapy in adults and

nurse realizes that the category of this medication is a/an: 1. methylxanthine. 2. anticholinergic. 3. mast cell stabilizer. 4. leukotriene modifier.	children over the age of 12 as an alternative to inhaled corticosteroid therapy. They are not used to treat an acute attack. Implementation Application Physiological Integrity
39.4 A 65-year-old male client who continues to smoke tells the nurse that he is fine because he only has chronic bronchitis. The nurse determines that this client is experiencing: 1. beginning stages of lung cancer. 2. chronic obstructive pulmonary disease. 3. chronic asthma. 4. emphysema.	Answer: 2 Rationale: Although one or the other may predominate, COPD typically includes components of both chronic bronchitis and emphysema, which are two distinctly different processes. Small airways disease, which is the narrowing of small bronchioles, is also part of the COPD complex. Through different mechanisms, these processes cause airways to narrow, increased resistance to airflow, and slow or difficult expiration. Assessment Analysis Physiological Integrity
39.5 A client who smokes has a chronic cough with sputum production. Which stage of COPD is this client is most likely experiencing? 1. 0 2. 1 3. 2 4. 3	Answer: 1 Rationale: In stage 0 of COPD, lung function is normal, but chronic cough and sputum production are present. Assessment Analysis Physiological Integrity
39.6 A client who was diagnosed with carbon dioxide retention has a pulse oximetry reading of 80% on room air. A nurse should obtain a physician's order to do which of the following interventions? 1. provide high volume oxygen 2. intubate 3. provide an oral airway 4. administer low volume oxygen and monitor respirations	Answer: 4 Rationale: Hypercapnia, which is elevated $Paco_2$ levels, is often chronic in clients who retain CO_2. In these clients, administering oxygen can actually increase the $Paco_2$, which leads to somnolence and acute respiratory failure. Low volume oxygen levels are needed, not high volume in this situation. While oxygen is the drug of choice for treating clients with COPD, close monitoring is necessary during oxygen therapy. Pulse oximetry is used to monitor oxygen saturation of the blood. Marked airway obstruction and hypoxemia often causes oxygen saturation levels less than 95%. Pulse oximetry may be continuously monitored to assess the need for supplemental oxygen. Intubation is not a nursing function. Initiation of oxygen therapy, not insertion of an oral airway is needed. Lower level, noninvasive interventions are initiated and evaluated first. Implementation Application Physiological Integrity
39.7 The nurse is assisting a client with stage 3 COPD with menu items for daily meals while in the hospital. Which of the following items is the most beneficial for this client? 1. spaghetti with marinara sauce 2. tuna noodle casserole 3. flank steak with broiled vegetables 4. vegetable lasagna	Answer: 3 Rationale: A diet high in proteins and fats without excess carbohydrates is recommended. This type of diet minimizes carbon dioxide production during metabolism because carbohydrates are metabolized to form CO_2 and water. Spaghetti, noodles, and lasagna are high in carbohydrates. Planning Application Physiological Integrity
39.8 The nurse is instructing a client to breathe so that positive pressure is maintained longer during exhalation. The technique the nurse is teaching this client is: 1. diaphragmatic breathing. 2. pursed-lip breathing. 3. controlled breathing. 4. huff breathing.	Answer: 2 Rationale: Pursed-lip breathing helps maintain open airways by maintaining positive pressures longer during exhalation. Implementation Application Physiological Integrity

39.9 The nurse is providing care to a client with cystic fibrosis. Which of the following interventions would help prevent the onset of an acute illness?
  1. Provide prophylactic anti-inflammatory therapy.
  2. Check for capillary blood glucose level.
  3. Restrict fluids.
  4. Immunize against communicable diseases.

Answer: 4
Rationale: Immunization against respiratory infections is vital to promote optimal health. Yearly influenza vaccine is recommended, along with measles and pertussis boosters as needed. Blood glucose level assessment will not prevent acute illnesses. Restricting fluids may put the client at higher risk for an illness. Anti-inflammatory therapy is not typically prescribed prophylactically and may actually mask early signs of infections.
Planning
Analysis
Health Promotion and Maintenance

39.10 The nurse is positioning a client with atelectasis. Which of the following positions is the most beneficial for this client?
  1. lung with atelectasis is lower than the lung without atelectasis
  2. prone
  3. supine
  4. lung without atelectasis is lower than the lung with atelectasis

Answer: 4
Rationale: Nursing care to prevent and treat atelectasis is directed toward airway clearance. Position the client with atelectasis on the unaffected side to promote gravity drainage of affected segment.
Implementation
Application
Physiological Integrity

39.11 A client is diagnosed with sarcoidosis. Appropriate teaching for this client should include: (Select all that apply.)
  1. smoking cessation.
  2. report any onset of shortness of breath.
  3. if not treated, death by respiratory failure will occur.
  4. limit dairy food intake.
  5. avoid anything that irritates the respiratory tract.

Answer: 1, 2, 5
Rationale: Sarcoidosis often resolves spontaneously; therefore, treatment is indicated only when symptoms are severe or disabling. Nursing care for clients with sarcoidosis is directed according to involved organ systems and related manifestations. Respiratory care is supportive and includes avoiding respiratory irritants and maintaining adequate ventilation. Refer for smoking cessation assistance as needed. Limiting dairy food intake is not required for this diagnosis.
Planning
Application
Health Promotion and Maintenance

39.12 A client is believed to have a pulmonary embolism that was not diagnosed after a lung CT scan. The nurse should begin preparing the client to have a:
  1. lung scan.
  2. chest x-ray.
  3. ECG.
  4. pulmonary angiogram.

Answer: 4
Rationale: Pulmonary angiography is the definitive test for pulmonary embolism when other, less invasive tests are inconclusive. It is possible to detect very small emboli with angiography. A contrast medium injected into the pulmonary arteries illustrates the pulmonary vascular system on x-ray. Another lung scan or chest x-ray would not be the next level of testing. An ECG is not indicated as the problem is respiratory in nature, not cardiac.
Planning
Application
Physiological Integrity

39.13 A client who is receiving heparin (Hepalean) is found to have an extremely high partial thromboplastin (PTT) time. Which of the following should be available to assist this client should bleeding occur?
  1. protamine sulfate
  2. Vitamin E
  3. magnesium sulfate
  4. Vitamin K

Answer: 1
Rationale: Keep protamine sulfate available for heparin therapy. Keep vitamin K available for warfarin (Coumadin) therapy. Bleeding or hemorrhage due to excess anticoagulant may require antidote administration to rapidly reverse anticoagulant effects.
Planning
Application
Physiological Integrity

39.14 A client with pulmonary hypertension has an elevated hematocrit level. The nurse's discharge instructions should include:
1. Instructions about phlebotomy.
2. Discussion of the need for long-acting calcium channel blockers.
3. Instructions about anticoagulant therapy.
4. Instructions about the use of oxygen at home.

Answer: 1
Rationale: Treatment for pulmonary hypertension focuses on slowing the course of the disease, preventing thrombus formation, and reducing pulmonary vasoconstriction. Oxygen is administered to reduce hypoxemia and improve activity tolerance. This may be a temporary measure during hospitalization. If polycythemia is present, phlebotomy is performed to reduce the viscosity of the blood.
Planning
Application
Physiological Integrity

39.15 A client with hypoxemia is not improving despite oxygen therapy. Which of the following is indicated for this client?
1. Tracheostomy
2. Neuromuscular blocking agent
3. Analgesics
4. Continuous positive airway pressure (CPAP)

Answer: 4
Rationale: When respiratory failure is caused by hypoventilation or usual oxygen delivery systems do not correct hypoxemia, a tight-fitting mask to maintain continuous positive airway pressure (CPAP) may be used. CPAP increases lung volume, opens previously-closed alveoli, improves ventilation of underventilated alveoli, and improves ventilation-perfusion relationships. A tracheostomy is an invasive and higher level intervention that is not indicated next. A neuromuscular blocking agent would decrease the respiratory effort, increasing the hypoxemia. Analgesics would be used to decrease pain, but do not impact hypoxemia.
Planning
Analysis
Physiological Integrity

39.16 An extubated client is demonstrating respiratory stridor. The nurse's best action is to:
1. continue the current treatment plan, because this is normal after extubation.
2. assess for the presence of the gag reflex.
3. prepare for reintubation.
4. increase oxygen flow via a nasal cannula.

Answer: 3
Rationale: Close observation for respiratory distress is vital following extubation. Inspiratory stridor within the first 24 hours indicates laryngeal edema, which may necessitate reintubation.
Planning
Application
Physiological Integrity

39.17 A client who is receiving positive end-expiratory pressure (PEEP) can be expected to:
1. breathe spontaneously.
2. be intubated.
3. wear oxygen via face mask.
4. wear oxygen via nasal cannula.

Answer: 2
Rationale: Positive end-expiratory pressure (PEEP) requires intubation and can be applied to any of the previously-described ventilator modes. With PEEP, a positive pressure is maintained in the airways during exhalation and between breaths. Keeping alveoli open between breaths improves ventilation-perfusion relationships and diffusion across the alveolar-capillary membrane. This reduces hypoxemia and allows use of lower percentages of inspired oxygen.
Planning
Analysis
Physiological Integrity

39.18 An intubated client is not exhibiting signs of improved oxygenation. The nurse should: (Select all that apply.)
1. prepare for an emergency tracheotomy.
2. assess for endotracheal tube placement.
3. assess for the need to suction to clear the airway.
4. insert an oral airway.
5. insert a nasal airway.

Answer: 2, 3
Rationale: Intubation and mechanical ventilation do not ensure adequate oxygenation and ventilation. Displacement of the endotracheal tube or obstruction by respiratory secretions impairs ventilation. The client is already passed the stage of oral or nasal airways and is intubated. Checking the tube placement or determining if the tube is clear of secretions are anticipated initial steps in evaluating the client's response to intubation.
Implementation
Application
Physiological Integrity

39.19 An intubated client is awake and begins to cry. The nurse's best action is to: 1. provide a neuromuscular blocking agent. 2. explain that the breathing tube is a temporary measure. 3. wipe the client's tears and leave the room. 4. turn off the lights so that the client can sleep.	Answer: 2 Rationale: Reassure the client that intubation and mechanical ventilation is a temporary measure to allow the lungs to rest and heal. Reinforce that the client will be able to breathe independently again. The client may fear continued dependence on mechanical ventilation. Leaving the client alone, or in a dark room may frighten the client. Administering a neuromuscular blocking agent would be based on a physician's order and is not indicated for all intubated clients. Implementation Application Psychosocial Integrity
39.20 A client has a nasal endotracheal tube. The nurse recognizes that this method of airway management will result in: 1. a greater chance of upper respiratory infection. 2. easier removal of secretions. 3. more discomfort for the client. 4. ability for the client to communicate orally.	Answer: 4 Rationale: Nasal endotracheal tubes are more comfortable (and therefore, better tolerated by clients) and can facilitate communication and oral hygiene. Because the tube is smaller, secretions will be more difficult to remove and there is an increased risk of lower respiratory infections. Planning Application Physiological Integrity

CHAPTER 40

40.1 The client's right femur was fractured and repaired at the diaphysis. When teaching, the client asks the nurse to explain the diaphysis. The nurse's best response is: 1. "Short bones like the femur are cuboid, spongy bone that, in medical terms, are called the diaphysis." 2. "Irregular bones like the femur are plates of compact bone that are also called the diaphysis." 3. "Flat bones like the femur are disc-shaped and, in medical terms, are called the diaphysis." 4. "Long bones like the femur have a midportion or shaft that is also called the diaphysis."	Answer: 4 Rationale: The femur is the long bone in the upper leg that consists of the midportion (diaphysis) and two broad ends. Cuboid, spongy bone; irregular bones; and flat bones describe other types of bones in the body. Implementation Application Health Promotion and Maintenance
40.2 The client is ordered to be on bed rest for two months. The nurse realizes that the client's bones will: 1. not be affected by the bed rest. 2. undergo increased osteoclast activity and bone resorption. 3. increase their osteoblastic activity to promote ossification. 4. be affected positively by the rest and be stronger as a result.	Answer: 2 Rationale: Bones that are not in use for a prolonged time promote bone resorption or bone loss. Bones that are in use and subjected to stress will increase their osteoblastic activity and develop bone ossification. Planning Application Physiological Integrity
40.3 A client is seen in the clinic for chronic low blood calcium. What effect will this have on bone health? 1. Bone resorption will be triggered in order to increase serum calcium levels.	Answer: 1 Rationale: Bone resorption occurs to increase serum calcium levels because calcium ions are required for transmission of nerve impulses, release of neurotransmitters, muscle contraction, blood clotting, gland secretions, and cell division. There are no other body structures that have adequate amounts of calcium to increase serum levels.

2. Bone production will occur in order to help increase the blood calcium. 3. Bones will not be affected because the calcium is low in the blood. 4. Bones will pull the needed calcium from other body structures.	Assessment Application Physiological Integrity
40.4 The client is recovering from orthopedic surgery on a fractured arm. The nurse realizes that for musculo-skeletal function, what type of muscle is needed? 1. cardiac 2. smooth 3. skeletal 4. a combination of skeletal and smooth	Answer: 3 Rationale: Skeletal muscle is the only muscle in the body that allows musculoskeletal function. Cardiac muscle is exclusive to the heart and smooth muscle is found in organs such as the intestines and is not under voluntary control. Smooth muscle is not needed for musculoskeletal function. Planning Application Physiological Integrity
40.5 Teaching the client about an electromyelogram (EMG) should include: (Select all that apply.) 1. Do not smoke for several hours before the test. 2. Do not take any medication prior to this test without physician approval. 3. The test measures nerve conduction along pathways. 4. The test measures electrical activity of skeletal muscles at rest.	Answer: 1, 2, 4 Rationale: The electromyelogram (EMG) measures the electrical activity of skeletal muscles at rest. When preparing the client for the testing, instruct the client to avoid behaviors that may influence the test. This includes smoking and medications. The physician must have the final determination regarding which medications can be allowed prior to the testing. Implementation Application Health Promotion and Maintenance
40.6 Put the following techniques of a musculoskeletal examination in the proper sequence. 1. Assess joints for swelling, pain, redness, warmth, crepitus, and range of motion (ROM). 2. Inspect and palpate the bones for any obvious deformity or changes in size, shape, or a painful response. 3. Measure the extremities for length and circumference, and compare limbs bilaterally. 4. Assess gait and posture.	Answer: 4, 2, 3, 1 Rationale: When performing an assessment of the musculoskeletal system, first review the client's gait and posture. Inspection is the next technique. Employ visual inspection on the bones for changes and irregularities. Use hands-on techniques to review the presence of swelling, pain, redness, warmth, crepitus, and range of motion (ROM). Finally, measure the extremities for abnormalities. Assessment Application Health Promotion and Maintenance
40.7 The nurse is teaching about an endoscopic examination of the interior surfaces of a joint during which surgery and diagnosis can also be accomplished. What is a correct name for this technique? 1. arthrocentesis 2. arthroscopy 3. arthrogenesis 4. arthrodonesia	Answer: 2 Rationale: The suffix –scopy refers to using a scope for examination, treatment, or diagnosis. Arthro- refers to the knee. Arthroscopy is endoscopic examination of the interior surfaces of a joint during which surgery and diagnosis can also be accomplished. Assessment Application Health Promotion and Maintenance

40.8 The client is about to have a magnetic resonance imaging (MRI) to diagnose a soft tissue abnormality of the lower leg. The nurse should immediately notify the physician about which of the following?

1. The client has a concern about what will be found on the MRI.
2. The client has a pacemaker.
3. The client has a history of hypertension.
4. The client did not eat breakfast due to earlier nausea.

Answer: 2

Rationale: The client will be prohibited from having an MRI due to the pacemaker. Metallic implants prevent the test because radio waves and magnetic fields are used. All tests have the capacity to promote client concern and anxiety. This is a normal behavior and does not require physician notification. The presence of hypertension and reduced dietary intake will not have an adverse impact on the MRI results.

Assessment

Application

Health Promotion and Maintenance

40.9 The nurse should prepare the client for standard x-rays of an arm by:

1. initiating a peripheral IV in the opposite arm.
2. finding out the client's allergies.
3. doing no special preparation.
4. cleansing the arm with antibacterial cleanser.

Answer: 3

Rationale: No special preparation is needed for standard x-rays. Routine x-rays do not require the client to have an IV inserted. Allergies will not impact routine x-ray studies. Cleaning the extremity is not warranted for the x-ray.

Assessment

Application

Health Promotion and Maintenance

40.10 A bone scan would most likely be ordered for a client when:

1. bone cancer is suspected.
2. a muscle mass near the bone is suspected.
3. a client complains of new onset pain in the area of the bone.
4. lab tests indicate normal calcium.

Answer: 1

Rationale: Bone scans show increased uptake of the radioisotope in osteomyelitis, osteoporosis, cancer, and some fractures. The bone scan would do little to provide a definite analysis of a muscle mass. New onset bone pain would require other initial evaluation studies.

Assessment

Application

Health Promotion and Maintenance

40.11 A 62-year-old female client is scheduled to have a DEXA exam as a screening tool. The most likely reason that the test has been ordered is:

1. to check for fractures.
2. to check the degree of osteoporosis.
3. to screen for osteomyelitis.
4. to evaluate bone cancer.

Answer: 2

Rationale: The bone density exam (DEXA) evaluates bone mineral density and the degree of osteoporosis. X-rays would be used to assess for the presence of fractures. Bone scans would be used in the evaluation of osteomyelitis and potential bone cancer.

Assessment

Application

Health Promotion and Maintenance

40.12 When caring for older adults, the nurse realizes that an age-related change in the musculoskeletal system is:

1. difficulty with dexterity after age 50.
2. vertebrae lengthen and thin, which leads to increased bone production.
3. decreased bone mass and calcium absorption, which lead to a chance for fractures.
4. pain when ambulating due to increased bone mass and minerals.

Answer: 3

Rationale: Normal aging is associated with a reduction in bone mass and calcium absorption. Bone production does not increase with aging. Pain with ambulation is not associated with increased bone mass. Difficulty with dexterity is not necessarily a usual occurrence after age 50.

Assessment

Application

Health Promotion and Maintenance

40.13 In clients who are experiencing musculoskeletal disorders and diseases, alkaline phosphatase (ALP) is assessed to:
1. establish true calcium levels.
2. evaluate the presence of bone diseases.
3. determine phosphorus levels.
4. diagnose muscle trauma.

Answer: 2
Rationale: Alkaline phosphatase (ALP) levels are assessed in clients who are experiencing musculoskeletal disorders in order to evaluate the presence of bone diseases. Blood tests other than ALP establish calcium and phosphorus levels, and diagnose muscle trauma.
Assessment
Application
Health Promotion and Maintenance

40.14 Creatine kinase (CK) is evaluated in clients who are suspected of having:
1. juvenile rheumatoid arthritis.
2. gout.
3. muscle disease.
4. bone tumors.

Answer: 3
Rationale: CK (the isoenzyme CK-MM) is elevated in muscle trauma and muscle disease. Juvenile rheumatoid arthritis is a systemic disease process that affects the body's joints and other systems; CK levels will not assist in its diagnosis. Uric acid levels are used to diagnose gout. The presence of bone tumors would be identified by radiological testing.
Assessment
Application
Health Promotion and Maintenance

40.15 A client is seen in the physician's office following several tests. The test results include elevated blood calcium, elevated alkaline phosphatase, elevated phosphorus, normal creatine kinase, and increased uptake of the radioisotope on bone scan. The nurse realizes that the most likely diagnosis is:
1. bone spurs.
2. rheumatoid arthritis.
3. osteoporosis.
4. bone cancer.

Answer: 4
Rationale: The test results are a likely combination in a client with bone cancer. The blood values described would be anticipated, because the bone levels would be reduced in the presence of a malignancy. The other conditions listed would not produce the same blood value alterations. Areas of disease will demonstrate an increase in uptake of radioisotopes on the scans. X-ray would be useful in diagnosis of bone spurs. Rheumatoid factor is used to diagnose rheumatoid arthritis.
Evaluation
Assessment
Health Promotion and Maintenance

40.16 A young adult is seen in the clinic complaining of pain in the left wrist. There is no deformity of the wrist, the left radial pulse is strong, and there is no history of a fall or injury. What does the nurse expect to see ordered?
1. an x-ray of both arms to ensure there is no injury present
2. rest and comfort measures for several days unless pain worsens
3. lab work to assess calcium and phosphorus levels
4. a computerized tomography (CT) scan of the wrist to check for soft tissue injury

Answer: 2
Rationale: Based on the history and objective findings, there is not a present need to order x-rays or lab work. A CT scan of a wrist is not expected. Initially, rest and comfort measures are best to see if the pain resolves. If the pain persists over several days or if other signs and symptoms emerge, a more aggressive approach would be expected.
Planning
Assessment
Health Promotion and Maintenance

40.17 A client comes to the emergency department complaining of right knee pain after being knocked down while playing basketball. The exam reveals the client experiences difficulty when stepping down on the right leg due to acute pain around the knee and slight swelling of the right knee. Initially, the nurse expects that:

Answer: 3
Rationale: This injury would not be considered an emergency if alterations in sensation, perfusion, and movement of the leg are present. Since these changes are not noted on assessment, hospitalization or surgery would not be indicated. The possible injury to the knee (likely cartilage injury) will be evaluated by a specialist and a decision will be made regarding the need for the MRI. An MRI would evaluate tears of a ligament or cartilage.
Planning
Assessment
Health Promotion and Maintenance

1. the client will be sent home with instructions to use ice for one week.
2. the client will be admitted to the hospital and seen by an orthopedic specialist.
3. the client will be scheduled to see an orthopedic physician and a tentative appointment for a magnetic resonance imaging (MRI) scan.
4. the client will be admitted to the hospital and scheduled for exploratory surgery.

40.18 A client's gait is considered normal during assessment if:
1. the client does not stumble, run into objects, or fall.
2. the gait is smooth and steady without limping.
3. the gait is slow and deliberate as if the client is gingerly pulling one side up to meet the other.
4. the gait is jerky and quick, which indicates the client has excellent motor control.

Answer: 2
Rationale: Alterations in gait can be difficult to assess. The nurse should watch the client walk from the front and from behind and look closely to see that gait is smooth and steady. Slow, jerky, or stumbling movements are abnormalities that warrant further evaluation. An ideal time to assess this process is when the client is first asked to come in to the examination room.
Assessment
Application
Health Promotion and Maintenance

40.19 The nurse is assessing the client's spine, and the assessment includes an abnormal finding. The nurse should conduct further assessment by asking the client to:
1. sit and then stand as the nurse observes the client from the front.
2. stand, bend back slowly, then to the right and left while the nurse looks from the back.
3. bend over, stand tall, and stretch arms over the head.
4. lie down on their abdomen so the nurse can look at the back more carefully.

Answer: 1
Rationale: The spine should appear straight when viewed from the back. The cervical and lumbar spine should appear concave and the thoracic spine should appear convex. Standing and sitting while observed will enable the examiner to see the spine from the appropriate views. Bending and stretching movements will not provide the best views for this assessment.
Assessment
Application
Health Promotion and Maintenance

40.20 The nurse assesses a client and finds that a grating sound is present when a joint is bent and straightened. The appropriate medical term that is used to describe this finding is:
1. grating.
2. grinding.
3. crepitation.
4. joint noise.

Answer: 3
Rationale: Crepitation is the proper term when a grating sound is present in a joint. Crepitation results when the joint articulating surfaces have lost their cartilage. The other terms do not a correctly describe the finding.
Assessment
Application
Health Promotion and Maintenance

41.1 The nurse is teaching older adults about risks for musculoskeletal trauma. Strategies the nurse should include are:
1. avoid falls at home by not using throw rugs.
2. avoid injury in motor vehicle accidents by not driving.
3. avoid fire by not cooking in the kitchen when alone.
4. avoid injury by not using assistive devices at home.

Answer: 1
Rationale: Throw rugs, cords, and other objects that impinge on traffic areas and improper use of assistive devices like canes and walkers increase the risk of falls at home for older adults. Advising the client to avoid cooking and driving are not realistic in the plan of care. Assistive devices are intended to promote independence and should be used by the client.
Implementation
Application
Safe and Effective Care Environment

41.2 The nurse should assess for signs and symptoms of possible compartment syndrome after: (Select all that apply.)
1. fasciotomy.
2. cast application to a limb.
3. crush injury to a limb.
4. fat embolism.

Answer: 2, 3
Rationale: Compartments within limbs can contain nerves, blood vessels, and support bones and are not able to expand due to fascia or a fibrous membranes. A cast applied too tightly over a limb area can exert external pressure that results in compression of a compartment; hemorrhage and edema within the compartment after a fracture or crush injury can cause the compression of a compartment. Fasciotomy is a treatment that can be used in the management of compartment syndrome. Fat embolism is a complication associated with long bone fractures or crushing injuries.
Assessment
Application
Physiological Integrity

41.3 After trauma to the musculoskeletal or nervous system, reflex sympathetic dystrophy can occur. The nurse would recognize this complication when:
1. the client complains of persistent pain, swelling, and decreased motion.
2. the client's cone has not healed by the usual time expected.
3. the client complains of leg swelling, pain, tenderness, and cramping.
4. the client complains of numbness beyond a cast and toes are pale with delayed capillary refill.

Answer: 1
Rationale: Persistent pain, swelling, and decreased motion describe client complaints for reflex sympathetic dystrophy. A cone that has not healed by the usual time expected describe nonunion or delayed union. Leg swelling, pain, tenderness, and cramping describe symptoms of deep vein thrombosis. Numbness beyond a cast and toes that are pale with delayed capillary refill describe symptoms of possible compartment syndrome.
Assessment
Application
Safe, Effective Care Environment

41.4 An elderly client was found at home on the floor. When trying to move, the client reported severe pain in the right hip. The admitting diagnosis is right hip fracture. Orders include Buck's traction and the nurse is about to initiate the order. The nurse should: (Place the statements in the correct order.)
1. set up the traction at the foot of the bed.
2. while the assistant holds straight traction, carefully attach the weight to hang at the foot of the bed.
3. have an assistant stand at the foot of the bed holding traction in a straight line.
4. secure the Buck's boot to the skin on the leg.
5. place the Buck's boot around the lower leg.

Answer: 1, 3, 5, 4, 2
Rationale: Applying or adjusting Buck's traction is a two-person procedure that must be planned step by step in order to prevent further injury and minimize client discomfort. First, set up the traction at the foot of the bed. Then, have an assistant stand at the foot of the bed holding traction in a straight line. The third step is to place the Buck's boot around the lower leg. Then, secure the Buck's boot to the skin on the leg. The final step is to carefully attach the weight to hang at the foot of the bed while the assistant holds straight traction.
Implementation
Assessment
Physiological Integrity

41.5 A client refuses physical therapy. The nurse's initial action is:

1. determine why the client is refusing and then help the client process their choices.
2. explain that the client must cooperate or the physician will be called.
3. write a nursing note on the chart stating that the client refused.
4. tell the client they are allowed to refuse one time only and from now on they must go.

Answer: 1

Rationale: Therapeutic communication is needed in order to find out why the client is refusing. Common reasons are fear and pain. Then, assist the client to meet needs related to fear or pain, answer questions the client has, and help the client to reach a more informed decision about therapy. Using threats to contact the physician are not appropriate or the most therapeutic. The client's responses and potential refusal of treatment will require documentation but are not the initial actions. The client retains ongoing rights to decline treatment.

Planning

Assessment

Psychosocial Integrity

41.6 A client has a cast applied to the right lower leg. Following the cast application, the nurse is monitoring for complications. Which assessment data leads the nurse to be concerned about a serious complication?

1. the right foot toes are pink, warm, and sensation is intact
2. complaint of numbness in the right foot and toes
3. itching under the cast
4. general discomfort in the right lower leg

Answer: 2

Rationale: Numbness should be reported right away. It may indicate pressure on nerves or blood vessels related to a tight cast. This can lead to compartment syndrome. The extremities exposed should be pink and warm with sensation. Itching and generalized discomfort are anticipated for the client who recently had a cast applied.

Diagnosis

Assessment

Safe, Effective Care Environment

41.7 A client is scheduled to have skeletal traction. The nurse realizes that:

1. weighted skin traction will be applied.
2. a surgical pin will be inserted into a bone and the traction will be applied to the pin.
3. a cast will be applied to the area and a traction device will be connected to the cast.
4. A cast will be placed while the nurse holds manual traction.

Answer: 2

Rationale: Skeletal traction requires the insertion of a pin directly into the bone. This insertion is completed under sterile conditions in the surgical environment. Skeletal traction is used at times when more weight or longer-term immobilization is desired to maintain proper alignment. The application of skin traction is used for short-term therapies and does not require the insertion of mechanical hardware.

Planning

Application

Physiological Integrity

41.8 In caring for a client with an external fixator device, the nurse will:

1. cleanse pin sites per orders to reduce the chance of infection.
2. adjust the tension on the pins whenever the client experiences pain.
3. explain that bathing in a tub can be resumed after three days.
4. encourage the client to keep the limb with the external fixator very still.

Answer: 1

Rationale: Cleansing pin sites as instructed is within the scope of nursing practice. Adjusting the device is outside the scope of nursing; this is a physician responsibility. Bathing (soaking in water) in a tub will not be permitted due to the chance of infection through pin sites. An external fixator is meant to increase the client's independence while maintaining immobilization.

Implementation

Application

Safe, Effective Care Environment

41.9 Surgery is necessary for clients with fractures that:

1. do not heal.
2. require direct visualization and repair.
3. cannot be immobilized with a cast.
4. are spiral.

Answer: 2

Rationale: Some fractures require surgical intervention to accomplish direct visualization of the fracture in order to repair. The surgical procedure is known as open reduction and internal fixation (ORIF) is not necessarily required for spiral fractures, those that cannot be immobilized by casting, or nonhealing fractures.

Assessment

Application

Safe, Effective Care Environment

41.10 A client has been very slow to recover from a fracture. The physician has ordered a treatment that will increase the migration of osteoblasts and osteoclasts to the fracture site. The nurse realizes that this treatment is:
1. open reduction and manipulation.
2. open visualization and debridement.
3. electrical bone stimulation.
4. fracture assimilation.

Answer: 3
Rationale: A treatment that will increase the migration of osteoblasts and osteoclasts to the fracture site is electrical bone stimulation. This is accomplished by applying an electrical current at the fracture site. Surgical intervention will not increase migration of osteoblasts and osteoclasts.
Assessment
Application
Physiological Integrity

41.11 The nurse is caring for a client who was admitted following a fight. The client had several direct blows to the face. The assessment reveals normal blood pressure (BP), elevated pulse (P-108), elevated respiratory rate (RR-24), and obvious deformity to the right side of the face. The most important priority for client care is:
1. frequently assess the blood pressure for signs of shock and initiate IV fluids.
2. monitor the elevated respiratory rate and maintain the airway.
3. monitor the elevated pulse rate and look for signs of pallor.
4. frequently assess for facial pain and administer pain medication prn.

Answer: 2
Rationale: Consider the potential risk for airway compromise with facial fractures. Help the client clear secretions from the oropharynx and report elevated respiratory rate (tachypnea) to the physician. Although IV fluids may be initiated, the client's assessment does not reflect a significant risk for shock. The injuries will cause the client to exhibit bruising and discoloration, not pallor. While the client will require an ongoing pain assessment and management, this is not the most important nursing action.
Assessment
Application
Safe, Effective Care Environment

41.12 The nurse is preparing a presentation about adult bone health at the local health fair. Which of the following statements should the nurse include?
1. Strong bones depend on calcium intake and weight-bearing exercise.
2. Avoiding obesity will guarantee healthy bones for adults.
3. Calcium supplements are necessary for adult bone health.
4. In order to maintain bone health, daily multivitamins are necessary.

Answer: 1
Rationale: Both calcium intake and weight-bearing exercise are needed for good adult bone health. Maintaining a healthy weight will promote the health of bones but it is not an absolute guarantee. The need for calcium supplementation and multivitamins is individualized. Supplement dosages will be determined in part by the client's dietary intake, age, and overall health status.
Implementation
Application
Health Promotion and Maintenance

41.13 In the RICE therapy plan, what do the abbreviations mean?
1. rest, ice, compression, and elevation
2. rest, ice, CT scan, and elimination of pain
3. rest, immobilization, CT scan, and elimination of pain
4. rest, immobilization, compression, and elevation

Answer: 1
Rationale: The four therapies included in RICE are: rest for the injured area, application of ice for 20 minutes four to eight times a day, compression by an ace wrap or device, and elevation to help reduce swelling and pain.
Implementation
Application
Physiological Integrity

41.14 A priority nursing diagnosis to consider for every client who has

Answer: 3
Rationale: Due to the loss of part of a limb, every client who has an amputation needs to be assessed to confirm or rule out the *Altered Body Image* nursing

undergone an above the knee amputation is: 1. *Risk for Infection* 2. *Altered Nutrition* 3. *Altered Body Image* 4. *Chronic Pain*	diagnosis. Risk for infection is an important nursing diagnosis in any post-operative client, but is not a specific priority in amputation. Nutrition should not be altered with this procedure. Pain will be present in the post-operative period but should not be chronic in nature. Assessment Application Psychosocial Integrity
41.15 The main nursing responsibility before and after applying traction to the leg is: 1. check the distal pulse. 2. check for pallor. 3. assess for pain. 4. assess for paresthesia.	Answer: 1 Rationale: It is important to assess for blood flow to the distal extremity before and after movement. Color, level of comfort, and alterations in sensation should also be included in the assessment but are not the highest priority. Assessment Application Safe, Effective Care Environment
41.16 When moving a client with a fracture of the leg, the nurse should: 1. make sure that the extremity is supported distal to the fracture. 2. disconnect the weights from the balanced traction setup. 3. support the extremity above and below the fracture. 4. support the leg directly under the fracture.	Answer: 3 Rationale: Support above and below the fracture site can decrease pain and muscle spasms. The other options of supporting the leg above the site or directly under the fracture site may increase spasm and pain. If traction is in use, weights would not be removed. Implementation Application Physiological Integrity
41.17 In the client who has had surgery to repair a fracture, there is a risk of fat embolus. The early sign(s) and symptom(s) of fat embolus is (are): 1. fever. 2. chest pain. 3. restlessness. 4. petechiae and tachycardia.	Answer: 4 Rationale: Petechiae and tachycardia are identifying characteristics of fat embolus. Respiratory manifestations and complications are later occurrences. Fever is a later finding. Assessment Application Physiological Integrity
41.18 When caring for a client after an orthopedic leg surgery, the method that should be used for urinary elimination is: 1. bedside commode. 2. fracture bedpan. 3. regular bedpan. 4. walk to bathroom with help.	Answer: 2 Rationale: The fracture pan is thinner and does not require the client to lift their hips as high as a regular bedpan would require. Following orthopedic leg surgery, most clients will not be able to get up to the bedside commode or walk to the bathroom. Implementation Application Physiological Integrity
41.19 Following hip replacement surgery, the client returns with an abductor splint in place. This means: 1. the splint will stay on except when bathing. 2. the splint is taken off while the client sleeps. 3. the splint is only needed when the client rolls onto their side to sleep. 4. the splint is optional after the day of surgery.	Answer: 1 Rationale: The legs must remain in abduction until healing is well underway. This prevents the hip prosthesis from being dislocated. The splint will stay on except when bathing. It would not be removed for turning or during sleep. Implementation Application Safe, Effective Care Environment
41.20 When teaching a client to use a walker, it is important to teach: 1. that using a rolling walker is more dangerous.	Answer: 2 Rationale: The walker should be lifted, advanced, and then the client should walk forward two steps. Pushing down on the walker and carrying the walker are

2. how to lift the walker, advance it, and then take two steps.
3. how to push down on the walker heavier on the affected side.
4. how to pick up and carry the walker except when the client needs to steady their gait.

potential safety hazards. A rolling walker may be more difficult to control and therefore increase the risk of falls.

Implementation
Application
Safe, Effective Care Environment

41.21 A situation that is common after amputation is phantom limb pain. How should the nurse help the client to deal with this?
1. Reorient the client to the present and explain that the limb has been amputated.
2. Acknowledge that phantom limb sensation and pain are not uncommon and encourage the client to talk about it.
3. Explain to the client that it is not possible to feel a limb that has been removed and that it is important to get past their denial.
4. Request that the physician order a referral to a psychiatrist in order to have the client deal with their limb loss.

Answer: 2
Rationale: Use therapeutic communication techniques to help the client understand that, while the phenomenon of phantom sensation and pain is not completely understood, it occurs for many amputees. It is real pain. Acknowledging its existence and promoting discussion will help the client to deal with the situation. Psychiatric intervention is not needed based on the presence of phantom limb pain, nor does the presence of this pain indicate that the client is disoriented.

Implementation
Application
Psychosocial Integrity

CHAPTER 42

42.1 An older female adult client is seen in the clinic and is surprised to find that she is shorter than she was a few years ago. The client thinks the nurse may have made a mistake. What is the best response by the nurse?
1. Teach the client that older adults often lose height based on poor posture, bone compression fractures, and their sedentary lifestyles.
2. Teach the client that osteoporosis and age-related loss of bone mass could be responsible for a decrease in height and that it would be good to talk with the physician about this.
3. Tell the client that she is wrong, and that nurses see this happen every day in old people.
4. Teach the client that old people are not active enough so eventually they have a decrease in their bone mass that they could have prevented.

Answer: 2
Rationale: Teach the client that osteoporosis and age-related loss of bone mass could be responsible for a decrease in height, and recommend talking with the physician about it. This is shared in a therapeutic manner. Height loss is not often related to poor posture, bone compression fractures, or sedentary lifestyles. It is not therapeutic to tell the client that they are wrong. It is also not therapeutic or correct to tell the client that old people are not active enough and that they could have prevented a decrease in bone mass.

Implementation
Application
Health Promotion and Maintenance

42.2 The nurse is teaching a client about risk factors for osteoporosis that can be changed, which include:
  1. lifestyle.
  2. race.
  3. gender.
  4. age.
	Answer: 1
	Rationale: Lifestyle changes like reducing alcohol intake, not smoking, ensuring adequate calcium intake in the diet or by supplement, and avoiding a high intake of diet soda with high phosphorus (which depletes calcium stores) can all be effective strategies. Race, gender, and age are nonmodifiable risk factors for osteoporosis.
	Implementation
	Application
	Health Promotion and Maintenance

42.3 Client care of an older adult with osteoporosis should:
  1. focus on diagnosis and medical management.
  2. focus on slowing or stopping the process and preventing complications.
  3. focus on treating the development of complications and client complaints.
  4. focus on research related to causes and the progression of the condition.
	Answer: 2
	Rationale: An interdisciplinary approach to osteoporosis is important, which involves identifying risk factors, diagnosing the condition, slowing or stopping the process, alleviating symptoms, and preventing complications. Because the diagnosis has already been made, care should not focus on diagnosis and medical management. Treatment of complications does not allow the client to have long-term optimal functioning; it is better to focus on preventing complications. Research may benefit future clients but does not meet the immediate needs of this client.
	Planning
	Application
	Health Promotion and Health Maintenance

42.4 A 52-year-old client is prescribed raloxifene (Evista) for the treatment of osteoporosis. The nurse realizes that this drug is used with postmenopausal women, and that it works by:
  1. inhibiting bone breakdown.
  2. inhibiting bone loss.
  3. stimulating osteoblast activity and increasing bone formation.
  4. preventing bone loss by mimicking what estrogen does for bone density.
	Answer: 4
	Rationale: Raloxifene (Evista) prevents bone loss by mimicking the role of estrogen in promoting bone density, but without the risks of estrogen therapy. Alendronate (Fosamax) and risedronate (Actonel) are from the class of drugs known as biphosphonates, which inhibit bone breakdown, preserve bone mass, and increase bone density in the hip and vertebrae. Teriparatide (Forteo) is a synthetic parathyroid hormone, administered subcutaneously to stimulate new bone formation and mass.
	Evaluation
	Application
	Physiological Integrity

42.5 The nurse is teaching a 68-year-old female client information about dietary calcium recommendations. Which dosage should be included in the nurse's teaching?
  1. 500 mg per day
  2. 750 mg per day
  3. 1000 mg per day
  4. 1500 mg per day
	Answer: 4
	Rationale: The client should consume 1500 mg of calcium per day; this amount follows the recommendation for adults over 65. For 19–50 years of age, 1000 mg is recommended. For 51–64 years of age, 1200 mg is recommended. Calcium supplements should be taken in divided doses for improved distribution (two to three times per day).
	Implementation
	Assessment
	Health Promotion and Maintenance

42.6 The nurse is providing information to a client about Paget's disease. Which of the following statements by the client about pathophysiology of the disease reflects understanding?
  1. "Metabolic activity remains the same but bone resorption ceases and bones become larger."
  2. "Because metabolic activity is compromised, excessive bone resorption occurs followed by no bone formation."
  3. "Metabolic activity is enhanced and no bone resorption occurs, followed by continuing bone formation."
	Answer: 4
	Rationale: In Paget's disease, excessive metabolic activity causes excessive bone resorption, which is followed by excessive bone formation; this progressive skeletal disorder is also known as osteitis deformans. The cause is not known but this disorder affects bones of the axial skeleton and may affect one or multiple bones.
	Evaluation
	Application
	Physiological Integrity

4. "Due to excessive metabolic activity, excessive bone resorption occurs followed by excessive bone formation."	
42.7 Clients with Paget's disease: 1. present with a long history of various areas of bone pain and a history of pain medication abuse. 2. are asymptomatic for years but can eventually develop bone pain in affected bones. 3. develop symptoms early and are tested by bone biopsy to diagnose the disorder. 4. are often diagnosed early due to a spike in serum alkaline phosphatase.	Answer: 2 Rationale: Paget's disease may remain asymptomatic but is often diagnosed from incidental x-rays that show the progressive bone changes. Paget's disease does not have early symptoms and is progressive in nature. Assessment Application Physiological Integrity
42.8 A client is diagnosed Paget's disease, and is experiencing mild symptoms. The nurse expects that the plan of care will include: 1. indomethacin (Indocin) and ibuprofen (Motrin) to stop progression of symptoms. 2. ibuprofen (Motrin) for discomfort and alendronate (Fosamax) if elevated test results indicate excessive bone resorption. 3. indomethacin (Indocin) for discomfort and calcitonin (Calcimar) to prevent bone formation. 4. ibuprofen (Motrin) and hip replacement surgery to prevent further osteoarthritis.	Answer: 2 Rationale: Ibuprofen (Motrin) is a commonly-used NSAID to control mild pain; alendronate (Fosamax), a bisphosphonate, is commonly used to retard bone resorption. Indomethacin (Indocin) is also a commonly-used NSAID for control of discomfort. The administration of two NSAID drugs will not stop the progression of Paget's disease and probably would not be taken together due to potential adverse effects. Calcitonin (Calcimar) is used to retard bone resorption, not bone formation. A surgical hip replacement would be used to treat advanced osteoarthritis as a result of long-term Paget's disease. Evaluation Assessment Phsyiological Integrity
42.9 A client with Paget's disease tells the nurse that she fears falling. The nurse should: 1. recognize that the fear of falling makes the client more prone to falls and facilitate the client's expression of thoughts. 2. tell the client not to worry; this fear will go away with results from proper medication. 3. recognize that the fear of falling is silly and tell the client to think more positively about their disease. 4. tell the client to stay in the house where they will be safer.	Answer: 1 Rationale: Therapeutic nursing care requires the nurse to assess the client's needs and provide appropriate interventions as indicated. The client's fears must be incorporated into the plan of care. The fears will impact the client's progression if they are not addressed. The client's fears should not be dismissed as silly. Advising the client to remain in the house is not realistic. Implementation Application Psychosocial Integrity
42.10 A client comes to the clinic complaining of severe pain in the right great toe that started at night. The most probable prognosis is: 1. a strain of the great right toe. 2. a fracture of the great right toe.	Answer: 3 Rationale: The onset of gout is usually at night and often involves the first metatarsophalangeal joint, although gout can affect other connective tissues. The pain from a strain or fracture would not be exclusive to the night time hours and have associated symptoms of swelling or possibly bruising. Rheumatoid arthritis often manifests with stiffness and pain in the morning.

3. gout. 4. rheumatoid arthritis.	Assessment Application Physiological Integrity
42.11 A client is experiencing symptoms of gout. The nurse expects which of the following diagnostic test(s) will be ordered to diagnose gout? (Select all that apply.) 　1. MRI of the right foot 　2. serum uric acid level 　3. complete blood count (CBC) 　4. CT of the right foot	Answer: 2, 3 Rationale: An elevated uric acid level greater than 7.5 mg/dL is almost always identified with gout. A complete blood count includes a white blood cell (WBC) count which shows a significant elevation during an acute attack of gout. An MRI and CT are expensive tests and would not be needed to diagnose gout but could be ordered to rule out other diagnoses if the typical indicators for gout are not discovered. Diagnosis Application Health Promotion and Maintenance
42.12 The nurse is teaching a client who has gout. Which of the following should be included in the teaching? 　1. Avoid drinking bottled water. 　2. Avoid eating cottage cheese. 　3. Avoid drinking milk. 　4. Avoid eating shellfish.	Answer: 4 Rationale: When a low-purine diet is advised by the physician, high-purine foods to avoid include: all meats and seafood, yeast, beans, peas, lentils, oatmeal, spinach, asparagus, cauliflower, and mushrooms. Alcohol and foods that have initiated an attack should be avoided. Liberal fluid intake is needed to promote urinary excretion of uric acid. Therefore intake of water would be encouraged. Dairy products such as milk and cottage cheese are not prohibited in gout treatment. Implementation Assessment Health Promotion and Maintenance
42.13 A client was just diagnosed with gout. The nurse expects that the client will likely be prescribed which of the following medications? (Select all that apply.) 　1. prednisone (Deltasone) 　2. acetylsalicylic acid (Aspirin) 　3. colchicine (ColBenemid) 　4. allopurinol (Zyloprim)	Answer: 1, 3, 4 Rationale: An oral form of prednisone (Deltasone) is used in acute gout to decrease inflammation. Colchicine (ColBenemid) is used in the treatment and prevention of further gout attacks. Colchicine helps to decrease joint pain in acute gout. It also works to prevent further attacks of gout by preventing crystal deposition within joints. Allopurinol (Zyloprim) lowers plasma uric acid levels and facilitates mobilizing tophi that occur in many cases of gout. Acetylsalicylic acid (Aspirin) is avoided in gout treatment because it may interfere with uric acid excretion. Planning Synthesis Physiological Integrity
42.14 The nurse is providing nutrition education to the residents of a senior center. The presentation addresses the implication of vitamin D deficiency and low serum levels of phosphorus. Based upon their knowledge, the nurse advises the participants that potential complications include: 　1. osteomalacia; due to low intake of calcium and vitamin D in the diet. 　2. osteosarcoma; due to lack of nutrients that allows mutation of cells. 　3. tophi formation due to low intake of nutrients needed for bone formation. 　4. osteomyelitis; due to lack of nutrients for muscle cells, which then become inflamed.	Answer: 1 Rationale: Once nonexistent in the United States, osteomalacia has increased among older adults and adults who follow vegetarian diets. A diet low in vitamin D, decreased production of vitamin D with inadequate sun exposure, impaired intestinal absorption of fats (vitamin D is a fat-soluble vitamin), and disorders that interfere with metabolism of vitamin D all contribute to osteomalacia. Osteosarcoma is a malignancy of the bone. Osteomyelitis refers to infection of the bone. Tophi are associated with gout and result from increased levels of uric acid. Gout may be exacerbated by diets high in purine content, along with alcohol intake. Implementation Application Health Promotion and Maintenance
42.15 The following lab results would likely be seen in a client who is diagnosed with osteomalacia: 　1. elevated serum calcium, and normal parathyroid hormone and alkaline phosphatase	Answer: 2 Rationale: Serum calcium may be normal or low, depending on the cause of the disease. Parathyroid hormone is frequently elevated as a compensatory response to low calcium in renal failure or vitamin D deficiency. Alkaline phosphatase is usually elevated in osteomalacia.

2. low or normal serum calcium, and elevated parathyroid hormone and alkaline phosphatase 3. low serum calcium, and normal parathyroid hormone and alkaline phosphatase 4. high serum calcium, and low parathyroid hormone and alkaline phosphatase	Assessment Application Physiological Integrity
42.16 The nurse expects to care for clients most often with which of the following types of arthritis? 1. gouty arthritis 2. rheumatoid arthritis 3. osteoarthritis 4. ankylosing spondylitis	Answer: 3 Rationale: Osteoarthritis (OA) is the most frequent type of arthritis and a leading cause of pain and disability in older adults. OA results from a degeneration of joints. Assessment Application Physiological Integrity
42.17 One of the first symptoms of osteoarthritis the nurse expects to note in the assessment is: 1. crepitus in the joint with movement. 2. pain when at rest. 3. inability to walk long distances due to fatigue. 4. pain and stiffness in one or more joints.	Answer: 4 Rationale: The onset of osteoarthritis (OA) is gradual and progressive. The symptoms that are noticed first are pain and stiffness in the affected joint or joints. Crepitus and pain at rest are late signs of OA in a joint. Inability to walk is not characteristic of OA; pain and stiffness may cause the inability to walk long distances. Assessment Application Physiological Integrity
42.18 A client has early onset osteoarthritis of the left knee. The nurse expects which medication will be ordered? 1. meperidine (Demerol) 2. prednisone 3. ibuprofen (Motrin) 4. hyaluronan (Synvisc)	Answer: 3 Rationale: NSAID drugs like ibuprofen (Motrin) may control discomfort in early stages of osteoarthritis (OA). Meperidine (Demerol) is a narcotic drug used for moderate to severe pain, but it there is a risk for dependence and may interfere with normal mentation due to possible euphoria. Oral prednisone is not recommended due to immunosuppression. Infrequently a corticosteroid is injected into the affected joint but is detrimental to the cartilage. Hyaluronan (Synvisc) is a treatment for advanced OA of a knee joint and may provide improvement of knee function for up to one year, but it is not used for early arthritis treatment. Planning Application Physiological Integrity
42.19 Impaired physical mobility is a major nursing diagnosis for clients with osteoarthritis (OA). Nursing activities related to this diagnosis include: 1. assessing the range of motion of affected joints in order to plan appropriate interventions. 2. encouraging consistently high activity levels in order to prevent other problems associated with OA. 3. encouraging taking care of own self-care needs in order to remain more active. 4. assessing the need for narcotic analgesics around the clock to prevent pain in activities of daily living.	Answer: 1 Rationale: A determination of the client's range of motion is needed to provide individualized care. Clients with osteoarthritis (OA) will need to build in periodic rest periods in order to decrease pain and accompanying symptoms. Realistic goals will need to be set for the client with OA. Simply encouraging the client to remain active does not provide comprehensive care. OA is a chronic condition and the use of narcotics could lead to dependence. Implementation Application Physiological Integrity

42.20 The nurse planning care for a client who was diagnosed with muscular dystrophy (MD) needs to remember that:

1. the cause is related to a lack of blood supply to nerves.
2. the treatment of MD is aimed at eliminating the cause by identifyng the specific organisms that cause the muscle infection.
3. the treatment is daily electrical muscle stimulus.
4. the pathophysiology of MD involves muscle degeneration, which affects activities of daily living.

Answer: 4
Rationale: The cause of muscular dystrophy (MD) is not definitively known. Electrical muscle stimulus treatments would not affect MD. It is a degenerative muscle disorder, not a nerve disorder, which affects ability to perform activities of daily living. This condition is not felt to be caused by infectious organisms.
Planning
Application
Physiological Integrity

CHAPTER 43

43.1 When assessing cognitive function, the nurse should evaluate the client's:

1. ability to smell items placed under the nose while eyes are closed.
2. orientation to time, place, person, and ability to recall recent and past events.
3. ability to walk with a smooth, steady gait.
4. level of consciousness.

Answer: 2
Rationale: Cognitive abilities refer to mental abilities with regard to orientation to time, place, person, and ability to recall recent and past events.. Assessing the client's ability to smell items that are placed under the nose while eyes are closed is the method used to test for cranial nerve 1, the olfactory nerve. Level of consciousness and gait are not reflective of cognitive ability.
Application
Assessment
Physiological Integrity

43.2 When testing cranial nerve XI (spinal accessory), the nurse should ask the client to:

1. shrug shoulders and turn their head against resistance.
2. stick out the tongue and move it from side to side.
3. taste foods and distinguish sweet from sour.
4. smell and identify correctly with one side of the nares blocked.

Answer: 1
Rationale: Cranial nerve 11, the spinal accessory nerve, is tested by asking the client to shrug shoulders and turn their head against resistance. Cranial nerve 12, the hypoglossal nerve, is tested by asking the client to stick out the tongue and move it from side to side. Cranial nerve 7, the facial nerve, is tested by asking the client to distinguish between different tastes. Cranial nerve 1, the olfactory nerve, is tested by having the client identify smells correctly with one side of the nose blocked.
Application
Assessment
Physiological Integrity

43.3 Normally a client can differentiate between soft and sharp and can feel vibrations accurately. To test sensory function the nurse should:

1. touch both sides of various parts of the body with a sharp and a dull object.
2. have the client distinguish which parts of the body are being touched.
3. ask the client to guess whether they are being touched with a paper clip or a needle.
4. touch a part of the body without the client looking and have them identify the area being touched.

Answer: 1
Rationale: Sensory function is best evaluated by touching both sides of various parts of the body with a sharp and a dull object. the correct way to test sensory function.
Assessment
Application
Physiological Integrity

43.4 When testing the client to determine if tremors are present, the nurse should assess for:

Answer: 3
Rationale: Tremors are rhythmic movements that can be seen with activity or at rest. The type of tremors observed is linked to specific disease processes. Fasciculations

1. shaking. 2. jerky movements. 3. rhythmic movements. 4. fasciculations.	are twitching movements associated with motor neuron disease. Jerky movements would be descriptive of cogwheel rigidity associated with Parkinson's disease. Shaking is a term associated with generalized response to stressors such as cold. Assessment Application Physiological Integrity
43.5 The nurse observes a client who has a lack of coordination, clumsy movements, and an unbalanced gait. What is this called? 1. flaccidity 2. paralysis 3. hemiparesis 4. ataxia	Answer: 4 Rationale: In ataxia, there is a lack of coordination, clumsy movements, and an unbalanced gait. Flaccidity, paralysis, and hemiparesis are abnormal conditions in which movement does not occur at all in a part or is impaired. Assessment Application Physiological Integrity
43.6 While performing the Romberg test, the nurse asks the client to stand with the feet together and eyes closed. What must the nurse observe for the test to be considered normal? 1. swaying side to side 2. minimal swaying for up to 20 seconds 3. balance sufficient to hold still without swaying 4. swaying to one side and the loss of balance	Answer: 2 Rationale: A normal result of a Rhomberg test would be the client displaying minimal swaying for up to 20 seconds. Some minor swaying may occur, but this swaying should not cause loss of balance. The nurse should stand close to the client to prevent falling. A positive Romberg's test would indicate that the client sways and is a sign of cerebellar dysfunction as in cerebellar ataxia. Assessment Application Physiological Integrity
43.7 When the nurse asks the client to walk heel-to-toe, on toes, and then on heels, what function is being checked? 1. cerebellar 2. cerebral 3. mid-brain 4. brainstem	Answer: 1 Rationale: The ability to follow the instructions, walk heel-to-toe, on toes, then on the heels provides information about the cerebellum. Assessment Application Health Promotion and Maintenance
43.8 The nurse recognizes normal cerebral spinal fluid (CSF) as: 1. yellow without sediment. 2. blood tinged without sediment. 3. clear and colorless. 4. pink without sediment.	Answer: 3 Rationale: Normal cerebral spinal fluid (CSF) is clear and colorless. Assessment Application Physiological Integrity
43.9 When the nurse is assessing muscle strength and movement, it is important to: 1. grade the posterior tibial pulses. 2. grade flaccidity. 3. observe to see whether strength and movement are bilaterally equal and strong. 4. ask the client to walk normally in a heel-to-toe sequence.	Answer: 3 Rationale: Always compare one side to the other side when an extremity is being assessed or two sides exist. Note whether there is a difference in strength or movement from side to side. Pulses relate to blood supply, not muscles. It is not possible to grade flaccidity. When muscles are flaccid, there is no movement. Asking the client to walk normally in a heel-to-toe sequence assesses gait, not muscle strength and movement. Assessment Application Health Perception and Maintenance
43.10 The client has lower motor neuron injuries. The nurse realizes that what type of reflexes are present? 1. decreased 2. increased 3. normal 4. exaggerated	Answer: 1 Rationale: The finding of abnormally decreased reflexes points to disorders or diseases in which there is lower motor neuron impairment. Assessment Application Physiological Integrity

43.11 When the client is supine and the head is flexed to the chest without pain, resistance, or flexion of the hips or knees, the nurse is observing:
1. doll's eyes sign.
2. Brudzinski's sign.
3. Babinski's sign.
4. Kernig's sign.

Answer: 2
Rationale: Brudzinski's sign is elicited by placing the client in a supine position and flexing the neck toward the chest. A positive result would be noted if the client has pain or flexes the hip or knees in response to the neck flexion. A positive response indicates meningeal irritation. Babinski's and Kernig's signs are other important signs to observe in neurologically impaired clients. When performing a test known as the Babinski's sign, a normal response (absence of Babinski's) is plantar flexion of the toes. An abnormal response is dorsiflexion of the big toe and often a fanning of the other toes. Test Babinski's sign by gently scraping the sole of the foot with a blunt object. To elicit the reflex, start the stimulus at the midpoint of the heel, and move upward and laterally along the outer border of the sole to the ball of the foot. Continue the stimulus across the medial side and off the foot. To assess for Kernig's sign, the client will easily and completely extend the leg when in the supine position; or when lying with the thigh flexed on the abdomen, the leg cannot be completely extended. This is a positive sign of meningitis. Doll's eyes sign tests for the direction the eyes move when the head is turned.
Assessment
Application
Physiological Integrity

43.12 Abnormal posturing in adults with a neurological problem includes: (Select all that apply.)
1. decorticate.
2. decerebrate.
3. delocalicate.
4. deflaccidobrate.

Answer: 1, 2
Rationale: Decorticate refers to abnormal posturing where the upper arms are close to the sides, the elbows, wrists and fingers are flexed, the legs are extended with internal rotation and the feet are plantar flexed. Decerebrate refers to abnormal posturing where the neck is extended; the jaw is clenched; the arms are pronated, extended, and close to the sides; the legs are extended straight out; and the feet are plantar flexed. Delocalicate and deflaccidobrate are not terms used to describe posturing in neurological abnormalities.
Assessment
Application
Safe, Effective Care Environment

43.13 When the nurse is assessing the functional health pattern of health perception-health management for a client with a neurological problem, which of the following questions is appropriate?
1. "Have you noticed any problems with chewing?"
2. "Are you having any problems with the ability to see, hear, taste, or smell?"
3. "Has there been any change in your pattern of urinary or bowel elimination?"
4. "Do you have any problems with balance, coordination, or walking?"

Answer: 2
Rationale: The functional health pattern of health perception-health maintenance addresses the client's view of their level of functioning and in performance of usual activities. Asking about problems with taste, sight, hearing, and smell addresses basic sensory functions that should be addressed first. Option 1 and option 3 address other functional patterns and body systems, and option 4 addresses mobility which could be musculoskeletal.
Assessment
Application
Health Perception and Management

43.14 A client is seen in the clinic for a neuromuscular diagnosis. What neurological test(s) help to diagnose such a disease?
1. single-photon emission computed tomography (SPECT)
2. positron emission tomography (PET)
3. magnetic resonance imaging (MRI)
4. electromyogram (EMG)

Answer: 4
Rationale: An electromyogram (EMG) measures the electrical activity of skeletal muscles at rest and during contraction. An EMG is useful in diagnosing neuromuscular disease. A SPECT is a nuclear scan which provides information about blood flow. PET scan is useful in diagnosis of heart disease and cancers by providing information about cellular function. MRI is an exam that uses magnetic fields to produce images of body structures.
Planning
Synthesis
Physiological Integrity

43.15 A client in the hospital critical care unit is being evaluated for brain death. What neurological test(s) help to determine brain death?
1. electroencephalogram (EEG)
2. computed tomography (CT)
3. evoked potentials
4. electromyogram (EMG)

Answer: 1
Rationale: An electroencephalogram (EEG) is part of the brain death protocol in hospitals. It can also be used to diagnose brain disease. The other tests do not measure the electrical activity of the brain. Computed tomography (CT) looks at the intracranial contents and can help distinguish hemorrhage, tumors, cysts, aneurysms, edema, ischemia, atrophy, and tissue necrosis. Evoked potentials measures nerve conduction along pathways to evaluate muscle contractions. An electromyogram (EMG) measures the electrical activity of skeletal muscles.
Planning
Synthesis
Physiological Integrity

43.16 A client is in the hospital with suspected intracerebral hemorrhage. The nurse realizes that the client will most likely have which neurological test ordered?
1. x-rays of the spine
2. computed tomography (CT)
3. evoked potentials
4. electroencephalogram (EEG)

Answer: 2
Rationale: A computed tomography (CT) scan can visualize intracerebral hemorrhages because the computer-assisted x-rays view several levels of cross-sections of the head. Evoked potentials and EEG look at electrical activity and would not be helpful in diagnosis of intracerebral hemorrhage. Spine x-rays provide information about bony structure of the spine, and would not be useful in diagnosis of intracerebral hemorrhage.
Planning
Synthesis
Physiological Integrity

43.17 A client is brought to the emergency department by the rescue squad. The client was thrown from a vehicle. There was questionable consciousness on the way to the hospital. What neurological tests does the nurse expect to see ordered?
1. magnetic resonance imaging (MRI) and computed tomography (CT)
2. computed tomography (CT) and positron emission tomography (PET)
3. x-rays of the skull and spine and computed tomography (CT)
4. computed tomography (CT)

Answer: 3
Rationale: It is always important to "clear" the cervical spine by completing x-rays with visualization of all seven cervical vertebrae. A skull x-ray combined with a CT scan to gain information on the presence of blood or clots is also important in this case, because ejection from a vehicle likely caused head trauma. MRI and PET scans may be helpful but should be combined with x-ray of the skull and spine.
Planning
Synthesis
Physiological Integrity

43.18 The nurse understands that age-related changes in the neurological system include a decreased number of brain cells, decreased cerebral blood flow, and decreased metabolism. An example of how this would affect home care for an older adult is:
1. the older adult will be distracted after a few minutes on the task.
2. the older adult will not be open to learning to do their own dressing change.
3. the older adult will be less reliable to complete self-care activities.
4. when too many stimuli are present, the older adult cannot process and answer in a timely fashion.

Answer: 4
Rationale: When too many stimuli are present, the older adult cannot process and answer in a timely fashion. Older adults do better when learning is limited to 30 minutes at a time but they can focus for longer than a few minutes. Older adults may have more readiness to learn when the learning topic is related to previously-learned information. There is no proof that the older adult is less reliable, but this needs to be assessed for each individual to determine reliability and ability.
Planning
Application
Safe, Effective Care Environment

43.19 The nurse describes Alzheimer's disease (AD) to a civic group as: (Select all of the following that apply.) 　1.　increases in incidence with age. 　2.　tends to run in families. 　3.　more common in men. 　4.　caused by a virus.	Answer: 1, 2 Rationale: Alzheimer's disease does tend to increase with age and is thought to have a familial link. AD is more common in females and the cause is unknown. Implementation Application Physiological Integrity
43.20 One of the most common neurological diseases is characterized by abnormal cell firing in the brain. What does this disease cause in clients? 　1.　loss of consciousness 　2.　seizures 　3.　decerebrate posturing 　4.　headache	Answer: 2 Rationale: Abnormal cell firing in the brain describes seizures, which can appear to affect different parts of the body and last different amounts of time. The symptoms of loss of consciousness and headache have multiple causes (trauma, medications, diet) but are not associated with abnormal cell firing. Decerebrate posturing is caused by serious brain injury, specifically to the cerebellum. Assessment Application Physiological Integrity

CHAPTER 44

44.1 A change in breathing pattern to alternating regular periods of deep, rapid breathing followed by periods of apnea is called _____ and is related to damage in the diencephalon region of the cerebrum. 　1.　apneustic respirations 　2.　neurogenic hyperventilation 　3.　Cheyne-Stokes respirations 　4.　ataxic respirations	Answer: 3 Rationale: Cheyne-Stokes respirations are a change in breathing pattern to alternative regular periods of deep, rapid breathing followed by periods of apnea and are seen in many client conditions in the clinical setting. Apneustic respiration is a term used to describe an abnormal pattern of breathing characterized by deep, gasping inspiration with a pause at full inspiration followed by a brief, insufficient release. Neurogenic hyperventilation is hyperventilation associated with brain or spine injury. Ataxic respirations are shallow irregular respirations associated with damage to the medullary respiratory center. Assessment Application Physiological Integrity
44.2 Brain death is the cessation of all brain functions. The criteria to establish brain death varies from state to state but generally recognized criteria include: (Select all that apply.) 　1.　absent motor and reflex movements. 　2.　pupils are equal and responsive to light. 　3.　flat electroencephalogram (EEG) on successive EEGs. 　4.　no spontaneous respiration.	Answer: 1, 3, 4 Rationale: Absent motor and reflex movements, flat electroencephalogram (EEG) on successive EEGs, and lack of spontaneous respiration are part of generally-recognized brain death criteria. Pupils that are equal and responsive to light is a sign of pupillary response and indicates brain function. Assessment Application Physiological Integrity
44.3 In the client with altered level of consciousness (LOC), the most appropriate intravenous fluid is: 　1.　45 normal saline. 　2.　isotonic or hypertonic. 　3.　dextrose 5% in water. 　4.　dextrose 5% and .45 normal saline.	Answer: 2 Rationale: Isotonic (.9 normal saline) or slightly hypertonic (Lactated Ringer's) IV solutions are used in the client with altered level of consciousness (LOC). Hypotonic solutions (such as D5W and .45% normal saline) will cause fluid to move into the cells and worsen cerebral edema. Highly hypertonic solutions will cause fluid to move out of the cells. Planning Synthesis Safe, Effective Care Environment
44.4 The nurse anticipates that unconscious clients without a cough reflex will require: 　1.　continuous pulse oximetry instead of intubation.	Answer: 4 Rationale: This client is at risk for impaired airway and aspiration. Oximetry would be done in addition to intubation. Frequent oropharyngeal suctioning will not adequately protect the airway and the suctioning will cause hypoxia. No unconscious client should be fed food or fluids.

2. frequent suctioning with a tonsil-tip suction device. 3. close observation as they are fed. 4. intubation and mechanical ventilation.	Planning Application Safe, Effective Care Environment
44.5 Following a craniotomy, the nurse should position the client in which position? 1. flat 2. high Fowler's (head of bed up 45 degrees) 3. low Fowler's (head of bed up 30 degrees) 4. sitting upright	Answer: 3 Rationale: Place the client's head at 30 degrees for optimal draining of cerebrospinal fluid and preventing increased intracranial pressure. Implementation Application Safe, Effective Care Environment
44.6 A client is in the emergency department following a head injury. The most accurate sign of developing increased intracranial pressure is: 1. elevated diastolic blood pressure. 2. decreasing level of consciousness. 3. decreasing respiratory rate. 4. pupils that are equal.	Answer: 2 Rationale: The brain is very sensitive to the level of oxygenation. As hypoxia develops, it will negatively affect the level of consciousness. Change in blood pressure is generally a widening pulse pressure. Change in respiratory rate is a late sign of IICP. Size, shape, and responsiveness of the pupils, not simply equality, should be assessed to determine if ICP is increasing. Assessment Synthesis Physiological Integrity
44.7 Decerebrate posturing is present in an unconscious client after a motor vehicle accident. The nurse assesses for decerebrate posturing again and expects to see that: 1. the arms and legs are hyperextended and arms are hyperpronated. 2. the arms are folded over the chest and spasms are rhythmic. 3. the arms are pulled inward and the head is turned to the side. 4. the arms and legs have tonic-clonic seizure activity.	Answer: 1 Rationale: Decerebrate posture is displayed by hyperextension of the arms and legs and hyperpronation of the arms. Decerebration is considered a sign that the client has a serious injury with a poor prognosis. The other options do not accurately describe decerebrate posture. Assessment Application Physiological Integrity
44.8 When assessing an adult after a fall, the nurse in the emergency department notes a dilated pupil on the right and a hematoma in the right temporal area. The nurse realizes that this likely means that: 1. the process affecting the pupil is occurring on the opposite side and is unrelated to the right temporal hematoma. 2. the process affecting the right pupil is temporary and soon both pupils will be equal in size. 3. the process causing the right pupil to dilate is a result of a metabolic process.	Answer: 4 Rationale: Generally, when a process is occurring locally, the pupil on the same side (ipsilateral) is affected. Assessment Application Physiological Integrity

4. the process affecting the pupil is occurring locally on the right side (ipsilateral pupil dilation).	
44.9 The nurse anticipates a medication order to halt status epilepticus. Which of the following medications is expected? 1. oral glucose 2. phenytoin (Dilantin) orally 3. gabapentin (Neurontin) and lamotrigine (Lamictal) 4. lorazepam (Ativan) IV	Answer: 4 Rationale: Lorazepam (Ativan) can be used IV to stop the seizure and is an appropriate treatment order. No drug would be given orally during status epilepticus, although glucose IV would be appropriate. The drug needs to be given IV in this situation and phenytoin (Dilantin) could be an option if ordered IV. The type of drug therapy used to treat epilepsy uses only one drug at a time. Implementation Application Physiological Integrity
44.10 Which of the following is the most important psychosocial need for a client with a seizure disorder? 1. self-care deficit 2. anxiety 3. altered body image 4. altered activity-exercise	Answer: 2 Rationale: The client's concerns will cause anxiety due to questions about the ability to work, drive a car, and feelings of embarrassment about having a seizure in public. The diagnoses of self-care deficit and altered activity-exercise are not psychosocial diagnoses. A client with a seizure disorder will generally not have any alteration in their physical appearance which would result in altered body image. Assessment Application Psychosocial Integrity
44.11 Traumatic brain injury (TBI) is the leading cause of death and disability in the United States. The nurse realizes that all of the following are causes of TBI. Place the answers in order from the most frequent to least frequent cause of TBI. 1. elevated blood alcohol 2. motor vehicle accidents 3. riding a motorcycle without a helmet 4. falls	Answer: 4,2,1,3 Rationale: Falls are the leading cause of TBI, followed by motor vehicle accidents, elevated blood alcohol, and riding a motorcycle without a helmet. Assessment Application Health Promotion and Maintenance
44.12 The client is hit by a swinging bat. This is an example of: 1. a penetrating head injury. 2. an acceleration injury. 3. a deceleration injury. 4. an acceleration-deceleration injury.	Answer: 2 Rationale: The bat creates an acceleration injury. A deceleration injury occurs when the head hits a stationary object. Acceleration-deceleration (contra-coup) occurs when the head hits an object and the brain rebounds within the skull. Penetrating injury occurs when an object disrupts the integrity of the head and skull. Assessment Application Physiological Integrity
44.13 The client was riding in a car that hit a tree. The head hit the windshield (coup) and then the brain rebounded within the skull toward the opposite side (contrecoup). This is: 1. a penetrating head injury. 2. an acceleration injury. 3. a deceleration injury. 4. an acceleration-deceleration injury.	Answer: 4 Rationale: In an acceleration-deceleration injury, two or more areas of the brain can be injured. A deceleration injury occurs when the head hits a stationary object. Penetrating injury occurs when an object disrupts the integrity of the head and skull. Acceleration injury occurs when the head is hit by a moving object, such as a swinging bat. Assessment Application Physiological Integrity
44.14 After a fall, the client is brought to the emergency department. There was a brief loss of consciousness, the client complains of headache, has vomited twice, has a dilated pupil on the	Answer: 3 Rationale: Classic signs of an epidural hematoma include a loss of consiousness followed by a brief lucid period before rapid deterioration. Because this injury involves a skull fracture that tears an artery, the client is bleeding uncontrollably into the head. Increased intracranial pressure and herniation will occur without

same side as a hematoma over the temporal area, and now is having a seizure. The nurse anticipates that:
1. this is a controlled situation once the seizure stops.
2. this is a serious situation in which a subdural hematoma is developing and requires surgery.
3. this is an emergency situation that is likely an epidural hematoma and requires surgery.
4. this is a typical situation seen with most clients who fall and will subside with observation.

prompt and timely intervention. A subdural hematoma would be manifested by drowsiness, confusion, and enlargement of the ipsilateral pupil within minutes of the injury. Hemiparesis and changes in respiratory pattern may soon follow. The assessments as stated indicate that the client will require immediate intervention and not simply observation.
Implementation
Synthesis
Physiological Integrity

44.15 The nurse is caring for a client on a medical unit who begins a tonic-clonic seizure. After a few minutes the seizure stops but repeats again after a minute. This pattern continues in which the client is having repeated tonic-clonic seizures and has lasted for more than 10 minutes. Place the following nursing actions into order from highest priority to lowest.
1. Hang an IV of normal saline to keep vein open.
2. Call respiratory therapy stat.
3. Call the physician stat.
4. Initiate oxygen via the nasal cannula at the bedside.

Answer: 4,2,3,1
Rationale: The client is in great danger of hypoxia and other complications if the seizure is not stopped. Initiate oxygen via the nasal cannula at the bedside. Call respiratory therapy stat so that a therapist can come to the aid of the nurse and help manage the airway and breathing. Call the physician stat in order to inform them of the emergent situation and to seek orders. Hang the IV of normal saline in anticipation that an open IV line will expedite administering the medication that will likely be ordered to stop the seizure.
Implementation
Synthesis
Safe, Effective Care Environment

44.16 The nurse is observing a client who is having a seizure that involves a blank stare, unresponsiveness to questions, and smacking of the lips. The seizure lasts less than a minute. The nurse categorizes the seizure as:
1. partial.
2. tonic-clonic.
3. absence.
4. status epilepticus.

Answer: 3
Rationale: Absence (or petit mal) seizures involve a blank stare, unresponsiveness to questions, and smacking of the lips. A partial seizure involves only one area of the brain. The symptoms displayed are reflective of the area affected and may be muscle contraction of a single body part if the motor cortex is affected. Sensory manifestations may be exhibited by hallucinations or abnormal sensations. Tonic-clonic seizures involve generalized contraction coupled with impairment of consciousness. Status epilepticus is a term used to describe repetitive seizures with only very brief calm periods in between.
Assessment
Application
Physiological Integrity

44.17 The client has a tonic-clonic seizure. During the seizure, the priority for nursing care is to:
1. obtain the vital signs.
2. insert a bite block to prevent the client from swallowing their tongue.
3. ask the staff to hold the client tightly.
4. protect the client from injury.

Answer: 4
Rationale: Protect the head and the rest of the body during the seizure. A bite block is not needed and may injure the client with forced insertion. The movements of the client should not be restrained because this can cause injury. The vital signs cannot be measured during a tonic-clonic seizure.
Planning and Implementation
Application
Safe, Effective Care Environment

44.18 The nurse realizes that medication ordered to control migraine headaches will be aimed at reducing the frequency and severity and to halt a headache in progress. Prophylactic therapy for migraines includes:

Answer: 1
Rationale: Propranolol hydrochloride (Inderal) is a beta-blocker that prevents dilation of vessels in the pia mater and inhibits serotonin uptake. Other drugs prescribed to prevent migraines include methylsergide maleate (Sansert), topiramate (Topamax), and valproic acid (Depakote). Sumatriptan (Imitrex) and zolmitriptan (Zomig) are taken once the migraine starts. Acetaminophen (Tylenol) is taken at the onset or during a migraine and helps some clients.

---

1. propranolol hydrochloride (Inderal). 2. acetaminophen (Tylenol). 3. zolmitriptan (Zomig). 4. sumatriptan (Imitrex).	Planning Application Physiological Integrity
44.19 The nurse is planning a seminar about headaches for a local civic group. The type of headache that has a strong familial connection, affects females three to one over males, and results in lost productivity is: 1. sinus. 2. migraine. 3. cluster. 4. stress.	Answer: 2 Rationale: Fifteen percent of the population is affected by migraines, which can last from a few hours to several days. Many require emergency department treatment. Cluster headaches are more common in men between the ages of 20 and 40. Stress or tension headaches are associated with stressful events and muscular contraction. Sinus headaches are associated with congestion in the frontal an maxillary sinuses and may be caused by allergy or infection. Implementation Application Health Promotion and Maintenance
44.20 The nurse is caring for a head-injured client with cerebral edema and increased intracranial pressure (IICP). To prevent further transient increases from occurring, the nurse should implement which of the following interventions? 1. Implement measures to help the client avoid coughing, sneezing, and straining. 2. Position the client in the supine position with the head of the bed at 30 degrees. 3. Initiate oxygen administration. 4. Initiate and monitor an IV with normal saline.	Answer: 1 Rationale: Coughing, sneezing, straining, and bending forward all cause transient increases in ICP and should be avoided in this situation. Keeping the client supine at 30 degrees, administering oxygen and providing an isotonic IV solution are all appropriate measures to care for this client, but are not helpful in preventing further increases in ICP. Planning and Implementation Application Safe, Effective Care Environment

CHAPTER 45

45.1 A client is admitted with signs of a stroke (CVA). On admission, vital signs were blood pressure 128/70, pulse 68, and respirations 20. Two hours later the client is not awake, has a blood pressure of 170/70, pulse 52, and the left pupil is now slower than the right pupil in reacting to light. These findings suggest: 1. impending brain death. 2. decreasing intracranial pressure. 3. stabilization of the client's condition. 4. increased intracranial pressure.	Answer: 4 Rationale: Rising systolic blood pressure, falling pulse, and a pupil that has become sluggish suggest increasing intracranial pressure (IICP). This is an emergency situation that requires notification of the physician intervention as the client's condition is becoming more unstable. Brain death is diagnosed by lack of brain waves and inability to maintain vital function. Assessment Synthesis Physiological Integrity
45.2 A hospitalized client has become unresponsive. The left side of the body is flaccid. The attending physician believes the client may have had a stroke (CVA). What is the nurse's priority intervention? 1. Move the client to the critical care unit. 2. Assess blood pressure. 3. Assess the airway and breathing. 4. Observe urinary output.	Answer: 3 Rationale: In any unconscious client, the airway must be protected. Assessment of the current airway and breathing status is of highest priority and will continue to be. Blood pressure and output monitoring as well as ensuring appropriate level of care are important interventions, but assessment of the client's ability to maintain an airway is the most vital. Assessment Synthesis Physiological Integrity

45.3 A client whose status is post-stroke (CVA) has severe right-sided weakness. Physical therapy recommends a quad cane. Which of the following is proper use of the cane by the client?

1. The client holds the cane in the left hand. The client moves the cane forward first, then the right leg, and then the left leg.
2. The cane is held in either hand and moved forward at the same time as the left leg. Then the client drags the right leg forward.
3. The client holds the cane in the right hand for support. The client moves the cane forward first, then the left leg, and then the right leg.
4. The client holds the cane in the left hand. The client moves the left leg forward first, then moves the cane and the right leg forward together.

Answer: 1
Rationale: Proper use of the cane is essential to fall prevention. The client should hold the cane in the left hand. The client should move the cane forward first, then the right leg, and then the left leg.
Assessment
Application
Safe, Effective Care Environment

45.4 The family of a client who has had a brain attack (CVA) asks if the client will ever talk again. The nurse should:

1. explain that the client's speech will return to normal with time.
2. explain that it is difficult to know how far the client will progress.
3. tell the family that nurses cannot discuss such issues. Tell them to ask the physician.
4. tell the family what they see today is all they can expect.

Answer: 2
Rationale: Therapeutic communication is needed. It is important to allow hope but be honest by not promising progress, since no one knows how much the client will improve. Progress may depend on the extent and the areas affected. The nurse does not know that speech will return in time. It is not therapeutic to tell the family to ask the physician, and it does not display a professional, caring attitude.
Implementation
Application
Physiological Integrity

45.5 The nurse is teaching regarding risk factors for stroke (CVA). The greatest risk factor is:

1. diabetes.
2. heart disease.
3. renal insufficiency.
4. hypertension.

Answer: 4
Rationale: Hypertension is the greatest risk factor for stroke, and should be controlled. Diabetes, heart disease, and renal insufficiency can all lead to stroke, however hypertension is the greatest risk.
Assessment
Application
Health Promotion and Maintenance

45.6 The nurse recognizes that the most common type of brain attack (CVA) is related to:

1. ischemia.
2. hemorrhage.
3. headache.
4. vomiting.

Answer: 1
Rationale: Eighty percent of all strokes are caused by ischemia. Hemorrhagic strokes are less common than ischemic strokes. Headache and vomiting may be symptoms associated with CVA, but not common causes.
Assessment
Application
Physiological Integrity

45.7 When caring for a client just admitted post-stroke (CVA) who has altered consciousness, the nurse should place the client in which position?

1. side-lying
2. supine

Answer: 1
Rationale: The side-lying position is the safest position to allow adequate drainage of fluids without aspiration.
Implementation
Application
Safe, Effective Care Environment

3. prone 4. semi-Fowler's	
45.8 The nurse must be alert to complications in the client who has just had a ruptured intracranial aneurysm. The nurse should assess the client for signs of: (Select all that apply.) 1. headache. 2. hydrocephalus. 3. rebleeding. 4. vasospasm.	Answer: 2, 3, 4 Rationale: Headache is a sign of a probable rebleed. Hydrocephalus, rebleeding, and vasospasm are the three major complications that a nurse must anticipate following a ruptured intracranial aneurysm. Assessment Application Physiological Integrity
45.9 The nurse is caring for a client with increased intracranial pressure (IICP). The nurse realizes that some nursing actions are contraindicated with IICP; which nursing action should be avoided? 1. Reposition the client every two hours. 2. Position the client with the head elevated 30 degrees. 3. Suction the airway every two hours per standing orders. 4. Provide continuous oxygen as ordered.	Answer: 3 Rationale: Suctioning further increases intracranial pressure; therefore, suctioning should be done to maintain a patent airway but not as a matter of routine. Maintaining client comfort by frequent repositioning as well as keeping the head elevated 30 degrees will help to prevent (or even reduce) IICP. Keeping the client properly oxygenated may also help to control ICP. Planning Synthesis Physiological Integrity
45.10 The client is exhibiting left-sided hemianopia following a stroke (CVA). The priority of nursing care is: 1. to train the client to scan the right side of the body. 2. to train the client to scan the surroundings. 3. to train the client to scan the left side of the body. 4. to explain that the client must pay more attention to what they are asked to do.	Answer: 2 Rationale: Vision has been lost from the left visual field, so scanning can help compensate for that and reduce risk of injury. The client is taught to scan the surroundings, not the affected or unaffected side of their body for potential hazards. Simply telling the client to pay more attention does not provide useful information to enhance safety. Planning Application Safe, Effective Care Environment
45.11 Prodromal manifestations prior to an intracranial aneurysm rupture could be recognized by the nurse as: (Select all that apply.) 1. visual deficits. 2. headache. 3. mild nausea. 4. dilated pupil.	Answer: 1, 2, 4 Rationale: Often intracranial aneurysms are asymptomatic until rupture but clients can complain of headache and eye pain, and have visual deficits and a dilated pupil. Nausea and vomiting is not usually associated with the prodromal manifestations of an intracranial aneurysm, but may occur with leaking or rupture. Assessment Application Physiological Integrity
45.12 Which of the following clients is at highest risk for a spinal cord injury? 1. 18-year-old male with a prior DWI arrest 2. 20-year-old female with a history of substance abuse 3. 50-year-old female with osteoporosis 4. 35-year-old man who coaches a soccer team	Answer: 1 Rationale: The three major risk factors for spinal cord injuries (SCI) are: age (young adults), gender (higher incidence in males), and alcohol or drug abuse. Females tend to engage in less risk-taking behavior than young men. Assessment Application Health Promotion and Maintenance

45.13 The nurse understands that when the spinal cord is injured, ischemia results and edema occurs. How should the nurse explain to the client the reason that the extent of injury cannot be determined for several days to a week?

1. "Tissue repair does not begin for 72 hours."
2. "The edema extends the level of injury for two cord segments above and below the affected level."
3. "Neurons need time to regenerate so stating the injury early is not predictive of how the client progresses."
4. "Necrosis of gray and white matter does not occur until days after the injury."

Answer: 2

Rationale: Within 24 hours necrosis of both gray and white matter begins if ischemia has been prolonged and the function of nerves passing through the injured area is lost. Because the edema extends above and below the area affected, so the extent of injury cannot be determined until after the edema is controlled. Neurons do not regenerate, and the edema is the factor that limits the ability to predict extent of injury.
Assessment
Synthesis
Physiological Integrity

45.14 A client is recovering following a carotid endarterectomy. The blood pressure has risen this morning to 168/60. The nurse should:

1. recheck the blood pressure and make sure the correct size cuff was used. Then compare the trend of blood pressure readings and call the physician now.
2. recheck the blood pressure every hour and report this change to the physician when they make rounds the next time.
3. record the blood pressure and find out who took this reading. Have that staff member demonstrate their blood pressure procedure and offer tips to obtain more accurate readings.
4. check the standing orders and see if there is a medication ordered prn for lowering blood pressure. If so, administer it and document the action.

Answer: 1

Rationale: Take a blood pressure reading manually to check technique, compare the results to the last several blood pressures recorded, and call the physician to report this blood pressure. Physicians typically have a range for maintaining the blood pressure following carotid endarterectomy, with standing orders for higher or lower blood pressures. If the blood pressure becomes higher, it is a danger and should be reported to the physician and documented in the client record along with orders received. Although the skill of the staff is important, it is a priority to notify the physician of the blood pressure reading so that treatment can begin. PRN antihypertensives may be ordered and administered, but physician notification after verification of the reading is the priority, so that further evaluation can occur.
Implementation and Evaluation
Synthesis
Safe, Effective Care Environment

45.15 A client with a spinal cord injury is recovering from spinal shock. The nurse realizes that the client should not develop a full bladder because what emergency condition can occur if it is not corrected quickly?

1. autonomic dysreflexia
2. autonomic crisis
3. autonomic shutdown
4. autonomic failure

Answer: 1

Rationale: Be attuned to the prevention of a distended bladder when caring for spinal cord injury (SCI) clients in order to prevent this chain of events that lead to autonomic dysreflexia. Track urinary output carefully. Routine use of bladder scanning can help prevent the occurrence. Other causes of autonomic dysreflexia are impacted stool and skin pressure. Autonomic crisis, autonomic shutdown, and autonomic failure are not terms used to describe common complications of spinal injury associated with bladder distension.
Assessment
Application
Safe, Effective Care Environment

45.16 While caring for the client with spinal cord injury (SCI), the nurse elevates the head of the bed, removes TED stockings, and continues to assess vital signs every 2–3 minutes while searching for the cause in order to prevent loss of consciousness or death. By practicing these interventions, the nurse is avoiding the most dangerous complication of autonomic dysreflexia, which is:

1. hypoxia.
2. bradycardia.
3. elevated blood pressure.
4. tachycardia.

Answer: 3
Rationale: Autonomic dysreflexia is an emergency that requires immediate assessment and intervention to prevent complications of extremely high blood pressure. Additional nursing assistance will be needed and a colleague needs to reach the physician stat.
Assessment and Intervention
Application
Safe, Effective Care Environment

45.17 A lumbar puncture (LP) is done on a client to rule out a spinal cord tumor. The cerebrospinal fluid (CSF) is xanthochromic, has increased protein, no cells, and clots immediately. What syndrome do these findings describe?

1. Glasgow's syndrome
2. Froin's syndrome
3. cord tumor syndrome
4. reflex syndrome

Answer: 2
Rationale: Froin's syndrome is seen with spinal cord tumors. A lumbar puncture, x-rays, CT scans, MRI, and myelogram are all common tests that are used to diagnose a spinal cord tumor. Glasgow's syndrome, cord tumor syndrome, and reflex syndrome are not terms associated with the symptoms of spinal cord tumor described.
Assessment
Application
Physiological Integrity

45.18 The nurse realizes that the goal of surgery for a client with a secondary metastatic spinal cord tumor is:

1. complete removal of the tumor and affected spinal cord tissue.
2. eradication of the tumor with excision and drainage.
3. tumor excision to reduce cord compression.
4. exploration to visualize the tumor and obtain a biopsy.

Answer: 3
Rationale: The tumor can exert pressure on the spinal cord, which interferes with function. In the case of secondary metastatic spinal tumor (which means a second site of cancer) and the metastasis (spread of cancer) the client outcome may be limited to preventing compression on the spinal cord and not totally removing the cancerous lesion. Complete removal along with along with affected spinal tissue or eradication by excision and drainage would not be likely due to the secondary nature of the tumor and the resulting disability. Biopsy can be accomplished without direct visualization.
Assessment
Synthesis
Physiological Integrity

45.19 A client with a spinal cord injury (SCI) has complete paralysis of the upper extremities and complete paralysis of the lower part of the body. The nurse should use which medical term to adequately describe this in documentation?

1. hemiplegia
2. paresthesia
3. paraplegia
4. quadriplegia

Answer: 4
Rationale: Quadriplegia describes complete paralysis of the upper extremities and complete paralysis of the lower part of the body. Hemiplegia describes paralysis on one side of the body. Paresthesia does not indicate paralysis. Paraplegia is paralysis of the lower body.
Assessment
Application
Physiological Integrity

45.20 The client is admitted with injuries that were sustained in a fall. During the nurse's first assessment upon admission, the findings are: blood pressure 90/60 (as compared to 136/66 in the emergency department), flaccid paralysis on the right, absent bowel sounds, zero urine output, and palpation of a distended bladder. These signs are consistent with:

Answer: 2
Rationale: Spinal shock is common in acute spinal cord injuries. In addition to the signs and symptoms mentioned, the additional sign of absence of the cremasteric reflex is associated with spinal shock. Lack of respiratory effort is generally associated with high cervical injury. The findings describe paralysis that would be associated with spinal shock in a spinal injured client. The likely cause of these findings is not hypovolemia, but rather spinal shock.
Assessment
Application
Physiological Integrity

1. paralysis.
2. spinal shock.
3. high cervical injury.
4. temporary hypovolemia.

CHAPTER 46

46.1 In order to care for adults with Alzheimer's disease (AD), the nurse recognizes which of the following as a common sign? (Select all that apply)
1. declining job skills
2. poor or decreased judgment
3. inability to be comfortable in social situations
4. obsession with organization

Answer: 1, 2, 3
Rationale: Poor or decreased judgment, memory loss that negatively affects job skills, difficulty completing familiar tasks, problems with language, disorientation to time and place, misplacing things, changes in mood or behavior, changes in personality, and loss of initiative are all warning signs of AD. These changes may make the client uncomfortable in social situations. It is important for the nurse to note the signs and look for combining signs in adults. Obsession with organization is not usually associated with Alzheimer's.
Assessment
Application
Physiological Integrity

46.2 The medication expected in the care of an Alzheimer's client is:
1. rivastigmine tartrate (Exelon).
2. adrenocorticotropic hormone (ACTH).
3. meperidine (Demerol).
4. acetaminophen (Tylenol).

Answer: 1
Rationale: Rivastigmine tartrate (Exelon) is used to improve the ability to carry out activities of daily living. It decreases agitation and delusions and improves cognitive function. Adrenocorticotropic hormone is a natural hormone, but it has no known ability to treat Alzheimer's. Demerol is a narcotic used to treat moderate to severe pain and would not be indicated in treatment of Alzheimer's. Tylenol is a nonsteroidal anti-inflammatory medication which would not be used routinely to treat Alzheimer's.
Implementation
Application
Physiological Integrity

46.3 The nurse is having a conversation with an older adult with Parkinson's disease. Which of the following would this client most likely exhibit during conversation with the nurse?
1. bubbly, spirited discussion
2. a low-pitched monotone voice
3. jumbled words that do not make sense
4. angry, loud talk

Answer: 2
Rationale: Voice amplitude is affected by the neuromuscular effects of Parkinson's disease. The voice becomes very monotone with progression of the disease. Clients will need to be reminded to speak loudly. Muscular ability may make communication difficulty, but the client will retain cognitive ability, so communication should make sense.
Assessment
Application
Psychosocial Integrity

46.4 A client who was diagnosed with Parkinson's disease is demonstrating bradykinesia. The nurse will likely observe the following actions in this client:
1. an increase in spontaneous movements that occur more slowly
2. active exercise and high energy as required to perform activities of daily living
3. very slow talk
4. a loss of spontaneous movement

Answer: 4
Rationale: Parkinson's disease creates a lack of spontaneous movement that affects starting to move and actually following through on the movement. High energy and active exercise is difficult for the client with Parkinson's. Clients with Parkinson's do talk slow, but the term bradykinesia refers to movement.
Assessment
Application
Physiological Integrity

46.5 Medication does not stop all symptoms with Parkinson's disease. The nurse notes tremors and muscle rigidity in an older adult client. Expected medication to combat these symptoms includes: (Select all that apply.)

Answer: 2
Rationale: Propranolol (Inderal) can be used to treat tremors. Acetaminophen (Tylenol), meperidine (Demerol), and nitroglycerin (Nitrobid) do not affect tremors.
Planning

1. acetaminophen (Tylenol).	Application
2. propranolol (Inderal).	Physiological Integrity
3. meperidine (Demerol).	
4. nitroglycerin (Nitrobid).	

46.6 An adult client has been diagnosed with Bell's palsy. The client asks if the facial paralysis and distortion will go away. The nurse should answer:

1. "About 80% of people recover completely within a few weeks to a few months, but there can be lasting effects."
2. "Everyone recovers from Bell's palsy in three to five weeks."
3. "Most people have permanent facial paralysis on both sides of the face."
4. "Most people have permanent facial paralysis on one side of the face."

Answer: 1
Rationale: About 80% of people recover completely from Bell's palsy within a few weeks to a few months, but there can be lasting effects. About 15% of clients recover some function but have some permanent facial paralysis.
Implementation
Application
Psychosocial Integrity

46.7 An adult woman comes to the clinic complaining of repetitive episodes of sudden severe pain on the right side of the face. The nurse expects that the diagnosis will be _____ and the medication treatment will be _____.

1. Parkinson's disease; propranolol (Inderal)
2. Bell's palsy; penicillin
3. trigeminal neuralgia; phenytoin (Dilantin)
4. myasthenia gravis; acetaminophen (Tylenol)

Answer: 3
Rationale: The cause of trigeminal neuralgia is not known but contributing factors are recent flulike illness, trauma or infection of the teeth or jaw, and arteriosclerotic changes of an artery close to the nerve. It is manifested by repetitive episodes of sudden severe pain on the affected side of the face. This symptom is not associated with Parkinson's disease, Bell's palsy, or myasthenia gravis.
Assessment
Application
Physiological Integrity

46.8 Huntington's disease has no cure and causes progressive chorea, speech problems, and dementia. When teaching the newly-diagnosed client about the disease, the client asks the nurse whether it can be passed on to future children. The nurse's best response is:

1. "Children will not be affected by the disease."
2. "The disease is passed on genetically in 75% of offspring."
3. "Each child will have a 50% chance of inheriting the gene."
4. "There may be genetic concerns that should be discussed with the physician."

Answer: 4
Rationale: Children have a 50% chance of inheriting the disease, so answer 3 provides correct information. However, nurses are not genetic counselors or physicians and should not share this diagnostic information. The nurse can follow up on concerns once the physician discusses the genetics.\
Planning
Synthesis
Health Promotion and Maintenance

46.9 The nurse is caring for a client with amyotrophic lateral sclerosis (ALS). The nurse realizes that the prognosis is:

1. poor. The disease rapidly progresses and is fatal.
2. good. The disease will progress over many years but the quality of life will be good.

Answer: 1
Rationale: The disease is characterized by weakness and wasting of muscles that are under voluntary control. There are no sensory or cognitive changes. Death usually occurs due to respiratory failure.
Planning
Application
Physiological Integrity

3. good. The disease progresses rapidly but can be halted by drug therapy. 4. excellent. The disease will progress slowly and can be controlled by medication.	
46.10 Once amyotrophic lateral sclerosis (ALS) is diagnosed, the priority nursing activity is to: 1. monitor for infection. 2. support the client and family to meet physical and psychosocial needs. 3. assist the client to avoid complications. 4. assist the client to adapt to the disease.	Answer: 2 Rationale: Support for the client and family should receive the highest priority for nursing intervention. It is also important to monitor for infection, and assist the client and family to avoid complications and adapt to the disease, but not as important as supporting the client and family to meet physical and psychosocial needs. Implementation Application Physiological and Psychosocial Integrity
46.11 Postpoliomyelitis syndrome is seen in about 50% of clients who had the poliomyelitis virus many years ago. While the pathophysiology is not understood, the nurse anticipates: 1. a new outbreak of polio with the need for a new immunization program. 2. caring for clients with respiratory complications who must be quarantined. 3. working with clients who have polio again. 4. caring for clients with cold intolerance, dizziness, headaches, urinary incontinence, and sleep disorders.	Answer: 4 Rationale: Clients who overcame the polio virus years ago will be faced with the postpoliomyelitis syndrome, which manifests as cold intolerance, dizziness, headaches, urinary incontinence, and sleep disorders. Presence of this postpoliomyelitis syndrome does not indicate that a resurgence of the disease polio is likely. The respiratory complications that may occur would be related to muscular weakness and would not require quarantine. Assessment Application Physiological Integrity
46.12 The nurse understands that tetanus is completely preventable by: 1. debriding the bite wound. 2. passive immunization. 3. active immunization. 4. administering antibiotics immediately after a bite.	Answer: 3 Rationale: Active immunization is achieved if a tetanus booster has been done every ten years. Debridment of the wound will not prevent infection. Antibiotics are used in the treatment of tetanus, but will not prevent it. Planning Application Safe, Effective Care Environment
46.13 A client with Guillain-Barre syndrome asks if they will get better. The nurse's best response is: 1. "Only time and prayer will tell." 2. "Do not worry about that right now." 3. "Recovery is not likely." 4. "Recovery will be slow but your chance of getting better is good."	Answer: 4 Rationale: Nontherapeutic responses do not address the client's concerns. Recovery is likely, but it can take weeks to years for recovery. Implementation Application Psychosocial Integrity
46.14 The nurse is assessing a client who was just admitted with the diagnosis Guillain-Barre syndrome. The nurse anticipates that the client will exhibit: 1. increased leg pain. 2. increased confusion. 3. increased intolerance to light. 4. increased muscular weakness.	Answer: 4 Rationale: As Guillain-Barre develops, muscle weakness with paralysis occurs from altered nerve conduction (motor nerves become demyelinated). Increased leg pain, confusion, and intolerance to light are not related. Assessment Application Physiological Integrity

46.15 A client is admitted to the hospital with a suspected case of botulism. The nurse realizes that the botulism infection was likely caused by which of the following scenarios?

1. The client ate infected dirt.
2. The client was injected with the poison.
3. The client ate food contaminated with the toxin.
4. The client had a dirty wound that developed this toxin.

Answer: 3
Rationale: Botulism takes several hours to develop after ingesting contaminated food. The contamination comes from improperly canned or cooked foods and especially home-canned vegetables and fruits, and smoked meats and fish.
Planning
Application
Health Promotion and Maintenance

46.16 A 30-year-old nurse who works on a busy medical-surgical unit has been diagnosed with multiple sclerosis (MS). The priority for this client is to:

1. work as hard as possible now because later, it may not be possible.
2. negotiate a regular schedule of working 8-hour dayshifts and consider applying for nursing positions that are less stressful and demanding.
3. continue to work as scheduled without making changes.
4. leave employment as a nurse due to the need for complete bed rest.

Answer: 2
Rationale: Multiple sclerosis (MS) is progressive and will be negatively affected by working long hours and enduring stressful shifts. It is important for this client to plan a schedule that is less demanding and move now to a work environment that is less stressful for adapting to life with MS.
Planning
Application
Physiological Integrity

46.17 The nurse anticipates the following medication administration for a client with multiple sclerosis (MS):

1. meperidine (Demerol).
2. MAO inhibitors.
3. adrenocorticotropic hormone (ACTH).
4. rivastigmine tartrate (Exelon).

Answer: 3
Rationale: Adrenocorticotropic hormone (ACTH) decreases inflammation and suppresses the immune system. Other drugs that are also helpful include azathioprine (Imuran), interferon, glatiramer acetate (Copaxone), and antidepressants. Demerol is a narcotic analgesic and would not be used to treat MS. MAO inhibitors are used to treat depression. Exelon is used in the treatment of Alzheimer's disease.
Planning
Application
Physiological Integrity

46.18 A surgical option for clients younger than 60 with myasthenia gravis (MG) is thymectomy. The nurse anticipates that _____ will obtain remission with the surgery.

1. 10%
2. 30%
3. 40%
4. 60%

Answer: 3
Rationale: While it may take several years, about 40% of clients who have a thymectomy will go into remission.
Assessment
Application
Physiological Integrity

46.19 A test that is used to diagnose myasthenia gravis (MG) is ordered by the physician. Because the test involves an injection of a drug that makes muscle strength improve for about five minutes the nurse realizes that this test likely is:

1. a Tensilon test.
2. a computed tomography (CT) scan of the legs.

Answer: 1
Rationale: The Tensilon test produces a five-minute increase in muscle strength. A computed tomography (CT) scan of the legs is not indicated for this client. The nerve stimulation study and the analysis of antiacetylcholine receptor antibodies are tests that can be done to help diagnose MG, but do not require a drug injection.
Planning
Application
Physiological Integrity

---

3. a nerve stimulation study. 4. analysis of antiacetylcholine receptor antibodies.	
46.20 The nurse is assessing a client with myasthenia gravis. Which of the following is characteristic of this disease? 　1. Visual problems may be an early symptom. 　2. Routine exercise provides an improvement in muscle strength. 　3. No improvement occurs in muscle strength with any treatment. 　4. Great improvement occurs in muscle strength with physical therapy.	Answer: 1 Rationale: The manifestations of myasthenia gravis correspond to the muscles involved. Initially, the eye muscles are affected and the client experiences either diplopia (unilateral or bilateral double vision) or ptosis (drooping of the eyelid). Although treatments such as glucocorticoid and immunosuppressant therapy may result in an increase in muscle strength, exercise tends to fatigue muscles, while rest will improve function. Assessment Application Physiological Integrity

CHAPTER 47

47.1 A client, recovering from a stroke, is demonstrating vision changes. The nurse realizes that this is because: 　1. the stroke occurred in the optic region of the client's brain. 　2. the brain interprets information received through the eyes. 　3. the client is experiencing another stroke. 　4. the client is unable to talk because of the stroke.	Answer: 2 Rationale: The primary functions of the eye are to encode the patterns of light from the environment through photoreceptors and to carry the coded information from the eyes to the brain. The brain gives meaning to the coded information, and interprets what is seen. Inadequate information is provided to determine the location of the infarct. There is no indication of the client's verbal abilities. The client's clinical manifestations are not consistent with another stroke. Diagnosis Analysis Physiological Integrity
47.2 While exiting a burning building, a client's eyebrows and lashes were burned. The nurse realizes that this client might experience: 　1. wound infections. 　2. fluid and electrolyte imbalance. 　3. foreign bodies in the eyes. 　4. itchiness as the hair grows back.	Answer: 3 Rationale: The eyebrows shade the eyes and prevent perspiration from entering the eyes. When stimulated, the eyelashes cause the blink reflex, which serves to protect the eyes from foreign body entry. Lack of eyelashes and eyebrows would not increase risk of wound infection or lead to fluid and electrolyte imbalance. Some discomfort might be experienced if hair growth occurs, but this is a minor concern compared to introduction of foreign bodies. Evaluation Analysis Physiological Integrity
47.3 While assisting a client with morning care, the client's left cornea was accidentally touched, which caused the client to blink and create tears. This response is considered: 　1. abnormal and should be reported to the physician. 　2. unusual but something that would clear up in time. 　3. a possible side effect of a medication. 　4. normal.	Answer: 4 Rationale: When the cornea is touched, purposefully or accidentally, the eyelids blink and tears are secreted. This is a normal response and is called the corneal reflex. Diagnosis Comprehension Health Promotion and Maintenance
47.4 The nurse notices that a client's pupils constrict when reading the consent form for medical treatment. This observation is considered:	Answer: 3 Rationale: The pupil constricts in response to bright light or when used for near vision as when reading. Visual changes, ability, or vision needs cannot be assessed with the limited information available.

1. evidence that the client has normal vision. 2. evidence that the client can read. 3. a normal pupillary response. 4. evidence that the client needs reading glasses.	Evaluation Comprehension Health Promotion and Maintenance

47.5 A client has sustained an injury to the inner layer of his left retina. The nurse realizes that this client will have difficulty with:
    1. tear production.
    2. blinking.
    3. reading.
    4. peripheral vision and color perception.
	Answer: 4
	Rationale: The retina is the innermost lining of the eyeball. It has an outer pigmented layer and an inner neural layer. The transparent inner layer is made up of millions of light receptors in structures called rods and cones. Rods enable vision in dim light as well as peripheral vision. Cones enable vision in bright light and the perception of color. Tear production and blinking are not controlled by the inner retina. Reading will still be possible with this type of injury.
	Assessment
	Application
	Physiological Integrity

47.6 A client with a right eye injury has received an eye patch. The nurse realizes that this client might experience difficulty with:
    1. depth perception.
    2. reading.
    3. light perception.
    4. color perception.
	Answer: 1
	Rationale: Depth perception depends upon visual input from two eyes that function well. Reading may be contraindicated if the treatment plan warns against the eyes moving. Light and color will still be discernable to the "good" eye.
	Diagnosis
	Analysis
	Physiological Integrity

47.7 During an eye examination, the nurse positions the client. After repeated attempts, the client is able to read all of the letters on the Snellen chart without difficulty at a distance of 15 feet. From this finding the nurse can determine that the client:
    1. has normal 20/20 vision.
    2. has normal reading vision.
    3. has visual impairments.
    4. has a normal pupillary reflex.
	Answer: 3
	Rationale: The client must stand closer than normal to read the chart. For people with normal vision, the distance from the viewed object at which the eyes require no accommodation is 20 feet. This point is called the far point of vision.
	Diagnosis
	Application
	Health Promotion and Maintenance

47.8 A client is found to need corrective lenses. Which of the following diagnostic tests was most likely used to determine this finding?
    1. computed tomography (CT) scan
    2. tonometry
    3. refractometry
    4. response to atropine eye drops
	Answer: 3
	Rationale: Refractive errors, with prescription for corrective lenses, are evaluated by retinoscopy and/or refractometry. Pupils must be dilated for accurate diagnosis. A computed tomography (CT) scan is used to assess structures. Tonometry is used to assess ocular pressure. The client's responses to atropine drops would not be used to evaluate the client's need for corrective lenses.
	Evaluation
	Application
	Health Promotion and Maintenance

47.9 The nurse is assessing a client's visual fields by covering the client's right eye with an opaque covering. The nurse should then:
    1. cover own right eye.
    2. cover own left eye.
    3. keep both eyes uncovered.
    4. turn the lights on in the room before conducting this examination.
	Answer: 2
	Rationale: Ask the client to cover one eye with the opaque cover while the nurse covers the eye opposite the client's. For example, if the client covers the right eye, the nurse should cover the left eye. The nurse must have normal fields of vision to perform this examination.
	Implementation
	Application
	Health Promotion and Maintenance

47.10 A 20-year-old client is demonstrating difficulty with near vision. The nurse realizes that this finding is:	Answer: 4 Rationale: Changes in near vision, especially in clients over 45, can indicate presbyopia, which is impaired near vision that results from a loss of elasticity of

1. consistent with the aging process. 2. normal in a 20-year-old client. 3. evidence of presbyopia. 4. evidence of hyperopia.	the lens related to aging. In younger clients, this condition is referred to as hyperopia or farsightedness. Diagnosis Analysis Health Promotion and Maintenance
47.11 The nurse notes that a client's left eye deviates inward while focusing on an object. This finding is consistent with: 1. presbyopia. 2. hyperopia. 3. strabismus. 4. myopia.	Answer: 3 Rationale: Strabismus is a weakening of the eye muscles that causes the eye to deviate inward toward the nose when focusing on an object. The cover-uncover test is used to assess for the condition. To conduct the test, hold a pen or a finger about 1 foot from the eyes and ask the person to focus on that object. Cover one of the client's eyes and note any movement in the uncovered eye. As the cover is removed, assess for movement in the eye that was just uncovered. Myopia is the term used for nearsightedness; presbyopia is impaired near vision resulting from a loss of elasticity of the lens related to aging. In younger clients, this condition is referred to as hyperopia (farsightedness). Assessment Analysis Health Promotion and Maintenance
47.12 A client who is using atropine eye drops is found to have a poor consensual light response. The nurse realizes that this finding is considered: 1. abnormal and should be reported to the physician. 2. normal because of the eye drops. 3. evidence of retinal degeneration. 4. evidence of optic nerve damage.	Answer: 2 Rationale: Some eye medications may cause unequal dilation, constriction, or inequality of pupil size. Morphine and narcotic drugs may cause small, unresponsive pupils, and anticholinergic drugs such as atropine may cause dilated, unresponsive pupils. Retinal degeneration is evidenced by an inability of the pupils to respond appropriately to light. Damage to the optic nerve would likely produce visual disturbances. Diagnosis Analysis Physiological Integrity
47.13 During the assessment of a client's outer eyes, the nurse suspects that the client has a hair follicle infection and elevated lipid levels. Which of the following did the nurse most likely assess in this client? (Select all that apply.) 1. xanthelasma 2. ptosis 3. exophthalmos 4. sty 5. yellow sclera	Answer: 1, 4 Rationale: Yellow plaques noted most often on the lid margins are referred to as xanthelasma and may indicate high lipid levels. An acute localized inflammation of a hair follicle is known as a hordeolum or a sty and is generally caused by staphylococcal organisms. Ptosis, or drooping of the eyelid, may be associated with stroke, neuromuscular disorders, or be congenital in nature. Expothalmos is an abnormal prominence of the eye and is associated with thyroid disease. Yellowing of the sclera is associated with liver diseases such as hepatitis or cirrhosis. Diagnosis Analysis Physiological Integrity
47.14 The client assessment reveals absence of the fovea centralis. The next examination that may be anticipated by the nurse is: 1. inspection of the red reflex. 2. inspection of the retina. 3. inspection of the macula. 4. inspection of the optic disc.	Answer: 3 Rationale: During the inspection of the macula, the macula should be visible on the temporal side of the optic disc. Absence of the fovea centralis is common in older clients; however, it may indicate macular degeneration, which is a common cause of loss of central vision. Red reflex should be visible when using the ophthalmoscope if it is properly positioned. Inspection of the retina and optic disc would not provide any further information in the presence of absent fovea centralis. Assessment Application Physiological Integrity
47.15 A client is having difficulty maintaining equilibrium. The nurse realizes that the portion of the ear involved with this symptom is: 1. the labyrinth. 2. the malleus, incus, and stapes.	Answer: 1 Rationale: The ears are divided into three areas: the external ear, the middle ear, and the inner ear. All three are involved in hearing, but only the inner ear is involved in equilibrium. The inner ear is also called the labyrinth. The auricle and tympanic membrane are part of the outer ear; the malleus, incus, and stapes are part of the middle ear.

3. the tympanic membrane. 4. the auricles.	Assessment Comprehension Physiological Integrity
47.16 A client with a sore throat is complaining of "troubles hearing." The nurse realizes that this client might be experiencing: 1. a sinus infection. 2. a middle ear infection. 3. infected tonsils. 4. an inner ear infection.	Answer: 2 Rationale: The mucous membrane that lines the middle ear is continuous with the mucous membranes that line the throat. The manifestations of a sinus infection or tonsillitis would not include auditory compromise. The inner ear is not indicated in this client scenario. Assessment Analysis Physiological Integrity
47.17 During a Weber test, a client is found to have increased hearing in the right ear. The nurse realizes that this finding is consistent with: 1. normal aging. 2. conductive hearing loss in the left ear. 3. possible build-up of cerumen or otitis media in the right ear. 4. perforated left ear drum.	Answer: 3 Rationale: During the Weber test, sound heard in, or lateralized to, one ear indicates either a conductive loss in that ear or a sensorineural loss in the other ear. Conductive losses may be due to a build-up of cerumen, an infection such as otitis media, or perforation of the eardrum on the affected side. Lateralization is not associated with normal aging. Diagnosis Analysis Physiological Integrity
47.18 A client is found to have small, raised lesions on the rim of the ear. This finding is consistent with: 1. hypertension. 2. gout. 3. heart disease. 4. kidney failure.	Answer: 2 Rationale: Small, raised lesions on the rim of the ear are known as tophi and indicate gout. Tophi are the result of uric acid crystal buildup. These lesions are not associated with hypertension, heart disease, or kidney failure. Diagnosis Analysis Physiological Integrity
47.19 An elderly client says, "I seem to be talking so much louder these days and I don't know why!" The nurse realizes that this client is experiencing: 1. loss of hair cells in the middle ear. 2. cochlea atrophy. 3. impacted cerumen. 4. stiffening of the middle ear structures.	Answer: 4 Rationale: One age-related change of the middle ear is the weakening and stiffening of muscles and ligaments, which decreases the acoustic reflex. Sounds made from one's own body and speech are louder and may further interfere with hearing, speech, and communications. Loss of hair cells in the middle ear, cochlea atrophy, and impacted cerumen would not produce the perception that the client is speaking louder. Diagnosis Analysis Health Promotion and Maintenance
47.20 A client is scheduled for diagnostic tests to determine the cause of his hearing and balance disorder. The diagnostic tests that could be used to help this client include: (Select all that apply.) 1. tonometry. 2. computed tomography (CT) scan. 3. caloric test. 4. auditory evoked potentials (AEP). 5. auditory brainstem response (ABR).	Answer: 3, 4, 5 Rationale: Diagnostic tests used to determine hearing and balance disorders include audiometry, auditory evoked potentials (AEP), auditory brainstem response (ABR), and the caloric test. Tonometry is used to measure intraocular pressures. CT scan would note abnormalities in organ structure, but not be helpful in identifying hearing and balance issues. Planning Analysis Physiological Integrity

48.1 A client who became blind in his left eye because of an industrial accident says, "I still have one good eye and I can still do a lot." The nurse realizes that this client is demonstrating signs of:

1. denial.
2. remorse.
3. anticipatory grieving.
4. acceptance.

Answer: 4

Rationale: Acceptance of the change from sighted to blind is characterized by releasing the hope that vision will be regained. Denial would be manifested by a refusal of the permanence of the condition. Anticipatory grieving involves feeling sorrow for an upcoming event. Remorse involves feeling apologetic about the events.

Diagnosis
Analysis
Psychosocial Integrity

48.2 The nurse is instructing a client on the self-instillation of eye drops for acute conjunctivitis. The most important step to instruct this client is:

1. proper hand washing before instilling the drops.
2. rub the eyes only when necessary.
3. insert contact lenses after the eye drops have been instilled.
4. reuse cotton swabs as needed.

Answer: 1

Rationale: Hand washing is the single most important measure to prevent transmission of infection to the eye. Rubbing the eyes and reuse of cotton swabs should be avoided as they can contribute to infection. Contact lenses should be avoided until the infection had resolved.

Implementation
Application
Physiological Integrity

48.3 A client is learning how to apply and care for a new set of contact lenses. Instructions for this client should include: (Select all that apply.)

1. distilled water is the best solution for the lenses.
2. wash hands before and after applying the lenses.
3. once applied, only remove when cloudy.
4. eye pain is a common complaint and should not be a concern.
5. contact eye physician if eyes become red or tear.

Answer: 2 and 5

Rationale: Contact lens care includes: hand washing; keeping the storage case clean; removing the lenses before sleep and storing them in the appropriate container; use appropriate wetting solution for the lenses; do not use homemade or solutions or water for the lenses; contact eye care professional if eyes become red, tear, experience a vision loss, or pain occurs; and do not share contact lenses or allow another person to "try on" lenses.

Implementation
Application
Physiological Integrity

48.4 A client comes into the clinic complaining of "black spots and a curtain dropping" in his right eye. The nurse realizes that this client is experiencing signs of:

1. conjunctivitis.
2. detached retina.
3. sty.
4. cataract.

Answer: 2

Rationale: Flashes of light, floaters, or the sensation of a curtain being drawn over the eye are indicators of retinal detachment. Conjunctivitis presents with pain, redness, and possible discharge. A sty would demonstrate swelling and tenderness. Cataracts manifest with opacity of the eye.

Diagnosis
Analysis
Physiological Integrity

48.5 A teenage client is diagnosed with a corneal abrasion. Which of the following should the nurse instruct this client?

1. Only share a towel with family members.
2. Gently rub the eyes when itchy.
3. Do not share or use another person's eye makeup.
4. Use the prescribed eye drops until the symptoms disappear.

Answer: 3

Rationale: Teach all clients about proper eye care, including the importance of not sharing makeup and towels, avoiding rubbing or scratching the eyes, and preventing trauma and infection. Rubbing the eyes may further cause trauma or injury. Prescribed medications must be taken as long as ordered.

Planning
Application
Health Promotion and Maintenance

48.6 A client with a left eye ectropion continues to experience eye dryness and corneal abrasions. This client might benefit from: 1. corrective lenses. 2. UV protective sunglasses. 3. contact lenses. 4. corrective surgery.	Answer: 4 Rationale: In ectropion, surgery may be performed to correct the defect, reduce the risk of damage to the eye, and improve cosmetic appearance. Corrective lenses, UV protection sunglasses, and contact lenses would not be beneficial in correcting the eversion of the lid margin. Evaluation Analysis Physiological Integrity
48.7 A client is hospitalized with blunt trauma to his left eye. To best minimize eye movement, the nurse should: 1. patch or provide an eye shield for both eyes. 2. place the client in a side lying position, with the eye up. 3. keep the bed position flat. 4. patch the unaffected eye.	Answer: 1 Rationale: Interventions for the client with blunt trauma to the eye include placing the client on bed rest in semi-Fowler's position and protecting the eye from further injury with an eye shield. The unaffected eye should also be patched to minimize eye movement. Planning Application Physiological Integrity
48.8 An elderly client with a mobility disorder is being discharged after having a cataract removed as an outpatient. The nurse should assess this client for their: 1. ability to read discharge instructions. 2. ability to provide eye drops postprocedure. 3. ability to drive. 4. ability to ambulate.	Answer: 2 Rationale: Assess for factors that may interfere with the client's ability to provide self-care postoperatively. A chronic condition such as arthritis that may affect the ability to administer eye drops may indicate the need to include a family member in teaching. A mobility disorder would not affect the client's ability to read discharge instructions. Driving and ambulation are not related to the postoperative care required for this client. Assessment Application Physiological Integrity
48.9 The nurse assesses a reduction in a client's peripheral vision. Which of the following additional measures is a priority during the assessment of this client? 1. cranial nerve assessment 2. neck range of motion assessment 3. intraocular pressure assessment 4. retina assessment	Answer: 3 Rationale: Open-angle glaucoma is painless, with gradual loss of visual fields. This loss of peripheral vision generally occurs so gradually that the client is often unaware of it, and it is often only detected during a comprehensive vision examination. Intraocular pressure is usually, but not always, elevated. Cranial nerve assessment, retinal assessment, and neck range of motion may all be performed as part of client assessment, however measuring intraocular pressure is the priority, so that glaucoma can be diagnosed and appropriately treated. Planning Application Physiological Integrity
48.10 A client with COPD is being treated for glaucoma. The medication that will most likely be prescribed for this client is a(an): 1. beta–blocker. 2. calcium channel blocker 3. antibiotic. 4. adrenergic agonist.	Answer: 4 Rationale: Beta-blockers alone may be contraindicated in glaucoma treatment in clients with COPD. An adrenergic agonist may be prescribed along with a beta-blocker or if beta-blockers are contraindicated, as for clients with heart failure, asthma, or COPD. Calcium channel blockers would not be useful in treating glaucoma. Glaucoma is not caused by infection, so antibiotics are not useful. Planning Analysis Physiological Integrity
48.11 A client is diagnosed with exudative macular degeneration. The client's primary recreation is reading. Which of the following can the nurse suggest to this client? 1. Find another activity that does not require reading. 2. Obtain books on tape or CD. 3. Spend more time with friends and family.	Answer: 2 Rationale: Activities that require close central vision, such as reading and sewing, are particularly affected by exudative macular degeneration. Many clients who are faced with impaired vision make conscious choices to maintain a positive attitude and lifestyle, and develop strategies that allow them to continue with activities that are important to them or provide pleasure. The nurse can help support and encourage these choices and selection of positive behaviors to maintain independence and self-worth. Implementation

4. Listen to music instead of watching so much television.	Application Psychosocial Integrity
48.12 A mother is concerned that her school-age child is having difficulty walking and seeing during the night. The nurse realizes that this client might be demonstrating signs of: 　1. early macular degeneration. 　2. detached retina. 　3. glaucoma. 　4. retinitis pigmentosa.	Answer: 4 Rationale: The initial manifestation of retinitis pigmentosa, which is difficulty with night vision, is often noted during childhood. As the disease progresses, there is slow loss of visual fields, photophobia, and disrupted color vision. The progression to tunnel vision and blindness is gradual; the client may be totally blind by age 40. The clinical manifestations that are described do not indicate early macular degeneration, detached retina, or glaucoma. Diagnosis Analysis Physiological Integrity
48.13 A client experiences an increase in ear pain when the auricle is pulled up and back. The nurse realizes that this client might be experiencing: 　1. otitis externa. 　2. otitis media. 　3. mastoiditis. 　4. otitis interna.	Answer: 1 Rationale: The pain of otitis externa can be differentiated from that associated with otitis media by manipulating the auricle. In external otitis, this maneuver increases the pain; whereas the client with otitis media experiences no change in pain perception. Otitis interna would not be manifested by pain on external manipulation. Mastoiditis is a complication of otitis media and is manifested by recurrent earache and hearing loss of the affected side. Assessment Analysis Physiological Integrity
48.14 A client is seen for hearing loss and odd popping noises in his left ear after "having a cold." This client is demonstrating signs of: 　1. otitis externa. 　2. serous otitis media. 　3. acute otitis media. 　4. otitis interna.	Answer: 2 Rationale: Typical manifestations of serous otitis media include decreased hearing in the affected ear and complaints of "snapping" or "popping" in the ear. Otitis externa is manifested by pain on manipulation of the external ear. Acute otitis media is manifested by pain and hearing loss, but without complaints of "snapping" or "popping." Otitis interna would be manifested by impairment of balance. Diagnosis Analysis Physiological Integrity
48.15 A client with chronic acute otitis media infections is having tympanostomy tubes placed. Post-tube placement instructions for this client should include: 　1. wash hair only with warm water. 　2. make sure showers are completed within 10 minutes. 　3. avoid gum chewing. 　4. avoid getting any water into the ears.	Answer: 4 Rationale: While the tube is in place, it is important to avoid getting any water in the ear canal because it may then enter the middle ear space. Avoiding the introduction of water into the ear rather than the length of showers and temperature of the water is the concern. Gum chewing may produce discomfort, but it is not as crucial as avoiding the introduction of water into the ear canal. Implementation Application Physiological Integrity
48.16 A client with chronic otitis media is diagnosed with a cholesteatoma. The nurse realizes that the treatment of choice for this client will be: 　1. nothing. It will resolve on its own. 　2. antibiotics. 　3. tympanostomy tubes. 　4. surgery.	Answer: 4 Rationale: Cholesteatomas are benign and slow-growing tumors that can enlarge to fill the entire middle ear. Untreated, the cholesteatoma can progressively destroy the ossicles and erode into the inner ear, and cause profound hearing loss. A cholesteatoma may require delicate surgery for its removal. If at all possible, radical mastoidectomy with removal of the tympanic membrane, ossicles, and tumor is avoided. Planning Analysis Physiological Integrity

48.17 A client is experiencing a severe episode of Ménière's disease. The medication to help reduce the sensation of spinning and nausea is:

1. hydrochlorothiazide (HydroDIURIL).
2. meclizine hydrochloride (Antivert).
3. diazepam (Valium).
4. droperidol (Inapsine).

Answer: 2
Rationale: Antivertigo/antiemetic medications such as meclizine hydrochloride (Antivert), prochlorperazine (Compazine), or hydroxyzine pamoate (Vistaril) are prescribed to reduce the whirling sensation and nausea. Hydrodiuril is a diuretic and would not be used to treat Ménière's disease. Valium is a benzodiazepine used for sedation and to treat anxiety. Inapsine is a tranquilizer and not the drug of choice.
Planning
Analysis
Physiological Integrity

48.18 The nurse is instructing a client who has a hearing and balance disorder. Which of the following should be included in these instructions? (Select all that apply.)

1. Change positions slowly.
2. Stand very still with the onset of vertigo.
3. Increase pace of ambulation.
4. Turn the whole body, rather than just the head.
5. Take antivertigo medication only when able to lie down.

Answer: 1, 4
Rationale: The following should be discussed with the client: change positions slowly, especially when ambulating; turn the whole body rather than just the head; sit down immediately with the onset of vertigo and lie down if possible; and take prescribed antiemetic and antivertigo medications. It is not necessary to only take antivertigo medication when able to lie down.
Implementation
Application
Physiological Integrity

48.19 During an assessment, a client without any health problems explains how his "ears ring" periodically. The nurse realizes that this assessment finding most likely is:

1. a preliminary symptom of a severe disease.
2. nothing.
3. pending drug toxicity.
4. aspirin overdose.

Answer: 2
Rationale: Tinnitus is the perception of sound or noise in the ears without stimulus from the environment. The sound may be steady, intermittent, or pulsatile and is often described as a buzzing, roaring, or ringing. Most tinnitus is chronic and has no pathologic importance. Tinnitus associated with drug toxicity, such as aspirin would not generally be described as periodic.
Diagnosis
Analysis
Health Promotion and Maintenance

48.20 An elderly client often responds incorrectly to questions or during general conversation. The nurse realizes that this client should be assessed for:

1. history of strokes.
2. level of education.
3. cognitive impairment.
4. hearing disorder.

Answer: 4
Rationale: Inappropriate responses due to a hearing deficit can cause others to perceive the client as having problems such as stroke or dementia. Level of education is unrelated to the issue of inappropriate responses.
Planning
Analysis
Health Promotion and Maintenance

CHAPTER 49

49.1 A female client tells the nurse that it was discovered that her inability to become pregnant is because of her husband's choice of underwear. The nurse realizes that this is because:

1. tight male underwear causes sperm to not produce.
2. tight male underwear impedes blood flow to the penis.
3. sperm is produced at 2 to 3 degrees below body temperature, and tight underwear may increase heat in the genital area.
4. of an "old wives' tale."

Answer: 3
Rationale: The optimum temperature for sperm production is about 2 to 3 degrees below body temperature. Sperm production is not directly related to underwear sizing. Sperm is not produced in the penis. There is truth in the client's statements, so this is not an "old wives' tale."
Evaluation
Application
Health Promotion and Maintenance

49.2 A male client was born with only one testis. The nurse realizes that this client most likely: 1. may need testosterone replacement therapy. 2. is sterile. 3. will need estrogen replacement therapy. 4. will have a normal level of sperm production.	Answer: 1 Rationale: The testes produce sperm and testosterone. With one testis, there will be a reduction in produced testosterone and sperm. The client will not be sterile if the remaining testicle is producing sperm. Estrogen replacement will not be indicated in the absence of a testicle. Evaluation Analysis Health Promotion and Maintenance
49.3 A male client has an infection of his epididymis. Because of this infection, the client will have a reduction in: 1. testosterone production. 2. mature sperm. 3. blood flow to the penis. 4. the ability to sustain an erection.	Answer: 2 Rationale: The epididymis is the final area for the storage and maturation of sperm. An infection in the epididymis does not impact testosterone production, blood flow to the penis, or the ability to sustain an erection. Diagnosis Analysis Physiological Integrity
49.4 Upon analysis of a client's semen, it is found that the client could have difficulty making his wife pregnant. This client's semen most likely contains what volume of sperm? 1. 300 million 2. 200 million 3. 100 million 4. 50 million	Answer: 4 Rationale: The total ejaculate of a healthy male contains from 100 to 400 million sperm. Sperm count of 50 million would likely not result in pregnancy. Evaluation Analysis Health Promotion and Maintenance
49.5 Upon semen analysis, it is determined that a client's sperm are not developing motility. The body structure that assists with this development is the: 1. prostate. 2. epididymis. 3. scrotum. 4. penis.	Answer: 2 Rationale: The spermatids elongate into a mature sperm cell with a head and a tail. The head contains enzymes essential to the penetration and fertilization of the ova. The flagellar motion of the tail allows the sperm to move. The sperm cells then move to the epididymis to mature further and develop motility. The prostate, scrotum, and penis do not play a role in the development of motility of the sperm. Evaluation Analysis Physiological Integrity
49.6 A male client's PSA (prostate-specific antigen) level is elevated. The nurse realizes that this client most likely will need which of the following diagnostic tests to accurately diagnose the presence or absence of cancer? 1. abdominal x-ray 2. biopsy 3. CT scan 4. small bowel examination	Answer: 2 Rationale: Prostate cancer is diagnosed and monitored by measuring prostate-specific antigen (PSA). The prostate may be examined by ultrasound to identify testicular torsion or masses, and by a prostate biopsy to accurately diagnose cancer. A CT scan, small bowel examination, and abdominal x-ray will not definitively diagnose the presence of prostate cancer. Planning Analysis Physiological Integrity
49.7 During a focused interview, a male client describes his erection and ejaculate in terms that are less than professional. The nurse should: 1. ask the client to refrain from using the terms. 2. ask the client to define the terms. 3. document the client's response in the terms used. 4. find another nurse to complete the assessment.	Answer: 3 Rationale: Men may be embarrassed to discuss health problems or concerns involving their reproductive organs; it is important for the nurse to ask questions in a nonthreatening, matter-of-fact manner. Consider the psychosocial and cultural factors that affect sexuality and sexual activity. Use words that the man can understand, and do not be embarrassed or offended by the words he uses. Documentation of the client's exact terms is necessary for accuracy. Intervention Comprehension Psychosocial Integrity

49.8 A 40-year-old male client is concerned with his inability to have an erection since he was prescribed an antispasmodic for a muscular back injury. The client's health history includes the use of hydrocortisone creams to manage a chronic integumentary condition. The nurse realizes that this client is experiencing:
1. a side effect of the antispasmodic medication.
2. age-related erectile dysfunction.
3. a psychological problem.
4. a reason to avoid sexual encounters.

Answer: 1
Rationale: The following drugs may cause sexual function problems: antihypertensives, antidepressants, antispasmodics, tranquilizers, sedatives, and histamine$_2$-receptor antagonists. A male at the age of 40 does not routinely experience erectile dysfunction. There are no indications that the client has psychological or emotional concerns that would contribute to his inability to have an erection.
Diagnosis
Analysis
Physiological Integrity

49.9 The nurse is preparing to examine a male client's reproductive organs. Which of the following should the nurse do in preparation for this examination? (Select all that apply.)
1. Secure a private examination room.
2. Use clean hands for the examination.
3. Ask the client to lie down on the exam table.
4. Ask the client to empty his bladder.
5. Make sure the room temperature is cool.

Answer: 1, 4
Rationale: Ask the client to empty his bladder, remove his clothing, and put on a gown or drape. The assessment may be done with the client sitting or standing. Expose only those body parts that are being examined to preserve modesty. Ensure that the examining room is warm and private. Put on gloves before beginning and wear them throughout the examination. A cool temperature may be uncomfortable to the client who is undressed.
Planning
Application
Health Promotion and Maintenance

49.10 An elderly male client comes into the emergency department for an edematous and painful scrotum. The scrotum transilluminates. The nurse realizes that this means the client's scrotum is filled with:
1. a mass.
2. blood.
3. urine.
4. serous fluid.

Answer: 4
Rationale: Swellings that contain serous fluid will transilluminate. Swellings that contain blood or tissue will not transilluminate. Urine would not be present in the scrotum.
Diagnosis
Comprehension
Physiological Integrity

49.11 The nurse is preparing to assess a female client's external genitalia. The structures that should be included in this assessment are the: (Select all that apply.)
1. vagina.
2. cervix.
3. clitoris.
4. labia majora.
5. labia minora.

Answer: 3, 4, 5
Rationale: The external genitalia collectively are called the vulva. They include the mons pubis, the labia majora and minora, the clitoris, the vaginal and urethral openings, and glands. The vagina and cervix are located internally.
Assessment
Knowledge
Health Promotion and Maintenance

49.12 A female client complains of severe menstrual cramps. The nurse realizes that the uterine structure responsible for this client complaint is the:
1. perimetrium.
2. myometrium.
3. endometrium.
4. cervix.

Answer: 2
Rationale: The myometrium is the middle layer and makes up most of the uterine wall. This layer has muscle fibers that run in various directions, and allow contractions during menstruation or childbirth and expansion as the fetus grows. The perimetrium is a serous layer, and the endometrium is the innermost layer that is shed during menstruation. Neither have muscle which is responsible for pain. The cervix is the pathway between the vagina and the uterus and is not responsible for the muscle contraction that causes menstrual cramps.

Assessment

Analysis

Health Promotion and Maintenance

49.13 A female client tells the nurse that she has been taking special vitamins to "increase the production of eggs" so that she can get pregnant. The nurse realizes that this client is: 　1.　being proactive in her attempts to become pregnant. 　2.　a healthy female and should not worry. 　3.　anxious about nothing. 　4.　misinformed.	Answer: 4 Rationale: A woman's total number of ova is present at birth. The nurse needs to explain this to the client and then further evaluate the types of vitamins the client has been taking. The client might have other health issues that hinder her ability to become pregnant. Evaluation Analysis Psychosocial Integrity
49.14 A young female client tells the nurse that she has a "thin, runny discharge" from her vagina every month, about halfway through her menstrual cycle. The nurse realizes that this client is describing: 　1.　normal cervical mucous changes. 　2.　evidence of a blocked vaginal gland. 　3.　sexual arousal response. 　4.　evidence of a sexually-transmitted disease.	Answer: 1 Rationale: In the menstrual cycle, as the maturing follicle begins to produce estrogen, around days 6 to 14, the proliferative phase begins. The amount of cervical mucus produced near the time of ovulation increases. Cervical mucus changes to a thin, crystalline substance, and forms channels to help the sperm move up into the uterus. Assessment Analysis Physiological Integrity
49.15 During an assessment, the client asks why the nurse is "feeling her armpit." Which of the following would be an appropriate response for the nurse to make to this client? 　1.　"I'm counting the ribs." 　2.　"Don't you feel your own armpits?" 　3.　"Breast tissue extends into this area." 　4.　"I'm assessing hair distribution in this area."	Answer: 3 Rationale: Various palpation patterns may be used as long as every part of each breast is palpated, including the axillary tail. The axillary tail is also called tail of Spence, which is the breast tissue that extends from the upper outer quadrant toward and into the axillae. Assessment Application Health Promotion and Maintenance
49.16 During an assessment of a female client's internal genitalia, the nurse feels a bulging along the client's posterior vaginal wall. The nurse realizes that this finding is considered a: 　1.　prolapsed uterus. 　2.　cystocele. 　3.　rectocele. 　4.　blocked gland.	Answer: 3 Rationale: Bulging of the anterior vaginal wall and urinary incontinence suggest a cystocele. Bulging of the posterior wall suggests a rectocele. Protrusion of the cervix or uterus into the vagina indicates uterine prolapse. The vagina does not contain glands, but rather is lubricated by mucous producing cells. The Skene's and Bartholin glands are located between the labia in the vestibule. Diagnosis Application Physiological Integrity
49.17 The nurse is unable to palpate a 60-year-old female client's ovaries. This finding is considered: 　1.　normal. 　2.　evidence of an infection. 　3.　abnormal and should be followed up with an ultrasound. 　4.　evidence of endometriosis.	Answer: 1 Rationale: The ovaries are not usually palpable 3 to 5 years after menopause. Assessment Comprehension Health: Physiological Integrity

49.18 A female client is scheduled for an ultrasound to study the uterus. The nurse should instruct this client to:
1. take a laxative the night before the test to clear the colon of feces.
2. restrict fluids.
3. take no food or fluids after midnight the day before the test.
4. increase fluid intake and to not void until after the test.

Answer: 4
Rationale: For an abdominal ultrasound, the client should be instructed to force fluids and instruct the female client to not void until the test is completed. This ensures a full bladder to lift the pelvic organs higher in the abdomen and improve visualization. Restricting food and clearing the colon of feces is not necessary as the colon does not obstruct view of the uterus.
Implementation
Application
Health Promotion and Maintenance

49.19 A specimen has been taken from a lesion on a male client's penis and is sent for dark-field examination. The nurse realizes that this lesion might be indicative of:
1. gonorrhea.
2. syphilis.
3. yeast infection.
4. chlamydia.

Answer: 2
Rationale: A specimen from a lesion believed to be caused by syphilis is examined microscopically using a dark-field examination to identify Treponema pallidum.
Gonorrhea and chlamydia are diagnosed by a culture of discharge from the penis. A review of clinical manifestations by a healthcare practitioner is typically used to diagnose a yeast infection.
Diagnosis
Comprehension
Health Promotion and Maintenance

49.20 An elderly female client complains about the growth of "hair on the chin." The nurse realizes that this complaint is consistent with:
1. increased estrogen production.
2. increased LH production.
3. decreased estrogen production.
4. decreased follicle stimulating hormone production.

Answer: 3
Rationale: The normal reduction in estrogen production associated with aging causes changes throughout the body, and includes loss of skin tone and growth of facial hair.
Evaluation
Analysis
Health Promotion and Maintenance

CHAPTER 50

50.1 A 35-year-old male is concerned about his inability to sustain an erection. Appropriate assessment questions the nurse can ask this client include:
1. employment history.
2. marital status.
3. substance use or abuse.
4. education level.

Answer: 3
Rationale: Most problems with erection are the result of any disease, injury or chemical substances such as prescribed medications, alcohol, nicotine, cocaine, marijuana, and others, that decrease blood flow in the penis. Marital status, employment status, and educational level are not associated with an inability to sustain an erection.
Planning
Application
Health Promotion and Maintenance

50.2 A 55-year-old client with a history of angina and who is being treated with nitroglycerin asks for a prescription to aid with erectile dysfunction. Which of the following should be done to assist this client?
1. Provide education about the medication once the prescription is provided.
2. Explain why the erectile dysfunction medication is not a good idea with the heart medication.
3. Remind the client to stop taking the heart medication when planning to take the erectile dysfunction medication.

Answer: 2
Rationale: The use of medications for erectile dysfunction are contraindicated for the client who is taking medications used to manage cardiac conditions. Sildenafil (Viagra) and vardenafil (Levitra) should not be taken by men who are also taking nitrate-based drugs. Tadalafil (Cialis) should not be taken if the man is also taking nitrates. Discontinuing cardiac drugs is not advisable. A behavioral health consult would not be the first or primary suggestion in this case as physical issues should be explored.
Planning
Comprehension
Physiological Integrity

4. Suggest a behavioral health consult to analyze the reason for the erectile dysfunction.	
50.3 A male client with type I diabetes mellitus and coronary artery disease is able to achieve an erection but cannot maintain it. Which of the following could be done to assist this client? 1. Discuss penile implant surgery. 2. Provide tadalafil (Cialis) teaching material. 3. Provide sildenafil (Viagra) teaching material. 4. Suggest an "O" ring.	Answer: 4 Rationale: Since the client has coronary artery disease, it is assumed that the client might be prescribed nitroglycerin for transient chest pain. Erectile dysfunction medications would be contraindicated in this case. The least invasive measure would be to provide or offer information about the "O" ring, which is a small band placed on the base of the penis that helps to maintain an erection. When managing an erectile dysfunction condition, the least invasive treatments should be employed first. Implementation Application Health Promotion and Maintenance
50.4 A female client asks the nurse for help because her husband has not been able to attain an erection in several months. Which of the following can the nurse do to help this client? 1. Assess for the most recent sexual practices. 2. Suggest that she seek psychiatric counseling. 3. Suggest that they both see a marriage counselor. 4. Provide a prescription for tadalafil (Cialis).	Answer: 1 Rationale: It is essential for healthcare providers to understand the client and partner's sexual pattern in order to provide appropriate, individualized care. It is premature to suggest marital or psychiatric counseling. Prescribing medications is beyond the nurse's scope of practice. Implementation Application Health Promotion and Maintenance
50.5 A client is recovering from a penile implant procedure. Which of the following should be included in the care of, and teaching about, the implant? (Select all that apply.) 1. Suggest wearing loose-fitting underwear. 2. Encourage the client to practice inflating and deflating the device during the recovery period. 3. Encourage the client to resume sexual activity within 3 weeks. 4. Remind the client to not inflate or deflate the device for at least 4 weeks. 5. Suggest wearing snug-fitting underwear and loose-fitting trousers to conceal the semi-erection.	Answer: 2, 5 Rationale: For a penile implant, teach the client and his partner how to use the pump, including how to inflate and deflate the device. Suggest that he practice inflation and deflation during the postoperative period. Suggest wearing snug-fitting underwear with the penis placed in an upright position on the abdomen and loose trousers. Provide information about length of healing, and that sexual activity may resume within 6 to 8 weeks following surgery. Practice using the pump will maintain the pump position and promote tissue growth around the implant. The type of clothing worn can improve the ability to conceal the semi-rigid prosthesis and decrease embarrassment. Recovery from surgery is necessary before resuming sexual activity. Planning Application Physiological Integrity
50.6 A male client is concerned about ongoing premature ejaculation. Which of the following can the nurse do to assist this client? 1. Review any newly-prescribed medications, and check for side effects. 2. Suggest that the client talk with the physician about medication choices.	Answer: 4 Rationale: Premature ejaculation is very responsive to medical management. The man can experiment with wearing condoms to decrease sensitivity. Using relaxation and guided imagery can delay sexual excitement. Mechanical devices, such as constrictive rings around the base of the penis, can help the man delay ejaculation and sustain an erection. Premature ejaculation is not generally a side-effect of medications. Implementation Application Health Promotion and Maintenance

3. Tell the client that the condition is temporary and will disappear in time. 4. Suggest that the client wear a condom with sexual activity.	
50.7 A client comes into the emergency department with complaints of an erection that has lasted for more than four hours. Which of the following should the nurse include in the client's assessment? 1. substance abuse 2. use of medications for erectile dysfunction 3. number of sexual partners 4. blood pressure	Answer: 2 Rationale: Men who use intracavernous injection therapy or tadalafil (Cialis) for erectile dysfunction are at risk for priapism. Substance abuse assessment and blood pressure measurements would be included in any admission process but do not have a direct influence on the sustained erection. Number of sexual partners is not related to the problem. Assessment Application Physiological Integrity
50.8 A male client who presents with the complaint of a "swollen" scrotum is found to have fluid within his scrotum. The nurse realizes that this finding is consistent with a: 1. hydrocele. 2. spermatocele. 3. variocele. 4. scrotal cancer.	Answer: 1 Rationale: A hydrocele, which is the most common cause of scrotal swelling, is a collection of fluid within the tunica vaginalis. A hydrocele may be differentiated from a solid mass by transillumination or ultrasound of the scrotum. A spermatocele is a mobile, usually painless mass that forms when efferent ducts in the epididymis dilate and form a cyst. A varicocele is an abnormal dilation of a vein within the spermatic cord. It is caused by incompetent or congenitally missing valves that allow blood to pool in the spermatic cord veins. The dilated vein forms a soft mass that may be painful. Scrotal cancer would be manifested by a solid mass rather than a fluid-filled area. Diagnosis Analysis Physiological Integrity
50.9 A 40-year-old male is diagnosed with epididymitis. The nurse realizes that the most likely causes of this disorder for this client are: (Select all that apply.) 1. unprotected anal intercourse. 2. undiagnosed congenital disorder. 3. gonorrhea. 4. urinary tract infection.	Answer: 1, 4 Rationale: In men older than 35, epididymitis is usually associated with a urinary tract infection or prostatitis. Men who practice unprotected anal intercourse may acquire sexually transmitted epididymitis. Urethritis, not epididymitis, would be consistent with gonorrhea. Dysuria would be the chief manifestation for the client who has a urinary tract infection. Congenital disorders are not associated with epididymitis. Diagnosis Analysis Physiological Integrity
50.10 A client who is being treated for epididymitis stops taking his antibiotics. The nurse realizes that this client is at risk for developing: 1. priapism. 2. orchitis. 3. hydrocele. 4. spermatocele.	Answer: 2 Rationale: Orchitis is an acute inflammation or infection of the testes. It most commonly occurs as a complication of a systemic illness or as an extension of epididymitis. Priapism, hydrocele, and spermatocele are conditions of the male reproductive system but are not associated with the presence of an infectious condition. Assessment Analysis Physiological Integrity
50.11 A client who is complaining of heaviness in his scrotum has learned that his serum lactic acid dehydrogenase level is normal. This information indicates that the client: 1. does not have testicular cancer. 2. has testicular cancer. 3. needs more diagnostic tests for testicular cancer. 4. has a spermatocele.	Answer: 3 Rationale: Elevations in serum lactic acid dehydrogenase levels are associated with the presence of testicular cancer, and may be significantly elevated when metastatic disease is present. This laboratory test is a less specific indicator of testicular cancer than the human chorionic gonadotropin and alpha-fetoprotein. The levels alone are not sufficient to make a diagnosis of cancer and should promote further testing. Levels of serum lactic dehydrogenase would not be useful in diagnosis of spermatocele. Diagnosis Analysis Physiological Integrity

50.12 A male client is diagnosed with stage 1 testicular cancer. The nurse realizes that the first step in the treatment for this client is:
1. radiation.
2. chemotherapy.
3. aspiration of the enlarged testicle.
4. surgical removal of the testicle.

Answer: 4
Rationale: Radical orchiectomy is the treatment used in all forms and stages of testicular cancer. The type and progression of the disease process will determine the remaining steps in the plan of treatment.
Planning
Application
Physiological Integrity

50.13 A client is diagnosed with asymptomatic inflammatory prostatitis. The nurse realizes that this diagnosis was made:
1. after examining prostate tissue.
2. by testing the serum PSA (prostate-specific antigen) level.
3. according to the client's symptoms.
4. after palpating the client's prostate gland.

Answer: 1
Rationale: Men with asymptomatic inflammatory prostatitis have no subjective symptoms, but are diagnosed when a biopsy or prostatic fluid examination is conducted.
Evaluation
Analysis
Physiological Integrity

50.14 The nurse is planning instructions for a client diagnosed with prostatitis. Which of the following should be included in these instructions? (Select all that apply.)
1. Increase fluid intake up to 3 liters per day.
2. Withhold voiding for as long as possible.
3. Adhere to a daily bowel movement regime.
4. Only take antibiotics when symptoms are present.
5. Remind the client that the condition does not cause cancer.

Answer: 1, 3, 5
Rationale: Teaching for the man with prostatitis focuses on symptom management. Men with acute and chronic bacterial prostatitis should be taught to increase fluid intake to around 3 liters daily and to void often. Regular bowel movements help to ease pain associated with defecation. Local heat, such as sitz baths, may be helpful to relieve pain and irritation. It is important to teach the man to finish the course of antibiotic therapy. Men with chronic prostatitis/chronic pelvic pain syndrome need to know that the condition is not contagious and does not cause cancer.
Planning
Application
Health Promotion and Maintenance

50.15 A 65-year-old male client complains of "problems emptying his bladder, especially at night." The nurse realizes that the client is demonstrating symptoms of:
1. urinary tract infection.
2. benign prostatic hypertrophy.
3. bladder cancer.
4. testicular cancer.

Answer: 2
Rationale: Benign prostatic hypertrophy (BPH) begins at 40 to 45 years of age, and continues slowly through the rest of life. It is estimated that more than half of all men over age 60 have BPH. Primary symptoms associated with benign prostatic hypertrophy are associated with voiding and difficulty starting the urine stream, dysuria, and nocturia. Testicular cancer would first be manifested by a growth in the testicle. Urinary tract infection may share the symptom of dysuria with BPH, but the client would not have difficulty starting urine stream. Bladder cancer may also have pain as a symptom, but is also accompanied frequently by hematuria.
Assessment
Analysis
Physiological Integrity

50.16 A client was diagnosed with benign prostatic hypertrophy. The nurse realizes that the blood pressure measurement of this client will be beneficial to determine:
1. the dose of finasteride (Proscar).
2. if surgery is indicated.
3. the volume of urine being retained in the bladder.
4. if the client can tolerate doxazosin mesylate (Cardura).

Answer: 4
Rationale: Excessive smooth muscle contraction in benign prostatic hypertrophy (BPH) may be blocked with the alpha-adrenergic antagonists such as doxazosin mesylate (Cardura) and tamsulosin (Flomax). These medications relieve obstruction and increase the flow of urine. They may cause orthostatic hypotension. The use of surgical intervention to manage BPH may not be used. The client's condition may initially be managed with pharmacotherapies. The volume of urinary residual does not have bearing in this question.
Planning
Application
Physiological Integrity

50.17 A client is planning to have surgery for the treatment of benign prostatic hypertrophy. The procedure that has the fewest postoperative complications is:
1. transurethral needle ablation (TUNA).
2. transurethral incision of the prostate (TURP).
3. perineal prostatectomy.
4. suprapubic prostatectomy.

Answer: 1
Rationale: The transurethral needle ablation (TUNA) system uses low-level radiofrequency through twin needles to burn away a region of the enlarged prostate. Shields protect the urethra. TUNA improves the flow of urine through the urethra and does not cause impotence or incontinence. Transurethral incision of the prostate (TURP) involves the insertion of a surgical instrument and optical device into the urethra to the prostate. Erectile dysfunction is not a common occurrence with this procedure; however, there may be retrograde ejaculation. Perineal prostatectomy removes the gland by way of a perineal incision. This procedure has a high incidence of complications including impotence and rectal injury. The suprapubic prostatectomy utilizes an abdominal incision. It involves greater blood loss and an increased risk of infection.
Evaluation
Analysis
Physiological Integrity

50.18 The nurse is instructing a client with benign prostatic hypertrophy about techniques to reduce urinary retention. These instructions should include:
1. encourage ingesting large amounts of fluids at one time.
2. urinate until all of the urine is drained from the bladder.
3. avoid alcoholic beverages.
4. over-the-counter cold remedies are permitted with other medications.

Answer: 3
Rationale: Client teaching for urinary retention should include: the manifestations of acute urinary retention; the risk of developing urinary retention increases with over-the-counter decongestant medications, or prescription medications such as antidepressants, anticholinergics, calcium channel blockers, antipsychotics, and medications to treat Parkinson's disease; avoid the intake of large volumes of liquid at any one time; how to use double-voiding technique; and limit liquids that stimulate voiding, such as coffee and alcoholic beverages.
Implementation
Application
Health Promotion and Maintenance

50.19 A 55-year-old male client has an abnormal digital rectal examination (DRE) with a PSA (prostate-specific antigen) level of 18 ng/mL. The nurse realizes that this client might be scheduled next for a:
1. CT scan of the spine.
2. a transrectal ultrasonography (TRUS).
3. a bone scan.
4. an MRI.

Answer: 2
Rationale: Transrectal ultrasonography (TRUS) may be used when the digital rectal examination (DRE) is abnormal or if the PSA (prostate-specific antigen) level is elevated. In the TRUS test, a small probe is inserted in the rectum. The probe gives off sound waves that make a picture of the prostate on a video screen. Guided by this picture, the physician inserts a narrow needle through the rectal wall into the prostate gland, and the needle removes a sample of tissue for examination. The bone scan, MRI, or CT scan may be performed at a later date to determine the presence of tumor metastasis.
Planning
Analysis
Physiological Integrity

50.20 A male client complains of "not being able to hold urine" especially when the bladder is very full or when lifting objects. Which of the following interventions by the nurse is indicated?
1. Suggest that the client ask the physician for medications to control this incontinence.
2. Suggest that the client restrict fluids.
3. Instruct the client how to do Kegel exercises.
4. Suggest the client wear a Texas catheter.

Answer: 3
Rationale: The symptoms being described by the client are consistent with incontinence. The treatment plan for incontinence should initially begin with the least invasive measures. Kegel exercises can be used to improve tone and eliminate or reduce stress incontinence. The use of a catheter is not indicated at this time.
Planning
Analysis
Health Promotion and Maintenance

50.21 A male client reports concern about his recent increase in breast tissue. The nurse can best assist this client by:

Answer: 2
Rationale: Any condition that increases estrogen activity or decreases testosterone production can contribute to gynecomastia. Conditions that increase estrogen activity include obesity, testicular tumors, liver disease, and adrenal carcinoma;

---

1. telling him that it is self-limiting and will go away in time.
2. reviewing the client's health history.
3. suggesting that the client has a mammogram to ensure he does not have breast cancer.
4. recommending a breast biopsy to find out the reason for the increase in breast tissue.

conditions that decrease testosterone production include chronic illness such as tuberculosis or Hodgkin's disease, injury, and orchitis. Drugs such as digitalis, opiates, and chemotherapeutic agents are also associated with gynecomastia. Dismissing the client's concerns is not therapeutic and until further evaluation is completed this could be potentially dangerous. Gynecomastia is usually bilateral. If it is unilateral, biopsy may be necessary to rule out breast cancer.
Implementation
Analysis
Health Promotion and Maintenance

CHAPTER 51

51.1 A female client tells the nurse that lately she "isn't interested in sex" but is concerned that her husband will divorce her. Which of the following would be an appropriate response for the nurse to make to this client?
1. "I'm sure it's nothing and will go away in time."
2. "There are other activities you and your husband can do together."
3. "Sex isn't that important in a marriage anyway."
4. "Let's talk more about how you are feeling right now."

Answer: 4
Rationale: This client is explaining inhibited sexual desire which can have physiological or psychological causes. Since the client states that lately she's had a disinterest in sexual activity, the nurse should not discount the client's feelings but rather encourage more communication about the situation. Advising the client that sex is not important to the marriage is placing a personal viewpoint on the client.
Implementation
Application
Psychosocial Integrity

51.2 A 55-year-old female client thinks she's "losing her mind" because of constant anxiety, inability to sleep, and headaches. The nurse realizes that this client is describing symptoms of:
1. pregnancy.
2. menopause.
3. normal menstruation.
4. chronic fatigue syndrome.

Answer: 2
Rationale: Vasomotor instability in menopause often results in hot flashes, palpitations, dizziness, and headaches. Other problems that result from vasomotor instability include insomnia, frequent awakening, and night sweats. The woman may experience irritability, anxiety, and depression as a result of these events. The clinical manifestations being exhibited are not typical of pregnancy, normal menstruation, or chronic fatigue syndrome.
Diagnosis
Analysis
Health Promotion and Maintenance

51.3 A female client who is experiencing menopause is "tired of the night sweats." Which of the following can the nurse suggest to help this client?
1. Ensure that the bedroom temperature is cool and limit sleeping attire.
2. Reduce fluid intake.
3. Suggest talking with the physician about a hysterectomy.
4. Exercise one hour before going to sleep.

Answer: 1
Rationale: The underlying cause of hot flashes is not known; however, many physiologic effects of menopause are responsive to nonpharmacologic methods of relief, such as lifestyle changes. Reducing fluid intake will not improve the symptoms the client is experiencing. Encouraging the client to look into surgical intervention is outside the scope of nursing practice. In addition, a hysterectomy will further reduce the client's natural estrogen levels. Exercise prior to retiring will act to further increase the client's ability to rest at night.
Implementation
Application
Health Promotion and Maintenance

51.4 A female client complains about increasing premenstrual symptoms over the past few years and thinks "something must be wrong." The nurse realizes that this client is experiencing:
1. early menopausal symptoms.
2. premenstrual dysphoric disorder.

Answer: 4
Rationale: Premenstrual syndrome (PMS) is seen less frequently during the teens and 20s, and reaches a peak in women in their mid-30s. Major life stressors, age greater than 30, and depression are risk factors associated with PMS. The manifestations being exhibited are not consistent with menopausal symptoms. There are no indications of interpersonal relationship concerns. Premenstrual dysphoric disorder is PMS of such severity that it has a psychiatric label. This

3. interpersonal relationship difficulties. 4. normal pattern of premenstrual syndrome.	severe form of PMS effects a small number of women and is not indicated by the client's complaints. Diagnosis Analysis Health Promotion and Maintenance

51.5 The nurse is assisting a client with ways to reduce the severity of the monthly menstrual discomforts associated with premenstrual syndrome. Information that can be reviewed with this client includes: (Select all that apply.)
  1. apply ice packs to the lower abdominal region.
  2. use abdominal breathing.
  3. balance exercise with rest.
  4. increase sodium intake.
  5. restrict caffeine intake.
	Answer: 2, 3, 5
	Rationale: Treatment plans that the woman with premenstrual syndrome (PMS) may find helpful focus on diet, exercise, relaxation, and stress management. Sodium should be restricted to minimize fluid retention. Caffeine restriction reduces irritability. Exercise is beneficial but rest is also necessary. Techniques for relaxation and stress management include deep abdominal breathing, meditation, muscle relaxation, and guided imagery. Heat, not ice, relieves muscle spasms and dilates blood vessels, which increases the blood supply to the pelvis and uterine muscles.
	Implementation
	Application
	Health Promotion and Maintenance

51.6 The mother of a 16-year-old female child voices concern to the nurse. The parent reports that the teen began menstruating at age 14 but has stopped for at least 5 months. Which of the following responses would be most appropriate for the nurse to make to this mother?
  1. "That's normal."
  2. "Have you thought about a pregnancy?"
  3. "It's probably psychological."
  4. "Have you noticed any other changes in diet, activity, or weight loss?"
	Answer: 4
	Rationale: Secondary amenorrhea, which is absence of menses for at least 6 months in a previously menstruating female, may also be caused by anorexia nervosa, excessive athletic activity or training, or a large weight loss. Other causes include hormonal imbalances and ovarian tumors. The condition being reported by the parent is not normal. It is inappropriate for the nurse to include potential diagnoses such as pregnancy and psychological concerns in the conversation. These conditions are not necessarily indicated.
	Implementation
	Application
	Health Promotion and Maintenance

51.7 A client is scheduled for an endometrial ablation for extreme uterine bleeding. Which of the following provides evidence that this client understands the long-term effects of this treatment?
  1. The client states that future menstrual cycles will be normal.
  2. The client states that pregnancy needs to be avoided for 6 months after the procedure.
  3. The client states that menstrual cycles and the option for pregnancy have ended.
  4. The client states that hormone replacement therapy will still be needed to regulate menstrual cycles.
	Answer: 3
	Rationale: In an endometrial ablation, the endometrial layer of the uterus is permanently destroyed using laser surgery or electrosurgical resection. It is performed in women who do not respond to pharmacologic management or D&C. The woman needs to understand that this procedure ends menstruation and reproduction.
	Evaluation
	Application
	Physiological Integrity

51.8 A client is diagnosed with uterine prolapse into the vagina. The factor that most likely contributed to this client's disorder is:
  1. multiple pregnancies.
  2. endometriosis.
  3. pelvic inflammatory disease.
  4. tumor.
	Answer: 1
	Rationale: Downward displacement of the pelvic organs into the vagina results from weakened pelvic musculature, which is usually attributed to stretching of the supporting ligaments and muscles during pregnancy and childbirth. Unrepaired lacerations from childbirth, rapid deliveries, multiple pregnancies, congenital weakness, or loss of elasticity and muscle tone with aging may contribute to these disorders.
	The presence of endometriosis, pelvic inflammatory disease, and tumors would not be likely causes of uterine prolapse.

	Diagnosis Analysis Physiological Integrity
51.9 A female client is diagnosed with "chocolate" cysts. The nurse realizes that these cysts are caused by: 　1. infection. 　2. use of oral contraceptives. 　3. endometrial overgrowth. 　4. hormone imbalance.	Answer: 3 Rationale: Endometrial cysts are caused by endometrial overgrowth and are often filled with old blood, which leads to the name "chocolate cysts." Endometrial cysts are the result of endometrial implants on the ovary and are associated with endometriosis. These cysts are not associated with infection, use of oral contraceptives, or hormone imbalance. Evaluation Application Physiological Integrity
51.10 A female client of child-bearing age is diagnosed with large uterine fibroids. Since the client wants to have children, the nurse realizes that treatment will most likely be: 　1. oral contraceptives. 　2. estrogen replacement. 　3. iron replacement therapy. 　4. leuprolide acetate (Lupron).	Answer: 4 Rationale: Leuprolide acetate (Lupron) is used to decrease the size of the tumor if surgery is contraindicated or not desired. Gonadotropin-releasing hormone (GnRH) agonists are also administered. The use of oral contraceptives and estrogen replacements will "feed" hormone-controlled tumors such as uterine fibroids. Iron replacement therapy is not appropriate for this client. Planning Application Physiological Integrity
51.11 A 25-year-old female is diagnosed with endometriosis. The nurse should include which of the following when teaching the client about this disorder? (select all that apply) 　1. It can be treated without any long-term effects. 　2. If children are desired, pregnancy should occur before the disease progresses. 　3. Laser ablation and birth control pills are the treatments for this condition. 　4. Leaving it untreated will not result in any long-term health issues.	Answer: 2, 3 Rationale: Endometriosis is a slowly progressive disease that is responsive to ovarian hormone stimulation. Because progressive scarring may interfere with the ability to conceive, women with significant endometriosis are encouraged to have children early if they wish to do so. Women who experience the effects of endometriosis may experience painful, lengthy, or heavy menstrual periods. These characteristics do constitute health issues for the client. Management of endometriosis may include drug (birth control pills) or surgical (laproscopy and laser ablation) intervention; however, these treatments do have long-term effects. Planning Analysis Physiological Integrity
51.12 A postmenopausal woman is diagnosed with cervical dysplasia caused by the human papillomavirus. The procedure that would both diagnose and treat the dysplasia is: 　1. Pap smear. 　2. colposcopy. 　3. cervical biopsy. 　4. loop diathermy.	Answer: 4 Rationale: A loop diathermy technique or loop electrosurgical excision procedure (LEEP) allows simultaneous diagnosis and treatment of dysplastic lesions found on colposcopy. This procedure is performed in the office, and uses a wire for both cutting and coagulation during excision of the dysplastic region of the cervix. Pap smears are used to diagnose the presence of cervical dysplasia. This is a diagnostic test, which is not used to manage conditions. Planning Analysis Physiological Integrity
51.13 A client is prescribed radiation treatments to the pelvic region after having surgery for cervical cancer. The nurse should instruct this client to: 　1. preserve the skin markings made for the radiation treatments. 　2. use an oil-based lotion on the skin area being radiated. 　3. skin burning is expected. 　4. pain is always associated with focused radiation.	Answer: 1 Rationale: Instruct the woman not to remove the markings used to localize the radiation beam to the target area. Markings are used in future radiation treatments. Non–oil-based lotions are recommended for tissue undergoing radiation. Skin burning and pain should not be considered normal and should be reported as possible complications from the radiation therapy. Planning Application Physiological Integrity

51.14 A female client is experiencing a reoccurrence of endometrial cancer. The nurse realizes that this client's treatment might include:
1. radiation therapy after surgery.
2. progesterone therapy.
3. partial abdominal hysterectomy.
4. chemotherapy.

Answer: 2

Rationale: Although the treatment of choice for primary endometrial carcinoma is surgery, progesterone therapy may be used for recurrent disease. About one-third of women respond favorably, primarily those with well-differentiated tumors. Chemotherapy is less effective than other forms of therapy, although cisplatin (Abiplatin) or combination chemotherapy may be used for women with disseminated disease. After the diagnosis is confirmed, a total abdominal hysterectomy and bilateral salpingo-oophorectomy is performed. A radical hysterectomy with node dissection is performed if the disease is stage II or beyond. Treatment with external and internal radiation may be performed as a preoperative measure or as adjuvant treatment in advanced cases.
Planning
Analysis
Physiological Integrity

51.15 A client who is recovering from a complete hysterectomy for endometrial cancer is concerned that she will not be able to continue a sexual relationship with her husband because of the related activity intolerance. Which of the following would assist this client?
1. Suggest other activities to participate with her spouse.
2. Suggest that she discuss her fears with a marriage counselor.
3. Remind her that she has successfully survived cancer surgery.
4. Suggest that she and her husband coordinate sexual activity with rest periods and pain-free periods.

Answer: 4

Rationale: Altered sexuality may result from a feeling of unattractiveness, fatigue, or pain and discomfort. The woman's partner may fear that sexual activity will be harmful. Encourage expression of feelings about the effect of cancer on their lives and sexual relationship. Verbalizing feelings helps relieves stress and maximizes relaxation. Suggest that the couple explore alternative sexual positions and coordinate sexual activity with rest periods and periods that are relatively free from pain. This creates a more favorable environment for satisfying sexual activity.
Implementation
Application
Psychosocial Integrity

51.16 A female client is concerned that she will develop ovarian cancer because her mother's grandmother had the disease. Which of the following factors will most reflect a potential reduction in risk factors for the client?
1. didn't start menstruating until age 10
2. has never had long-term antibiotic therapy
3. had her first child at the age of 20
4. has asymptomatic menstrual cycles

Answer: 3

Rationale: Family history is a significant risk factor, with a 50% risk of developing the disease if two or more first- or second-degree relatives have site-specific ovarian cancer. Risk factors also include having no children or giving birth after age 35, exposure to talc or asbestos, endometriosis, pelvic inflammatory disease, and living in a western civilized country. Protective factors include long-term contraceptive use, having a child before the age of 25, tubal ligation, breastfeeding, and hysterectomy.
Evaluation
Analysis
Psychosocial Integrity

51.17 A client who was just diagnosed with cervical cancer does not want to have surgery. An alternative treatment for this client is:
1. chemotherapy.
2. radiation therapy.
3. vitamin therapy.
4. hormone replacement therapy.

Answer: 1

Rationale: While surgery is the treatment of choice for ovarian cancer, chemotherapy may be used to achieve remission of the disease. Chemotherapy is not curative for ovarian cancer. Radiation therapy using external-beam or intracavitary implants is performed for palliative purposes only and is directed at shrinking the tumor at selected sites. Hormone and vitamin therapies will not provide treatment for ovarian cancer.
Planning
Application
Physiological Integrity

51.18 A mass is found on a mammogram of a 42-year-old female client. The mass is diagnosed as a cyst upon ultrasound. The nurse realizes that the best course of action for this client is:

1. suggest the "watch and wait" approach.
2. reduce caffeine intake.
3. apply warm soaks to the cyst.
4. a surgical biopsy is needed to rule out cancer.

Answer: 4
Rationale: When a woman presents with a breast mass, nursing responsibilities include taking a careful history and facilitating follow-up care. If a palpable mass is present, it is important to ask how long the lesion has been present and whether the woman has noticed any pain associated with the mass, any change in its size, and any changes in association with the menstrual cycle. In many cases, definitive diagnosis of the breast disorder requires surgical biopsy to rule out cancer. During the diagnostic process, the nurse can provide emotional support and education about diagnostic and therapeutic procedures, self-care and comfort measures, and resources to help the woman cope with the experience.
Planning
Application
Physiological Integrity

51.19 A female client is recovering from breast cancer surgery that included axillary node dissection. The nurse realizes that this client is at risk for developing:

1. lymphedema.
2. metastasis.
3. anemia.
4. postoperative wound infection.

Answer: 1
Rationale: Axillary node dissection is generally performed during surgery for all invasive breast carcinomas to stage the tumor. This surgery can cause lymphedema, nerve damage, and adhesions, as well as alter immune system functioning. Removal of the lymph nodes does not increase risk of metastasis or anemia. Post operative wound infection is a risk even if node dissection is not performed.
Diagnosis
Analysis
Physiological Integrity

51.20 A client who was just diagnosed with breast cancer is scheduled for a lumpectomy. The nurse believes that the client is demonstrating signs of anticipatory grieving because the client is:

1. joking with her hospital roommate.
2. making calls to her girlfriends.
3. doing a crossword puzzle.
4. sitting quietly, occasionally crying.

Answer: 4
Rationale: Breast surgery, even lumpectomy, alters the appearance of the breast. This loss is expressed through grief. The nurse should listen attentively to expressions of grief and watch for nonverbal cues such as failure to make eye contact, crying, or silence. Not all women will express grief clearly; sometimes unspoken grief is the most painful. Grief is relieved only when expressed in a nonthreatening environment. The behaviors seen in the client are consistent with grief. Joking, socializing, and working on crossword puzzles are not obvious signs of grieving.
Evaluation
Application
Psychosocial Integrity

CHAPTER 52

52.1 A male client tells the nurse that he is not concerned about sexually transmitted diseases because he is in a monogamous relationship. The nurse realizes that this client would benefit from education because:

1. he currently has a sexually transmitted disease.
2. all sexually active persons are at risk for a sexually transmitted disease.
3. sex means different things to different people.
4. he is having difficulty with sperm production.

Answer: 2
Rationale: Every sexually active person is at risk for sexually transmitted infections (STIs), and some of these diseases can be life-threatening, particularly for women and infants.
Planning
Application
Health Promotion and Maintenance

52.2 A female client is having difficulty accepting the diagnosis of a sexually transmitted disease because she has "been on the pill" for years. Information the nurse can provide to aid this client is that:

1. skipping doses could have caused the disease.

Answer: 4
Rationale: Oral contraceptives do not protect against sexually transmitted diseases. By making the vaginal environment less acidic, oral contraceptives can predispose women to infection. The type of oral contraceptive used or inconsistency of dose does not increase risk of STD.
Implementation
Application
Health Promotion and Maintenance

2. she possibly needs to change the type of birth control pill being used. 3. some diseases are virulent and the pill will not protect her. 4. oral contraceptives do not protect against sexually transmitted diseases.	
52.3 A male client is "relieved" to learn that he has a sexually transmitted disease and is not HIV positive. Which of the following would be an appropriate response for the nurse to make to this client? 1. "Having a sexually transmitted disease does predispose the body to be infected with HIV if exposed to the virus." 2. "You are lucky." 3. "I told you not to be concerned." 4. "You would know if you had HIV."	Answer: 1 Rationale: The emergence of HIV/AIDS has created a kind of "epidemiologic synergy" among all sexually transmitted infections (STIs). Other STIs facilitate the transmission of HIV/AIDS, and the immune suppression caused by HIV potentiates the infectious process of other STIs. Individuals who are infected with STIs are 2 to 5 times more likely than uninfected individuals to acquire HIV if they are exposed to the virus. The other responses do not provide the client with necessary information about HIV risk. Implementation Application Health Promotion and Maintenance
52.4 A female client who was just diagnosed with a sexually transmitted disease is beginning treatment. The nurse should remind the client to: 1. avoid all sexual activity in the future. 2. begin birth control pills to prevent future disease transmission. 3. be pleased that she was not diagnosed with HIV. 4. inform all sexual partners about the diagnosis so they can also be treated.	Answer: 4 Rationale: For treatment to be effective, sexual partners of the infected person must also be treated. Implementation of safe sex practices, rather than avoidance of all sexual activity is a more appropriate action. Birth control pills will not prevent disease transmission. Minimizing the client's diagnosis is not therapeutic. Implementation Application Health Promotion and Maintenance
52.5 A female client is seen for a new onset of blisters on the labia majora. The nurse realizes that this client is experiencing: 1. a drug reaction. 2. first episode of a herpes virus infection. 3. prodromal symptoms of the herpes virus. 4. latency period of the herpes virus infection.	Answer: 2 Rationale: The first outbreak of herpes lesions is called first episode infection, and has an average duration of 12 days. The latency period is a time, during which time the person remains infectious even though no symptoms are present. Prodromal symptoms of recurrent outbreaks of genital herpes can include burning, itching, tingling, or throbbing at the sites where lesions commonly appear. Lesions of the type described are not commonly associated with drug reactions. Assessment Analysis Physiological Integrity
52.6 A client with genital herpes is experiencing increased pain with urination. The nurse should suggest that the client: 1. drink more water. 2. drink more cranberry juice. 3. drink more orange juice. 4. restrict fluids.	Answer: 1 Rationale: Drinking additional fluids also helps dilute the acidity of the urine; however, fluids that increase acidity, such as cranberry and orange juice, should be avoided. Implementation Application Physiological Integrity
52.7 A male client is concerned about a "smooth growth" that appeared on his penis. The nurse suspects this client is experiencing which type of genital wart?	Answer: 3 Rationale: There are four types of genital warts: condyloma acuminata, keratotic warts, papular warts, and flat warts. Papular warts are smooth lesions that also develop on keratinized skin. Condyloma acuminate are cauliflower-shaped

1. condyloma acuminata 2. keratotic wart 3. papular wart 4. flat wart	lesions that appear on moist skin surfaces such as the vagina or anus. Keratotic warts are thick, hard lesions that develop on keratinized skin such as the labia major, penis, or scrotum. Flat warts are slightly raised lesions, often invisible to the naked eye, also develop on kertinized skin Assessment Analysis Physiological Integrity

52.8 After the removal of genital warts, the male client says, "Now I can have sex again." Information that the nurse should provide to this client includes:
  1. efforts to prevent reinfection now that he is cured of the warts.
  2. the need to always use a chemical barrier to avoid impregnating his partner.
  3. ask every partner if they have a diagnosed sexually transmitted disease.
  4. remind to always use a condom with sexual activity.
	Answer: 4
	Rationale: Even though there is no known cure for human papillomavirus, which is the causative agent for genital warts, the client needs to be reminded to protect himself and any sexual partners from the transmission of the virus.
	Implementation
	Application
	Health Promotion and Maintenance

52.9 A female client continues to develop vaginal infections. Which of the following can the nurse provide to assist this client? (Select all that apply.)
  1. "Wear only nylon underwear."
  2. "Be sure to wash the perineal region daily and as necessary throughout the day."
  3. "Avoid wearing tight jeans or pants."
  4. "Douche daily."
  5. "Use condoms when engaging in sexual activity."
	Answer: 2, 3, 5
	Rationale: Preventive measures for vaginal infections include educating women about personal hygiene practices and safer sex. Women need to avoid frequent douching and wearing nylon underwear or tight pants. Unprotected sexual activity, particularly with multiple partners, increases the risk of vaginal infections.
	Planning
	Application
	Health Promotion and Maintenance

52.10 A female client is complaining of a "watery" vaginal discharge with a "really strong fishy" odor. The nurse suspects that this client is experiencing:
  1. bacterial vaginosis.
  2. yeast infection.
  3. trichomoniasis infection.
  4. genital warts.
	Answer: 1
	Rationale: Bacterial vaginosis is the most common cause of vaginal infection in women of reproductive age. The primary manifestation is a vaginal discharge that is thin and grayish-white, and has a foul, fishy odor. Yeast infections present with a thick, cheesy discharge. Trichomoniasis presents with a frothy, yellow-green discharge with a strong odor. Genital warts are growths.
	Assessment
	Analysis
	Physiological Integrity

52.11 A female client says that she has been using "the medication for a yeast infection" but it is not "getting any better." The nurse realizes that this client most likely:
  1. has not used the medication long enough.
  2. might be using a treatment that is not appropriate for the cause.
  3. is not using the medication correctly.
  4. is not washing her hands before applying the medication.
	Answer: 2
	Rationale: Some antifungal agents are available without prescription, which can lead to self-medication with the incorrect agent or allow repeated infections to go unreported.
	Evaluation
	Analysis
	Physiological Integrity

52.12 A female client is seen for a recurrence of a vaginal infection. The nurse realizes that this client might benefit from instruction about:
1. personal hygiene.
2. wearing tight underwear.
3. saving some of the prescribed medication for use when symptoms return.
4. avoiding sexual contact until the infection heals.

Answer: 4
Rationale: The nurse should instruct this client to avoid sexual contact until treatment is completed. Treatment of the infected woman and her sex partner as well as sexual abstinence is necessary to prevent reinfection. Avoiding tight clothing and personal hygiene practices should be included, but avoiding sexual contact is the best method of prevention of reoccurrence. Saving unused prescription medication is never recommended. Clients should be taught to complete the entire course of medication therapy.
Planning
Application
Physiological Integrity

52.13 A female client who was just diagnosed with chlamydia says, "I thought I was really sick. This isn't anything." Which of the following should the nurse respond to this client?
1. "You're right. This is minor."
2. "You're lucky that you only need treatment and not your partner."
3. "This is one cause of sterility and ectopic pregnancy in women."
4. "Most men have this disease anyway."

Answer: 3
Rationale: If chlamydial infections in women are not treated, they ascend into the upper reproductive tract and cause such complications as pelvic inflammatory disease (PID), which includes endometritis, salpingitis, and chronic pelvic pain. These infections are a major cause of infertility and ectopic pregnancy, which is a potentially life-threatening disorder in women. Complications of chlamydial infections in men include epididymitis, prostatitis, sterility, and Reiter's syndrome.
Planning
Application
Physiological Integrity

52.14 A male client is diagnosed with epididymitis. The nurse realizes that the sexually transmitted disease known to cause this disorder is:
1. gonorrhea.
2. syphilis.
3. chlamydia.
4. genital herpes.

Answer: 1
Rationale: In men, gonorrhea can cause acute, painful inflammation of the prostate, epididymis, and periurethral glands and can lead to sterility. Syphilis, chlamydia, and genital herpes do not generally cause epididymitis.
Assessment
Analysis
Physiological Integrity

52.15 A female client is being seen for her first prenatal visit. The nurse should be prepared to conduct which of the following diagnostic tests for this client? (Select all that apply.)
1. screening for chlamydia
2. screening for a yeast infection
3. screening for syphilis
4. screening for gonorrhea

Answer: 1, 3, 4
Rationale: Diagnosis of gonorrhea is based on cultures from the infected mucous membranes, examination of urine from an infected person, and a Gram stain to visualize the bacteria under the microscope. Pregnant women are routinely screened during their first prenatal visit. Pregnant women are also screened for the presence of syphilis. Chlamydia testing is also recommended by the CDC for pregnant women. Vaginal yeast (Candidiasis) is part of the normal flora and are only problematic if overgrowth occurs.
Planning
Application
Health Promotion and Maintenance

52.16 A female client has the complaint of a "weird rash" on her hands and feet. Which of the following should the nurse include in the care of this client? (Select all that apply.)
1. Conduct a complete sexual history assessment.
2. Ask if the client has experienced a foul-smelling vaginal discharge.
3. Find out if the client has experienced a chancre sore on her mouth or genital area.
4. Ask the client if she uses a public gym for working out.
5. Ask the client how long the rash has been present.

Answer: 1, 3, 5
Rationale: The primary stage of syphilis is characterized by the appearance of a chancre and by regional enlargement of lymph nodes; little or no pain accompanies these warning signs. The chancre appears at the site of inoculation, which is typically the genitals, anus, mouth, breast, or finger, from 3 to 4 weeks after the infectious contact. In women, a genital chancre may go unnoticed, and disappear within 4 to 6 weeks. In both primary and secondary stages, syphilis remains highly infectious, even if no symptoms are evident. Manifestations of secondary syphilis may appear anytime from 2 weeks to 6 months after the initial chancre disappears. These symptoms can include a skin rash, especially on the palms of the hands or soles of the feet, mucous patches in the oral cavity; sore throat; generalized lymphadenopathy; condyloma lata on the labia, anus, or corner of the mouth; flulike symptoms; and alopecia. These manifestations generally disappear within 2 to 6 weeks, and an asymptomatic latency period begins. Foul smelling vaginal drainage is not consistent with the other symptoms of syphilis, but other infections such as yeast. Syphilis is a sexually transmitted disease and is not associated with use of public facilities to exercise.

Assessment
Application
Physiological Integrity

52.17 A client who was just diagnosed with syphilis is allergic to penicillin. The nurse realizes that the first choice of drug to treat this client is:
1. amoxicillin (Amoxil).
2. doxycycline (Adoxa).
3. erythromycin (Erythrocin).
4. amoxicillin and clavulanate (Augmentin).

Answer: 2
Rationale: Clients who are allergic to penicillin are given oral doxycycline (Adoxa). The length of therapy depends on the estimated duration of infection. If the client cannot tolerate doxycycline, oral erythromycin (Erythrocin) is substituted. Amoxicillin (Amoxil) and amoxicillin and clavuanate (Augmentin) are contraindicated in those with penicillin allergy.
Planning
Analysis
Physiological Integrity

52.18 A female client complains of a fever and foul-smelling vaginal discharge. Upon a gynecological examination, the client has pain when the cervix is palpated. The nurse realizes that this client should have a diagnostic test for:
1. ectopic pregnancy.
2. syphilis.
3. yeast infection.
4. many sexually transmitted diseases.

Answer: 4
Rationale: Pelvic inflammatory disease is usually polymicrobial (caused by more than one microbe) in origin; gonorrhea and chlamydia are the common causative organisms. Ectopic pregnancy, syphilis, and yeast infection would not have cervical pain as an associated symptom.
Planning
Application
Physiological Integrity

52.19 A female client, who missed two previous appointments, is seen for a continued infection that caused pelvic inflammatory disease. Which of the following instructions should the nurse include in the teaching session?
1. the need to keep appointments and to complete all prescribed medications
2. methods to enhance personal hygiene
3. the need to stay on birth control pills while being treated
4. the reason to avoid all sexual activity while being treated

Answer: 1
Rationale: The nurse should explain the need to complete the treatment regimen and the importance of follow-up visits. If the client or partner fails to take all of the medication as prescribed, the infection may not be completely cured. Noncompliance and recurrence are common, particularly if follow-up appointments are not kept. Teaching proper hygiene and safe sex practices are important, but the question is focusing on the client's noncompliance with scheduled follow-up. Use of barrier methods of contraception should be stressed as a method of preventing transmission.
Implementation
Application
Physiological Integrity

52.20 A client has been diagnosed with herpes simplex II. The nurse provides information to the client about the disorder. Which of the following statements by the client indicates the need for further teaching?
1. "I will have this disease for life."
2. "When I become pregnant, this condition can affect my pregnancy, labor, and delivery."
3. "I can only give this to my partners when my blisters are present."
4. "It is important to keep the lesions clean and dry."

Answer: 3
Rationale: Herpes can be transmitted when the client is "active" as well as when no outward signs and symptoms are present. The condition does not currently have a cure. The condition may play a role in the pregnancy, especially with regard to labor and delivery. The lesions must be kept clean and dry to promote healing and to reduce the chance of infection.
Evaluation
Analysis
Health Promotion and Maintenance